A Professional Study and Resource Guide for the CRNA

Second Edition

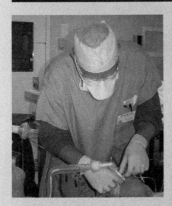
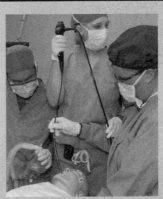
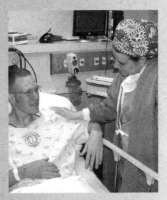
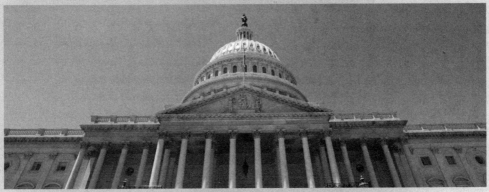

Scot D. Foster, CRNA, PhD, FAAN
Margaret Faut Callahan, CRNA, DNSc, FAAN

American Association of Nurse Anesthetists
222 South Prospect Avenue
Park Ridge, IL 60068-4001

Copyright © 2011 American Association of Nurse Anesthetists

Printed in the United States of America

Last digit indicates print number: 10 9 8 7 6 5 4

The author(s) and publisher have done everything possible to make this book accurate, up to date, and in accord with accepted standards at the time of publication. The authors, editors, and publisher are not responsible for errors or omissions or for consequences from application of the book, and make no warranty, expressed or implied, in regard to the contents of the book. Any practice described in this book should be applied by the reader in accordance with professional standards of care used in regard to the unique circumstances that may apply in each situation.

Library of Congress Cataloging-in-Publication Data

A professional study and resource guide for the CRNA / edited by Scot D. Foster, Margaret Faut Callahan. -- 2nd ed.
    p. ; cm.
 Includes bibliographical references and index.
 ISBN 978-0-9700279-8-6
 I. Foster, Scot Douglas. II. Faut-Callahan, Margaret. III. American Association of Nurse Anesthetists.
 [DNLM: 1. Nurse Anesthetists. 2. Anesthesia--nursing. 3. Health Knowledge, Attitudes, Practice. 4. Nurse's Role. WY 151]

 617.9'6--dc23

    2011045535

Dedication

This text is dedicated to the contributions of Mr John F. Garde, CRNA, MS, FAAN, former executive director of the American Association of Nurse Anesthetists (AANA). John passed away in 2009, having established an unparalleled legacy of service to the nursing profession. For many Certified Registered Nurse Anesthetists (CRNAs), he will remain the epitome of what we envision as the consummate professional and leader in healthcare. The value of this text will undoubtedly be enhanced when recalling John's contributions to CRNAs worldwide. He remains one of our finest examples of the professional spirit.

John's career spanned nearly a half century. He graduated from the Alexian Brothers Hospital School of Nursing and St Francis Hospital School of Anesthesia, La Crosse, Wisconsin. John received his undergraduate degree in psychology from the University of Detroit and a master's degree in physiology from Wayne State University School of Medicine. He was associate professor and chair, Department of Anesthesia, at Wayne State University, College of Pharmacy and Allied Health Professions. He became education director of the AANA in 1980 and executive director in 1983, retiring in 2000.

The CRNA community has long recognized John's leadership contributions. He was elected the first male and youngest president of the AANA in 1972. The Association honored his contributions in 1981 with the Helen Lamb Outstanding Educator Award and in 2000 with AANA's most coveted honor, the Agatha Hodgins Award for professional leadership. These honors recognized John's influence in moving nurse anesthesia programs into graduate schools in colleges and universities and the establishment of the AANA's formidable federal policy role manifested in the development of the AANA Office of Federal Government Affairs based in Washington, DC. John's tenure as an active political leader in the AANA and executive director included other accomplishments of vision such as the establishment of the council system of governance, the recognition of the Council on Accreditation of Nurse Anesthesia Educational Programs by the Department of Education, the formulation of several for-profit subsidiaries, and development of the AANA Foundation and the historical archives of the Association.

Few CRNAs appreciate the expansive influence of the AANA as a healthcare leader within the national and international nursing community. John was at the forefront of these efforts as he guided development of the International Federation of Nurse Anesthetists and served on the boards of directors of the Nursing Organization Liaison Forum and the National Federation for Specialty Nursing Organizations. He was also a charter member of the Josiah Macy Jr Foundation Committee for the Promotion of the Quality of Specialty Nursing Practice. For these and other contributions to nursing, John was one of the first CRNAs to be elected to the prestigious American Academy of Nursing in 1994—a group of noted nursing leaders recognized for formulating national healthcare policy based on cutting-edge nursing science.

John's professional contributions continued unabated after his retirement. He served as the interim executive director for the National League for Nursing Accreditation Commission, interim executive director for the American Psychiatric Nurses' Association, and interim executive director for the American Academy of Nursing. At the time of his death, John was serving as interim executive director for the AANA. Soon after, John was elected to the ANA Hall of Fame, attesting to the extraordinary scope of importance of his life's work.

Although John's legacy of leadership will be noted for many things, I believe as the two most important were his role as mentor and his personal commitment to the value of quiet humility. During his tenure as a school director at Wayne State University, his ability to mentor and nurture new CRNAs for leadership positions was long noted. Many of John's graduates have become AANA committee and council members and chairs, noted authors and scientists, doctorally prepared CRNAs, AANA presidents, association executives, business entrepreneurs, school directors, and AANA representatives to such organizations as the Joint Commission and state boards of nursing. This profound gift for mentoring and development of others was mirrored at the AANA where John attracted a professional staff of unparalleled talent and commitment to service.

Most appealing about John's leadership style was his humble and gracious demeanor. He presided over some of the most expansive and positive legislative change for CRNAs of the last half century while letting others take credit. He was always there to provide subtle direction and historical perspective on issues, but never sought the spotlight. He offered alternatives that most often became solutions, yet deferred articulation to elected leadership. He always had time for every AANA member and treated each one with the same regard and attention he gave to Association leaders. His attention was given totally and completely to the member.

In Chapter 1 the authors discuss the indomitable spirit of CRNAs and their role as leaders in healthcare. The conclusion to that narrative provides an apt reflection of John's many gifts to us all personally and professionally: "Professionalism is both a state of mind and commitment to action. It exemplifies the knowledge that our clinical work is possible only when others understand and value our service. To reach that goal requires active, lifelong commitment for which we are collectively and individually responsible. Professionalism demands that CRNAs project and promote the best of what our profession has to offer and care unselfishly for people and the values we share. It requires a global vision that incorporates the views of others and meets the requirements of all stakeholders and does so in a way that demands attention and respect for its value in solving problems and promoting optimal care.

"The constellation of professional skills required of every CRNA involves active participation in workplace affairs, issue forums, public relations efforts, interdisciplinary networking, and community involvement. Through these efforts, nurse anesthetists will become better informed, more effective at managing change, more satisfied with their career choices, and more adaptable to the changing healthcare environment. Most importantly, professionalism is a requisite for all CRNAs today and tomorrow, because ultimately, it is the only means to ensure our continued leadership in the world community of healthcare."

It is with great honor and thanks that we dedicate this book to the indomitable legacy of John F. Garde, CRNA, MS, FAAN.

Scot D. Foster, CRNA, PhD, FAAN
Senior Editor

Preface

After nearly a decade, we are proud to offer the second edition of *A Professional Study and Resource Guide for the CRNA*. The original text proved to be a valuable educational resource for students, as it remains the single compendium of information for understanding the whole of our professional experience and responsibility as nurse anesthetists. Although the text is aimed primarily to students in graduate programs, the practicing CRNA will also find relevance in the comprehensive chapters on departmental management, recertification, asserting influence in healthcare policy, and professional advocacy.

In this new edition, the editors and authors have attempted to better balance theory with realities of practice. That is, students will have more ready access to information that can be put into practice in pragmatic ways. The biggest change in the professional socialization chapter is the addition of role formation (Benner's work) to the traditional concepts of socialization, both of which drive the development of emerging professionals and can help guide their growth and development throughout their careers. This fundamental change is apparent throughout the book for example, more practical information on how to apply clinical evidence to patient care, and in regard to ethics, how the CRNA can be better prepared to manage ethical decision making. The chapter on reimbursement has undergone major change to lessen its focus on the "how to" a practitioner might need to more illustrative examples of exactly how the reimbursement system works. The chapter on information management now stresses how management principles can drive the practice environment to genuine qualitative change and improvement. The chapter on improving quality has undergone a major rewrite that more accurately reflects the role and function of current stakeholders, which have changed dramatically over the decade.

Certainly one of the difficulties in approaching this text is the issue of content currency. For instance, given the rate at which health policy changes and the multitude of nuances and political factors that shape a final policy product, we encourage the reader to periodically consult a variety of additional sources provided by the AANA, such as the Federal Government Affairs Hotline. This is especially relevant for the chapters mentioned above, as they concentrate on the Affordable Patient Health Care Act. Given that many of the provisions are yet to be implemented, further congressional action could substantially change what was available at press time.

We hope not to lose sight of a common thread that unifies this text: the message that our professional growth and future standing as leaders in healthcare changes by the minute and involves much more than clinical preparation for providing anesthesia care. It is only through the process of intelligent maturation as professionals that we can sustain our leadership, our standing in healthcare and the grateful thanks of patients we serve.

Scot D. Foster, CRNA, PhD, FAAN
Margaret Faut Callahan, CRNA, DNSc, FAAN

Contributors

Scot D. Foster, CRNA, PhD, FAAN
Senior Editor
Academic Vice President and Provost
Samuel Merritt University
Oakland, California

Margaret Faut Callahan, CRNA, DNSc, FAAN
Associate Editor
Dean and Professor, College of Nursing
Marquette University
Milwaukee, Wisconsin

Gene A. Blumenreich, JD
Former General Counsel
American Association of Nurse Anesthetists
Boston, Massachusetts

Marcia Sue DeWolf Bosek, RN, DNSc
Associate Professor
University of Vermont Department of Nursing
Burlington, Vermont

Lee S. Broadston, ABA, COBS
Senior Healthcare Practice and Policy Analyst
President and CEO
Waconia, Minnesota

Nancy Bruton-Maree, CRNA, MS
Program Director
Raleigh School of Nurse Anesthesia/University of North Carolina at Greensboro
Raleigh, North Carolina

Ronald F. Caulk, CRNA, FAAN
Former Executive Director
International Federation of Nurse Anesthetists
Cave Creek, Arizona

Susan S. Caulk, CRNA, MA
Former Director of Continuing Education, Certification, and Recertification
American Association of Nurse Anesthetists
Cave Creek, Arizona

Ira P. Gunn, CRNA, MLN, FAAN
Consultant
El Paso, Texas

David E. Hebert, JD
Principal
The DEH Group, LLC
Washington, DC

Larry G. Hornsby, CRNA, BSN
Senior Executive Vice President
AmSol USA
Moody, Alabama

Betty J. Horton, CRNA, PhD, FAAN
Education Consultant
Education Committee Chair, International Federation of Nurse Anesthetists
Tower Hill, Illinois

Michael J. Kremer, CRNA, PhD, FAAN
Professor and Director, Nurse Anesthesia Program
Rush University College of Nursing
Chicago, Illinois

Jeanne Learman, CRNA, MS
Staff CRNA
St Joseph Mercy Health System,
Ann Arbor, Michigan

Sandra M. Ouellette, CRNA, MEd, FAAN
Past President
International Federation of Nurse Anesthetists
Winston-Salem, North Carolina

Karen Plaus, CRNA, PhD, FAAN
Executive Director
National Board on Certification and Recertification for Nurse Anesthetists
Park Ridge, Illinois

John C. Preston, CRNA, DNSc
AANA Senior Director of Education and Professional Development
American Association of Nurse Anesthetists
Park Ridge, Illinois

Diana Quinlan, CRNA, MA
Former Chair, Peer Assistance Advisors Committee of the AANA
Retired Emeritus
St Maarten, Dutch West Indies

Rita M. Rupp, RN, MA
Senior Staff Specialist
Policy and Board Affairs (1988-2005, retired)
American Association of Nurse Anesthetists
Overland Park, Kansas

Janet M. Simpson, JD
President
Holbrook and Osborn, PA
Overland Park, Kansas

Mitchell H. Tobin, JD
President
Tobin Consulting, LLC
Park Ridge, Illinois

Sandra K. Tunajek, CRNA, DNP
Consultant
Self-employed
Charlotte, North Carolina

James R. Walker, CRNA, DNP
Director and Associate Professor
Graduate Program in Nurse Anesthesia
Baylor College of Medicine
Houston, Texas

Wynne R. Waugaman, CRNA, PhD, FAAN
Professor
University of Southern California
Los Angeles, California

Christine S. Zambricki, CRNA, MS, FAAN
Deputy Executive Director
American Association of Nurse Anesthetists
Washington, DC

A Professional Study and Resource Guide for the CRNA

Scot D. Foster, CRNA, PhD, FAAN, and
Margaret Faut Callahan, CRNA, DNSc, FAAN, editors

Table of Contents

The Essence of Professionalism

CHAPTER 1
Defining Work and the Professional Spirit

Scot D. Foster, CRNA, PhD, FAAN
Betty J. Horton, CRNA, PhD, FAAN

Key Concepts

- Certified Registered Nurse Anesthetists (CRNAs) are advanced practice nurses certified to practice the nursing role of anesthesiology in all 50 states. Anesthesia practice is not a delegated act of medicine, but rather, a constellation of highly complex nursing skills described by a scope of practice and recognized and regulated by an appropriate state agency.

- As of 2010, the education of CRNAs is at the graduate level using college/university-based theoretical and clinical sciences to prepare CRNAs to provide patients the full range of anesthesia services. A continued commitment to graduate education is anticipated since both the Council on Accreditation of Nurse Anesthesia Educational Programs and the American Association of Nurse Anesthetists support doctoral degrees for entry into practice by 2025.

- Professionalism is a multidimensional set of behavioral attributes, the fundamental core value of which is integrity. Integrity is an understanding and commitment to exhibit honest, forthright, ethical, value-driven behavior that exemplifies skills of critical thinking, broad-based perspectives, evaluation of consequences, and competent justification.

Continues on next page.

Key Concepts (continued)

- Professionalism requires attention not only to developing clinical skills, dedication to patient care, and achieving positive patient outcomes, but also a commitment to serve the public's interest as well as one's own interest expertly and unselfishly. Professionals advocate knowledgeably and act responsibly.

- Advocacy is a fundamental responsibility of the professional CRNA. Avenues of advocacy include participation in issue forums, public relations, development of and maintenance of communication networks external to the profession, active involvement in legislative and regulatory activity, community service, and the education of new generations of CRNAs.

The singular goal of this text is to capture in words the spirit of pride, issues in practice, and ideals of professionalism exemplified in the work of the Certified Registered Nurse Anesthetist (CRNA). George Matthew Adams once wrote: "It is the spirit of a person that hangs above him like a star in the sky. People identify him at once, and join with him until there is formed a parade of men and women, thus inspired. No matter where you find this spirit working, whether in a person or an entire organization, you may know that Heaven has dropped a note of joy into the world."

It is within that context that we introduce one of the most exciting and demanding of all advanced practice nursing roles: the nurse anesthetist.

History of Nurse Anesthesia

It is still surprising for many to learn that nurse anesthetists have provided anesthesia services in the United States since the 19th century. In fact, the development of the nurse anesthesia profession followed the discovery of ether by William Morton, a dentist.[1] The discovery of ether was a watershed event in history that allowed patients to undergo dental and surgical procedures without pain. Thus, the discovery of ether was a critical step leading to the practice of modern anesthesia and surgery, where lengthy and complex surgical procedures are common.

After ether was discovered, a need was soon seen for a category of healthcare worker to assume responsibility for the safety of patients, because the administration of ether anesthesia resulted in unconsciousness as well as pain relief. Nurses were already experienced in providing care and protection to unconscious patients, and anesthesia care soon became an added responsibility to the general duties of nurses in the United States.[2] By the late 1880s some nurses began to specialize in anesthesia and became known as nurse anesthetists.[3]

The first educational programs for nurse anesthetists were established in 1909, preceding the development of anesthesiology as a role for physicians, which began following World War II.[3] Throughout the next 90 years, the education of nurse anesthetists changed dramatically from certificate training programs to degree-granting programs. By January 1, 1998, the Council on Accreditation of Nurse Anesthesia Educational Programs (COA) implemented a requirement that all accredited nurse anesthesia educational programs offer extensive clinical and didactic experiences leading to the award of a master's degree or higher. In 2004, additional standards were adopted for doctoral degree programs.

More than 44,000 nurse anesthetists administer approximately 32 million anesthetics to patients in the United States each year. According to the American Association of Nurse Anesthetists (AANA),[4] CRNAs are the primary anesthesia providers in rural America, affording these underserved areas obstetrical, surgical, and trauma stabilization capabilities. CRNAs administer all types of anesthesia for a wide array of procedures—from minor surgical procedures to major, complex, surgical interventions. They practice in every setting in which anesthesia is delivered, including traditional hospital surgical suites; obstetrical delivery rooms; critical care access hospitals; offices of dentists, podiatrists, ophthalmologists, plastic surgeons, and pain management specialists; ambulatory surgical centers; all permutations of managed care organizations; military installations; public health service centers; US military healthcare facilities; and Veterans Administration facilities. CRNAs also provide clinical support services outside of the operating rooms in MRI units,

5

cardiac catheterization labs, and in cardiopulmonary resuscitation. Many other CRNAs are involved in administration, education, consultation, or research.

Currently, the demand for CRNAs far exceeds available supply, and, despite the continuous and positive growth of the profession, surgical demand continues to outpace available services in most areas of the country. According to an extensive CRNA Manpower Study from the National Center for Nursing Research in 1990,[5] the number of CRNAs required by the year 2010 would exceed 35,000, an increase of 40% more than the 25,000 needed in 1990. It is becoming apparent that these numbers were conservative estimates as we witness the continued growth and demand for CRNA services. By 2003, an increase in the number of CRNAs who were retiring, combined with only a modest increase in graduation rates, had contributed to the overall demand for anesthesia services.[6] The need for more CRNAs was confirmed by 2 other 2003 studies conducted by anesthesiologists. The first study from the Cleveland Clinic[7] noted that an increasing enrollment in nurse anesthesia programs might help to alleviate shortages, but more graduates were needed to offset substantial anticipated retirement rates and declining work efforts of those approaching retirement. The second study by Rowland[8] noted that staffing shortages were likely to be persistent and affect every location. As a result, anesthesiologists' income and CRNAs' salaries had increased in almost every market.[8]

The ongoing increase in the numbers of nurse anesthetists graduating was also noted by the American Society of Anesthesiologists (ASA) in a November 2004 report.[9] Based on the numbers of nurses in training, the author noted that even larger numbers were expected to graduate in the following 2 years. The author also noted that the decline in numbers entering nurse anesthesia programs in the 1990s occurred at the same time as the decline in numbers entering anesthesiology residences. He attributed the current increase in student registered nurse anesthetists to optimism about their career opportunities. At the same time, a decline in recruitment of physician anesthesiology residents was evident in the face of a continuous growth of the US population.

Finally, in research conducted for the AANA, Merwin, Stern, and Jordan[10] reported that the supply of CRNAs had increased, stimulated by shortages of CRNAs, to maintain a constant age in the CRNA population. The researchers projected that the average age of CRNAs would continue to increase in the near future despite increases in the number of CRNAs trained. They also forecasted that the supply of CRNAs in relation to surgical procedures would increase in the near future. These facts, coupled with an increasing surgical demand from a burgeoning geriatric population, offer bright prospects and potential for new CRNAs entering nurse anesthesia practice.

The profession of nurse anesthesia has been richly documented in a variety of other texts. These publications provide a compelling account of the work of CRNAs since the 1870s. Virginia S. Thatcher's 1953 publication, *History of Anesthesia with Emphasis on the Nurse Specialist,*[1] stands as the first public recognition of nurse anesthetists. The definitive history of CRNAs, *Watchful Care: A History of America's Nurse Anesthetists* by Marianne Bankert,[3] was published in 1989. Evan Koch, CRNA, MSN, and Lee C. Fosburgh, MLIS, MA, highlighted pertinent historical information in "Justifiably Proud: A Brief History of Nurse Anesthetists," a chapter in *Principles and Practice of Nurse Anesthesia,*[11] which was published in 1999. Evan Koch also contributed a chapter, "Nurse Anesthesia: A History of Challenge," in *Nurse Anesthesia*,[12] which was published in 2010.

Professional Definitions

A CRNA is a licensed registered nurse who is educationally prepared at the graduate level and certified as competent to engage in the practice of anesthesiology, which is defined as the art and science of rendering a patient insensible to pain by the administration of anesthetic agents and related drugs. Anesthesia and anesthesia-related care represents those services that anesthesia professionals provide upon request, assignment, and referral by the patient's physician or other healthcare provider authorized by law, most often to facilitate diagnostic, therapeutic, and surgical procedures. In addition to general or regional anesthesia techniques or sedation techniques required for surgery, a referral or request for consultation or assistance may be for management of pain associated with obstetrical labor and delivery, management of acute and chronic ventilatory problems, or management of acute and chronic pain through the performance of selected diagnostic and therapeutic blocks.[13]

CRNAs are responsible and accountable for their individual professional practice and are capable of exercising independent judgment within the scope of their education (credentials), demonstrated competence (privileges), and licensure.[14] CRNAs are recognized in all 50 states by state regulatory (licensing) bodies, primarily boards of registered nursing. The practice of CRNAs is a recognized role within the profession of nursing and is not a medically delegated act. In order to be a CRNA an individual must have:

- Obtained unrestricted state licensure as a registered professional nurse.

- Graduated with at least a master's degree from a nurse anesthesia educational program accredited by the Council on Accreditation of Nurse Anesthesia Educational Programs.
- Successfully passed the certification examination administered by the Council on Certification of Nurse Anesthetists.
- Complied with criteria for biennial recertification, as defined by the Council on Recertification of Nurse Anesthetists. These criteria include evidence of (1) current licensure as a registered nurse, (2) substantial anesthesia practice as a CRNA, (3) 40 hours of appropriate continuing education, and (4) verification of the absence of mental, physical, and other problems or conditions that could interfere with the practice of anesthesia.[15]

Scope of Practice

The scope of practice of CRNAs encompasses the professional functions, privileges, and responsibilities associated with nurse anesthesia practice. These acts are nearly always performed in collaboration with other qualified and legally authorized professional healthcare providers who may include surgeons, anesthesiologists or other consulting physicians, nurses, therapists, or technicians who assume distinct and specialized roles required for comprehensive, perianesthetic patient care. Collaboration is a process that involves 2 or more parties working together, each contributing his or her respective expertise. Collaboration must necessarily exist whether a CRNA works in an anesthesiologist-led anesthesia care team (ACT) or as an independent practitioner.

The terms *supervision* and *medical direction* most often describe a relationship between a nurse anesthetist and a physician, dentist, podiatrist, or other healthcare

7

professional with whom the nurse anesthetist collaborates to varying degrees. The specifics of these terms exist on a continuum, if they exist at all, in a particular state or region. On one end of the continuum, a CRNA's scope of practice could potentially encompass a broad range of discretionary, independent practice rights as determined by the appropriate state regulatory agency and authorized only by the general consent of another licensed provider as established by state law. On the other end of the continuum, a CRNA's scope of practice may be limited by state or local medical staff bylaws to only approved activities (privileges). The variation in these practice roles can be substantial and requires graduating nurse anesthetists to carefully evaluate any potential limitations imposed on their scope of practice. Finally, the term "collaboration" does not imply a mandated supervisory role by an anesthesiologist. Other chapters in this text provide details on state and federal requirements for supervision or medical direction if and where they occur.

Nurse anesthetists administer anesthesia and anesthesia-related care in 4 general categories: (1) preanesthetic preparation and evaluation; (2) anesthesia induction, maintenance, and emergence; (3) postanesthesia care; and (4) perianesthetic and clinical support functions. A nurse anesthetist's scope of practice is detailed in Table 1.1, and additional, more specific information can be found in the Guidelines for Granting Clinical Privileges to CRNAs in the *Professional Practice Manual for the Certified Registered Nurse Anesthetist.*[16]

Educational Preparation of Nurse Anesthetists

From the first call in 1933 for educational standards by Gertrude Fife, president of the National Association of Nurse Anesthetists, to today, nurse anesthesia programs have become increasingly sophisticated and reflective of the higher education academy. As of August 2011, there are 112 accredited programs nationwide, all of which offer a graduate degree upon completion of a rigorous course of clinical and academic study. Approximately 56% of programs are housed within a department of nursing and the balance within schools of allied health, medicine, or other related health disciplines. Today there are more than 5,325 student registered nurse anesthetists enrolled in programs whose permanent, regular faculty have master's or doctoral degrees in nursing, education, and the physical, biological, and clinical sciences. Each year, more than 2,000 students graduate from these programs and become eligible for certification.

Program length is a minimum of 24 months, although 90% of all programs require a 27- to 36-month period of enrollment. Each program provides an extensive curriculum that combines academic theory and research-based clinical practice that, in many programs, approximates 2,400 hours of actual anesthetic clinical time.[17] Required coursework common to all programs includes upper-level anatomy, physiology and pathophysiology, chemistry, biochemistry and physics, pharmacology, basic and advanced practice principles, equipment, technology, pain management, clinical conferences, and professional issues. The clinical curriculum prepares the student for the full scope of current practice in a variety of work settings including a variety of procedures, techniques, and anesthesia practices. In addition, curricula require educational experiences in some form of research activity or other mode of scientific inquiry as well as advanced theoretical principles of nursing practice and health policy. Specific

Table 1.1. CRNA Scope of Practice[13]

Performing and documenting a preanesthetic assessment and evaluation of the patient, including requesting consultations and diagnostic studies; selecting, obtaining, ordering, or administering preanesthetic medications and fluids; and obtaining informed consent for anesthesia

Developing and implementing an anesthetic plan

Initiating the anesthetic technique, which may include general, regional, and local and sedation

Selecting, applying, and inserting appropriate noninvasive and invasive monitoring modalities for continuous evaluation of the patient's physical status

Selecting, obtaining, or administering the anesthetics, adjuvant drugs, and fluids necessary to manage the anesthetic

Managing a patient's airway and pulmonary status using current practice modalities

Facilitating emergence and recovery from anesthesia by selecting, obtaining, ordering, or administering medications, fluids, and ventilatory support

Discharging the patient from a postanesthesia care area and providing postanesthesia follow-up evaluation and care

Implementing acute and chronic pain management modalities

Responding to emergency situations by providing airway management, administration of emergency fluids or drugs, or using basic or advanced cardiac life support techniques

Additional responsibilities that are within the expertise of the individual CRNA including administration/management, quality assessment, education, research, committee appointments, interdepartmental liaison, clinical/administrative oversight of other departments

The functions listed above are a summary of CRNA clinical practice and are not intended to be all inclusive. A more specific description of CRNA functions and practice parameters is detailed in the *Professional Practice Manual for the Certified Registered Nurse Anesthetist.*

curricular requirements for program accreditation are available in the Standards for Accreditation of Nurse Anesthesia Educational Programs.[18]

Although admission criteria vary among programs, minimum requirements of the COA mandate that students (1) possess baccalaureate degrees, (2) maintain current licensure as registered nurses, and (3) complete at least 1 year of experience as registered professional nurses in acute care in which they have had the opportunity to develop as independent decision makers and demonstrate psychomotor skills and the ability to use and interpret advanced monitoring techniques based on a knowledge of physiologic and pharmacologic principles.

Most often, successful applicants have acquired extensive clinical backgrounds as professional nurses in coronary, respiratory, postanesthesia, and surgical intensive care units; emergency departments; or as members of trauma or cardiac surgical teams. The specifics of appropriate clinical experiences, in addition to those required by the COA, are the prerogative of the program. This and other general information about the role of nurse anesthesia, a listing of all accredited programs, and educational program standards can be found on the Internet at www.aana.com or by email at info@aana.com. Many individual programs also maintain their own specific websites that detail educational philosophy, curricula, admission requirements, and other items of interest to prospective candidates.

The Challenge of Professionalism

For CRNAs who have spent the greater part of their professional careers as educators, it becomes increasingly clear that the success of the educational endeavor hinges directly on the accomplishment of 2 objectives. The first, which is generally the easier of the two and requisite to clinical practice, is to equip students with the skills and abilities to conduct and manage a safe, high-quality anesthetic. The second objective, which is equally vital but often far more difficult to achieve, is to imbue students with a clear and functional appreciation for the responsibilities of professionalism—specifically, to inculcate the values that are the foundation of effective patient care and anesthesia services as well as values that promote the well-being, public image, longevity, and the leadership role of nurse anesthetists.

The difficulty in meeting this educational challenge stems from a variety of sources. First, the concept of professionalism is not easy to understand because the term has been applied so broadly and indiscriminately that a clear, unambiguous conceptual picture is often hard to formulate. The issue is further clouded because contemporary literature has yielded few new interpretations or salient applications of professional behaviors that would be useful to new students socializing into the profession. Most critically, students spend a great deal of time, necessarily perhaps, sequestered in operating rooms and have little opportunity to engage with students in other programs or CRNAs in practice. Consequently, far too many graduates fail to experience the socializing influence of CRNA role models and don't learn the value of their social commitment to the public or their own professional well-being.

Historical Evolution of the Professions

An informed understanding of professionalism should be based on historical perspectives. The professions were derived largely from those who sought to teach or to profess. Originally, members of the professions were meant to take the vows of a religious order, but by the 17th century the term "professionalism" had been secularized to mean the achievement of due qualification.[19] From this developed the idea that persons claiming membership in the professions profess to know better than others the nature of certain matters and to know better than their clients what aids them or their affairs.[20] Origins of professionalism were initially associated with the clergy; however, the professions separately organized when religion was no longer a predominant social force. Gradually, professions became formally associated with the universities of medieval Europe, which most clearly resembled the more contemporary training schools for the traditional professions of law, medicine, and theology.

Stein and Kristenson[19] noted that professional occupations were learned through apprenticeships or short training courses. Because both theory and practice had always been considered dual components of the learned professions, the advent of apprenticeships put renewed emphasis on the practice component. Professional candidates placed themselves under the able tutelage of a minister, lawyer, or doctor and hoped by observation and imitation to be subsequently admitted to professional status.

In the American colonies, early professional education came primarily from the great European universities because of a lack of colonist faculties or organized professional schools. Slowly the American colonists began to develop their own system of higher education from which would eventually emerge the professional school. This effort was greatly aided by the establishment of professorial chairs and special professorships in traditional academic disciplines.

Proprietary schools (staffed by teaching practitioners) were also developed during this time to help provide greater numbers of professionals. The overall quality of many of these schools was dubious at best. They did provide employment for what many considered a proliferation of doctors and lawyers so ill-trained that they could not find gainful employment elsewhere. Proprietary schools did contribute in small part to the development of professional education by emphasizing didactic instruction and relying less on apprentice-type learning by experience; however, the actual contributions of proprietary schools to the curricular integrity of professional educational programs remains a point of historical contention.

It was not until after the US Civil War that the scope and sophistication of professional schools began to fully develop. Medical practice drew increasing respectability by incorporating scientific principles and new research gleaned largely from European physicians. The medical curricula became more comprehensively based on new developments in chemistry and biology that would offer solid scientific foundations. Lawyers would come to value the need for more balanced educational approaches incorporating longer, more formalized internships under qualified mentors. Even professional faculty in schools of theology were beginning to incorporate some of the newer modes of scholarship adapted from the German models of professional education. These activities ushered the movement of professional schools into the university setting and away from the more disorganized and often ethically specious proprietary schools.

The occupations of engineering and certain of the social sciences and healthcare fields were becoming recognized and accepted as professions subsequent to the move of those disciplines into more formal educational frameworks. Because of the diverse missions of emerging types of institutions of higher education, the land-grant institutions, for instance (eventually state universities), began to recognize agriculture and home economics as professional occupations. With the advent of state competence examinations, practice regulatory authorities, accreditation mechanisms, and performance standards, professional schools became more credible and reliable providers of professional services.

Responsibilities of Professionalism

The student and practitioner should be reminded that abilities to practice anesthesia within the scope of what is termed a "professional capacity" is not a right afforded unconditionally. Conceptually, the traditional professions were recognized as occupational groups who, in time, gained the recognition and trust of the public for services that were highly valued by society. Consequently, professional recognition was an earned right granted solely and exclusively by the public in exchange for certain services and conduct. Society retained the right to deny recognition of any professional service provider when those services no longer met the needs, expectations, or standards of the public. Too often, professional healthcare providers are under the mistaken notion that their rights to practice are afforded directly by statute or some particular licensing or regulatory body; however, these bodies are merely social conventions designed to operationalize public policy. Although this notion may appear of little importance, it should remind us that we practice anesthesia because we have earned the confidence and trust of the public. If the quality, scope, and vigilance attendant to our work fails, so may the ability to claim professional status.

Chief among the responsibilities for which the public holds CRNAs responsible (in exchange for the designation, benefits, and prerogatives of professional practice) is that professional activities should accrue benefit to the public, not the profession. Subsequently, the primary goal of any profession should be public service. In cases in which a professional organization comes to value its financial interest over public interest, it is likely the profession will risk regulatory sanction or worse.

Most sociologists concur that the critical features of any definition of professionalism are a mastery of skill and competence acquired by rigorous clinical training, a research-based theoretical education, and an ethical code of behavior. Research has demonstrated that the boundaries of accepted behavior for nurse anesthetists are set by unwritten moral codes[21] (Table 1.2). In addition to the unwritten code, the AANA maintains a formal code of ethics espousing "right" behaviors based on a published set

---

Table 1.2. Moral Code of Nurse Anesthesia in the United States[21]

Patient care values must be honored.

Nurse anesthetists must be honest.
  Admit mistakes.
  Be able to say, "I don't know."
  Accept personal responsibility for actions.
  Tell the truth at all times.

Nurse anesthetists are loyal.
  Allegiance to the larger group of nurse anesthetists
  Supportive of individual colleagues in a crisis
  Supportive of accomplishments of colleagues

Nurse anesthetists believe in equal opportunities for individuals.
  Equality for gender and sexual orientation
  Equality for race and religion

Nurse anesthetists do not anesthetize family members except in an emergency.

The Essence of Professionalism

Table 1.3. Criteria for Qualification as a Profession[23]

The professional is engaged in a full-time occupation that comprises his or her principal source of income. Professionals have a strong motivation or calling to the occupation manifested by a lifetime commitment.

The professional possesses a specialized body of knowledge and skills acquired during a prolonged period of formal education and training.

The professional makes decisions on behalf of a client by means of a clearly defined yet broad foundation of theoretical knowledge and expertise in clinical application.

The professional has a service orientation. This service implies diagnostic skill, competent application of general knowledge to the special needs of the client, and an absence of self-interest or self-promotion.

The profession's service to the client is assumed to be based on the objective needs of the client and independent of the particular sentiments that the professional may have about the client. This promises a "detached" diagnosis and withholding of moral judgment about the client's revelations or diagnosis.

The professional demands autonomy in actions and judgment and subscribes to standards judged by a panel of peers. Legal protection is sought through political influence.

Professional associations are formed, which define criteria of admission, educational standards, licensing, entry examinations, and areas of jurisdiction for the profession. Ultimately, the professional association's function is to protect the autonomy of the profession; it develops reasonably strong forms of self-government by setting rules or standards for the profession.

13

---

of values or principles that the profession reveres. The code is a value-based guide for CRNAs to use as a framework for establishing and maintaining professional relationships with patients, coworkers, institutions, and external agencies.[22]

Although there is some degree of difficulty encountered in definitions of professionalism, most people agree there is need for criteria that designate when any particular work group evolves to the level of professional status. Table 1.3 provides a listing of commonly accepted characteristics of and qualifications for designation as a profession.

Pellegrino[24] provides a humanistic perspective of what constitutes a profession. He states that the philosophical grounding of a true profession lies in the special kind of interpersonal relationship it requires between its practitioners and those who seek their assistance. Tenets of his approach include the need for healthcare providers to understand the following:

- Patients exist in a special and compromised state of vulnerability.
- Patient needs that the professions address are of the most sensitive kind, including mortality, freedom, human values, and rights.

- The provider must always uphold the values of dignity and privacy.
- Patients trust the provider will use knowledge only in their best interest.

Pellegrino[24] states:

> To be a professional is to make a promise to hope, to keep that promise, and to do so in the best interest of patients. It is to accept the trust the patient must place in us as a moral imperative, one that the ethos of the marketplace or competition does not expect us, in our society, to honor. The special nature of the helping and healing professions is rooted in the fact that people become ill and need to trust others to help them restore health.

Based on Pellegrino's definition, nurse anesthesia is a true profession that values the relationship between CRNAs and their patients. These patient care values include individualized care, serving as a patient surrogate, protective care, surveillance and vigilance, and using touch to communicate caring.

It is obvious that when the provider-patient relationship is threatened, certain social and political activities are required to maintain it. Thus, the definition of professionalism is necessarily segmented into activities that address some element of the social covenant previously described. These activities can take the form of social advocacy, public education, community building, elevating standards, or influencing public policy, to name only a few.

Once the commitment is made to engage in these activities, CRNAs will find themselves immediately exposed to some element of scrutiny, public exposure, controversy, and stress from interdisciplinary conflict. Initially they may find themselves relatively uneducated about issues and needs, naive in affairs of diplomacy, and perhaps even ineffectual in debate and argument. However, in the same way that clinical skills are honed, skills of advocacy and service can also be developed. In fact, when substantive change occurs as a result of advocacy, there are accrued benefits of personal satisfaction, increased self-confidence, and a sense of personal worth and value, as well as broader visions for future change and direction.

In short, professionalism is a commitment to serve expertly and unselfishly, to advocate knowledgeably, and to act responsibly. It is a process that both exposes and promotes the philosophical underpinnings and value of work. It is through the process of exposing what we value about our work that our work will be valued by others who gain service from it. Professionalism is manifested in a variety of ways including clinical competence; however, clinical competence alone is an insufficient ingredient to secure the continued success of nurse anesthetists as viable entities in the marketplace or leaders in healthcare. Success demands more: It demands professionalism.

Abuses of Professionalism

It should be evident to the most naive observer of the professional landscape that the traditional privileges and social status of the professions have been slowly eroded during the past several decades. Whether the discipline be law, medicine, religion, nursing, or managed care, one can cite numerous examples that account for the downturn in public esteem the professions once enjoyed. Reasons are generally attributable to a decreasing sensitivity of providers to public need, resistance to change in the public interest, commercialization, unaffordable cost for fewer and lower-quality services, and projection of professional interests (especially financial) over those of the public.

As a result, the consumer has been reasonably effective in initiating needed change, although many feel the hardest choices and most difficult work lie ahead. Examples of these public concerns and advocacy efforts include the desire for public reports comparing healthcare providers, prohibiting payment in the instance of tragic "never events," mandating access to care, rights of redress for poor quality or rationed care, and provision of affordable health insurance. Consequently, state and federal legislators are contemplating legislative efforts to reverse trends the public has determined are not in their best interest. Those include caps on certain legal fees in medical liability cases, eliminating anticompetitive practices that restrict nonphysician access to patients, exclusion of prescription allowances, and lack of ability to sue HMOs for substandard, unavailable, or uncompensated care.

Healthcare professionals should remain mindful of the core concepts of professionalism even when tempted by the forces of a competitive marketplace to do otherwise. Clearly, providers must recommit to traditional professional values that wisely emphasize their moral obligations and the changing needs of contemporary society.

Values Held by CRNAs

Values held by a group of people are part of the unique culture that binds them together. Certain values are learned, shared, and transmitted to younger generations of a group as guides for thinking, decisions, and actions.[25] Furthermore, the shared values and behaviors in a culture are often a result of coping with common problems. This has certainly been true for the culture of nurse anesthesia. In fact, nurse anesthetists have unconsciously developed characteristic attitudes and behaviors that have proven successful in dealing with external challenges to the profession throughout its history (Table 1.4).

15

Table 1.4. Dominant Rules of Behavior of Nurse Anesthetists in the United States[21]

Is able to control and manage stressful clinical situations.
Makes independent judgments quickly.
Accepts a high degree of responsibility.
Belongs to a professional organization (AANA).
Is committed to lifelong learning of scientific facts.
Demonstrates self-confidence.
Is effective in using assertiveness to facilitate role as patient advocate.
Engages in political activities.
Enjoys short-term patient care.
Functions effectively and calmly in life-and-death situations.
Is organized, with meticulous attention to detail.
Possesses intelligence and current knowledge.
Is technically skilled, efficient, and clinically competent.
Upholds patient care values.
Is willing to work hard and dedicate long hours to the job.

Table 1.5. Dominant Cultural Values of Nurse Anesthesia in the United States[21]

Achievement: education and personal life
Autonomy: right to be self-governing
Continuing education: commitment to lifelong learning
Education: control and standard setting
Group cohesiveness: institutional and professional organization
Identity as a CRNA: a way of life
Membership in the AANA: strength in numbers
Political activism: state and national
Technology: efficiency and safety

Nurse anesthetists share the vast majority of American values. These values include achievement, goal attainment, assertiveness, materialism, technology, equal rights, action orientation, and reliance on scientific facts.[25] However, nurse anesthesia differs from the American culture in valuing group cohesiveness over individualism and equality for race, gender, religion, and sexual orientation.

Importantly, there are dominant shared cultural values held among nurse anesthetists that set the group apart from other nurses (Table 1.5). These values are autonomy, education, continuing education, achievement, group cohesiveness, identity as CRNAs, membership in the AANA, political activism, and technology.[21]

The Core Value of Integrity

Fundamental to any definition of professionalism for either students or clinicians is the principle of integrity. In its most broadly applicable form, integrity is an understanding of and commitment to honest, forthright, value-driven behavior. The definition implies that any action taken by a clinician must be characterized by an intent to achieve excellence and to do so ethically. Actions taken, or in the case of CRNAs, clinical

decisions made or collegial behaviors demonstrated, should always reveal elements of critical thinking, broad-based perspectives, careful evaluation of consequences, and competent justification. Actions that reveal themselves as self-centered, cursory, ill-timed, or myopic are usually characteristic of decisions made absent of any genuine commitments that value integrity.

Integrity in Student Life

For students, academic integrity is of paramount importance. That is, students should be resolved to pledge all intellectual resources to the process of learning. They should enter an educational program as an informed consumer and be clear as to their motivation and capability for pursuing a career in nurse anesthesia. Students should make a studied analysis of their educational needs, choose an appropriate learning environment, and work diligently toward certification.

During a student's enrollment, faculty measure the student's commitment to academic integrity in a variety of ways: optimal classroom preparation and study, meeting deadlines, well-executed planning and organizational skills, self-motivated inquiry, self-discipline, and exceeding minimal performance standards both in the classroom and the clinical area. Clearly, the experience of many educators has repeatedly confirmed the observation that a graduate is only as good as the quality effort he or she expends in pursuit of educational goals. The success students attain as clinicians is a function largely of the personal expectations and standards they set for themselves. Subsequently, the veracity, commitment, and honesty to self with which students approach challenges of graduate education remain primary keys to success.

Another way in which all students should demonstrate their commitment to professional responsibility is by attending educational conferences available to them. Repeatedly, the observation is made that the students who actively seek opportunities to participate in state and local educational programs are those who continue to actively and productively participate in affairs of both the state and national organizations of the AANA. In addition to clinical education sessions, AANA meetings provide opportunities to learn about advocacy issues, speak publicly, network with colleagues, perhaps manage educational programming, and, importantly, learn about the values and culture that CRNAs promote. For example, Horton[21] found that honesty is highly valued as a philosophical concept in the nurse anesthesia culture. Practitioners consistently base patient care decisions and actions on honesty, which is believed to foster safe patient care. Honesty guides CRNAs' thinking, decision making, and behavior in both education and practice. Admitting mistakes, accepting responsibility for personal actions, and telling the truth at all times are part of the culture.

Integrity in Professional Life

The most fundamental professional responsibility of CRNAs is to maintain clinical competence through a variety of mechanisms such as continuing education seminars, in-house educational conferences, and attendance at local, state, and national meetings of the AANA and other qualified sponsors. It is incumbent on CRNAs to make certain that their scope of practice and expertise is constantly undergoing productive change and expansion in order to maintain skills required for the marketplace and optimally enhance patient care.

In the clinical area, a commitment to maintaining competence is a form of behavioral integrity measured by the extent and manner in which CRNAs use their knowledge in the best interests of patients; avoid breeches of patient confidentiality; and deal interpersonally with patients in an informed, supportive, and unambiguous manner. Ultimately, it is about maintaining the highest possible standards of care.

Clinical skills are only as good as a provider's ability to communicate effectively to both patients and other providers. Without effective communication skills, there is high probability that the provider will not be seen as an effective team member or patient advocate. Furthermore, unskilled communications are usually the hallmark of those who lack any fundamental appreciation of the tenets of responsible interpersonal skills. Too often the professional arrogance of healthcare providers results in written and oral communication that is misinformed, demonstrates an egregious lack of respect for others, and is often characterized by a total lack of skill for diplomacy or reasoned debate. This type of behavior is the antithesis of productive professionalism. It should always be of concern to students and

17

CRNAs that their professional credibility as clinicians hinges as much on their facility to communicate and project an appropriate, caring, and sensitive demeanor as it does on clinical skill.

Avenues of Professional Advocacy

CRNAs have long revered their ability to practice with relative autonomy, to conduct patient care activities in ways they believe are most appropriate, and to participate fully in the healthcare system as respected providers. However, these privileges have neither been without cost nor will they be available in the future without continued participation by all CRNAs in activities that strengthen their public image and promote a legislative agenda designed to secure their practice rights and privileges. As will be revealed in later chapters, CRNAs have long been involved in such legislative and policy efforts via the AANA, the professional organization boasting a membership of approximately 90% of all CRNAs in the United States.

Many CRNAs have developed substantial skills in formally advocating a professional agenda that advances both patient care and issues affecting their own personal well-being. Countless numbers of CRNAs participate daily in a variety of nonclinical activities that enhance the standing, credibility, and value of CRNAs to the healthcare community. What is key for CRNAs to appreciate about advocacy is that there is a necessary role for everyone to assume. Providing quality patient care, although important, is not sufficient alone to maintain the leadership role of CRNAs in healthcare at the local and national levels.

The extent to which CRNAs become involved in professional advocacy efforts will change to accommodate activities that require more skill and dedication of time, yet there are tremendous personal and professional rewards in achieving goals that promote the welfare of all involved. Above all, the continued ability of CRNAs to compete as major healthcare providers and to maintain the substantial professional prerogatives they currently enjoy depends directly on their personal assumption of their share of work to maintain them. In the game of high-stakes competition, expansive market flux, a dwindling resource base and ever-increasing demands for better outcomes and more cost-effective work production, there will be no "Big Brother" to care for your needs, ensure your job security, or nurture your development. Big Brother is us!

Participation in Issue Forums

Important advocacy efforts in which CRNAs may find their niche include local departmental meetings at the work site, hospital committees, or community service organizations. CRNAs should always include attendance at state and national meetings of the AANA. It is of paramount importance that CRNAs "be at the table" when planning, negotiation, and decision making occur.

Public Relations

There are no more important activities than those directed at helping the public, policy makers, and colleagues understand the nature and value of your work as a CRNA. Invite a legislator into the operating room to observe interactions with patients, sponsor community health fairs, write articles for your local newspaper, and take every opportunity to participate on talk radio or in television clips. Always respond to inaccuracies of the press regarding your work. Establish a regular press contact and function as their primary source of information about CRNAs and anesthesia. Above all, communicate your message in an informed, accurate, and responsible way.

External Networks

Advocating for CRNA work includes getting the message to other persons and organizations who share your philosophies and interests. Some of the most valued relationships CRNAs have established with state and national political leaders were formed through years of acquaintance as neighbors. CRNAs have established other valued communication and project networks as members of consulting teams, city administration bureaucracies such as school or utility boards, and state boards of nursing; as representatives to other nursing groups; as expert witnesses; as liaisons to corporate healthcare leaders; and in countless other ways. Remember, on the most basic level, personal relationships with local facility administrators are the first and best liaisons to establish. Additionally, involvement with external groups demonstrates your personal willingness to be part of the solution and not part of the problem.

Legislative and Regulatory Activity

Some CRNAs will be called upon to assume more formal relationships with policy makers to formulate or influence legislation or regulation that affects CRNA practice. Functional roles may include working directly with legislative or agency staff in state government such as the board of nursing and administrative code offices, insurance commissioners, heads of other state health regulatory agencies and boards, and congressional representatives and staff at the federal level. Almost every state organiza-

tion of nurse anesthetists retains a professional lobbying firm whose activities depend heavily on CRNA involvement to achieve legislative or policy goals. Remember that optimum function of professional lobbyists is not possible without the direct involvement of CRNAs. Legislators want to hear directly from you about how issues affect you and your patients.

Serving the Community

Much of the provision of healthcare in the future will be decentralized and take place within the community as opposed to in large medical centers. Consequently, CRNAs need to be involved in community health projects that best expose their skills and value to society. Many CRNAs have become actively involved in teaching the public cardiopulmonary resuscitation, staffing immunization clinics, or offering missionary or volunteer work on federal or private ventures to foreign countries that provide surgical services to the underprivileged.

Professionalism and the Responsibilities of Teaching

It has long been appreciated that the need for education lies at the core of the human enterprise. History has demonstrated repeatedly that education is the critical component for transmitting social values, norms, and cultural traditions from generation to generation. On a more pragmatic level, education secures a competent work force and ensures a productive society and thriving economy. Education is of paramount importance to the CRNA for these reasons, in addition to enhancing patient outcomes.

It is critical that CRNAs in all practice settings consider providing student registered nurse anesthetists some teaching-related service. These services may come in various

19

forms, but all have immense value in the preparation of the next generation of CRNAs. The growth of programs and maintenance of national manpower requirements is singularly dependent on access of students to clinical sites where they can gain clinical experiences. For some CRNAs, participation in education and teaching may include an invitation to a student to observe or practice clinically in a hospital, outpatient surgery center, physician's office, or other environment in which the CRNA acts as a formal instructor or mentor. CRNAs may also serve as regular teaching faculty or clinical coordinators for established programs of nurse anesthesia. Hundreds of CRNAs who are not able to provide access to their clinical sites volunteer to lecture to students or participate in continuing education programs for CRNAs and students. Through these efforts and commitments to education, accredited programs of nurse anesthesia have increased the number of clinical sites from only a few a decade ago to more than 2,000 today. As market demand continues to flourish for CRNAs, more clinical sites will be needed for supervised educational experiences, especially in community-based sites such as outpatient surgery centers and physician's offices in addition to major medical centers.

Summary

Historical events have strongly influenced the development of values, attitudes, and behaviors that are accepted as appropriate for nurse anesthetists. Some of the values originate from American culture, and other values are held by the larger group of nurses. Certain values such as honesty and protective care are part of the unique culture of nurse anesthesia that binds CRNAs together. These values are the philosophical foundation underlying the provision of effective patient care, anesthesia services, and professionalism.

Professionalism is both a state of mind and a commitment to action. It exemplifies the knowledge that our clinical work is possible only when others understand and value our service. To reach that goal requires active, lifelong commitment for which we are collectively and individually responsible. Professionalism demands that CRNAs project and promote the best of what our profession has to offer and care unselfishly for people and the values we share. It requires a global vision that incorporates the views of others and meets the requirements of all stakeholders and does so in a way that demands attention and respect for its value in solving problems and promoting optimal care.

The constellation of professional skills required of every CRNA involves active participation in workplace affairs, issue forums, public relations efforts, interdisciplinary networking, and community involvement. Through these efforts, nurse anesthetists will become better informed, more effective at managing change, more satisfied with their career choices, and more adaptable to the changing healthcare environment. Most importantly, professionalism is a requisite for all CRNAs today and tomorrow, because ultimately, it is the only means to ensure our continued leadership in the world community of healthcare.

References

1. Thatcher VS. *History of Anesthesia with Emphasis on the Nurse Specialist.* Philadelphia, PA: JB Lippincott; 1953.

2. Robb IH. *Nursing: Its Principles and Practices for Hospital and Private Use.* Toronto: J. A. Carveth & Co; 1893:331-340.

3. Bankert M. *Watchful Care: A History of America's Nurse Anesthetists.* New York, NY: Continuum Publishing; 1989.

4. American Association of Nurse Anesthetists. Certified Registered Nurse Anesthetists (CRNAs) at a Glance. http://www.aana.com. Accessed March 30, 2010.

5. Study of Nurse Anesthetists Manpower Needs. Washington, DC: US Government Printing Office: National Center for Nursing Research; 1990.

6. Shortage of certified registered nurse anesthetists limits access to healthcare. American Association of Nurse Anesthetists [press release]. April 22, 2003.

7. Schubert A, Eckhout G, Tremper K. An updated view of the national anesthesia personnel shortfall. *Anesth Analg.* 2003;96(1):201-214.

8. Rowland RG. Are you prepared for a shortage of anesthesia providers? It may be time to review your contract-negotiation strategies. *Healthc Financ Manage.* 2003;57(3):66-70.

9. Grogono AW. Resident numbers and graduation rates from residencies and nurse anesthetist schools in 2004. *ASA Newsletter.* 2004;68(11).

10. Merwin E, Stern S, Jordan L, Bucci M. New estimates for CRNA vacancies. *AANA J.* 2009;77(2):121-129.

11. Koch E, Fosburgh LC, Justifiably proud: a brief history of nurse anesthetists. In: Waugaman WR, Foster SD, Rigor BM, eds. *Principles and Practice of Nurse Anesthesia.* 3rd ed. Norwalk, CT: Appleton and Lange; 1999:3-17.

12. Koch E. Nurse anesthesia: a history of challenge. In: Nagelhout JJ, Plaus KL, eds. *Nurse Anesthesia.* 4th ed. St. Louis, MO: Elsevier Saunders; 2010:1-27.

13. Scope and standards for nurse anesthesia practice. In: *Professional Practice Manual for the Certified Registered Nurse Anesthetists.* Park Ridge, IL: American Association of Nurse Anesthetists; 2007.

14. Qualifications and capabilities of the Certified Registered Nurse Anesthetist. In: *Professional Practice Manual for the Certified Registered Nurse Anesthetist.* Park Ridge, IL: American Association of Nurse Anesthetists; 2007.

15. Criteria for recertification. Park Ridge, IL: National Board of Certification and Recertification for Nurse Anesthetists; 2008.

16. Guidelines for granting clinical privileges to CRNAs. In: *Professional Practice Manual for the Certified Registered Nurse Anesthetist.* Park Ridge, IL: American Association of Nurse Anesthetists; 2007.

17. Summary of NCE/SEE performance and transcript data. Park Ridge, IL: Council on Certification of Nurse Anesthetists; 2008.

18. Standards for Accreditation of Nurse Anesthesia Educational Programs. Park Ridge, IL: Council on Accreditation of Nurse Anesthesia Educational Programs; 2004.

21

19. Stein HD, Kristenson AL. *The Professional Schools and the University: The Case of Social Work.* New York, NY: Council on Social Work Education; 1970:2.

20. Hughes EC. Professions, proceedings of the American Academy of Arts and Sciences. *Daedalus.* 1963;4:665-668.

21. Horton BJ. *Nurse anesthesia as a subculture of nursing in the United States.* [dissertation]. Ann Arbor, MI; 1998.

22. Code of ethics. In: *Professional Practice Manual for the Certified Registered Nurse Anesthetist.* Park Ridge, IL: American Association of Nurse Anesthetists; 2007.

23. Schein EH. Professional education: some new directions. In: *Carnegie Commission Report on Higher Education.* New York, NY: McGraw-Hill; 1972: 7-14.

24. Pellegrino ED. What is a profession? *J Allied Health.* 1983;12(3):168-176.

25. Leininger MM. The tribes of nursing in the USA culture of nursing. *J Transcult Nurs.* 1994;6(1):18-21.

Key References

1. *Professional Practice Manual for the Certified Registered Nurse Anesthetists.* Park Ridge, IL: American Association of Nurse Anesthetists: 2007.

2. Bankert M. *Watchful Care: A History of America's Nurse Anesthetists.* New York: Continuum Publishing; 1989.

22

Study Questions

1. What are the dominant cultural and patient care values CRNAs share? How do they contribute to the professionalism of nurse anesthetists?

2. Discuss the value of the unwritten moral codes that are part of the nurse anesthesia culture. How do they compare with the AANA's written code of ethics?

3. Discuss the issue of autonomy, what it means, and its relevance to any healthcare discipline or role in today's healthcare environment.

4. Identify the basic tenets of professional work groups as they evolved historically and determine the extent to which they are applicable today. How have historical events influenced the development of nurse anesthesia?

5. List and discuss your perception of a professional. What does it mean to you and how is it manifested in your school experience or professional life?

6. What association is there between professional behavior and its convergence with your personal views on responsibilities of leadership?

7. Discuss potential avenues for expressing your own skills of professional advocacy. In what ways do you advocate for patients, yourself, colleagues, affiliations, etc, on a daily basis?

CHAPTER 2

The Socialization and Professional Roles of Certified Registered Nurse Anesthetists

Wynne R. Waugaman, CRNA, PhD, FAAN
Margaret Faut Callahan, CRNA, PhD, FAAN
Larry Hornsby, CRNA, BS

Key Concepts

- Professional socialization is the essence of how nurses become nurse anesthetists by developing skills, knowledge, professional behavior, and career commitment during the educational process.

- Personal motivation is a key factor in promoting professional membership and the lifetime continuance of the professional career.

- Professional socialization and career commitment of nurse anesthetists are facilitated by early exposure to professional role models during clinical education.

- Age, gender, culture, and race or ethnicity all influence professional socialization.

- The use of research in evidence-based practice will substantially influence Certified Registered Nurse Anesthetist (CRNA) practice in the 21st century.

Continues on next page.

Key Concepts (continued)

- To enhance their value to the healthcare team, CRNAs must develop new skills to become versatile professionals and must strengthen their clinical management and leadership roles.

- Emerging roles for CRNAs include opportunities as acute care and pain management specialists, business entrepreneurs, administrators, alternative therapy experts, blended or combined advanced practice nurses, educators, researchers, writers, and legislators.

Opportunities for new work roles and professional positions will continue to evolve for Certified Registered Nurse Anesthetists (CRNAs) by virtue of their rich education and practice experience. This expansion will evolve within the context of a new focus in healthcare—that of basing care on a model of wellness, rather than disease. This raises logical questions about our future, considering the fact that much of our work is based on care models designed to ameliorate or palliate disease. How will CRNAs in the future accommodate these changes? How will we move nurse anesthesia care into a community-based model of service? To explore a new vision of practice and service, we must carefully analyze trends in healthcare and give critical attention to new and pervasive market influences and the rapidly changing US demographic. In short, student registered nurse anesthetists will socialize into the profession of nurse anesthesia in a markedly changed environment from that which existed several decades ago.

Professional Socialization

The concept of professional socialization describes how nurses are "molded" into their new roles as nurse anesthetists by developing knowledge, skills, behavior, and career commitment appropriate to the profession. This process occurs during the educational period and is influenced by both intentional and unplanned circumstances of the academic environment. Professional socialization is the process of becoming a nurse anesthetist through exposure to experiences members regard as prerequisites for inclusion in the profession. Socialization involves active membership in the professional group and acquisition of the cultural attributes of the profession.[1] Personal motivation is a key factor in promoting professional membership and a lifetime commitment to a professional career.

The process of professional socialization enables graduate students to identify with and acquire behaviors and attitudes of the CRNA group to which they are seeking membership. This includes assuming the group's organizational goals, social mission, and knowledge advancement.[2,3] Critical components of professional socialization include learning the technology and language of the profession, internalizing values and norms, and integrating the professional role into one's professional identity and other life roles.[4]

Numerous models and conceptual frameworks have been used to study the socialization process in nurses. Waugaman and Lu[5] adapted the multidimensional model of Simpson[1] to study the socialization process of nurse anesthetists. This model describes professional socialization as consisting of 3 analytically distinct dimensions or categories of variables: education or the imparting of occupational knowledge and skills, development of occupational orientations, and forming personal relatedness to the occupation. The first 2 dimensions are mainly cognitive, and the third dimension is motivational. Each dimension comprises 1 or more scales that describe the components of each dimension (Table 2.1).

A change in any of the dimensions does not necessarily influence another. For example, a temporary decline in professional commitment to the job itself may occur because of changing family roles, while the identifying features important to the work role remain stable.[5] In other words, life experiences can influence some of the variables that influence socialization, but these are temporary effects.

Professional socialization and career commitment among nurse anesthetists are facilitated by early exposure to professional

27

Table 2.1. The Dimensions and Scales of Professional Socialization of Nurse Anesthetists

Dimension	Scale
Education	Orientation to nurse anesthesia
Cognitive occupational orientations	Holistic vs bureaucratic view of patient care Administration and supervision Collegialism
Relatedness to the professional role	Attraction to nurse anesthesia Socioeconomic rewards Commitment to nurse anesthesia Self-identification as a nurse anesthetist

role models during clinical education.[6] The emphasis in nurse anesthesia education on practical experience during the curriculum enables students to visualize their professional roles with a high degree of realism very early in the program. Role modeling by nurse anesthetists and anesthesiologists throughout the program is a valuable tool of professional socialization.[3] The mentoring role is especially important in the helping professions because of the interdependent working conditions among these professionals. Educational program content; design; and faculty, practitioner, and mentor role models all play vital roles in the professional socialization of nurse anesthetists. These factors directly influence the degree to which students are socialized into the profession, and the continuation of the socialization process influences the degree of professional career commitment as people mature from nurses to nurse anesthetists.[3]

In general, the process of professional socialization of nurse anesthetists has been especially important in the development of the specialty profession of nurse anesthesia. Clearly, it is because of this process that CRNAs have built a formidable national professional organization representing 95% of all practicing CRNAs. It is also because of the socialization process that the American Association of Nurse Anesthetists (AANA) has emerged as a potent lobbying group influencing myriad state and national issues that have had profound and beneficial effects for individual practitioners and patients alike.

Socialization Versus Formation

A recent study by the Carnegie Foundation for the Advancement of Teaching noted the need for rapid and vast changes in nursing education in order to meet the healthcare needs of society.[7] The key recommendations that are important for nursing entry into practice should be considered in advanced practice nursing as well. The recommendations include making transitions:

1. From a focus on covering decontextualized knowledge to an emphasis on teaching for a sense of salience, situated cognition, and action in particular situations.

2. From a sharp separation of clinical and classroom teaching to an integration of both types of teaching.
3. From an emphasis on critical thinking to an emphasis on clinical reasoning and multiple ways of thinking.
4. From an emphasis on socialization and role taking to an emphasis on formation.

The final recommendation suggests that emphasis be placed on formation of the student with regard to identity and self-understanding as he or she moves into a professional role. This is an important aspect of moving a nurse to a nurse anesthetist role, and student registered nurse anesthetist and faculty must intentionally "use these transformational experiences, focusing on the formation of professional identity rather than on socialization."[7] Both formation and socialization experiences are needed in nurse anesthesia education and practice.

Nursing Intellectual Capacity

In addition to the challenges of role socialization, nurses work in a constantly changing environment. Nursing is no longer task-based and has become a knowledge-based profession.[8] Simpson[8] notes that often, nursing intellectual capacity is measured in numbers, which is not the only factor in a knowledge-based profession.

Corso[9] noted "This movement was inspired by the rapid growth of what has been termed the knowledge economy, a greater reliance on human ideas, services, and information technology than seen in the manufacturing and production-oriented industrial economy of the past." Knowledge, rather than numbers, is the key to understanding the needs of a rapidly changing healthcare environment. The importance of building nurse anesthesia intellectual human capacity through rigorous educational experiences is essential.

Maintaining Professionalism

Fasoli[10] reflected on the changing healthcare environment and the increased use of technology, which often detracts from independent thinking and leads to "deprofessionalization." Fasoli wrote "As technical complexity increases in an organization, professionals are drawn in to deal with the increased demand for highly skilled, more "complex" workers. Therefore, professionals are more likely to work within an organization, versus independently, as the work increases in complexity (the number of different elements that must be dealt with simultaneously), uncertainty (predictability of the elements and their behavior), and interdependence (interrelationships between elements)."[10] As complexity increases, concerns arise that bureaucratization will promote a decrease in independent, professional decision making. This change risks a profession digressing to a job or task orientation. Nurse anesthetists must resist such changes in the practice environment.

Student Registered Nurse Anesthetists

Student registered nurse anesthetists, unlike some other professional students, identify with their professional role very early in their professional education. Of the US student registered nurse anesthetists enrolled during the 1998-1999 academic year, 67% reported thinking of themselves as nurse anesthetists within the first 6 months of their graduate program. By 24 to 30 months of enrollment, 95% identified completely with the nurse anesthetist professional role.[11] Many factors influence the professional socialization process, including age, gender, culture, and race or ethnicity.

29

As the population continues to change, the nursing and nurse anesthesia population will also change. To meet the educational needs of future student registered nurse anesthetists, faculty must evaluate how curricular and instructional design influences the degree of professional socialization attained, particularly in minority cultures. Even more fundamental is the fact that nurse anesthesia faculty must appreciate the values and cultural mores of diverse groups, especially as they relate to learning style. Without this, faculty may inadvertently impede professional socialization and student learning by imposing teaching methods deemed successful for the dominant culture, but unproved for diverse populations. Demonstration of cultural competence in teaching is key to enhancing recruitment and retention in diverse populations in graduate specialty nursing, particularly nurse anesthesia.

Waugaman and Lu[5] found, in their study of professional socialization of more than 1,000 US student registered nurse anesthetists, that culture, race, and ethnicity correlated significantly ($P < .05$) with the dimensions of the professional socialization process (See Table 2.1) for all nondominant student registered nurse anesthetist groups, when compared with the "dominant" group (European Americans). The 4 nondominant groups were identified for the purposes of this study as Asians and Pacific Islanders, Hispanics, African Americans, and Native American and Alaskan Natives. Overall, Asians and Pacific Islanders in this study responded more positively to the traditional process of professional socialization. Hispanic student registered nurse anesthetists who were surveyed had a statistically significant negative response compared with all other cultural groups to the educational dimension, which describes the skills and knowledge of nurse anesthesia practice. Asians and Pacific Islanders surveyed valued collegialism and were more likely to pursue administrative and supervisory roles than were African Americans. Hispanics had a statistically significant negative response to the dimension of personal relatedness, which identifies the relationship of the individual to the occupation through status identification, professional commitment, attraction to the job, and socioeconomic rewards. The profound negative response by Hispanic students also suggests that professional recruitment and retention of this ethnic group into nursing, specifically advanced practice nursing specialties, may be more difficult than for some of the other groups.

Emerging cultures are changing the US demographic and that, in turn, profoundly influences both the education and practice of all advanced practice nursing specialties. The 2009 US Census Bureau reports that by 2050, the country will be more ethnically and racially diverse and much older.[12] Furthermore, minority groups are expected to become the majority by 2042, increasing to 54% of the population by 2050. Half of all children are expected to be from minority groups by 2023.

The Hispanic American population is expected to triple between 2008 and 2050, representing an increase from 15% to 30% of the total US population. The single-race white population is expected to decrease to approximately 46% by 2050. The black population is expected to grow by 15% by 2050. Asian Americans will account for 9.2% of the population in 2050.[12]

Among the remaining race and ethnic groups, American Indian and Alaskan Native populations are projected to rise from 4.9 million to 8.6 million, or from 1.6% to 2% of the total population. The Native

Hawaiian and Other Pacific Islander population is expected to more than double, from 1.1 million to 2.6 million. The number of people who identify themselves as being of 2 or more races is projected to more than triple, from 5.2 million to 16.2 million.[12]

In 2030, one fifth of US residents will be 65 years and older. By 2050 this number is expected to climb to 88.5 million, double the older population in 2008. More striking is the fact that the population of individuals 85 years and older will triple by 2050.[12]

Entering students are often older and enter nursing as a mid-life career change. The ratio of men to women (40:60) in nurse anesthesia is vastly different from the generic nursing population. Factors of age and sex also influence professional socialization. According to a study by Waugaman and Lohren,[11] in the US population of student registered nurse anesthetists, older students (> 40 years old) responded less positively to the scales comprising the dimensions of socialization than younger student registered nurse anesthetists. Older students were less related to the occupation through status identification, commitment, and attraction to nurse anesthesia as a career. Students more than 40 years old were less concerned with the socioeconomic rewards of the profession as a component of socialization when compared with students less than 30 years old. Older students also expressed the belief that age is a factor in how they respond to their educational process, in how instructors evaluate them, and in their own ability to provide patient-centered anesthesia care.[11] Male student registered nurse anesthetists strongly associated with characteristics typified in bureaucratic organizations, such as following rules and regulations, the importance of technology, distancing oneself from patients, and the importance of proper physical care irrespective of the patient's feelings.[11] Men also were more oriented toward assuming administrative and supervisory roles, while women were more focused on holistic care and providing culturally congruent anesthesia care.

Nursing Shortage and the Impact on Nurse Anesthesia

The general population of nurses and nurse anesthetists is aging. Overall, nursing opportunities are expected to grow by more than 581,500 new jobs by 2018 according to the Bureau of Labor Statistics.[13]

Buerhaus and colleagues[14] estimate that, despite the economic downturn of 2008 and 2009, there will be a shortage of more than 260,000 nurses by 2025. This figure represents one of the greatest nurse shortages in US history. Because of the nursing shortage and the demand for more nurses in primary care due to the Patient Protection and Affordable Care Act of 2010, nurses may elect to pursue this career pathway.[15]

The Effects of Graduate Education on Socialization

Educational programs have a profound influence on the socialization of CRNAs. During the educational program, students are first exposed to a very different culture than they are used to as practicing, highly experienced intensive care nurses. Often, students entering nurse anesthesia programs undergo tremendous adjustments to graduate study. For many students, sitting in a classroom each day for one or more academic terms when accustomed to active clinical practice is difficult at best. Some students may have been away from the academic setting for a decade or more and must develop new study habits to ensure success in graduate school.

31

Table 2.2. Increase in Nurse Anesthesia Educational Programs, Graduates, and Clinical Sites from 1999 to 2010

	1999	2010	Increase %
Nurse anesthesia educational programs	83	110	33
Graduates	948	2,375	150
Clinical sites	619	2,200	255

For a variety of reasons, a nurse anesthesia educational program is unlike most other forms of higher education in that it mixes a highly rigorous academic curriculum with demands for accomplished performance in a high-stress clinical environment. Furthermore, many students of nursing come to the educational experience unprepared for the demands of critical thinking. It is common for many nurses to have assumed a role in the course of their daily work as master technicians, and for the most part, observers and recorders of patient problems. They are not, by and large, prepared to be problem solvers and to think through multidimensional problems in systematic ways to yield usable solutions. The concept that they will be ultimately responsible for all decisions regarding a patient's care is often foreign because they have depended on physicians to assume that role. In addition, there is a substantial amount of new, didactic information that they are required to sort through, prioritize, and recall in appropriate circumstances. These are major stressors for students embarking on the process of socializing to new roles as anesthetists.

Graduate education in nurse anesthesia demands that students be self-motivated, independent thinkers. Pedagogic teaching styles, in which teachers impart knowledge to passive students, are essentially nonexistent. Specialist education requires that students take primary responsibility for learning under expert guidance, developing skills of critical thinking and integration of theory into practice. Nurse anesthetists must learn to apply useful theoretical principles to clinical practice in order to make rational, justifiable decisions relative to patient care problems. Instruction requires that students be actively engaged in learning through independent study, small group discussions, case analysis presentations, research presentations, and a vast amount of reading from books and periodicals. Education imparts the values of socialization through self-discipline, resourcefulness, responsibility, and setting standards of academic and clinical performance.

In January 2010, there were 110 accredited nurse anesthesia educational programs.[16] In 2010, the COA had reviewed and approved more than 2,200 clinical sites. Furthermore, there were 4 programs in capability review. Table 2.2 demonstrates the substantial increase in nurse anesthesia programs, graduates, and clinical sites from 2000 to 2010. In 2010 there were no program closures and the turnover in program administrators decreased to 15% compared with 22% in 2005. In 2010, US Nurse Anesthesia programs admitted 2,852 applicants, and 4,152 qualified applicants were not offered admission. Fifty-six percent of programs offer a graduate degree in nursing,

34% in nurse anesthesia, and the remaining 10% in a variety of related disciplines.[16]

The Influence of Healthcare Changes on CRNA Roles

A number of factors are predicted to substantially influence healthcare and nursing practice in the 21st century. Chinn[17] predicted that these changes will be largely related to the technology explosion, an evolution of drastic disease trajectories, increasing scarcity of healthcare resources, and an increasing demand for new and still unmet services. Other sources of change affecting nursing will come from the increased use and management of information, movement of care to outpatient and home environments, demand for evidenced-based care, emerging quality measurement mandates, and heightened compliance requirements for clinical credentialing and privileging. In addition, the passage of the Patient Protection and Affordable Care Act of 2010 will provide healthcare coverage for more than 30 million Americans who had previously limited or no access to healthcare.[15] The need for CRNAs has never been greater.

What will these changes imply for the evolving clinical role of nurse anesthetists in the future? How will CRNAs need to change in order to remain competitive and viable in the marketplace?

- *Education:* CRNAs in the future will need substantially more formal preparation in the social demographics of their patients in order to provide culturally competent care. There must be more curricular attention given to biomedical engineering and information management to master new clinical technology and database-driven mechanisms for clinical decision making. There will be increasing use of human simulation as an instructional technique and more attention given to engendering skills of critical thinking and incorporation of intellectual standards.

- *Practice:* CRNAs will be required not only to maintain their scope of practice, but also to expand it to areas of acute and chronic pain management, critical care, and home delivery of care to chronically ill patients requiring pain blocks and specialized ventilatory care. Some CRNAs will be examining potential roles in administration of alternative therapies such as herbal preparations and aromatherapy, acupuncture, hypnosis, and massage techniques. All CRNAs increasingly will be required to document anesthesia care in ways that demonstrate competence, productivity, and quality. They will have to learn to manage and interpret a new generation of monitoring modalities that dimensionally display vital organ function. They will be administering anesthesia services increasingly more often as sole providers, using physicians in consultant roles.

- *Credentialing:* CRNAs will eventually be required to recertify by simulated testing or other means to demonstrate clinical competence beyond initial certification. Graduate education for all practitioners will likely be a requirement in all states for the next generation of providers.

- *Surgery:* All CRNAs should be aware of how changes in surgical technique influence demand for their services. What are the implications for CRNAs of the increasing use of endoscopic techniques in surgery, specialized catheter access procedures, laser technology, and advanced imaging procedures? Coupled with frequent changes

33

in the numbers and types of cases that qualify for reimbursement in general, how will the nature of CRNA services necessarily change?

- *Work setting:* CRNAs will be increasingly employed under contractual arrangements that do not include the traditional package of employee benefits. CRNAs will be hired on the basis of proven expertise. They must be mobile and functionally cross-trained to assume a variety of care roles. Care settings increasingly will use community-based clinics, physician offices, schools, skilled nursing facilities, and the home environment.

- *Communication:* CRNAs will be required to demonstrate increasingly sophisticated communication skills that facilitate critical thinking, effective problem solving, negotiation, and fulfillment of organizational goals, primarily within some form of integrated managed-care organization.

- *Professional advocacy:* In order to remain competitive, all CRNAs must be able to demonstrate some effectiveness in advocacy efforts that promote their own well-being and that of their patients. These are skills that are learned through systematic study of the profession within the social context.

Emerging Professional Roles

In addition to clinical roles, CRNAs often assume employment roles in pharmaceutical or manufacturing companies or a host of other public and private agencies that deal with healthcare products and services. The unique educational background and clinical expertise of CRNAs make them particularly well-suited to positions in education, marketing, or sales with companies that man-

ufacture and sell anesthesia equipment, devices, and pharmaceutical agents and adjuncts used in anesthesia practice. Some nurse anesthetists have assumed positions as advisors to public and private agencies such as the Food and Drug Administration. These professional contributions by CRNAs enhance public awareness of CRNA services as well as promote the importance of our role in healthcare planning and delivery.

CRNAs are involved increasingly in creating and managing entrepreneurial enterprises. CRNA-owned practices, group or individual, have proven track records of success. Some CRNAs have become successful as educational conference or seminar providers, and others have developed and marketed computer software. Consulting for organizational and management entities, the legal profession, or educational institutions is frequently a full-time or part-time professional option for qualified CRNAs. Advanced degrees in education, business, finance, and economics often provide the skills and experiences on which to base entrepreneurial efforts.

The field of administration has been embraced by countless nurse anesthetists who serve as department managers, chief nurse anesthetists, or directors of clinical services. These professionals are responsible for general administrative management, budgeting, resource procurement and distribution, human resource activities, and frequently, institutional committee work including quality management. CRNAs have also assumed positions in educational administration. These professional opportunities include deanships or other academic administrative roles, department or division chair positions, and program directorships. Nurse anesthesia administrators in higher education must be well-versed in accreditation and certification requirements in nurse anesthesia, graduate and university policies, and public and case law, all of which have an impact on higher education. Educational administrators are responsible for developing and deploying the curriculum, recruiting and retaining students, and in most cases, demonstrating accomplishment in service, teaching, and research.

Increasingly, CRNAs in the academy as well as in clinical practice are becoming involved in the promulgation of research, either as full-time or part-time professionals. CRNAs with doctoral degrees in the basic sciences are more likely to conduct research in a basic science laboratory, often using animal models. Some CRNAs prefer applied research that involves testing and evaluation of clinical theories and modes of practice and therapy. Clinical studies may include testing anesthesia products or equipment or managing clinical trials of new pharmaceutical agents or other relevant clinical applications. Opportunities are available for nurse anesthetists to complete degree or certificate programs in clinical research, enabling them to participate in and lead the conduct of clinical drug trials.

CRNAs who have doctoral degrees in behavioral sciences or education may prefer to conduct research that evaluates educational models and theories applied to nurse anesthesia practice or professional behavioral adjustments such as socialization. Since nurse anesthesia education has moved into the graduate framework, most curricula include some course preparation in theory and research. Some programs offer research opportunities for master's degree level students, and other programs reserve this experience for doctoral students. However, the conduct of research need not be reserved for doctoral students and doctorally prepared CRNAs. Practicing CRNAs are frequently and actively involved in the research programs of the department in which they are employed.

Professions are often measured by their scholarly works and peer-reviewed publications and not exclusively by the quality of their clinical practice.[6] More CRNAs are required to conduct original research and write for publications to enhance the professional standing of the nurse anesthesia community as a valued contributor to the body of anesthesia knowledge and, in turn, raise the level of consumer awareness and value placed on nurse anesthesia services. Although nurse anesthesia is the oldest nursing specialty, for many years it had the smallest number of publications (textbooks and journals) compared with other nursing specialties. During the first decade of the 21st century, great strides were made in this area. CRNAs have a professional obligation to share new knowledge with colleagues and consumers so that all can benefit from their findings or message. This dissemination of knowledge is a link to the next generation, our legacy.

A Different Path: CRNAs as Entrepreneurs

Nearly 80% of all CRNAs in the United States are employed by healthcare facilities or physician groups. In these types of employment relationships, salary and benefits are not usually delineated by formal contract, but rather in a work agreement, by professional appointment, or some other type of informal arrangement that defines, at minimum, the employee's salary, benefits, and perhaps work hours. Formal credentialing and privileging documents usually are part of this package. These detail the extent of the employee's ability to provide care according to his or her education and experience. Within these arrangements, employees typically have an

35

implicit understanding that they work within the policies, procedures, and salary and benefit structure designed by the employer and/or medical staff. In short, there is little room for discussion or negotiation of terms involved in the work offered. Consequently, the traditional contract, per se, is rare in these work settings.

There are, however, many CRNAs who are working, not as employees, but as contracted professionals either in solo or group practice, as employees of other CRNAs or anesthesiologists, or as contracted employees to another independent individual, group, or agency who may, in turn, be under contract to a larger facility. These types of employment arrangements are most often described in detailed contracts between the parties involved.

Generally these types of entrepreneurial practitioners provide anesthesia services for a global fee to a facility or other provider that may be collecting reimbursements from public or private third-party payers or the facility or hospital with which they are contracting. Contractors work most often for a set salary and no benefits, although, of course, those details can be addressed differently in the contract. In short, contracting CRNAs work in a host of different employment arrangements for generally higher wages because they assume no claim to benefits as employees do. They do not enjoy the typical protections of due process (unless otherwise specified in the contract), and they are mobile in providing their services and are immediately available. In certain contracting situations, the wages are higher because the contractor assumes substantial overhead costs (eg, billing services, insurance, supplies, equipment).

Alternative employment arrangements generally involve contracted services. This discussion is not comprehensive in scope or meant to constitute legal advice, but rather to provide a "flavor" for the role of what is commonly referred to as the *independent provider* or *solo practitioner*. CRNAs who enter into contracted services should consider retaining the services of a professional accountant and attorney to ensure their rights and protection.

The number of contracted, professional workers in anesthesia will likely increase in the future, parallel to trends in the US workforce outside healthcare, in which highly skilled, specialized, and mobile professionals are sought to fill temporary needs. This is done in order for business and industry to remain flexible, attentive to changing market demand, and cost efficient.

Who Seeks This Type of Employment Arrangement?

Perhaps the better question to ask is this: What opportunities and responsibilities does this type of arrangement provide? First and foremost, it requires that a CRNA be fully confident in his or her abilities to practice independently, that is, capable of making decisions alone or with other professional consultants if they are available. It also requires that the CRNA be prepared in the full scope of practice, because CRNAs with limited skills are of little use to a surgeon or facility. It demands that the CRNA be able to handle all risk categories of patients. The CRNA should be well-acquainted with the standards of care of the profession, use good judgment in determining what is in the best interest of the patient, and always act or intervene within the boundaries of experience and qualification. Finally, CRNAs must be effective communicators, because without this skill, they are unlikely to be able to secure productive or long-lasting contractual relationships.

CRNAs often cite this type of work arrangement as providing them with greater latitude to select practice environments, assume a great range of responsibilities for anesthesia services, become more autonomous in decision making and, in short, exercise their full potential as anesthesia providers. There are also benefits of potentially higher wages, but with those benefits come increased responsibilities to provide coverage and to work hours that are not confined to typical "shift" rotations. With new business responsibilities comes the need to find individual insurance coverage, coverage for family, and potentially, for employees. Also associated with business management or ownership are numerous overhead costs that often do not occur to an employed worker. Clearly, with any great potential, there can be considerable risk. In order to enter the work of contracted employment, preparatory study, planning, and hard work in projecting potential success and roadblocks are vital first steps.

Negotiation

One of the most often cited barriers to CRNAs exploring entrepreneurial practice arrangements is that they feel ill at ease with their negotiating skills. Many believe that there is some well-kept secret about the true art of negotiation when, in fact, every CRNA has some ability to negotiate, and many have great expertise. In our everyday lives, we all negotiate with siblings, parents, and friends to watch a particular movie, dine at a favorite restaurant, or do something to return a favor. So why should we be so passionate about these situations and feel so inept when faced with the prospect of negotiating a pay raise with the boss or a contract with a facility? Perhaps it is fear of the unknown.

CRNAs who wish to pursue these entrepreneurial opportunities will find strong support and rich resources within the AANA. CRNAs who have pursued private practice are most willing to share their expertise and assist.

Summary

Nurse anesthetists have been leaders in healthcare for more than a century, and our roles have continually evolved to meet societal needs. As CRNAs, we must be visionary in identifying our future professional directions and make deliberate choices that move us toward those realities. It is not sufficient to react to challenge and opportunity or expect that change will not occur. We must be proactive in designing the future. For nurse anesthetists, there is no status quo. We must be evolving in a continual, planned, and creative way.

Nurse anesthetists must be ready for what Gladwell[18] names as the "tipping point." These critical points occur when an idea or movement reaches the point of making an impact and there is no returning to the status quo. The profession of nurse anesthesia has already witnessed many key "tipping points" such as when anesthesia was determined to be the legitimate practice of nursing, or when CRNAs were first granted direct reimbursement for services, which ultimately provided for the financial stability of the profession. A more recent tipping point was the publication of evidence that CRNAs provide safe, quality anesthesia care and demonstrated the cost-effectiveness of CRNAs.[19,20]

Furthermore, in a landmark study[21] published by the Institute of Medicine entitled "The Future of Nursing: Leading Change, Advancing Health," advanced practice nurses, including CRNAs, are cited as integral parts of a transformed healthcare

37

system. The study determined that barriers to full scope of practice for CRNAs and other advanced practice nurses must be removed. The specific recommendations[21] in the report are:

1. Nurses should practice to the full extent of their education and training.
2. Nurses should achieve higher levels of education and training through an improved education system that promotes seamless academic progression.
3. Nurses should be full partners with physicians and other healthcare professionals in redesigning healthcare in the United States
4. Effective workforce planning and policy making require better data collection and an improved information infrastructure.

This is the ultimate "tipping point" in the acceptance of nurse anesthetists in expanded, respected, and essential roles in healthcare. As we look to the future, CRNAs must be prepared to accept expansion of roles and practice opportunities that a dynamic healthcare system will require.

References

1. Simpson IH. *From Student to Nurse: A Longitudinal Study of Socialization.* Cambridge, UK: Cambridge University Press; 1979:3-326.
2. Schlotfeldt RM. Structuring nursing knowledge: a priority for creating nursing's future. *Nurs Sci Q.* 1988; 1(1):35-38.
3. Waugaman WR. From nurse to nurse anesthetist. In: Waugaman WR, Rigor BM, Katz LE, Bradshaw HM, Garde JF, eds. *Principles and Practice of Nurse Anesthesia.* Norwalk, CT: Appleton & Lange; 1987:3-5.
4. Cohen HA. Authoritarianism and dependency: problems in nursing socialization. In: Flynn B. *Current Perspective in Nursing Social Issues and Trends.* St Louis, MO: Mosby; 1980.
5. Waugaman WR. Lu J. From nurse to nurse anesthetist: the relationship of culture, race, and ethnicity to professional socialization and career commitment of advanced practice nurses. *J Transcult Nurs.* 1999;10(3):237-247.
6. Waugaman WR. From nurse to nurse anesthetist: effects of professional socialization on career commitment [dissertation]. University of Pittsburgh; 1991.
7. Benner P, Sutphen M, Leonard V, Day L. *Educating Nurses: A Call for Radical Transformation.* San Francisco, CA: Jossey-Bass; 2009.
8. Simpson R. Information technology: building nursing intellectual capacity for the information age. *Nurs Admin Q.* 2007;31(1):84-88.
9. Corso JA. Rethinking traditional methods for measuring intellectual capital. *Nurs Admin Q.* 2007;31(1):13.
10. Fasoli DR. The culture of nursing engagement: a historical perspective. *Nurs Adm Q.* 2010;34(1):18-29.
11. Waugaman WR. Lohren DJ. Abstract A43: Factors influencing status identification as a nurse anesthetist among graduate students. AANA Foundation poster abstracts [abstract]. *AANA J.* 1999;67(6):527.
12. US Bureau of the Census. US Interim Projections by Age, Sex, Race, and Hispanic Origin: 2000-2050. http://www.census.gov/population/www/projections/usinterimproj/. Accessed December 12, 2009.

38

13. Bureau of Labor Statistics. Occupational employment projections to 2018. http://www.bls.gov/opub/mlr/2009/11/art5full.pdf. Accessed November 17, 2010.

14. Buerhaus PI, Staiger, DO, Auerbach DI. *The Future of the Nursing Workforce in the United States: Data, Trends, and Implications.* Boston, MA: Jones and Bartlett Publishers; 2008.

15. Patient Protection and Affordable Care Act. http://www.govtrack.us/congress/bill.xpd?bill=h111-3590. Accessed November 17, 2010.

16. Gerbasi F. Council on Accreditation of Nurse Anesthesia Educational Programs 2010 Annual Report. Park Ridge, IL: American Association of Nurse Anesthetists; 2010.

17. Chinn PL. Looking into the crystal ball: positioning ourselves for the year 2000. *Nurs Outlook.* 1991;39(6):251-256.

18. Gladwell M. *The Tipping Point: How Little Things Can Make a Big Difference.* New York, NY: Little Brown and Company; 2002.

19. Dulisse, B, Crowmwell J. No harm found when nurse anesthetists work without supervision by physicians. *Health Aff.* 2010;29(8):1469-1475.

20. Hogan PF, Seifert RF, Moore CS, Simonson BE. Cost effectiveness analysis of anesthesia providers. *Nurs Econ.* 2010;28(3):159-169.

21. Institute of Medicine. The Future of Nursing: Leading Change, Advancing Health. http://www.iom.edu. Accessed November 17, 2010.

39

Study Questions

1. What is professional socialization and how does it influence how CRNAs view their profession?

2. How do age, gender, culture, race, and ethnicity factors influence the professional socialization of nurse anesthetists?

3. How will changes in healthcare affect CRNA roles in the future?

4. What are examples of extended or emerging CRNA roles beyond that of clinician?

5. What are the advantages of pursuing the extended nontraditional roles available in nurse anesthesia?

6. Discuss among peers your perceptions of how the roles and responsibilities of employed CRNAs may be different from those of contracted CRNAs.

CHAPTER 3

American Association of Nurse Anesthetists: The Role of the Professional Organization

Scot Foster, CRNA, PhD, FAAN
Rita M. Rupp, RN, MA

Key Concepts

- The American Association of Nurse Anesthetists (AANA) is the single professional organization in the United States that represents the interests of Certified Registered Nurse Anesthetists (CRNAs). Its mission is to promote the full scope of practice for CRNAs and promote healthcare policy that supports nurse anesthesia practice.

- The AANA is based in Park Ridge, Illinois. The national headquarters supports approximately 115 full-time staff members. In addition, the Federal Government Affairs Office in Washington, DC, has 7 staff members.

- The national Association staff works under the direction of the executive director, who follows the directives of the Board of Directors. All Board members, including officers, are elected by member CRNAs.

- The AANA membership represents approximately 90% of all CRNAs.

- State organizations of the AANA are independent organizations supported by national dues that access a variety of support services from the national Association on issues related to state and federal government affairs, practice, managed care and reimbursement, public relations, education, continuing education, research, and membership.

Many have claimed that the collective strength and influence of nurse anesthetists in the healthcare arena today has been largely the result of 2 factors. First and foremost is the quality of anesthesia services provided by Certified Registered Nurse Anesthetists (CRNAs), and second, the strength of the professional association of CRNAs, the American Association of Nurse Anesthetists (AANA). Given birth and guided by such legendary figures as Agatha Hodgins, Helen Lamb, Hilda Salomon, Adeline Curtis, and Gertrude Fife, the AANA has evolved into a professional organization of substantial influence. This chapter charts that growth since 1931 and acquaints the student registered nurse anesthetist with the organizational structure of the AANA, the role members play in its continued development, and the services accrued from active participation in Association business.

A Philosophical Perspective

Professional organizations, regardless of the discipline with which they are associated, play a unique and demanding role in society. Often the roles they assume are complex, multifaceted, and seemingly contradictory; yet they have become the necessary vehicle by which professional healthcare providers are able to promote their interests, interface with the public, maintain relationships with external healthcare agencies, and effectively influence health policy in both state and federal legislatures.

There are several basic tenets that every student of nurse anesthesia should come to appreciate about professional organizations. First, organizations are established by members for the pursuit of collective goals that serve the self-interest of the provider. Organizations such as the AANA would not exist if not for the support and mandate of its members; therefore, organizational goals should be based largely on the basic tenets, philosophies, and values of its membership. Second, professional organizations cannot exist apart from the underlying fabric of social norms and values. As stated in the initial chapter of this book, professions exist only at the behest of society; that is, they are given the rights and privileges of practice because they remain accountable to the public. Consequently, professional organizations are required to walk a fine line between member and consumer interest. It is largely this ambiguity that can result in the perception by the public of overriding self-interest on the part of the profession. If not managed with great care, this situation can lead to public skepticism and mistrust. This results in increased public advocacy via legislative action intended to shift the balance back toward the public good. When a profession fails its public responsibility, society will usually demand and obtain change.[1]

Some have claimed that professional organizations are inherently in conflict with the greater good of society and as such should be abolished. However, for all the justification that could support this argument, few alternatives have been suggested to adequately substitute for the work of professional organizations. The fact remains that a strong, visionary professional association is one of the best means of securing the rights and privileges of practice for its members. All CRNAs should appreciate, however, the need to maintain the delicate balance between self-interest and the public good.

The AANA remains unique in several respects when compared with other professional organizations. The AANA was among the first nursing specialty organizations to be recognized within nursing. Few other professional specialty organizations in nursing can claim its tenure, experience, or stature. The AANA also claims an active membership of 90% of all CRNAs in the country.[2] This statistic, we believe, is paralleled in few other professional organizations of healthcare providers. Given the fact that CRNAs are not required to join the professional organization to practice, it would appear obvious that most CRNAs value the role and productivity of the AANA.

Finally, the success of the AANA may be predicated on the unique relationship between its members, the executive office, and its elected leadership. Decision making relative to AANA business is encouraged at every level. Individual members have direct access to communicate with their elected state or national leaders, and they exercise direct voting privileges; that is, membership sentiment is not funneled through a delegate system in which individual opinions may be diluted or distilled into a group or consensus opinion. Therefore, CRNAs remain singularly individual in their ability to participate and be heard on issues affecting their practice.

Historical Development

In 1926, the first meeting of the Lakeside Hospital alumnae group of nurse anesthetists was held in Cleveland, Ohio. There, Agatha Hodgins announced her vision of establishing a national association of nurse anesthetists. Before this time, a few states had had varying success with establishing small groups of CRNAs in which to discuss difficult cases, yet none were organized to the extent that they could claim a national following. Hodgins maintained the philosophy that nurse anesthesia should not be considered a part of nursing service, rather a part of general hospital service. On several occasions she approached the American Nurses Association (ANA) in regard to

nurse anesthetists being recognized within that group. However, the ANA failed to approve the proposition and required more study of the Hodgins proposal. Headstrong and tiring of inattention by the ANA, Hodgins called CRNAs around the country to convene at Lakeside Hospital "for the purpose of considering the organization of the nurse anesthetists group." Forty-four CRNAs from 12 states agreed to form the National Association of Nurse Anesthetists (NANA) and to continue their efforts to affiliate with the ANA.

Over the next several years, Hodgins again attempted affiliation with the ANA but to no avail. Its board of directors finally rejected the proposal of the NANA, stating that affiliate membership could be accomplished through regular, established channels at the state level. Few of NANA's early leaders were surprised at this outcome, none less than Hodgins, who by now was in ill health and left a small, fledgling organization still without the national recognition she fervently sought.[3(pp65-73)]

By 1933, NANA had still not convened its first national meeting and suffered from general disarray organizationally. However, Gertrude Fife, the recently elected president of the organization, was encouraged by John Mannix, a department of anesthesia administrator at Lakeside Hospital, to seek recognition from the American Hospital Association (AHA). Given the fact that this group readily recognized the value of nurse anesthetists to their hospitals, the AHA invited NANA to present its first national meeting in conjunction with them. Fife stated, "We were going to put on the first convention. Who was going to make out the program? We had very little time. And Mannix said that we had to meet . . . we had to put that convention on. And, consequently, Helen Lamb and Walter Powell

43

44

came to Cleveland and we made out the program over my kitchen . . . my dining room table. The three of us."[3(p76)] And so a renewed, vibrant, and committed organization of nurse anesthetists met for the first time in Milwaukee, Wisconsin, from September 13 to 15, 1933. By the close of the first annual meeting of NANA, Gertrude Fife, the newly reelected president of the association, declared, "I feel that we are making history and that we are laying the foundation for a fine organization that will be a great benefit to the future of the work."[3(p78)]

After this meeting, Fife was faced with the first and most important issue facing nurse anesthetists: education. She called for a committee to investigate all schools of nurse anesthesia with the objective of creating a list of "accredited" schools. In addition, she called for the establishment of National Board Examination for Nurse Anesthetists. With this agenda set for NANA in 1933, the members continued to move forward.[3(p80,81)] In 1939, the organization's name was changed to the American Association of Nurse Anesthetists. In 1955, the US commissioner of education recognized the AANA as the national accrediting authority for nurse anesthesia education. This was a milestone for the AANA, as recognition afforded students of accredited programs eligibility for federal funds such as grant or loan programs.[3(p139)]

Mission, Values, Philosophy, and Objectives

The mission of the AANA has guided the development of its strategic plan and operational priorities. According to the AANA strategic framework, the mission of the Association is "Advancing patient safety and excellence in anesthesia." The strategic planning process of the organization is ongoing. The AANA Strategic Framework document details a vision, mission, core values, motto statements, organizational goals, and outcome statements. The planning document is updated periodically through environmental scanning (also referred to as "enviroscanning"), a process of looking at and identifying internal and external factors that affect the profession. Participation in this ongoing process involves the AANA Board, committees, Foundation, and subsidiaries; councils; state associations; and AANA members through discussions at meetings and input received through the AANA annual membership survey. The strategic framework document is published on the AANA member website.[4]

The Bylaws and Standing Rules of the AANA state: "The members of this professional association are dedicated to the precept that its members are committed to the advancement of educational standards and practices, which will advance the art and science of anesthesiology and thereby support and enhance quality patient care."[5]

Since the founding of the Association, the objectives of the AANA have changed very little from those presented at the first Annual Meeting. As required by law in Illinois, the objectives appear in the original certificate of incorporation of the AANA notarized October 11, 1939, and filed with Edward J. Hughes, then Illinois secretary of state, on October 17, 1939. The certificate is renewed annually. The objectives were amended at the AANA 1978 Annual Meeting (Table 3.1).

Responsibilities and Qualifications of Membership

The ability of CRNAs to become involved in their professional Association is not without cost and responsibility. Foremost

---

Table 3.1 Objectives of the AANA[5,6]

1. To promote continual high-quality patient care

2. To advance the science and art of anesthesiology

3. To develop and promote educational standards in the field of nurse anesthesia

4. To develop and promote standards of practice in the field of nurse anesthesia

5. To facilitate effective cooperation between nurse anesthetists, anesthesiologists, and other members of the medical professions, the nursing profession, hospitals, and agencies representing a community of interest in nurse anesthesia

6. To publish scientific journals, bulletins, and other publications pertinent to the objectives of the Association

7. To maintain informational and statistical data for reference and assistance in matters pertaining to the profession or its practice

8. To provide opportunities for continuing education in anesthesia

9. To provide members with direction pertaining to governmental policy, legislation, or judicial decisions of importance to anesthesia

---

(Reprinted with permission from the AANA.)

is the responsibility each CRNA has to carefully assess his or her professional commitment by making the decision whether to become an active, dues-paying member. This decision should be based largely on careful study of what services the professional Association can provide to the member and the extent to which the individual CRNA shares the values, philosophy, and objectives promoted by the membership. Active membership requires that all CRNAs who become involved in Association activities be conversant with current issues in order to effectively engage in discussions and decision-making activities. As students will soon realize, most CRNAs have little problem voicing their opinions; however, as with any professional organization, the quality of those decisions is predicated largely on an informed position, one that not only serves the individual member but also recognizes the needs and priorities of colleagues and stakeholders in our services who are external to the organization.

There are 5 categories of active membership, which are explained in Table 3.2. Qualifications for active membership are graduation from an accredited program in nurse anesthesia; successful completion of the Certification Examination; and compliance with Association guidelines, standards, or other qualifications set forth in the bylaws of the Association. Students who are enrolled in accredited programs of nurse anesthesia are eligible for student associate membership at a fraction of the cost of full membership. One-third of the current dues for membership in the AANA is allocated

45

Table 3.2. The 5 Categories of Active Membership in the AANA[5]

A. Categories. There shall be five categories of Active membership:

1. Active certified—Individuals who have been granted initial certification by the Council on Certification of Nurse Anesthetists. Once certified, membership is automatic for the remainder of said fiscal year and then only until the individual is eligible for membership as an Active recertified member.

2. Active recertified—Individuals who are currently recertified by the Council on Recertification of Nurse Anesthetists.

3. Active nonrecertified—Individuals who are required to be recertified but are not currently recertified and desire to enjoy the rights and privileges of Active membership. Individuals who are actively practicing anesthesia may not remain in this category of membership for a period to exceed two years or one recertification period following the date of expiration of their recertification. Individuals who are not actively practicing anesthesia may remain in this category. Upon recertification, Active nonrecertified members shall become Active recertified members.

4. Life—This is a closed category of membership comprised of individuals who have held this category of membership since August 31, 1976, and will do so for the remainder of their lifetime. Life members shall be granted the category of Active membership for which they qualify. Life members shall be exempt from payment of dues.

5. Emeritus—Individuals who have held Active membership for a minimum of 25 years, who desire to enjoy the privileges of Active membership, but have retired from the practice of anesthesia.

(Reprinted with permission from the AANA.)

to the state association in which the CRNA resides. Membership in the AANA constitutes automatic recognition of membership of the CRNA in his or her respective state organization. The privileges and rights of members will be addressed in a later section of this chapter and in Table 3.3.

Organizational Structure and Function

The AANA was incorporated on October 17, 1939, in Illinois and designated as a tax-exempt organization by Subsection 501(C)(6) of the Internal Revenue Service. The AANA's education and research foundation was incorporated on July 15, 1981, and designated as a tax-exempt organization by Subsection 501(C)(3) of the Internal Revenue Code.

The AANA Bylaws are essentially the AANA's working constitution and dictate how the Association operates. The bylaws consist of 22 articles that have a number of important subheadings, called sections, which further detail important facts about the Association and its policies. Articles address areas such as the different classes of membership available, decision-making procedures, the responsibilities of the AANA's elected officials, and configurations of committees and function of their members.

Proposed amendments to the AANA Bylaws must be submitted in writing by 5 active members to the Association's executive director not less than 90 days before the next Annual Meeting. Proposed amendments must be referred to the Bylaws

Table 3.3. Benefits and Services Provided to AANA Members[5]

Heightened public awareness of the profession
- Greater professional recognition and identity
- National public relations campaign to educate the public regarding the role of nurse anesthetists
- Patient information brochures and videotapes for use by practicing CRNAs

Support regarding business and clinical practice issues
- Consultative assistance on employment practices, clinical practice issues, and quality-of-care issues
- Guidance on regulatory and institutional accreditation issues
- National representation with relevant external health agencies
- Practice publications, such as monographs and position statements
- AANA Peer Assistance hotline

Government affairs activities
- Input on important issues through AANA's Washington, DC, and Park Ridge, Illinois, offices
- Coordination and liaison with regulatory bodies such as the Centers for Medicare & Medicaid Services and the Department of Health and Human Service
- AANA Government Relations hotline
- Tracking and analysis of state legislation and regulations in more than 25 subject areas
- Strategic consultation and issue briefings to state associations and their lobbyists and attorneys
- Response to questions concerning state legislative and regulatory requirements and provisions
- PAC advocacy for nurse anesthesia causes
- Lobbying on federal and state CRNA issues
- Coordination of grassroots efforts
- Prominent Washington presence for Association on Capitol Hill
- Legislative coverage in the *AANA NewsBulletin*
- "Day on the Hill" activities in conjunction with Mid-Year Assembly
- Presence at Washington, DC, fundraisers
- One of nation's most influential PACs

Publications that inform and educate
- Information on the latest scientific and educational advancements in the bimonthly *AANA Journal*
- News on healthcare policy and other nurse anesthesia issues in the monthly *AANA NewsBulletin*
- A calendar of AANA continuing education program events
- Opportunities for CRNAs to have articles published in the *AANA Journal* and *AANA NewsBulletin*

Continues on page 48.

47

Table 3.3. Benefits and Services Provided to AANA Members (continued)

Informative meetings
- Networking opportunities
- Reduced registration fees for AANA members
- Annual Meeting that is the largest gathering of CRNAs and colleagues of its kind
- Annual Assembly of States that focuses on state association management and national issues
- Annual Assembly of School Faculty especially for anesthesia educators
- Mid-Year Assembly focusing on state leadership and government affairs issues and providing firsthand exposure to the AANA's healthcare lobbying efforts
- Hands-on, practice-oriented programs in the AANA Learning Center

Support for nurse anesthesia education
- Ensuring adequate supply of CRNAs
- Funding student scholarships through the AANA Foundation
- Printed materials, speaking engagements, and exhibits aimed at recruiting nurses into the nurse anesthesia profession
- Standards for CRNA education
- Procurement of government funding for CRNA education
- Identification of sources for student scholarships and/or loan programs
- Faculty development programs
- CRNA scholarships for advanced education

Quality and patient safety
- Support for credentialing mechanisms that serve the public's trust
- Establishment of standards and guidelines for practice
- Provision of patient education information
- Participation in national organizations focused on healthcare quality and patient safety initiatives
- Publication of *Quality Review in Anesthesia* newsletter

Continuing education activities
- Maintenance of continuing education records for recertification
- Participation in coalition activities with other healthcare organizations
- Access to C-TACS, the credit and transcript automated communication system
- Access to your CE records via the Internet
- Review and approval of continuing education programs
- Provision of school transcripts
- Provision of alumni reports for program directors

Support for research
- Research forum program
- Consultation for research activities
- Funding of research proposals through the AANA Foundation
- Workshops for researchers
- State of the Science sessions at the AANA Annual Meeting

Continues on page 49.

48

Table 3.3. Benefits and Services Provided to AANA Members (continued)

Other member services
- AANA bookstore and resource center
- Inclusion in AANA database of CRNAs eligible for Medicare reimbursement
- Group and individual health insurance programs, including health savings accounts
- Home and auto insurance program
- Disability income protection and life insurance
- AANA MasterCard credit card
- Partial payment of the biennial recertification fee
- Annual nurse anesthesia practice and employment survey
- Estate planning seminars sponsored by the AANA Foundation
- Archives to record historical contributions of CRNAs and the AANA

AANA online services
- www.CRNAcareers.com
- Speaker databank
- *AANA Journal* Course online (6 CE credits)
- Credential verification
- Membership renewal
- Online voting for general election

AANA Insurance services
- Professional liability insurance for CRNAs in virtually every practice setting
- Online insurance application and renewal process

(Reprinted with permission from the AANA.)

Committee for review and recommendations and then are forwarded to the membership at least 30 days before the Annual Meeting. For adoption, amendments to the Bylaws require an affirmative vote of two-thirds of members who are present and voting at the Annual Business Meeting.

The AANA Foundation

The AANA Foundation was formed in 1981. Its mission is to advance the science of anesthesia through education and research, and its vision is to "serve as the leading resource for assuring safe anesthesia care through education and research."[7] The core values of the Foundation are knowledge, integrity, excellence, and stewardship. The Foundation's governing body, the Board of Trustees, consists of 14 CRNA members and 2 public members. Included among the 14 CRNAs are the AANA president-elect, AANA vice president, and the AANA executive director. The responsibility of the Board of Trustees is to direct the various activities of the Foundation, specifically to work in cooperation with the AANA to meet its mission of promoting research in areas of professional development and outcomes. The executive director of the Foundation reports directly to the Board of Trustees as a result of the 2006 realignment of the AANA with the organizational affiliates and staff reorganization (Figure 3.1).

Foundation activities include a grants program for research in anesthesia, student scholarships, fellowships to assist CRNAs to attain graduate degrees, and cutting-edge workshops that advance the practice of anesthesia in clinical settings. From inception through August 2010, the Foundation has awarded 675 scholarships (totaling $871,000), 118 fellowships ($495,000) to assist CRNA students in pursuit of doctor of philosophy and doctor of nursing practice (DNP) degrees, 166 research grants to CRNAs ($456,000), and 31 student research grants ($23,000). The Foundation has supported 1,100 poster presentations. Additionally, the Foundation sponsors workshops in research funding, estate planning, regional anesthesia, and evidence-based practice. Also, the Foundation recognizes leaders in research, philosophy, and advocacy each year.

There are many ways donors can support the Foundation, including annual gifts, planned gifts, endowments, scholarship sponsorship, corporate donations, or attending special events. Major donors are recognized through the Friends for Life and Gertrude Fife Society recognition programs. From inception of the AANA Foundation through 2010, 258 Friends for Life and 67 Gertrude Fife Society members were honored.

National Headquarters

The AANA executive office moved from Cleveland to Chicago in 1937.[3(p129)] After being situated in downtown Chicago for many years, the office moved to 216 Higgins Road in Park Ridge, Illinois, a northwest suburb of Chicago, in 1980. In 1992, because of limited space, expanding staff, and increased member services, the AANA purchased a 43,000 square-foot building at 222 S Prospect Ave, in the downtown area of Park Ridge. This new building nearly tripled the size of the AANA's national headquarters, allowing the housing of all member services, the AANA archives, and AANA organizational affiliates at 1 site, including a new learning center from which continuing education seminars became available to members on a variety of clinical and professional topics. Until 2004, the International Federation of Nurse Anesthetists was also housed at the Prospect Avenue address.

Because of the increased attention given to federal-level issues affecting nurse anesthetists, the AANA recognized a need to have continuous representation in Washington, DC. In 1991, the AANA established a Federal Government Affairs Office to increase nurse anesthetists' visibility nationally and to deal with relevant practice issues. The AANA was recognized by *Fortune* magazine in 1999 as having one of the most effective lobbying organizations in Washington, DC, among major healthcare associations.[8(p206)]

Departmental Organization

In 2005, a major internal staffing reorganization was implemented. As of August 2010, there are 8 divisions: Executive Affairs, Federal Government Affairs, State Government Affairs, Professional Practice, Finance and Administrative Services, Communications, Research, and Educational and Professional Development (see Figure 3.1). Each division is led by a senior director who reports to the executive director, and ultimately, to the Board. Within each of these divisions are member service sections. The executive staff serves in many capacities, including staff functions connected with each of the standing and ad hoc committees of the Association. The Park Ridge AANA executive office consists of approximately 115 professional and clerical staff members. The Washington, DC, office has a professional staff of 7, headed by the senior director of federal government affairs,

Figure 3.1. American Association of Nurse Anesthetists Functional Staff Structure, August 2010

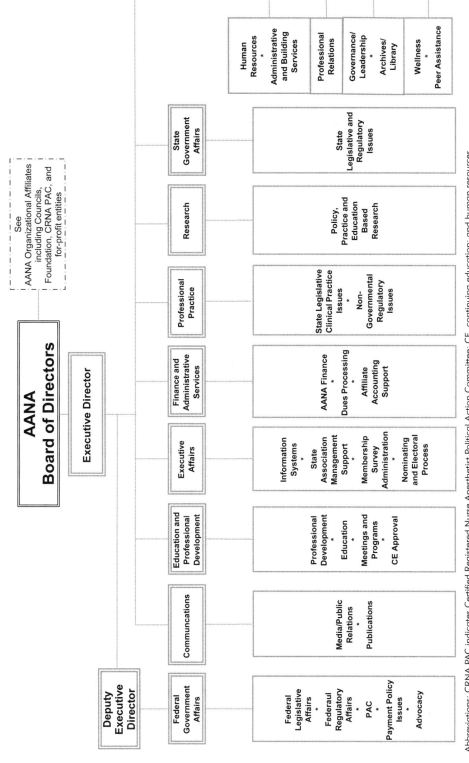

Abbreviations: CRNA PAC indicates Certified Registered Nurse Anesthetist Political Action Committee; CE, continuing education; and human resources. (Reprinted with permission from the AANA.)

51

working on behalf of members regarding a wide variety of federal issues that have an impact on nurse anesthesia practice.[9(p9)]

Organizational Affiliates

In 2006, as part of the functional reorganization, an AANA Organizational Affiliates category status was created, which depicts the staffing and organizational relationship of the AANA with the following entities: the AANA Foundation; AANA Association Management Services; CRNA Political Action Committee (CRNA-PAC); the Council for Public Interest in Anesthesia; the Council on Accreditation; and the National Board of Certification and Recertification for Nurse Anesthetists (inclusive of the Council on Certification and the Council on Recertification, Figure 3.2).

The AANA executive director remains responsible for the administrative functions of the national office and reports directly to the Board of Directors. The executive director, a position created by President Lucy Richards in 1948,[3(p129)] is responsible for keeping minutes of all AANA meetings, attending meetings of the Board of Directors and the Executive Committee, and any other activities designated by the president. The executive director has no voting privileges on the Board of Directors. He or she provides advice and guidance on policy formulation, maintains professional AANA staff, negotiates and renews necessary service contracts for the AANA, oversees all financial decisions for the national office at the direction of the Board, and provides leadership to educational, legal, and legislative entities of the AANA, as well as serving as a representative of the AANA to external organizations.

Council Configurations and Relationships

The council structure was established in the AANA Bylaws in the mid-1970s to assure the public that certification, recertification, accreditation, and public interest functions of the discipline of nurse anesthesia were separate from and not unduly influenced by the national Association. These bylaws allowed for the establishment of 4 separate, independent councils: the Council on Certification of Nurse Anesthetists, the Council on Recertification of Nurse Anesthetists, the Council on Accreditation of Nurse Anesthesia Educational Programs, and the Council on Nurse Anesthesia Practice (subsequently restructured as the Council for Public Interest in Anesthesia). The councils were made solely responsible for their own internal affairs, including the election of officers and the direction of financial activities. The councils did not report to the Association president or executive director, with the exception of a shared evaluation and oversight of the staff director by the respective council and AANA executive director. Membership on the councils includes CRNAs, students, physicians, and lay representatives, appointed or elected according to their own internal set of bylaws. Most professional healthcare organizations of similar type to the AANA have made provisions within their operational bylaws to establish these requisite bodies, which, although supported financially in part or whole by the professional organization, do not interfere with their basic functions. Communication between the AANA and the councils has taken place through a formal liaison committee of council chairs and Association officers to facilitate discussion of issues of mutual concern.

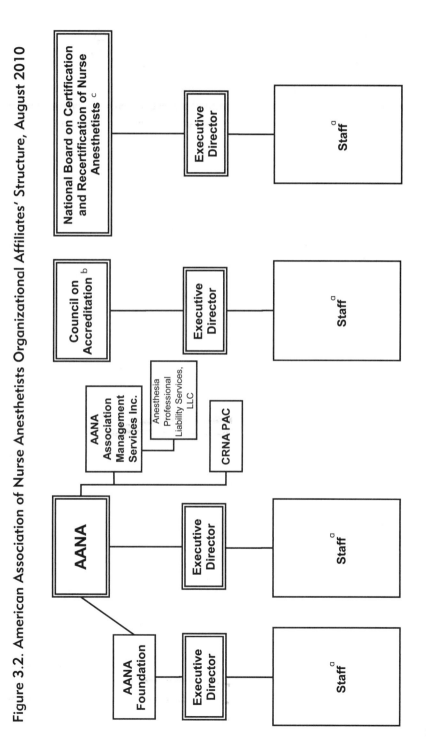

Figure 3.2. American Association of Nurse Anesthetists Organizational Affiliates' Structure, August 2010

[a] Under staffing agreement with AANA
[b] Accreditation-related education activities under agreement with AANA
[c] Includes Council on Certification of Nurse Anesthetists (CCNA) and Council on Recertification (COR)
CRNA PAC indicates Certified Registered Nurse Anesthetist Political Action Committee; AANA Association Management Services.
(Reprinted with permission from the AANA.)

In 2005, as part of the AANA internal staffing reorganization, dialogue was initiated with the councils to work with them in determining their staffing needs. It was also observed at that time that there were discrepancies between the original description of the councils' structure and functions in the AANA Bylaws and the councils' actual structures and functions delineated within the councils' own bylaws, policies, and procedures. As a result of the deliberations and discussions among the councils, the AANA Board of Directors, and the AANA executive director, the following outcomes were achieved:

- Recognition and service agreements with the 4 councils were completed in 2007. As part of the agreements, the staff director of the respective council reports solely to the council[9(14)] (see Figures 3.1 and 3.2).
- In 2007, the Council on Certification of Nurse Anesthetists and the Council on Recertification of Nurse Anesthetists were separately incorporated under a newly formed not-for-profit corporation, the National Board of Certification and Recertification for Nurse Anesthetists (NBCRNA).[9,10]
- By agreement, both the Council on Accreditation of Nurse Anesthesia Educational Programs and the Council on Public Interest in Anesthesia would remain under the AANA structure as autonomous and independent councils but will not be separately incorporated.[9]
- In 2008, the AANA Bylaws were amended to recognize the 4 autonomous councils and to authorize the AANA to enter into agreements with the councils. All references as to purpose, function, and structure of the councils were deleted from the AANA Bylaws in order to make the bylaws

consistent with the current state of council affairs.[10]

National Board of Certification and Recertification for Nurse Anesthetists

As mentioned, the NBCRNA consists of 2 councils: the Council on Certification of Nurse Anesthetists and the Council on Recertification of Nurse Anesthetists. Its objectives are to revise credentialing criteria to meet professional and patient safety needs; develop and implement electronic transmission of forms, as well as the eligibility and verification of credentialing; and determine future areas of growth for certification and recertification. The members of the Council on Certification and Recertification are the directors of the NBCRNA.[11(p18)] Two external agencies accredit the councils' certification and recertification programs. These are the National Commission for Certifying Agencies and the American Board of Nursing Specialties.

Council on Certification of Nurse Anesthetists

The Council on Certification of Nurse Anesthetists consists of individuals representing the community of interest involved in the process of certification of nurse anesthetists. The purpose of this council is to formulate and adopt requirements, guidelines, and prerequisites for certification and for eligibility to take the Certification Examination. The council is also responsible for administering each Certification Examination and evaluating the candidate's performance. The council grants initial certification to those candidates who successfully complete the certifying examination and who meet the other criteria for eligibility.

Council on Recertification of Nurse Anesthetists

The Council on Recertification of Nurse Anesthetists consists of individuals representing the community of interest involved in the process of recertification of nurse anesthetists. Its purpose is to formulate and adopt criteria for eligibility for recertification of CRNAs based on participation in approved continuing education activities and other recognized activities conducive to professional proficiency. The council is also responsible for formulating and adopting criteria for recertification requirements as recommended by the AANA Continuing Education Committee.

Council on Accreditation of Nurse Anesthesia Educational Programs

The Council on Accreditation of Nurse Anesthesia Educational Programs (COA) consists of individuals representing the community of interest involved in the accreditation process of educational programs. The purposes of the COA are to (1) advise, formulate, and/or adopt standards, guidelines, procedures, and criteria for the accreditation of nurse anesthesia educational programs, subject to review and comment by all constituencies that are significantly affected by them and (2) accredit entry into nurse anesthesia practice educational programs. In essence, the COA is the body responsible for ensuring to the public that educational programs of nurse anesthesia are of high quality, as evidenced by compliance with a set of minimum educational performance standards. The COA is recognized by the US Department of Education and the Council for Higher Education Accreditation to conduct accreditation activities for nurse anesthesia educational programs at the master's, post-master's certificate, and doctoral degree levels. The COA is also specifically recognized to accredit distance education, a designation not currently possessed by all nursing and nursing-related accrediting agencies.[11(p17)]

Doctoral Education of Nurse Anesthetists

From the mid-1980s through the late 1990s, the AANA and the COA assessed the need and feasibility of practice-oriented doctoral degrees for nurse anesthetists. In October 2004, the American Association of Colleges of Nursing (AACN) adopted its Position Statement on the Practice Doctorate in Nursing, which envisioned a practice doctorate as a requirement for all advanced practice nurses for entry into practice by 2017. In 2005, the AANA Board of Directors convened an invitational summit to discuss interests and concerns surrounding doctoral preparation of nurse anesthetists. In 2006, an AANA Task Force on Doctoral Preparation of Nurse Anesthetists was appointed and charged with developing options relative to doctoral preparation of nurse anesthetists for the AANA Board to consider. In April 2007, following extensive work of the AANA Task Force, which involved numerous meetings, surveys, and open hearings, the AANA Board received the final report of the task force, which included 4 options for consideration. In June 2007, the Board unanimously adopted the following option of the 4 options submitted by the Task Force: "The AANA supports doctoral education for entry into nurse anesthesia practice by 2025."[11] Following the action of the AANA, the COA voted to endorse the position. The COA noted that, although doctoral-level education for nurse anesthetists will be a requirement for individuals entering the

55

profession in and after 2025, as it is currently proposed all certified and practicing nurse anesthetists on that date will be grandfathered and their ability to remain certified will not depend on possessing or earning doctoral-level preparation. The COA, in making this endorsement, noted that the endorsement is for any type of doctoral preparation and not strictly practice doctorate preparation. The COA's Research and Practice Doctoral Task Force will continue to explore the implications of doctoral-level education requirements for CRNAs.[10(p14),11(p17)]

Council for Public Interest in Anesthesia

In response to increasing interactions between the communities of interest in anesthesia, the general public, and external healthcare organizations, the AANA Board of Directors in 1974 appointed an Ad Hoc Council on Nurse Anesthesia Practice. In 1975, the council was officially established and named the Council on Nurse Anesthesia Practice. In 1988, it was renamed the Council for Public Interest in Anesthesia and charged with the responsibility of monitoring issues that affect the public interest in matters regarding nurse anesthesia practice and serving as the appellate review body for matters related to accreditation, certification, recertification, and the AANA's continuing education approval program. Beginning in 2006, the Council, through an agreement with the AANA, assumed responsibility for the management and implementation of the AANA Wellness Program, which includes assuming oversight of the peer assistance advisors' activities. The peer assistance advisors will continue functioning as a member resource as envisioned by the AANA— handling requests from CRNAs, coworkers,

supervisors, program directors, students, family members, and disciplinary bodies concerning substance misuse. Few other professional healthcare organizations have addressed the issue of public accountability in the manner of referring such issues to an autonomous body. This action again serves to ensure that public interest issues are not subordinated to the self-interest of the professional organization.[11(p16)]

On August 7, 2010, the AANA membership adopted a bylaw amendment proposed by the AANA Board of Directors that dissolved the Council for Public Interest in Anesthesia.[12]

Subsidiary

The AANA Association Management Services, Inc (AAMS), is an AANA subsidiary that provides a source of nondues revenue for the Association as well as services to the general membership. The nondues revenue it generates helps reduce the amount of dues charged to AANA members, and the services it provides meet essential needs of AANA members. This subsidiary has 3 divisions, which provide publishing services, medical malpractice insurance, and housing services for AANA members.

The publishing division, AANA Publishing, Inc, produces the *AANA Journal* and various other publications of the Association. The *AANA Journal* disseminates original research and information on current issues, and it serves as a source of information for persons interested in the art and science of anesthesia and the role and functions of the nurse anesthetist.

The insurance division, AANA Insurance Services, Inc (formerly Anesthesia Professional Liability Services), has been providing professional liability insurance for members since 1989. AANA Insurance Services provides insurance primarily for those members who are self-employed or work as independent contractors. In addition to having insurance coverage available for members in virtually every practice setting (including students), AANA Insurance Services is a resource for insurance information to help address any professional liability issue or problem that a member may have. AANA Insurance Services' agents are appropriately licensed and undergo continuing education to maintain their positions.

The housing division within the AAMS provides a hotel reservation service to AANA members when they travel to AANA meetings or for personal reasons. The AAMS has approximately 30 full-time staff and is wholly owned by the AANA. Its relationship to the AANA and other organizational affiliates is depicted in Figure 3.2.

Elected Leadership

Board of Directors

The affairs of the AANA are conducted and led by an elected Board of Directors. The Board consists of the president, president-elect, vice-president, treasurer, and 7 regional directors. Officers serve for 1 year, and directors serve a 2-year term. To be eligible to serve as a director, an individual must have served at least 1 term as an officer or director of a state association and must have been active in state or AANA affairs. The Nominating Committee presents a slate of candidates for the Board of Directors at the Mid-Year Assembly. All CRNA members are allowed to vote for all officers and directors regardless of the region in which they hold membership. The newly elected Board of Directors is introduced to the membership at the Annual Business Meeting in August.

The Board of Directors is the administrative governing authority of the AANA. It receives and considers the reports of committees and directs the president to prepare an annual report reviewing the work of the preceding year, which is submitted to the AANA membership. The Board of Directors assumes many other responsibilities on behalf of the Association, including the responsibility of contracts and all budgetary and related financial matters, promoting position statements, promulgating clinical standards, managing the Association standing committees, and maintaining a liaison with myriad external governmental and professional agencies. The Executive Committee of the Board of Directors is composed of the president, president-elect, vice-president, and treasurer, and manages the affairs of the AANA between meetings of the Board.

Committees

The appointed committees of the AANA include Program, Bylaws, Continuing Education, Education, Finance, Government Relations, Minutes, Practice, and Public Relations. Committee members are appointed by the president with approval of the Board of Directors. All committees consist of at least 3 active members appointed for a 1-year term by the president, who designates their committee chair subject to the approval of the Board of Directors. The committees conduct their business as directed by the AANA strategic framework, with input and guidance from the Board. Committees usually meet 2 to 3 times each year, often in conjunction with other major Association-related meetings.

The elected committees of the Association are the Nominating Committee and the Resolutions Committee. Election of these 2 committees is by mailed ballot, in conjunction with the election of officers and regional directors. The Nominating

57

Committee is responsible for slating and determining eligibility of candidates for the AANA Board of Directors and the elected committees. Members of the Resolutions Committee submit resolutions, which are signed by at least 5 active members, to the executive director no less than 90 days before the AANA Annual Meeting. (A resolution is a written "main motion" that contains subject matter potentially having an important impact on the policies of the AANA.) At the Annual Meeting, the Resolutions Committee holds an open hearing during which all submitted resolutions may be discussed. The Board of Directors is responsible for implementing any resolutions approved by the general membership.

Conducting the Business of the Association

In addition to the daily activities of the national office, the business of the Association is conducted largely via primary meetings of different membership segments of the Association. These include the Assembly of School Faculty, Fall Assembly of States, Mid-Year Assembly, and Annual Meeting. All members are invited to attend and fully participate in these activities.

Assembly of School Faculty

The Assembly of School Faculty takes place twice a year, once in February and again in conjunction with the Annual Meeting. Participants generally include program directors, associate directors, physician and CRNA faculty, PhD faculty, educational advisors, students, and other interested individuals. Participants of the assembly discuss affairs pertinent to the conduct of educational programs, including current issues, standards, legal implications, legislative trends, clinical practice, teaching/instruction, and re-

search. The meeting is conducted by the AANA Education Committee.

Assembly of States

The Assembly of States is held each year in the fall. Attendees of this meeting include the Board of Directors, members of the standing AANA committees, officers and board members of affiliated state associations, and other interested members. Assemblies usually take place over an extended weekend and are held to disseminate information on current issues affecting practice and to provide other programming to assist state organizations in the conduct of their business. Both the Assembly of School Faculty and Fall Assembly of States provide ample open forums during which any member may speak about issues of his or her concern.

Mid-Year Assembly

Each year the AANA hosts a Mid-Year Assembly in the Washington, DC, area to provide opportunity for CRNAs to meet their elected national congressional delegation and to directly lobby the AANA federal legislative agenda. These sessions also present nationally and internationally recognized political and bureaucratic leaders as speakers in addition to providing instructional workshops for CRNAs to improve their lobbying skills. This meeting provides an opportunity for participants to experience a rare behind-the-scenes look at the legislative process and learn firsthand about federal legislative activities and how important CRNAs are to the process of shaping national healthcare legislation.

Topics discussed at this meeting include healthcare reform, Medicare reimbursement for anesthesia services, and federal policies and law affecting healthcare cost, access, and quality as well as current issues affecting practice patterns of CRNAs. Most CRNAs attending the meeting meet personally with their members of Congress on the final day of the conference to discuss their positions on proposed legislation. Much of the assembly is given to preparing CRNAs on the issues and how to best deal with congressional members and staff during face-to-face meetings.

Annual Meeting

One of the most popular meetings the AANA holds is its Annual Meeting, which typically lasts for 5 days in early to mid-August in a major metropolitan city. Attendance at this meeting typically exceeds 3,000, of which approximately 1,000 are students. Members cite many benefits of attending the Annual Meeting, such as earning continuing education credits from more than 100 scientific sessions, networking with fellow CRNAs, observing the latest in technology and equipment, hearing nationally and internationally known speakers, and sharing ideas and positions with colleagues and elected leaders of the profession.

The meeting includes an entire day of activities for students, including the Anesthesia College Bowl and student luncheon. The student program is managed by the Education Committee and its elected student representative.

In addition, the meeting includes the AANA Opening Ceremonies, general business session, bylaws hearings, scientific sessions and workshops, focus sessions concentrating on special issues, exhibits, receptions, and the Annual Banquet, which draws sold-out crowds.

State Organizations

State associations are formed by members who live and work in a particular state and are recognized by the Board of Directors as a duly incorporated entity. State associations are responsible for organizing their own committees, electing state officers, and handling their own financial affairs. States are supported financially by state membership dues, which the AANA collects and pays back to the state association. Officer and board configurations of state associations are similar to the national organization. State organizations deal with many local issues, such as CRNA access to hospitals and other healthcare institutions, clinical privileges, and ability to receive adequate reimbursement from a variety of payers. Activity of the state association depends largely on the volunteer effort of CRNAs and is of primary importance to the profession, because most of the legislative activity affecting CRNA practice is conducted at the state level. Furthermore, an active state association is vital for optimal function of the AANA Federal Government Affairs office. Without the state level contacts and networks that state organizations have with their elected state executive and legislative leaders, the national legislative agenda of the AANA would be much less effective. Participation by CRNAs in their state association is usually considered the point of entry into activities and offices at the national level.

Members from each state association maintain contact with the national office by providing them annually with a list of its officers, committee members, and current bylaws. Officers and members of individual state associations often contact executive office staff, seeking advice and counsel on issues related to practice, government affairs, education, public relations, and membership.

59

National Association Membership Services

There are many reasons to become a member of the AANA or to renew membership annually. Table 3.3 provides a list of the benefits CRNAs enjoy through active participation in the AANA. It is also important to recognize that AANA membership provides another substantial benefit to interested members. Because the AANA is a voluntary organization, it values and requires the active participation of members on its standing committees and in its ad hoc work groups, continuing education programs, consultant activities, and the AANA Foundation, to mention only a few. These opportunities provide invaluable experiences for CRNAs to expand their own professional development and skill base as administrators, managers, team members, educators, researchers, and leaders by working together to achieve organizational goals. Then CRNAs bring back benefits of these experiences to the workplace, which undoubtedly enhance their potential for promoting the interests of nurse anesthesia more effectively, expanding their own personal and professional roles, or even achieving promotion. There is no doubt that these voluntary experiences play a vital role in socializing CRNAs into a more satisfying professional role.

Summary

As the healthcare field continues to grow and change, so does the AANA, thanks to its loyal members, who continue to serve with the dedication, enthusiasm, and perseverance characteristic of its founding members. The AANA is a unique organization that owes its success to the support of 90% of the nation's CRNAs, who make up its membership. Each CRNA has something of importance to contribute to the AANA, and the diversity among its members is a vital key to its continued growth and success. To meet the challenges of the future, we must remain an informed and unified organization that serves all its members and extends its promise of quality and caring service to the public.

References

1. Malone BL. Clinical and professional leadership. In: Hamric AB, Spross JA, Hanson CM, eds. *Advanced Nursing Practice: An Integrative Approach.* Philadelphia, PA: Saunders; 1996.

2. Certified Registered Nurse Anesthetists (CRNAs) at a glance. American Association of Nurse Anesthetists website. http://www.aana.com. Accessed January 12, 2010.

3. Bankert M. *Watchful Care: A History of America's Nurse Anesthetists.* New York, NY: Continuum Publishing; 1989.

4. American Association of Nurse Anesthetists Strategic Framework. American Association of Nurse Anesthetists website. http://www.aana.com. [membership required]. Accessed October 2, 2008.

5. Bylaws and Standing Rules of the American Association of Nurse Anesthetists. Park Ridge, IL: American Association of Nurse Anesthetists Inc; 2008. http://www.aana.com. Accessed October 2, 2008.

6. *Professional Practice Manual for the Certified Registered Nurse Anesthetist.* Park Ridge, IL: American Association of Nurse Anesthetists Inc; 2007. http://www.aana.com. Accessed January 12, 2010.

7. About the AANA Foundation. American Association of Nurse Anesthetists website. http://www.aana.com. Accessed January 13, 2010.

8. Birnbaum JH. Follow the money. Hard money. Soft money. Lobbying money. Which buys the most influence in Washington? *Fortune.* December 6, 1999; 140(11):206-208. http://money.cnn.com. Accessed January 12, 2010.

9. Inside the Association: AANA internal staff reorganization. *AANA NewsBulletin.* March 2005;59(3):9. http://www.aana.com. Accessed October 2, 2008.

10. Formation of NBCRNA announced. *AANA NewsBulletin.* 2007;61(9):1,7. http://www.aana.com. Accessed August 27, 2010.

11. AANA Annual Reports, 2007-2008. American Association of Nurse Anesthetists website. http://www.aana.com. Accessed October 2, 2008.

12. Amendments to AANA Bylaws and standing rules at the Annual Business Meeting. AANA Annual Business Meeting. Seattle, WA. August 7, 2010. *AANA NewsBulletin.* 2010;64(9). http://www.aana.com. Accessed August 26, 2011.

Study Questions

1. Discuss the philosophical questions and potential conflicts that could arise relative to the dual mission of a professional organization serving the interests of both patients and providers. Give examples.

2. Discuss issues or problems you have observed as a student that CRNAs have in the workplace and conjecture ways in which the AANA or state organizations could help solve the issues.

3. Design a plan of action and rationale that you would use to convince a fellow CRNA of the value of and need for membership in the AANA.

4. Describe the organizational relationship of the 3 councils to the AANA and the rationale for why they are constituted in such a manner.

CHAPTER 4

The International Federation of Nurse Anesthetists

Ronald F. Caulk, CRNA, FAAN
Sandra M. Ouellette, CRNA, MEd, FAAN

Key Concepts

- The International Federation of Nurse Anesthetists (IFNA) is an international organization of nationally registered nurses with special education in nurse anesthesia.

- Standards as approved by the IFNA are the ultimate mandate internationally for educational preparation and clinical and ethical behavior of the nurse anesthetist.

- Nurses participate in the delivery of anesthesia services in 107 countries and participate in 70% to 80% of all cases of anesthesia administered in the world.

- It is in the best interest of the IFNA to align itself with established international organizations whose goals and programs are consistent with the aims of the IFNA.

- The IFNA represents the second of only 7 international nursing specialties to be recognized by the International Council of Nurses.

- Future effectiveness of international professional organizations lies in their ability to provide international solutions to local problems.

Continues on next page.

Key Concepts (continued)

- The IFNA educational, practice, and ethical standards stand as an international witness for the globalization of a profession in both preparation and practice.

- The IFNA is the only international nursing organization to establish international standards.

- Each member country of the IFNA exists in its own political and legal environment, and any assistance given must take those elements into consideration.

In 1978, two European nurse anesthetists, Jan Frandsen of Denmark and Hermi Löhnert of Switzerland, attended the Annual Meeting of the American Association of Nurse Anesthetists (AANA). Their interest in international cooperation among nurse anesthetists and the AANA's agreement planted the seed for what would become the International Federation of Nurse Anesthetists (IFNA).

This chapter describes the historical development, philosophy, objectives, and functions of the IFNA. Qualifications for membership, organizational structure, and educational and research activities are addressed. Future directions and the value of the federation to the profession conclude the chapter.

History of the International Federation of Nurse Anesthetists

It was not until 1978 that nurse anesthetists began to realize that they were a worldwide entity. Sparked by the interest of Löhnert and supported by the AANA Board of Directors, the idea of international cooperation began. From this concept, the IFNA was born. The IFNA, which represents 45,000 active practicing nurse anesthetists worldwide, is a growing organization whose members practice in both developed and developing countries.

The first International Symposium for Nurse Anesthetists, cosponsored by the AANA and the newly formed and then-called Schweizerische Fachvereinigung für Nichtärztliche Anästhesisten (Swiss Association for Nonphysician Anesthetists), convened in Lucerne, Switzerland, in June 1985, and was attended by 250 nurse anesthetists from 11 countries. At a meeting of the official country representatives, the decision was made that another international

symposium should be held in 3 years. The Symposium Organizing Committee was formed to plan the next symposium, and the representatives requested that country organizations bid to host the symposium. This committee was composed of a representative from Switzerland, the Netherlands, Denmark, Germany, and the United States and held its first organizational meeting in Roskilde, Denmark, in February 1986. The offer of the Netherlands Association to host the international symposium in 1988 was accepted. When the 2nd International Congress of Nurse Anesthetists convened in Amsterdam, the Netherlands, 511 nurse anesthetists from 16 countries attended.

At the 1987 March meeting of the Congress Organizing Committee and country representatives, several European associates had already proposed the possibility of developing an international organization. It was decided that each representative would discuss the feasibility of an international organization with his or her board of directors. The AANA Board of Directors suggested that Ronald Caulk, CRNA, FAAN, the AANA representative to the Congress Organizing Committee, prepare a feasibility questionnaire to determine the objectives of such an organization. The questionnaire asked the nurse anesthesia leaders of each country organization to determine what they felt would be the goals, purpose, objectives, and composition of such an organization. The questionnaire was distributed to all official country representatives, and the results were presented at the Amsterdam meeting.

The responses to questionnaires indicated that the country representatives shared the same goals and objectives. The concept of forming an international organization was greeted with great enthusiasm at the Amsterdam meeting, and plans were made to

65

continue to move ahead with the formation of an international organization. The name of the International Congress changed to World Congress for Nurse Anesthetists, and the committee name changed to the Congress Planning Committee (CPC).

In September 1988, the first organizational meeting of the proposed international organization was held in Teufen, Switzerland. The meeting was chaired by Löhnert, and Caulk was appointed secretary. The name of the organization and the philosophy were adopted. Caulk presented definitions of society, association, alliance, organization, and federation. It was decided that membership would be by national organizations and that "federation" best described the intent of the proposed organization.

Federation was defined as the act of federating or uniting in a league; the formation of a political unity, with a central government by a number of separate states, each of which retains control of its own internal affairs; a league or confederation; a federated body formed by a number of states, societies, unions, and so on, each retaining control of its own internal affairs.

It was the decision of the representatives that Switzerland be the site of the proposed federation.[1] Subcommittees were formed to discuss structure and bylaws, membership, dues, functions, and objectives. Structure, bylaws, and dues and the official languages were planned. The dues were established at 0.50 Swiss francs per active member of each member organization.[1] The original dues structure was changed in 2004 to 3 Swiss francs per country member for high-income countries, 1.25 Swiss francs for middle-income countries, and 0.75 Swiss francs for low-income countries. This change was implemented to allow all countries the opportunity to be a member of the

IFNA.[1] The official language would be English, with German and French being established as "working languages."[1] Working languages have since been removed from the bylaws. Membership in the IFNA presented a major obstacle because not all countries present utilized nurses solely for administration of anesthesia, and subcommittees regarding categories of membership and conditions of membership were appointed to prepare recommendations for the March 1989 meeting in Oslo, Norway.[1] Objectives and functions developed and agreed on at this meeting are listed as Articles IV and V in Table 4.1. It was agreed that a World Congress would be planned every 3 years.[1]

In March 1989, the CPC and representatives from various countries met to resolve the membership issue and the completed draft of the constitution (bylaws), which a committee of 4 had outlined. Since internationalism was new to the group, leaders had sought the advice and support of the International Council of Nurses (ICN) during the planning and development of the organization.

In May 1989, Sandra M. Maree, CRNA, AANA president, and Caulk, then the AANA representative to the CPC, attended the ICN 19th Quadrennial Congress in Seoul, Korea. The purpose of attending the meeting was to study the history of the organization and to attend the business session of the Council of National Representatives (CNR). It was believed that lessons learned from this nearly 100-year-old organization would undoubtedly be beneficial in the formation of the IFNA.[1] It was at this meeting that the CNR adopted a resolution to recognize internationally organized nursing specialties.

In June 1989, country representatives met in Teufen, Switzerland, to finalize and

Table 4.1. IFNA Bylaws[2]

Article I
Name and description
The name is the International Federation of Nurse Anesthetists (IFNA). It is a federation of national nurse anesthetist associations that have been formally admitted for membership and that have complied with the dues for membership. The IFNA is organized and functions unrestricted by consideration of nationality, race, creed, color, politics, sex, or social status.

Article II
Philosophy
The IFNA is an international organization of nationally registered nurses with special education in nurse anesthesia. The members of this professional organization are dedicated to the precept that its members are committed to the advancement of educational standards and practices, which will advance the art and science of anesthesiology and thereby support and enhance quality patient care.

Article III
Purpose
The purpose of the IFNA is to promote assistance in the development of strong national nurse anesthesia associations.

Article IV
Objectives
To promote cooperation between nurse anesthetists internationally
To develop and promote educational standards in the field of nurse anesthesia
To develop and promote standards of practice in the field of nurse anesthesia
To promote opportunities for continuing education in anesthesia
To assist nurse anesthetists' associations to improve the standards of nurse anesthesia and the competence of nurse anesthetists
To promote the recognition of nurse anesthetists
To establish and maintain effective cooperation between nurse anesthetists, anesthesiologists, and other members of the medical profession, as well as hospitals and agencies representing a community of interest in nurse anesthesia

Article V
Functions
To promote continual high-quality patient care
To serve as the authoritative voice of nurse anesthetists and nurse anesthesia internationally
To provide a means of communication among nurse anesthetists throughout the world
To promote the independence of the nurse anesthetist as a professional specialist in nursing
To advance the art and science of anesthesiology

Continues on page 68.

This table is a summary of the complete document, which is available from IFNA headquarters.

Table 4.1. IFNA Bylaws (continued)

Article VI
IFNA languages
The official language of IFNA is English.

Article VII
Definition of nurse anesthetist
A nurse anesthetist is a person who has completed a program of basic nursing education and basic nurse anesthesia education and is qualified and authorized in his/her country to practice nurse anesthesia.

This table is a summary of the complete document, which is available from IFNA headquarters.

adopt the proposed bylaws and to review country applications for IFNA membership. Eleven countries were admitted as charter members. The first meeting of the IFNA Board of Directors was held on June 10, 1989. Caulk served as acting chair for the formal acceptance of the proposed bylaws and the election of officers. The bylaws were adopted and officers elected. Löhnert was the first president. Other officers included Caulk, vice president; Hanna Birgisdottir, Iceland, secretary; and Svein Olaussen, Norway, treasurer. Committees were formed, and arrangements were made for incorporation in Switzerland. Switzerland was selected as the IFNA's home for several reasons: political neutrality, monetary stability, geographic location, and the fact that it was also the home of ICN, the World Health Organization (WHO), the International Red Cross, and other international organizations.

After the formation of the organization, the Board of Directors set out to address the objectives. During the first year, the IFNA Board of Directors requested the Education Committee to develop international educational standards for nurse anesthetists.[3] The decision to develop the educational standards was intended to address the

IFNA objectives based on the fact that the educational standards worldwide were very diverse. These standards were adopted in 1990. The following year, the Education Committee developed international standards of practice that were adopted by the IFNA Board of Directors in 1991.[4] The code of ethics was adopted in 1992.[5] It was not until 1997 that the IFNA leadership learned from the Center for Quality Assurance in International Education (CQAIE) that the IFNA was the only international nursing organization to adopt such standards. At this organizational meeting it was agreed that Löhnert be recognized as the IFNA's founder based on his initial concept of an international symposium and his active participation in the founding of the IFNA.

In November 1990, IFNA President Caulk and Vice President Löhnert visited the ICN and the WHO in Geneva, Switzerland. The purposes of the visit were to thank the ICN for its assistance and support in the development of the IFNA and to learn more about the process for ICN recognition of international nursing specialties. The purpose of the visit to the WHO was to introduce the IFNA to the offices of the nongovernmental organizations and nursing. Table 4.2 provides the year, city, and attendance figures for 9

Table 4.2. Attendance at the IFNA World Congress

Year	City	Anesthetists in attendance
1985	Lucerne, Switzerland	250
1988	Amsterdam, Netherlands	511
1989	Oslo, Norway	1,100
1994	Paris, France	2,606
1997	Vienna, Austria	1,700
2000	Chicago, IL, United States	4,000
2002	Helsinki, Finland	1,047
2006	Lausanne, Switzerland	1,278
2010	The Hague, Netherlands	1,012

Table 4.3. IFNA Member Countries and Year of Admission

Member country	Year of admission	Member country	Year of admission
Austria[a]	1985	Jamaica	1997
Benin	1994	Luxembourg	2005
Cambodia	1997	Morocco	1997
Croatia	1999	Netherlands	1995
Democratic Republic of the Congo	1992	Nigeria	1993
		Norway[a]	1985
Denmark	1997	Poland	1998
Finland[a]	1985	Serbia	2008
France[a]	1985	Slovenia[a]	1985
Gabon	1994	South Korea[a]	1985
Germany[a]	1985	Spain	1992
Ghana	1993	Sweden[a]	1985
Great Britain	1995	Switzerland[a]	1985
Hungary	1999	Taiwan	1999
Iceland[a]	1985	Tunisia	2003
Indonesia	2006	Uganda	1996
Italy	2001	United States[a]	1985
Ivory Coast	1994		

IFNA indicates International Federation of Nurse Anesthetists.
[a] Charter countries.

69

of the 10 IFNA International Congresses. When the first Congress met, 11 countries were represented. By the 1994 Congress in Paris, 47 countries were involved. After the 2010 Congress, the IFNA will sponsor a congress every 2 years. In 2012 the Congress will be held in Slovenia, and in 2014, it will be held in Tunisia.

Since the IFNA was founded, membership has grown at a rapid pace. Table 4.3 lists the 34 countries that were members as of 2008. In 1995, the executive office of the

IFNA was established at the AANA headquarters in Park Ridge, Illinois, with Caulk as the first executive director. Pascal Rod became the second executive director of the IFNA in 2004, and the office was moved to Paris, France.

Definition and Role of Nurses in Anesthesia Delivery Worldwide

The IFNA is an international organization of nationally registered nurses with special education in nurse anesthesia. A nurse anesthetist is a person who has completed a program of basic nursing education and basic nurse anesthesia education and is qualified and authorized in his/her country to practice nurse anesthesia. Member countries of the IFNA are dedicated to the precept that

their individual members are committed to the advancement of educational standards and practices, which will advance the art and science of anesthesiology and thereby support and enhance quality patient care. The IFNA vision and mission statements are listed in Tables 4.4 and 4.5.

There has been and remains some confusion about nurse anesthesia worldwide. The role varies from country to country and continent to continent. Throughout mainland Europe, nurse anesthetists commonly practice in an "anesthesia care team" setting. This setting consists of physician anesthetists (or anesthesiologists) supervising the nurse anesthetists. The ratios for this supervision vary from 1:2 to 1:3 and are generally accepted as being cost-effective in both the cost of education and the provision

Table 4.4. The IFNA Vision Statement[6]

The International Federation of Nurse Anesthetists (IFNA) is the authoritative voice for nurse anesthetists and nurse anesthesia, supporting and enhancing quality anesthesia care worldwide. As professionals, nurse anesthetists are recognized for their significant contribution to global health care as nurses, practitioners, teachers, administrators, researchers, and consultants. The IFNA participates in the formulation and implementation of health care policy and the recognition of nurse anesthetists as essential and cost-effective health care providers.

Adopted November 17, 2000.

(Reprinted with permission from the IFNA.)

Table 4.5. The IFNA Mission Statement[7]

The International Federation of Nurse Anesthetists (IFNA) is an international organization representing nurse anesthetists serving the public and its members. The mission of the federation is dedicated to the precept that its members are committed to the advancement of educational standards and practices which will advance the art and science of anesthesiology and thereby support and enhance quality anesthesia care worldwide. The IFNA establishes and maintains effective cooperation with institutions that have a professional interest in nurse anesthesia.

Adopted November 17, 2000.

(Reprinted with permission from the IFNA.)

of anesthesia services. There is an agreement as to the respective roles, and the team works in harmony. The overall educational preparation of the nurse anesthetist lasts, on average, 18 months.[8]

In recent times there has been much discussion about the role of the "anesthetic nurses" who were used in the past to assist the physician anesthetist. Although they have been utilized in several areas of the world, more often they are found in the United Kingdom, Australia, New Zealand, Canada, and Hong Kong. Whether called a discussion or debate, current interest involves the role today and the future of the anesthetic nurse. It is the understanding of the IFNA that the role of the anesthetic nurse was originally to assist the physician anesthetist and that the educational preparation of the anesthetic nurse was approximately 22 weeks. It is the belief of the IFNA that if nurses are utilized for the preoperative and postoperative preparation of the patient and if they perform venous and arterial cannulation, induction and emergence of anesthesia, intubation, and extubation, and if they are left alone for any reason, they should be appropriately educated. In addition to a defined scope of practice and appropriate educational background, there should be recognition for practice as well as oversight in the recognition of the educational process and credentialing. The IFNA is not concerned about whether these countries utilize nurse anesthetists. If nurses are being utilized in such a manner, however, the IFNA is concerned that their scope of practice is defined and the educational process is sufficient to support anesthesia practice and patient safety.

In the United States, nurse anesthetists practice in all 50 states, Puerto Rico, and the District of Columbia. Although it is a common belief that all nurse anesthetists in the United States are independent practitioners and in competition with physician anesthesiologists, current practice does not support this perception. Seventy-five percent of all nurse anesthetists in the United States practice in the anesthesia care team model. Most independent practitioners provide anesthesia services in rural areas where there are no physician anesthesiologists.

In the United States, nurse anesthetists are registered nurses with a baccalaureate degree who have successfully completed a nurse anesthesia educational program at the master's degree level. In 2025, entry-level educational requirements for nurse anesthetists will be at the doctoral level. Nurse anesthesia educational programs are accredited by the Council on Accreditation of Nurse Anesthesia Educational Programs. This council is recognized by the US Department of Education as the official accrediting agency.

Following graduation, nurse anesthetists must successfully complete the National Certification Examination for Nurse Anesthetists administered by the Council on Certification of Nurse Anesthetists before using the credential Certified Registered Nurse Anesthetist (CRNA). Nurse anesthetists then remain certified through a recertification process every 2 years. The Council on Recertification of Nurse Anesthetists oversees this process. Nurse anesthetists provide more than 65% of the anesthetics administered in the United States and are the sole anesthesia providers in approximately 67% of all rural hospitals.

Nurse anesthetists and other nonphysician anesthetists in less developed countries or in countries in transition play a major role in the provision of anesthesia services. Many of these countries have very few physician anesthesia providers, and some have none. Most physician providers are

71

located in universities and teaching hospitals as educators and team leaders. Outside of the teaching setting, nurse anesthetists provide 90% to 100% of the anesthesia services. Because of the practice setting and the situations in which they practice, there is concern about the educational preparation and continuing education opportunities for these individuals. The IFNA is also concerned about the ratios of anesthesia providers in these countries. Whereas Scandinavian countries enjoy ratios of approximately 1:3,000 of anesthesia providers to populace, and the United States and central Europe have approximately 1:7,000, some countries in Africa and Southeast Asia have ratios of 1:200,000 to greater than 1:300,000.

Qualifications for Membership in the IFNA

Because it is a federation, IFNA membership is by country. It is the belief that it takes a strong country organization to effectively address issues involving nurse anesthesia practice. While many nurse anesthetists are organized within their countries, some have organized in order to apply for membership in the IFNA.

Within a country, one national nurse anesthetist association or federation of nurse anesthetists may become a member of the IFNA. When neither of these exists, a separate nurse anesthetist section or chapter of a national association composed of other healthcare workers may become a member. Member-country organizations are controlled by nurse anesthetists, speak for nurse anesthetists on nurse anesthesiology matters, and are the most representative of nurse anesthetists in the country, according to the IFNA definition of nurse anesthetist (See Table 4.1).

Each national nurse anesthetist association has the right to define its own membership at the national level. Where there is more than 1 small group of nurse anesthetists within a region, nurse anesthetists may form a regional organization for representation in the IFNA.

Duties of the member country associations include communication with the executive director of the IFNA regarding names and addresses of officers, number of members, and bylaws of the country organization. Representatives of member associations are responsible for seeing that dues are paid. They also report to the CNR once a year, respond to requests for information from the board, and make recommendations to the CNR regarding amendments to the bylaws, policies, or position statements of the IFNA.

Nonnurse anesthesia provider organizations may apply for associate membership in the IFNA. These members may participate at meetings of the CNR as observers with the right to speak but no voting privileges. Dues for associate membership are one half the regular membership dues. As of 2010, Tunisia is the only associate member country in the IFNA.

IFNA Organizational Structure

The IFNA's business is governed by bylaws, which were approved initially in 1989. Several revisions to the bylaws have occurred since adoption. A summary of the current bylaws is found in Table 4.1. A complete copy of this document can be obtained from IFNA headquarters.

Committees are the backbone of the IFNA. It is through committee activity that projects are developed, planning is accomplished, and research is promoted. Committee members are selected by the IFNA president with the approval of the CNR.

The IFNA CPC is responsible for planning the IFNA World Congress. Other duties of the CPC are listed in Table 4.6. The country selected to host the World Congress appoints a National Organizing Committee.

An IFNA World Congress is a professional highlight for nurse anesthetists internationally. Objectives of the World Congress are to (1) provide a forum whereby major trends and issues of interest to the international community of nurse anesthetists are discussed by peers and experts; (2) share and disseminate new knowledge and professional experiences as related to topics of interest of nurse anesthetists; (3) provide an opportunity for nurse anesthetists occupying similar positions in different countries to gather to discuss matters of mutual interest; and (4) strengthen collaboration between nurse anesthetists internationally to improve standards for nurse anesthesia education, continuing education, and practice at a high scientific level.[9]

Educational Activities of the IFNA

A major focus of the IFNA has been improving anesthesia education and safety throughout the world. In keeping with that focus, education, practice, and ethical standards were adopted between 1990 and 1992. A standard represents what the prudent nurse anesthetist in similar circumstances must exercise. Standards as approved by the IFNA are the ultimate mandate internationally for educational preparation and clinical and ethical behavior of the anesthetist.

The preamble to the IFNA Educational Standards for Preparing Nurse Anesthetists is given in Table 4.7. The standards were revised in 1996 and 1999. The preamble to the IFNA Standards of Practice appears in Table 4.8. These standards were revised in 1996. The preamble to the IFNA Code of Ethics appears in Table 4.9; that document was adopted in May 1992. Complete copies of these documents can be obtained from the IFNA headquarters.

In addition to standards, the Education Committee also prepared monitoring guidelines. In contrast to standards, guidelines are not mandated. They are suggested or advised. Table 4.10 presents the 1998 revised Patient Monitoring Guidelines,[10] now called Patient Monitoring Standards. During the 1991 World Congress, a first attempt was made to ascertain whether nurse anesthesia teachers would be interested in establishing a forum at the World Congress that related to their interests. The initial forum consisted of 45 representatives from the following 13 countries: Tunisia, France, Poland, Sweden, Norway, Switzerland, Korea, Finland, Austria, Slovenia, the Netherlands, Denmark, and the United States. The forum did not provide for simultaneous interpretation from the language of presentation. Nonetheless, the participants were eager to continue with the concept. The first IFNA Teachers' Session was held at the 4th World Congress. It was so successful that this session was expanded and is now a permanent part of the World Congress.

The IFNA headquarters continues to receive many requests for information on starting new programs. In response to this need, the IFNA Education Committee prepared a document in 1996 titled "Guidelines for Starting a New Program and Sample Curriculum." It was revised in 1998. Members of the Education Committee from Sweden, Taiwan, Norway, Ghana, and the United States are available for consultation to countries wanting to start a program. Because the IFNA's goal is to provide competent, safe anesthesia care, its guidelines state that only nurses who have completed a program of instruction in nurse anesthesia

---

Table 4.6. Duties of the IFNA Congress Planning Committee

1. Plan, organize, implement, and evaluate the International Federation of Nurse Anesthetists (IFNA) World Congress in collaboration with the NOC, or National Organizing Committee.

2. Participate with the NOC in planning the IFNA World Congress with regard to the education and venue activities and including social and culture activities in the spirit of international cooperation, socialization, education, and exchange of experiences.

3. Establish a checklist for the Congress Planning Committee and NOC which lists the organizational tasks connected with the planning, organizing, implementing, and evaluating the IFNA World Congress.

4. Maintain effective communication and collaboration between the IFNA, the NOC, and the IFNA Executive Director and Board of Officers and Executive Committee.

5. Ensure continuity of IFNA traditions in relation to the scientific program and ambiance of the IFNA World Congress.

74

Table 4.7. IFNA Educational Standards for Preparing Nurse Anesthetists

Preamble
Nurse anesthetists are prepared and utilized in many countries throughout the world to provide, or assist in the provision, of quality anesthesia services to patients. The following position on Educational Standards for Preparing Nurse Anesthetists is written to accommodate the major variance in the scope of nurse anesthesia practice within these countries as they relate to national organizational membership in the International Federation of Nurse Anesthetists (IFNA). Rather than writing minimal and optimal standards, the Education Committee of the IFNA has chosen to build such flexibility within a single set of standards. It is believed that such standards will have the capability to foster a responsible basis for preparing nurse anesthetists competent to provide anesthesia services, which adheres to qualitative standards and assures patient safety, comfort, and well-being while providing flexibility that allows for the identification of new goals and facilitates their achievement as scopes of practice grow and change in the years to come.

Definition of a nurse anesthetist
A nurse anesthetist provides, or participates in the provision of, advanced specialized nursing and anesthesia services to patients requiring anesthesia, respiratory care, cardiopulmonary resuscitation, and/or other emergency, life-sustaining services wherever required. Advanced specialized nursing and anesthesia services incorporate the biological and behavioral sciences into practice as they relate to patients and their families.

(Reprinted with permission from the IFNA.)

Table 4.8. IFNA Standards of Practice[4]

Preamble

The International Federation of Nurse Anesthetists (IFNA) is an international organization of registered nurses with special education in nurse anesthesia. A nurse anesthetist is a person who has completed a program of basic nursing education and basic nurse anesthesia education and is qualified and authorized in his/her country to practice anesthesia. The member countries of this professional organization are dedicated to the precept that their members are committed to the advancement of educational and practice standards, which will advance the art and science of nurse anesthesiology and thereby support and enhance quality patient care.

A characteristic of any profession is its responsibility to the public for developing standards, whereby the quality of practice rendered by its members can be judged. Establishing standards is essential in upgrading practice, and they are developed and subscribed to by all members based upon the profession's philosophy, theory, science, principle, and research. Standards provide a means to evaluate the practice and provide the practitioner with a level of expectation and a framework within which to operate.

Purpose of standards

While nurse anesthetists' services are utilized in many countries throughout the world, anesthesia practice may vary from one country to another or from one geographic location to another within a country because of requirements or limitations imposed by local law or institutional characteristics. Additionally, the practice of the nurse anesthetist is governed by policies, rules, and regulations as established by the health care institution in which the anesthesia care is being provided. The standards are descriptive, providing a basis for evaluation of the practice and reflecting the rights of those receiving anesthesia care.

(Reprinted with permission from the IFNA.)

Table 4.9. IFNA Code of Ethics[5]

Preamble

The fundamental responsibility of the nurse anesthetist is to provide or participate in the provision of advanced specialized nursing and anesthesia services to patients requiring anesthesia, respiratory care, cardiopulmonary resuscitation, and/or other emergency, life-sustaining services wherever required. Advanced specialized nursing and anesthesia services incorporate the behavioral and biological sciences into practice as they relate to patients and their families. Inherent in anesthesia nursing practice is respect for life, dignity, and rights of man. It is unrestricted by considerations of nationality, race, creed, age, sex, politics, or social status.

The purpose of a code of ethics is to acknowledge a profession's acceptance of the responsibility and trust conferred upon it by society and to recognize the international obligations inherent in that trust. The International Federation of Nurse Anesthetists Code of Ethics is devised from the premise that as healthcare professionals, nurse anesthetists must strive, both on an individual and collective basis, to pursue the highest possible ethical standards.

(Reprinted with permission from the IFNA.)

Table 4.10. IFNA Patient Monitoring Guidelines[10]

Anesthesia safety is the goal of anesthesia delivery worldwide. Parameters that enhance safety include professional knowledge, vigilance, constant monitoring, and changes in the anesthetic plan based upon patient responses to the anesthetic.

Included in the International Federation of Nurse Anesthetists Standards of Practice is standard IV, which addresses monitoring. It states, "the nurse anesthetist will monitor psychological and physiological responses, interpret and utilize data obtained from the use of invasive and noninvasive monitoring modalities, and take corrective action to maintain or stabilize the patient's condition, and provide resuscitative care." The nurse anesthetist will monitor, record, and report the patient's physiological and psychological signs and provide resuscitative care that includes fluid therapy, maintenance of airway, and provision of assisted or controlled ventilation.

Patient monitoring guidelines are intended to assist the nurse anesthetist in providing consistent, safe anesthesia care. While these guidelines are intended to apply to patients undergoing general, regional, or monitored anesthesia care, they do not apply to epidural analgesia or labor or pain management. These guidelines may be exceeded in any or all respects at any time at the discretion of the anesthetist. In extenuating circumstances, the nurse anesthetist must use clinical judgment in prioritizing and implementing these guidelines. If there is reason to omit a monitored parameter, the reason for the omission should be documented on the record.

Ventilation:
Purpose: To assess adequate ventilation of the patient.
Guideline: Ventilatory adequacy shall be assessed by palpation or observation of the reservoir breathing bag, chest movement, and auscultation of breath sounds. Ventilation should be continuously assessed by the use of a precordial or esophageal stethoscope. Correct placement of an endotracheal tube must be verified by auscultation and chest excursion. When available, spirometry, ventilatory pressure monitors, and end-tidal CO_2 monitoring should be used. When a patient is ventilated by mechanical ventilator, the integrity of the breathing circuit must be monitored by a device that is capable of detecting disconnection.

Oxygenation:
Purpose: To assess adequate oxygenation of the patient.
Guideline: Adequacy of oxygenation shall be monitored by observation of skin color, color of the blood in the surgical field, and arterial blood gas analysis as indicated. The use of pulse oximetry is encouraged on all patients. During general anesthesia, the oxygen concentration delivered by the anesthesia machine shall be continuously monitored with an oxygen analyzer with a low oxygen concentration limit alarm. An oxygen supply failure alarm system shall be used to warn of low oxygen pressure in the anesthesia machine.

(Reprinted with permission from IFNA. These guidelines are now called Patient Monitoring Standards.)

Table 4.10. IFNA Patient Monitoring Guidelines (continued)

Circulation:
Purpose: To assess adequacy of the patient's cardiovascular system.
Guideline: Circulation shall be assessed by at least one of the following measures: digital palpation of pulse, auscultation of heart sounds, continuous intra-arterial pressure monitoring, or pulse oximetry. Skin color and capillary refill should be monitored. Blood pressure and heart rate shall be determined and recorded at least every 5 minutes. An electrocardiogram (EKG) continuously displayed from induction through emergence is highly encouraged.

Body Temperature:
Purpose: To assess changes in body temperature.
Guideline: During every anesthetic, there shall be readily available a means to measure body temperature. When changes in temperature are anticipated, the temperature shall be measured.

Neuromuscular Function:
Purpose: To assess neuromuscular function.
Guideline: When neuromuscular blocking drugs are used, neuromuscular function shall be assessed by respiratory strength, hand grip, sustained head lift, and negative inspiratory force. Assessment of neuromuscular function by a nerve stimulator is strongly recommended.

Anesthesia Equipment:
Anesthesia equipment should be selected to ensure appropriate delivery of available anesthetics and maintenance of physiological parameters adequate for organ preservation. Equipment should be checked thoroughly each day, and an abbreviated check of all equipment shall be completed before each anesthetic.

Nurse Anesthetist:
Continuous clinical observation and vigilance are the cornerstone for anesthesia safety. The nurse anesthetist shall be in constant attendance of the patient until care has been accepted by another qualified individual.

(Reprinted with permission from IFNA. These guidelines are now called Patient Monitoring Standards.)

77

or who are supervised nurse students within such educational programs should be allowed to provide or participate in the provision of anesthesia services.

The IFNA established the IFNA Education and Research Foundation on November 24, 2002. The purpose of this foundation is to support the education of non-physician anesthetists (nurse anesthetists) nationally and internationally. It exists to support education and continuing education programs worldwide and to promote nurse anesthesia research nationally and internationally. The foundation meets annually. Foundation officers include president (IFNA first vice president), vice president (IFNA Education Committee representative), treasurer (IFNA treasurer), and secretary (IFNA executive director). The foundation has supported research and sponsored 3 continuing education offerings in Africa. Applications for grants from the foundation are due no later than March 1 of each year.

IFNA's Research in Action

In response to a challenge in 1990 by Miriam Hirschfeld, chief scientist for nursing at the WHO, the IFNA set out to document the existence, role, education, and recognition of nurse anesthetists worldwide. Maura S. McAuliffe, CRNA, PhD, was appointed the IFNA official nurse anesthesia researcher to collaborate with the WHO on an ongoing international study, Nurse Anesthesia Worldwide: Practice, Education and Regulation.

The study surveyed WHO member countries and ICN member organizations. The first 2 phases of the study were completed in 1994, and the third and final phase concluded in 2000. Results were presented each of those years at the World Congress. The results of the first 2 phases of this study were astonishing, even to the IFNA. The results indicated that nurses were participating in the delivery of anesthesia services in 107 countries. It was even more surprising to learn that nurses were participating in 70% to 80% of all anesthesia administered in the world. In many of the less developed countries, results indicated that nurses are providing 90% to 100% of all anesthesia services. This valuable study was funded by the AANA Council on Recertification of Nurse Anesthetists (USA) and the IFNA.[8]

Of concern to the IFNA was the finding that many ministries of health and nursing leaders were unaware of who was providing anesthesia services within their respective countries. Of even greater concern was the discovery that many of these anesthesia providers have no formal education, are not officially recognized, and are pleading for continuing education opportunities.

Liaisons With Other International Organizations

It is clear today that it is in the best interests of the IFNA to align itself with established international organizations whose goals are consistent with and whose programs dovetail with the stated aims of the IFNA. To a degree, the IFNA's eventual success depends on its ability to become associated with the international organizations and programs it supports. This vision led the IFNA leaders to approach organizations with the widest possible constituencies for mutual support and affiliation.[11]

European Economic Community

One of the IFNA's objectives in having an early priority for defining standards of practice and education was to provide member countries with a document they could use to help upgrade education or practice. Specifically, defined standards could be used in planning for the anticipated formation in 1992 of the European Economic Community, which is now known as the European Union (EU). The official committee in charge of developing rules for nursing within the EU is the Advisory Committee for Training in Nursing (ACTN), with members appointed by governments of the EU. Each country appoints 3 representatives, 1 health authority, 1 nurse practitioner, and 1 nurse educator to ACTN.

In 1977, general care nursing education was defined by a specific sectarian directive and adopted by the Council of Ministers. Nursing specialties were not and currently are not addressed. Any new country members of the EU must agree to this directive. The EU Directorate XV, in charge of the inner market and free movement of professions, employs a permanent secretary for ACTN to whom the IFNA submitted the IFNA Standards of Practice. The permanent secretary responded that "the Commission services consider that such initiatives contribute to facilitate the recognition of professional qualifications with the Community Directives called the 'General System' (Directive 89/48/CEE and 92/51/CEE) which concern the recognition of specialized nurses' certifications." The professional self-regulation at the European level could be useful for competency authorities in the course of applying for recognition under the above directives in so far as if a professional has received an education in accordance with standards defined by the profession, that could signify that he or she has reached a certain level of professional competency. The IFNA maintains close contact with the permanent secretary of the ACTN.

In 1971, the Standing Committee for Nursing was formed, after the ICN meeting in Dublin, with Marie-Paul Florin (France) serving as the first president. The first formal meeting of the committee was held in Brussels, Belgium, and the organization was the official liaison with the European Community Commission. The committee is composed of nursing leaders from EU national nurses associations that are members of ICN. The committee works collaboratively with ACTN and makes recommendations but does not have any authority. It is anticipated that in the future the Standing Committee of Nursing will have more influence. The IFNA does work collaboratively with the committee, however.

The Council of Europe is the official committee of the EU and all European countries except for Russia. This council has in the past developed recommendations for the European level and developed the guidelines concerning nursing specialties that the IFNA used as reference in establishing the IFNA Educational Standards. Currently the council follows the decisions of the EU.

Another organization in which IFNA participates is the European Network of Nursing Organizations. This organization is composed of members from EU and non-EU countries and addresses nursing and nursing specialty issues. It is a branch of the Standing Committee for Nursing.

The IFNA Executive Director and other European nurse anesthetists have taken an active role in the discussion of nursing specialties and continue to monitor and participate in activities regarding nursing specialties in the EU. Establishing the definition of a nursing specialty is difficult in that what is recognized as a nursing specialty in one country is not recognized as a nursing specialty in another. The post-basic nursing education for the specialties also varies from country to country. Within Europe, nursing and nurse specialty organizations influence the decision-making process for the profession, but all regulations are determined by the EU ministries of health. The IFNA affords an appropriate forum for nurse anesthetists from various countries to cooperate and collaborate in these efforts.

Although the IFNA is frequently asked for assistance with career placement in other countries, it is not a role or function of the IFNA. Membership in the IFNA does not imply that reciprocity is available. Outside the EU, there are many requirements such as working visas, licensure as a nurse, recognition of nurse anesthesia education, and language proficiency examination before a nurse anesthetist can work in a foreign country. There are exceptions, but generally, information regarding employment abroad can be obtained from the respective ministry of health.

International Council of Nurses

Nurses' involvement in an early women's movement organized at the national and international level helped to coalesce nursing organizations in the United States and to form the ICN. A group of nurses had attended the 1899 meeting of the International Council of Women in London and decided that a need existed for an analogous international organization of nurses; a committee of these nurses met in July 1900, adopted a constitution, and elected officers, thereby forming ICN. At the time of formation, membership consisted of individual nurses from various countries. The first meeting of the ICN was held in Buffalo, New York, in 1901.

Because only 1 representative national group could join the US National Council of Women—which was affiliated with the International Council of Women—the American Federation of Nurses (AFN) was formed in 1900. The AFN linked 2 nursing organizations: the Nurses' Associated Alumnae—a loose association of graduates of various nursing schools—and the American Society of Superintendents of Training Schools.

By 1904, it was decided that the ICN should be a federation of national organizations representing nurses in each country, rather than a membership consisting of individual nurses. Accordingly, the AFN was invited, along with the German Nurses Association and the National Council of Nurses of England, to become charter members of the ICN. The American Nurses Association (ANA) was formed in 1911 as the representative organization of the Nurses' Associated Alumnae of the United States. After the AFN disbanded in 1913, the ANA became the official US representative to the ICN.

The ICN has grown substantially over the years—it currently has a membership of 129 countries and includes 126 of the 192 nations belonging to the WHO. Of the 66 countries missing, several are in the Middle East, where nursing associations are just now developing. The ICN conducts an international congress for nurses quadrennially. It was to the ICN that the IFNA planning committee turned for assistance in its formation. Although the ICN has been made up principally of national organizations representing nurses in general, it has devised a mechanism for the recognition and affiliation of international specialty nursing organizations.

The ICN Professional Services Committee defined qualifications for specialty organizational affiliation, which include the requirement that such organizations have membership from 2 organizations representing 50% of the 7 global areas adopted by the ICN (ie, representation from 4 of these global areas; the IFNA had representation only from 3). The problem was that the ICN North American voting area consisted of 2 countries: Canada and the United States. With Canada not having nurse anesthetists, it was impossible for the IFNA to meet ICN requirements.

In 1995, the ICN restructured the voting regions, including the reorganization of the European organizations and the addition of Mexico and the Caribbean basin to the North American voting area. In 1996, Mexico became a member of the IFNA, and in 1997 Jamaica became an IFNA member. With the addition of these 2 members to the IFNA, the ICN requirement of organizational representation from 4 of the global areas was met. In 1996 ICN officially recognized IFNA as having affiliate status. The IFNA was the second of only 3 international nursing specialties to be recognized by ICN at that time. Today the following 7 organizations have ICN affiliate status: European Federation of Nursing Associations; Council on International Neonatal Nurses; IFNA; International Federation of Perioperative Nurses; International Society of Nurses in Cancer Care; International Skin

Care Nursing Group; and World Federation of Critical Care Nurses. The IFNA continues to enjoy this relationship on a formal basis and attends CNR meetings as an observer.

World Health Organization

The IFNA has made contact with nurse anesthetists in a number of countries. The breadth of usage of nurse anesthetists includes both developed and developing countries. Because IFNA aims to foster and promote high-quality nurse anesthesia education and practice wherever nurses provide these services, it would be an important step to gain recognition or affiliation with the WHO.

Persons involved in assisting developing countries to achieve adequate health delivery systems have questioned using nurses rather than physicians for anesthesia services. Two reasons apply. First, physicians from these countries who trained elsewhere in anesthesia often do not return to their native countries to practice; even if trained in their own countries, they often emigrate elsewhere to practice. Nurses appear less prone to emigrate. The second reason is that the precarious economic status of many developing countries suggests that nurses would be the more cost-effective anesthesia provider and, as is evident in all IFNA member countries, would practice throughout the country, wherever need exists.

In general, it appears to be the WHO's primary aim to promote a strong primary care and disease prevention program in developing countries as a means to gain the most benefit for money spent. Although not often considered a primary care modality, anesthesia cuts across the various types of healthcare. Obstetrics, for example, is regarded as a primary care component, despite its involving high-risk patients and tertiary care; thus, access to selected anesthesia services in this healthcare area is essential to minimize both maternal and neonatal morbidity and mortality.

Furthermore, anesthesia may be required to assist in preventing or correcting infection, disease, traumatic injury, or congenital defects that, although not necessarily life-threatening initially, may over time cause disability and dependency and threaten life if untreated. Blindness, cleft lip or palate, conditions leading to deafness, and fractures with bone displacement exemplify such conditions.

It was at the first meeting with the WHO, in November 1990, when Caulk and Löhnert obtained an appointment with Miriam Hirschfeld, the WHO's chief scientist for nursing, that the question of establishing a relationship or liaison with the WHO was discussed. Hirschfeld, somewhat unfamiliar with nurse anesthetists and their practice, requested that additional information be furnished to her on the number of nurse anesthetists worldwide, the countries in which they are used, and the roles they fulfill. Unfortunately, other than for the 11 member organizations, such information was virtually unknown to the IFNA. The IFNA had only unsubstantiated reports that nurses were involved in the provision of anesthesia services elsewhere.

Occasion for another meeting with Hirschfeld arose when she came to be the keynote speaker at the International Nursing Research Conference in October 1991. Maura McAuliffe, CRNA, PhD, FAAN, then a doctoral student at the College of Nursing, University of Texas-Austin, and Caulk were present. At a subsequent meeting with Hirschfeld during the conference, it was discussed and proposed that a worldwide study of nurse anesthetists be

81

conducted. Hirschfeld agreed that the WHO would collaborate in the study. Funding was obtained, and the study is now complete. Although the IFNA is not yet recognized as a nongovernmental organization, it does maintain an informal relationship with the WHO.

Center for Quality Assurance in International Education

The Center for Quality Assurance in International Education (CQAIE) is a consortium of higher education associations and quality assurance and competency bodies located at the National Center for Higher Education in Washington, DC. The center is dedicated to monitoring quality issues in the globalization of US higher education and provides assistance in the development and improvement of quality assurance systems throughout the globe. In 1996, the center became the secretariat of a new global organization of business, government, education, and the professions dedicated to issues of quality and access in education and training that crosses national borders: the Global Alliance for Transnational Education (GATE).[12]

Marjorie Peace Lenn, MEd, EdD,[13] executive director of the CQAIE, presented the keynote address at the IFNA 5th World Congress in April 1997. Lenn outlined for the group action steps for establishing a profession nationally or regionally. She also stressed that the dynamics of globalization leave no professional time to dwell in myopia without rendering the profession irrelevant in a changing world. According to her, the future effectiveness of international professional organizations lies in their ability to provide international solutions to local problems or to be effective across borders as well as within borders. The IFNA concurs with this statement and continues to work with this organization. It is through the CQAIE that IFNA leaders have become aware of international trade agreements, such as the North American Free Trade Agreement, and the World Trade Organization with respect to trade in services affecting professional mobility. Many international organizations participate in CQAIE activities that include international accreditation and certification. Although the IFNA has not developed accreditation and certification internationally, it is an issue that will most probably be addressed in the future. The IFNA has been an organizational member of the CQAIE since 1997, and its representatives have both presented and participated at CQAIE and GATE meetings.

Table 4.11. Action Steps for Establishing a Global Profession

Act as an international witness for the need for professional standards in nurse anesthesia.

Interact effectively with appropriate regional and international organizations.

Act as liaison to other globalizing professions.

Consider development of an International Federation of Nurse Anesthetists (IFNA) quality assurance process for nurse anesthesia educational and professional development programs.

Monitor and record its own progress through research, publication, and international forums.

World Federation of Societies of Anaesthesiologists

A featured speaker at the 5th World Congress of IFNA in Austria was Dr Anneke Meursing, honorary secretary, World Federation of Societies of Anesthesiologists (WFSA). As a follow-up to this congress, IFNA representatives were asked to meet with the Executive Committee of the WFSA.

On June 30, 1998, the IFNA president, executive director, and 2 members of the Education Committee (Sandra M. Ouellette, CRNA, MEd, FAAN, United States, and Jeanne Capron, France) met with members of the WFSA Executive Committee in Braunfels, Germany. The purpose of the meeting was to explore the possibility of forming a liaison with the WFSA. Meursing suggested that 2 members of the IFNA Education Committee attend the meeting since many of the organizations' mutual interests involve education and continuing education in less-developed countries. The meeting focused on education and continuing education primarily in the less-developed countries and what the 2 organizations could do jointly to assist with these issues. Although it was emphasized by physician leaders that the WFSA is a physician-based organization and views anesthesiology as a physician-based specialty, the existence and contributions of both nurses and clinical officers in various parts of the world was acknowledged. Overall, the meeting was cordial and productive. It provided the IFNA with an opportunity to establish a working relationship with the WFSA.

In May 1999, Ouellette, serving as IFNA Education Committee chair, joined Meursing in Blantyre, Malawi. The purpose of the trip was to participate in the 6th Anaesthesia Refresher Course Seminar and the inauguration of the Association of Anaesthetists of Malawi. The IFNA sponsored another continuing education offering in Ghana in 2005 and partially sponsored a speaker for a seminar in Rwanda in 2006.

International Hospital Federation

In 1998, IFNA Executive Director Caulk and Glen Ramsborg, CRNA, PhD, met with the then director general of the International Hospital Federation (IHF), Errol Pickering to discuss the role of the IHF and its relationship with other international organizations. The IFNA was encouraged to become an organizational member of the IHF and to participate in IHF activities. In 1998, the IFNA became an organizational member of the IHF and was encouraged to submit articles on nurse anesthesia for the IHF journal. Caulk prepared an article about the IFNA, which was published in *World Hospitals and Health Services,* the official journal of the IHF.[11] This journal has a worldwide circulation. Although the predominant membership of the IHF is hospital administrators, the IHF addresses all issues in healthcare.

International Society for Quality in Health Care

The International Society for Quality in Health Care (ISQUA) is an independent, global organization with the following objectives: (1) promotion of quality improvement on a continual basis in healthcare internationally in both the public and private sectors; (2) development and maintenance of internationally agreed-upon terminology of quality improvement; (3) organization of meetings on a regional and global basis; (4) provision of an internationally agreed method of accreditation for courses in quality improvement and related matters; (5) promotion of research in quality

83

improvement in healthcare; and (6) maintenance of relationships with other relevant international and regional organizations.

Membership of the ISQUA includes many international professional organizations, national and regional accrediting bodies, and individuals participating in quality assurance. The Joint Commission formed an international arm called the Joint Commission International. In July 1999, Caulk attended the World Symposium on Improving Health Care Through Accreditation in Barcelona, Spain. This symposium was cosponsored by the Fundacion Avedis Donabedium, a Spanish accreditation body, and by Underwriters Laboratories, and endorsed by the EU-sponsored External Peer Review Techniques Group and the ISQUA. This was the first such meeting attended by a leader of the IFNA. International standards for hospital accreditation were proposed at this meeting. Of concern to the IFNA is the fact that such standards address not only the standards for anesthesia departments but also the credentials of "qualified anesthesia providers" within the department. The initiation of international standards met with mixed reviews, especially for the developing and less-developed countries, where the cost for the accreditation of one hospital could well be the entire annual healthcare budget.

When discussing ISQUA activities, the IFNA was advised that organizational membership in the ISQUA provided the only method for representation and addressing of issues affecting anesthesia services. Although some IFNA members have individual membership, it is only through organizational membership that the profession has an international voice. The IFNA became an organizational member of the ISQUA in 1999.

Globalization of the Professions

The topic of Lenn's[13] keynote address at IFNA's 5th World Congress of Nurse Anesthetists in 1997 was "Nurse Anesthesia and the Globalization of the Professions." In this address, Lenn stated that there is an eagerness at the World Congress to accentuate differences in national practice rather than to celebrate similarities in international practice. She believes that since the IFNA has adopted international standards, it is well on its way to globalization of the nurse anesthesia profession. At the heart of professional practice is a core of common standards that, if adopted across borders and regions, defines the profession of nurse anesthesia in ways that not only protect regulation and mode of practice but also provide the world's people the best in anesthesia care.

The IFNA's educational, practice, and ethical standards stand as international witness for the globalization of a profession in both preparation and practice.[2-4] The global marketplace and new technology are contributing to the rapid globalization of higher education. Issues of quality, purpose, and responsibility abound in the new borderless educational arena, posing new challenges to the regulatory communities of accreditation, certification, and licensure, the 3 pillars of quality and competency assurance among the professions of the world.

Table 4.11 lists action steps for the IFNA in establishing a global profession. The IFNA remains committed not only to globalization of the nurse anesthesia profession but also to national and regional development of the profession. With the IFNA being the only international nursing organization to establish international standards, it will continue to work toward daily application of the standards in anesthetic care worldwide.

IFNA: Accomplishments, Needs, Future

Since its founding in 1989, the IFNA has accomplished many goals. Recognized strengths include adopted standards and increased networking among other international organizations interested in healthcare.

As with any fairly new organization, the IFNA has some weaknesses that it must strive to overcome. Lack of financial support is one of its major problems. Many member countries are the size of some of the smaller states within the United States, and the number of nurse anesthetists in these countries is small. Many member countries have been financing their own representatives to the IFNA meetings, with money from the IFNA budget going only to those that cannot undertake any sponsorship. There is a need to identify sources of revenue for the organization and the IFNA Education and Research Foundation whereby donations can be accepted and used for some of the IFNA's planned activities and research. It would also be helpful if the IFNA could sponsor scholarships or find other means by which nurse anesthetists could receive financial aid to obtain additional education so as to better prepare them as educators and leaders within their countries.

The IFNA is not without potential for some internal political issues. National pride runs strong within each member country. Although the IFNA encourages global thinking, protection of one's own turf occasionally arises. Intent and desire to work together as equals are evident, but member nurse anesthesia organizations differ in size, in age, and in the development the specialty has attained. The principal fiscal support for the organization must come from the larger and longer-established organizations. This has the potential to leave the perception that 1 or 2 larger groups may attempt to dominate the group. Despite an organizational structure that can lend support to each member country, each must be sensitive to others' needs and offer support or assistance only when requested. Each country exists in its own political and legal environment, and any assistance given must take those elements into consideration.

Summary

This chapter has centered on the first decade of IFNA activities. The extent to which the IFNA will be successful in the future depends on member countries' support for the goals of the IFNA and on the IFNA's ability to align itself with the organizations and programs it supports.

The speed of transportation and communication has made us all world citizens. It is only through IFNA that we have the best opportunity to fulfill our professional obligations to our world community. We believe the future is bright for both the IFNA and the people we serve.

As we move forward in the 21st century, it is evident that the IFNA needs more international research. Although the IFNA international study in the late 1990s provided much needed information (Table 4.12) and worldwide publication for nurse anesthesia,[14,15] it is apparent that nurse anesthetists will need to be included as contributors to future healthcare and healthcare planning.

85

Table 4.12. Nurse Anesthesia Worldwide: Practice, Education, and Regulation[14]

The World Health Assembly, in 1977, determined that all Member Governments should have as their primary goal to achieve by the year 2000, a level of health that would allow their citizens to enjoy an economically and socially productive life. The main strategy for "Health for All by the Year 2000" is the development of a health system infrastructure, starting with primary health care, for the delivery of countrywide services that reach the whole population. Primary care includes maternal and child services and the identification and appropriate treatment of common acute diseases and injuries. The skills and resources required to provide these aspects of primary health care often involve relatively simple, yet life-saving or disability prevention procedures, such as is used in the management of acute labor and delivery complications of the mother and fetus, or the simple reduction of a displaced fracture of a leg or arm. These services, however, cannot be provided humanely without anesthesia.

In many countries, anesthesia is provided by nurses—a little known fact. This international study of nurse anesthesia was conducted to provide information with respect to the quantity and quality of anesthesia care delivered by nurses in countries in all regions as designated by The World Health Organization. This study provides information that can serve as a basis for future planning of anesthesia manpower resources and education.

Study Methods and Findings: In Phase I of the study, surveys were translated into five languages and mailed to Ministries of Health (164 countries); National Nursing Organizations (154 countries); and leaders in Nursing Administration (76 countries). The surveys asked if, in their countries, nurses gave or assisted in the giving of anesthesia, and requested respondents to provide names and addresses of nurse anesthetists who could participate in Phase II of the study. **Phase I Results:** Respondents from 107 countries (59% of all WHO member states) reported that nurses give anesthesia in their countries; 9 countries reported that nurses assist in the giving of anesthesia. In 18 countries the evidence was inconclusive, although it is highly likely that nurses in many of these countries give anesthesia. Respondents from 112 countries provided names and addresses of 624 nurse anesthetists.

In Phase II of the study, surveys containing items addressing anesthesia practice (80 items), education (16 items), and regulation (17 items) were translated into 4 languages and mailed to each of the 624 nurse anesthetists in Phase I of the study. **Phase II Results:** Respondents (n=299) from 92 countries validated the findings from Phase I. The Phase II subjects reported that nurse anesthetists provide as much as 77% of the anesthesia in urban areas and 75% of anesthetics in rural areas of their respective countries. The respondents reported that in the hospitals where they work, nurse anesthetists provide 85% of all anesthetics for cesarean sections; administer drugs to induce anesthesia (77%); perform tracheal intubation (74%); administer spinal anesthesia (57%); epidural anesthesia (44%); manage anesthetized patients intraoperatively (79%); perform tracheal extubation (77%); and manage patients in the immediate postoperative period (54%). Fifty-seven per cent of the respondents reported they were required to have a physician anesthetist supervise their work (most were from the European region), 43% of the sample reported having no such requirement. All respondents had a formal

Continues on page 87.

Table 4.12. Nurse Anesthesia Worldwide: Practice, Education, and Regulation[14] (continued)

course of study in anesthesia; however, many had to travel to other countries to receive their education. Fifty per cent reported that continuing education was not available. Respondents (74%) reported that hospital policies as well as governmental regulations (60%) guide their practice of nurse anesthesia.

Improved access to continuing education and supportive legislation were most frequently cited as changes that would improve the anesthesia practice of nurses. An additional finding was that although nurse anesthetists currently provide much, and in some countries virtually all the anesthesia, their contribution to health care often goes unrecognized by their governments. If "Health for All" is to be achieved by any nation, fiscally responsible health care systems that maximally utilize the services of qualified classes of health care providers must be instituted. National health care policy-makers should be made aware that nurse anesthetists currently provide much of the anesthesia care world-wide, and the most cost-effective and efficient anesthesia care includes the utilization of nurse anesthetists. To maximally utilize these health care providers, nurse anesthesia educational programs should be expanded, and supportive legislation should be initiated.

Maura S. McAuliffe, CRNA, PhD
Beverly Henry, RN, PhD, FAAN

(Reprinted with permission from the IFNA. http://www.ifna-int.org/ifna/e107_files/downloads/Practice.pdf)

87

References

1. Caulk R, Maree SM. A new beginning: the International Federation of Nurse Anesthetists. *AANA J.* 1990;58(3):158-164. http://www.ifna-int.org/ifna/page.php?16.

2. International Federation of Nurse Anesthetists Bylaws. 2000:1-11.

3. International Federation of Nurse Anesthetists. Educational standards for preparing nurse anesthetists. International Federation of Nurse Anesthetists. 1990:2-8.

4. International Federation of Nurse Anesthetists. Standards of practice. International Federation of Nurse Anesthetists. 1996:2-11.

5. Code of ethics. International Federation of Nurse Anesthetists. 1992:2-4.

6. Vision statement. International Federation of Nurse Anesthetists. 2000:1 http://www.ifna-int.org/ifna/page.php?16

7. Mission statement. International Federation of Nurse Anesthetists. 2000:1. http://www.ifna-int.org/ifna/page.php?16

8. Aker JG. Rupp RM. Standards of care in anesthesia practice. In: Foster SD, Jordan LM, eds. *Professional Aspects of Nurse Anesthesia Practice.* Philadelphia, PA: FA Davis Co; 1994:89-112.

9. International Federation of Nurse Anesthetists. *Congress Planning Committee Policy Procedure Manual.* 1997:1-46.

10. Patient monitoring guidelines. IFNA. 1999:2-4.

11. Caulk RF. The International Federation of Nurse Anesthetists (IFNA), an introduction. *World Hosp Health Serv.* 1998;34(2):11-14.

12. Caulk RF. The International Federation of Nurse Anesthetists (IFNA). *CRNA Forum.* 1992;8(2):3-19.

13. Peace Lenn MP. Nurse anesthesia and the globalization of the profession. *AANA J.* 1997;65(5):444-449.

14. McAuliffe M, Henry B. Countries where anesthesia is administered by nurses. *AANA J.* 1996;64(5):469-479.

15. Henry B, McAuliffe M. Practice and education of nurse anaesthetists. *Bull World Health Organ.* 1998;77(3):267-270.

Study Questions

1. The work of the IFNA in the last decade is a good example of collaboration with other healthcare organizations that have a worldwide influence. Why is this collaboration necessary or desirable?

2. What are the primary objectives of the IFNA? How do they relate to those of AANA?

3. What is a federation, and why is it a workable organizational framework for the IFNA?

4. Contact several international organizations of nurse anesthetists who are members of the IFNA and explore the ways in which their scope of practice compares with your own. How do they plan on further developing practice standards in their country?

Understanding the Responsibilities of Clinical Practice

CHAPTER 5

State Governmental Regulation of Nurse Anesthesia Practice

Mitchell H. Tobin, JD

Key Concepts

- State laws and regulations concerning nursing developed in the 20th century. Although state regulation of nursing initially dealt with registered nurses, from the 1970s to the present, most states adopted explicit statutory and regulatory provisions concerning advanced practice registered nursing roles such as "nurse anesthetist."

- Advanced practice registered nurses (APRNs) such as nurse anesthetists have sometimes encountered difficult battles in defining scope of practice in state laws and regulations; this is in part a result of organized medicine having successfully defined the practice of medicine broadly in state laws and regulations before formal recognition of nursing practice.

- Although state laws and regulations often set forth requirements nurse anesthetists must meet to be recognized or to practice, local institutional policies and procedures often affect practice significantly as well. Facilities (such as hospitals) have wide latitude to impose policies more restrictive than state law.

- The primary sources of state statutory and regulatory recognition for nurse anesthetists are state nursing statutes and board of nursing regulations. Other state statutes and regulations, such as state hospital or ambulatory surgical center regulations, can also have important practice implications.

Continues on next page.

Key Concepts (continued)

- The manner or type of statutory and regulatory recognition of nurse anesthetists varies considerably from state to state. In addition, the qualifications a nurse anesthetist must possess to practice, as well as how scope of practice is addressed, are not uniform in every state.

Formal state regulation of nursing practice in the United States is so entrenched that it is easy to assume it always existed. State laws and regulations concerning nursing, however, are a 20th century phenomenon. To understand why and how nurse anesthetists are formally recognized in states today, it is necessary to first explore the development of state regulation of medicine, then nursing.

Spurred by the efforts of the American Medical Association (AMA), Texas passed the first modern medical practice act in 1873.[1] The enactment of this state law was significant, because it heralded the beginning of an era in which physicians would have to obtain a license to practice medicine. The legitimacy of compulsory licensure for physicians did not go unchallenged, however. There were those who did not believe government had the right to require healthcare professionals to be licensed to practice. The US Supreme Court put the issue to rest in the 1889 case of *Dent v West Virginia*.[2]

In this case, the court upheld the constitutionality of the West Virginia Medical Practice Act. In doing so, the court relied on the Tenth Amendment to the US Constitution, which states: "The powers not delegated to the United States by the Constitution, nor prohibited by it to the States, are reserved to the States respectively, or to the people."[3] The Tenth Amendment is the source of the states' "police power," or right to regulate public health, welfare, and safety. As *Dent v West Virginia* confirmed, states have the authority as part of their police power to regulate and license healthcare professionals. Following the *Dent* decision in 1889, states moved quickly to adopt compulsory licensure laws for physicians. By 1905, 39 states had enacted medical practice laws that required physicians to obtain a license before practicing medicine.[4]

Medical licensure led the way for formal state regulation of nursing. As Bullough[4] noted, because organized medicine had already fought the battle concerning the legitimacy of state licensing laws, nursing's path was easier. Furthermore, medicine's efforts in state legislatures constituted a guide for the political actions necessary for adoption of state nursing laws.

Basic state regulatory terms are explained in Table 5.1. It is important to understand these terms, because they represent the building blocks states use to recognize nursing professionals. State nurse anesthetist associations should become conversant with the particular administrative procedures in their respective states. It is difficult to effectively play the rulemaking "game" without understanding the rules.

The fact that medical licensure preceded nursing's regulatory attempts also had negative implications. Physician medical practice laws defined the practice of medicine broadly. As Bullough[4] stated:

> [A]uthors of the early registration laws and those who worked on subsequent revisions in the early twentieth century assumed that medicine was the only health profession, and the language they used in the registration statutes often reflected that assumption. This meant that nursing and the other health professions had to consciously avoid that area previously carved out by medicine or, if they intruded therein, had to be prepared to face a battle. The nursing profession, as a result, avoided challenging the position of medicine. Only recently have things begun to change.

Development of Nursing Licensure

With medical licensure well established, the stage was set for formal state regulation of

Table 5.1. Basic State Regulatory Terms

Jurisdiction. A geographic area having the power to adopt, implement, and enforce laws. All states are jurisdictions, as are entities such as the District of Columbia, Puerto Rico, and the US Virgin Islands.

Law. See statute.

Statute. Also known as a *law*. Statutes are enacted, that is, passed, by state legislatures. The level of specificity of statutes varies. They are often general, leaving the specifics to administrative regulations. Every state has a primary law governing nursing practice. The law is usually called the "nurse practice act," "nursing practice act," or a similar designation.

Regulation. Also referred to as a *"rule."* Regulations are specific written policies adopted by an administrative agency. States typically have a law (often known as the "administrative procedure act") that sets forth the procedures state administrative agencies must follow to adopt regulations. Commonly, an administrative agency must publish a regulation, accept written comments, and hold hearings before the regulation can be finalized. Specific administrative rulemaking procedures, however, vary from state to state. In some states, for example, there are legislative oversight committees composed of state legislators who review proposed rules. The particular powers of such committees vary. An oversight committee may or may not have the power to reject a rule that an administrative agency has adopted; in other states, the committee may have the power to only recommend whether a rule should be adopted or not. In still other states, there are administrative oversight commissions or similar bodies whose task is to review proposed regulations and recommend whether the regulations should be adopted or modified.

State administrative agencies derive their rulemaking authority from an enabling law. An enabling law is one in which the state legislature delegates to an administrative agency the authority to adopt regulations to implement the law's purposes. The nurse practice act in every state is an enabling statute, in that it commonly authorizes the state board of nursing or similarly named entity to adopt regulations to implement the nurse practice act's provisions. In a few jurisdictions, board of nursing rules sometimes must be either jointly promulgated or adopted with the state board of medicine.

Once finalized, regulations generally have the force of law. To be valid, however, regulations must be consistent with the enabling statute under whose authority they were adopted. To the extent a regulation is inconsistent with an enabling law, the law will control. Regulations often contain a severance or savings clause that states that to the extent any particular provision of the regulations proves invalid, the remainder of the regulations will still be in effect.

Rule. See regulation.

nursing. Bullough[4] identified these 3 primary phases in the development of nursing regulation in the United States:

- 1903-1938: Enactment of nurse registration acts in numerous states.
- 1938-1971: State legislatures began defining the scope of nursing practice.
- 1971-present: Increasing state recognition of advanced practice nursing specialties (such as nurse anesthesia) of registered nurses (RNs).

First Phase

In 1903, North Carolina enacted the first nurse registration act in the United States.[4] The act provided that, beginning in 1904, only persons that the North Carolina Board of Examiners certified could be listed as RNs.[4] By 1923, similar laws had been passed in all states and the District of Columbia.[5] Greenlaw[5] identified 4 weaknesses that characterized these laws:

(1) These laws were title protection or "certification" laws in nature. The laws regulated the titles "registered nurse" and "RN" rather than the practice of nursing itself. Nurses who had not registered with the state as "registered nurses" could still practice as long as they did not refer to themselves as registered nurses or use the title RN. (2) The nursing boards created to implement registration laws often had physician members as well as nurses. As late as 1938, 17 state nursing boards still included at least one physician. (3) The registration laws required minimal educational requirements. As of 1938, 19 states did not require graduation from high school as a prerequisite of nursing registration. (4) Nursing practice was not defined in the registration laws. Registered nurses were defined exclusively by their qualifications rather than the functions they performed.

Second Phase

In 1938, New York passed the first mandatory nursing licensure law.[4] As Hadley[6] notes, the law contained 2 attributes that became the hallmark of all modern nursing statutes: a definition of what constitutes nursing practice and a prohibition against unauthorized practice. Bullough[4] states,

It was necessary to specify the scope of practice of the occupation that was being protected against encroachment. The older nursing laws made it illegal for an unauthorized person to use the title 'registered nurse,' but not illegal for such a person to practice nursing. Once the new mandatory laws made it illegal for an unauthorized person to practice nursing, a definition of the scope of practice had to be written into those laws.

The New York definition of the practice of nursing became a model for many other states. The New York statute defined the practice of nursing as[4]:

A person practices nursing within the meaning of this article who for compensation or personal profit (a) performs any professional service requiring the application of principles of nursing based on biological, physical and social sciences, such as responsible supervision of a patient requiring skill in observation of symptoms and reactions and the accurate recording of the facts, and carrying out of treatments and medications as prescribed by a licensed physician, and the application of such nursing procedures as involve understanding of cause and effect in order to safeguard life and health of a patient and others; or (b) performs such duties as are required in the physical care of a patient and in carrying out of medical orders as prescribed by a licensed

97

physician, requiring an understanding of nursing but not requiring the professional service as outlined in (a).

The New York definition did not refer to advanced nursing practice per se or identify specific advanced roles such as nurse anesthesia. Formal recognition of advanced practice would not emerge in the states for some time to come.

By 1946, 10 states had adopted a definition of nursing.[4] In 1955, while the trend to define nursing practice and adopt mandatory licensure laws gained momentum, the American Nurses Association (ANA) adopted a model definition of nursing.[4] Like the seminal New York law of 1938, the ANA model definition did not refer to advanced practice nursing or identify specific roles such as nurse anesthesia. The ANA's model definition of nursing practice stated:

> [P]ractice of professional nursing means the performance for compensation of any acts in the observation, care, and counsel of the ill, injured, or infirm, or in the maintenance of health or prevention of illness of others, or in the supervision and teaching of other personnel, or the administration of medications and treatments as prescribed by a licensed physician or dentist; requiring substantial specialized judgment and skill and based on knowledge and application of the principles of biological, physical, and social science. The foregoing shall not be deemed to include acts of diagnosis or prescription of therapeutic or corrective measures.

The ANA's definition of nursing practice became the new model for state nurse practice acts (NPAs). Fifteen states adopted the definition verbatim, and 6 states adopted the language with slight modifications.[4] Bullough[4] criticized the definition's specific exclusion from nursing practice of "acts of diagnosis or prescription of therapeutic or corrective measures." It is notable that this disclaimer was made by the ANA, not the AMA. Although a reasonable assumption might be that the nurses believed the disclaimer necessary to avoid medical opposition to the new practice acts, there is little evidence of overt pressure by physicians. In effect, organized nursing surrendered without any battle over boundaries.[4]

Greenlaw[5] writes that the disclaimer was troublesome for nurses who were already practicing independently. She also notes that the disclaimer failed to take into account that many nurses were currently performing acts constituting diagnosis and treatment. To reconcile discrepancies between the definition of nursing and existing practice, joint statements were often adopted by nursing, hospital, and medical organizations and associations. The joint statements typically specified activities qualified nurses could perform in certain settings. Interestingly, the joint statements were usually considered authoritative even though they were not legislatively authorized.[5]

Third Phase

The third and current phase of state regulation of nursing involves an increasing recognition of the role of RNs such as Certified Registered Nurse Anesthetists (CRNAs) practicing in an advanced role. Bullough[4] noted that factors influencing this growing formal recognition for nursing specialties were discussed and encouraged by a special committee appointed by the secretary of the US Department of Health, Education and Welfare in 1971. The special committee's report supported an extended scope of function for RNs. Bullough[4] stated that in "response to that request and to those forces that stimulated it, the state nurse practice act began to change."

Some of the factors Bullough[4] noted that influenced the growth of specialty nursing included upgrading of educational standards, increased complexity of practice because of developments in science and technology, and an aging population that required competent and affordable care. She also noted that the women's movement was a factor, because it helped reduce the sexual stereotyping that classified medicine as men's work and nursing as women's work. More men entered nursing specialties such as nurse anesthesia, and nurses in general assumed functions previously performed exclusively by physicians.

Another significant impetus for the third phase of nursing practice legislation was the ANA's amending of its model nursing definition in 1970. The ANA definition now stated that a professional nurse may also perform such additional acts, under emergency or other special conditions, which may include special training, as are recognized by the medical and nursing professions as proper to be performed by a professional nurse under such conditions, even though such acts might otherwise be considered diagnosis and prescription.[5]

The reference to "additional acts" performed "under emergency or other special conditions" marked a recognition, albeit somewhat oblique, that RNs with advanced education (such as CRNAs) existed and were practicing. The ANA's choice of language was unfortunate, however. The definition required that the additional acts be ones recognized by both the "medical and nursing professions." This implied that nursing could not legitimately be the sole arbiter of appropriate advanced nursing practice and needed medicine's consent to do so.

In 1990, the ANA's model nursing practice act no longer contained the reference to "additional acts" or the requirement that such acts be ones recognized by both the medical and nursing professions.[7] The ANA's 1990 model practice act in section 201[d],[7(p8)] defined *professional nursing practice* as encompassing "the full scope of nursing practice and includes all its specialties and consists of application of nursing theory to the development, implementation, and evaluation of plans of nursing care for individuals, families, and communities. Professional nursing practice requires substantial knowledge of nursing theory and related scientific, behavioral, and humanistic disciplines. Professional nursing practice includes, but is not limited to. . . ."

As of 1990, the ANA's model definition of nursing practice contained explicit reference to nursing's "specialties." As of that time, it had been the ANA's longstanding philosophy that NPAs should not refer to specific areas of specialized nursing practice, such as nurse anesthesia. In the comments section to its 1990 model nursing practice act, the ANA stated explicitly that acts "should not provide for recognition of particular clinical specialists in nursing or require certification or other recognition or credentialing beyond the minimum qualifications established for licensure. Standards for specialized areas of practice and the certification of individuals as competent to practice in specialized areas is the domain of the professional association."[7(p9)]

The ANA's current Model Practice Act, last revised in 1996, includes both a broad definition of nursing, as well as specific recognition of APRNs, including CRNAs.[8] This represents a shift from the ANA's previous philosophy of not mentioning specific advanced practice nursing roles in the ANA's

99

Model Practice Act. In the discussion section to its Model Practice Act, the ANA states that, while previous ANA model practice acts regulated only RN practice, the current act's intent is to regulate licensed practical/vocational nurses, RNs, and APRNs under one statute. Consistent with the ANA's policy that all of these nurses should be regulated under a common scope of nursing practice, the model practice act is intended to include APRNs in the definition of "nursing," allowing boards of nursing to "make professional distinctions in tasks by levels of practice."[8]

The ANA's Model Practice Act (section 2[I]) now defines nursing in part as "the performance of any acts to care for the health of the patient that require substantial, specialized or general knowledge, judgment and skill based upon principles of the biological, physical, behavioral and social sciences as defined through rules promulgated by the Board of Nursing.... The Board of Nursing shall determine the skill level and scope of practice for each type of nurse licensed under this Act."[8]

In addition, the Model Practice Act (section 2[B]) now includes a definition of *advanced practice registered nurse* as "a registered professional nurse who has specialized knowledge, education and skills to provide health care as determined appropriate by the Board of Nursing through administrative rule making and by fulfillment of all qualifications outlined in this Act. They are registered professional nurses with national certification as deemed appropriate by the Board of Nursing, and include nurse practitioners, nurse anesthetists, nurse-midwives and clinical nurse specialists."[8]

The ANA believes that a broad, general definition of nursing scope remains necessary to provide "expansiveness and flexibility [that] allows the profession—not the [board of nursing]—to define the practice."[8(p12)] This also allows nursing educators to "re-tool and restructure programs to reflect health care delivery needs and not the requirements of licensure and, if necessary, to redesign the requirements for each level of practice."[8(p12)]

The trend in recent years has been for states to increasingly grant specific recognition to APRNs practicing in identifiable nursing roles, such as CRNAs, nurse practitioners, nurse-midwives, and clinical nurse specialists. Later in this chapter we explore this phenomenon in detail as it relates to CRNAs. As is reflected in the changes to the ANA model practice acts, many aspects of the ANA's philosophy on state regulation of nursing have changed over time, along with state trends.

Most APRNs have applauded the trend toward specific recognition in state NPAs or board of nursing (BON) regulations, as opposed to exclusive reliance on broad definitions of nursing. As Greenlaw[5] states, "Nurses relying upon broad statutory language do not always feel confident that their practice will go unchallenged by physicians and, indeed, challenges have occurred."

States continue to defer in great measure to professional organizations regarding certification of APRNs, as well as accreditation of educational programs. Greenlaw[5] notes:

> In the mid-1970s, when the states began to recognize advanced nursing practice through statutory and regulatory provisions, the states also began to require that nurses in advanced practice obtain certification by the appropriate national nursing specialty organizations.... [This] can be viewed as a reasonable compromise between the authority of the state and the function of the professional association. The state is not usurping the functions

of the professional associations; rather, the state, exercising its power to safeguard the public, is giving statutory recognition, or deferring, to the role of the professional associations.

Debate Over Mandatory Licensure

Mandatory licensure of RNs and physicians is so well established that its necessity might seem a given. This is not the case, however, as many commentators have debated whether mandatory licensure per se should be eliminated. Licensure is the most restrictive type of state-granted credential. Mandatory licensure laws require individuals to obtain a license before practicing a specified profession. The scope of practice of the profession is commonly defined. Persons who do not possess the requisite license may neither use the title of the profession (eg, RN) nor practice the profession as it is defined. In this sense, mandatory licensure laws protect both titles and practice. Unauthorized practice is commonly punishable by sanctions handed down by the state administrative board that oversees the profession (eg, the BON). Depending on the specifics of state law, sanctions may include letters of reprimand, license suspension or revocation, fines, or other appropriate penalties. Criminal sanctions may also apply.

The primary rationale for mandatory licensure laws is the protection of the public's health and welfare and not individual professions. It has been argued that patients are sometimes unable to obtain sufficient information to adequately judge healthcare practitioner competence and therefore benefit by licensure. Furthermore, patients arguably do not possess the knowledge to accurately gauge the risks to their health from inadequate or incompetent care.

Clayton[1] argues that "[b]y setting minimum standards for the qualifications and training required of health care personnel, licensure laws attempt to control the quality of health care. Competent health care is, in turn, more likely to preserve the health and well being of patients and to save society the costs of unnecessary injuries and deaths that may result from bad medical care."

Despite its purported benefits, mandatory licensure has been criticized, as Clayton[1] notes. Commentators have questioned whether it actually improves patient care and have expressed concerns about its economic impact. Furthermore, by granting a monopoly over the practice of a profession to those individuals who meet state-defined standards, the state in effect outlaws competition by other individuals who might also deliver good medical care even though they cannot satisfy the criteria required for licensure. State licensing boards have also been accused of being slow to accept changes in technology, are prone to establishing professional practice standards that bear little relationship to an applicant's actual ability to take care of patients, and are overly protective of licensed professionals' vested interest in maintaining their own privileged status. State disciplinary and licensure bodies are also criticized for having little success in controlling professionals who either do not practice competently or practice in an unethical fashion. Licensure, it has been argued, contributes to high healthcare costs and reduces innovation and consumer choice. Alternatives to licensure, such as a voluntary accreditation system or a complete abolition of licensure, have been suggested.[1]

Gunn[9] has also discussed the criticisms of mandatory licensure. She points out that some have argued for allowing institutions such as hospitals to assume the

101

responsibility for screening healthcare professionals and eliminating government involvement. Gunn states, however, that opponents of institutional licensure have cited the possibility that institutions may sacrifice quality to assure fiscal soundness and profits, thereby engaging in marginal or unsafe care. Other major concerns about institutional licensure include the fear that there would be no consistency of healthcare standards or qualifications of providers, such as educational requirements; decreased geographic mobility for providers; and no way for consumers to make truly informed choices about their care. At least in part because of criticism of the proliferation of mandatory licensure, some states now require groups seeking passage of mandatory licensure legislation to demonstrate why licensure, rather than registration, certification, or no regulation, is necessary.[1] Despite criticisms of mandatory licensure, no state has eliminated licensure for either RNs or physicians. Mandatory licensure appears here to stay, absent a profound shift in how states view this area.

State Recognition and Regulation of CRNA Practice

As with RNs in general, formal state recognition of nurse anesthetists followed well-established practice. It is important to bear in mind that CRNA practice was widely regarded as legal and legitimate long before states formally regulated the profession. For the most part, formal state recognition and regulation of CRNAs have ratified existing practice rather than reshaping the parameters of the profession. On a day-to-day basis, institutional policies and procedures sometimes have a greater impact on practice than state statutes and regulations. An example of this practical re-

ality is regional anesthesia practice. Although no state laws or regulations prohibit CRNAs from administering regional anesthesia, some hospitals have institutional policies prohibiting CRNAs from administering regional anesthesia.

This example demonstrates another facet of state laws and regulations. Merely because a particular activity may be legal under state law does not compel institutions to permit practitioners to engage in the activity. In other words, employers such as hospitals and private anesthesiologist groups have wide latitude to impose policies more restrictive than state law. Employer policies may not violate antitrust, civil rights, and other types of laws potentially applicable to the workplace, but such laws often provide less protection than the unwary employee suspects. Although institutional and employer policies often have a more immediate impact on practice than state law, this does not mean state statutes and regulations are irrelevant. First, state NPAs and BON regulations often specify qualifications CRNAs must possess to practice. Second, although state statutes and regulations often do not restrict actual practice in significant ways, the potential for such restriction always exists. CRNAs must always be vigilant concerning proposed legislation or regulations that affect practice.

In addition, CRNAs must be alert to statutory or regulatory proposals to mandate anesthesiologist supervision. Currently some states require that CRNAs be "supervised" by a "licensed physician." No state, however, specifically requires in either its NPA or BON regulations that the supervising physician be an anesthesiologist. The supervision issue is a subject of continuing debate between state nurse anesthetist associations and their anesthesiologist counterparts. Anesthesiologist societies continually insist that CRNAs are technicians who should be supervised by anesthesiologists to ensure quality care. The American Association of Nurse Anesthetists (AANA) disagrees and opposes any statutory or regulatory proposal requiring that CRNAs be supervised by anesthesiologists. It is important to preserve the right of CRNAs to choose the practice situation in which they are most comfortable. Once anesthesiologist supervision is mandated in a statute or regulation, that choice is lost or seriously compromised, particularly for those who would like to be self-employed.

Significance of Non-Nursing Statutes and Regulations

To the extent that CRNAs are specifically regulated in a state's statutes and regulations, the most significant provisions concerning the type and manner of nurse anesthetist recognition usually appear in a state's NPA or BON regulations. Other state statutes and regulations can affect nurse anesthesia practice, albeit in less obvious ways. For example, virtually every state has hospital licensing regulations commonly promulgated and adopted by the state department of health. Hospitals must comply with these regulations to receive a license to provide patient care. Hospital licensing regulations frequently contain provisions concerning anesthesia. For example, some hospital licensing regulations require that CRNAs perform anesthesia under the supervision of a physician. Suppose such a provision appeared in the hospital licensing regulations of a state that did not specifically require physician supervision in its NPA or BON regulations. A hospital would nevertheless have to require physician supervision of CRNAs in order to comply with the state's hospital licensing requirements. To do otherwise would jeopardize the hospital's state

license. Individual CRNAs and state nurse anesthetist associations cannot afford to restrict their attention to proposals amending state nursing statutes and regulations. An anesthesiologist supervision requirement in a state's hospital licensing regulations would have as much potential for damage as one found in a state's NPA or BON regulations.

There is considerable reason to believe that CRNAs are potentially more vulnerable to restrictions in state facility licensing regulations than in BON regulations. Boards of nursing are typically much less inclined to entertain proposals to restrict CRNA practice than are state departments of health that regulate hospitals and ambulatory surgery centers. Departments of health are less likely than nursing boards to understand the nature of nurse anesthesia practice.

The preceding discussion illustrates that there are state statutes and regulations other than nursing statutes and regulations that can affect CRNAs. Individual states sometimes use different names for the various statutes, regulations, and regulatory agencies that can affect CRNAs. In addition to an NPA, most states have at least the generic equivalent of the following nonnursing statutes and regulations.

Medical Practice Acts/Board of Medicine Regulations

Medical practice acts or their generic equivalents are the state laws setting forth the scope of practice for physicians. In a few states, BON regulations are jointly developed or approved with the state board of medicine.

Hospital Licensing Statutes and Regulations

Although many states do not have a hospital licensing statute, virtually every state has

103

hospital licensing regulations, that is, regulations with which hospitals must comply to be licensed. These regulations are commonly promulgated by a state's department of health.

Ambulatory Surgery Center Licensing Statutes and Regulations

Although relatively few states have ambulatory surgery center (ASC) licensing laws, most states have ASC regulations. As with hospital licensing regulations, ASC regulations are usually promulgated and adopted by a state's department of health.

Trauma Center Statutes or Regulations

Some states have specific statutes or regulations concerning trauma centers; those that do tend to emulate the guidelines of the American College of Surgeons (ACS). These guidelines are problematic in some respects. In Level I and II trauma centers, the ACS guidelines require that anesthesia services must be available in-house 24 hours a day.[10] Although this requirement may be fulfilled by a CRNA or an anesthesiology resident, when CRNAs or residents are used, a staff anesthesiologist must be promptly available and present for all operations. In Level III trauma centers, the anesthesia services requirement may be fulfilled by either anesthesiologists or CRNAs, but CRNAs are required to be under physician supervision. To the extent that state regulation of trauma centers increases, CRNAs must prevent widespread adoption of the objectionable features of the ACS guidelines.

The 2006 ACS guidelines for Level I trauma centers contain an explicit reference to CRNAs, affirming the validity of CRNA practice in those centers.[10]

Dental Practice Acts/Board of Dentistry Regulations

These statutes and regulations are relevant because they frequently contain specific provisions concerning anesthesia. It is very common for states to require dentists who use anesthesia in the office to have advanced anesthesia education and training and obtain a special permit, even if the dentist uses a CRNA to administer the anesthesia. Dentists who use CRNAs or anesthesiologists to administer anesthesia should be exempted from advanced anesthesia education and training requirements. Although a handful of states have such exemptions, most do not. CRNAs who work with dentists, therefore, particularly in dental offices, should make certain that such dentists meet any applicable state requirements. In addition to requirements concerning who may administer anesthesia in the dental office, there are often equipment requirements as well.

A final caveat concerning CRNAs and dentists is relevant. As noted previously, state-imposed supervision requirements concerning CRNAs vary. States having supervision requirements sometimes specifically state that CRNAs can work under dental supervision. Other states, however, merely state that CRNAs must practice under the supervision of a licensed physician. Taken literally, this would preclude CRNAs from working with dentists absent physician supervision. In some states, however, it may be possible to argue that the term *licensed physician* in the context of CRNA supervision was intended to include dentists as well as medical doctors. This is a legally intricate argument that can be made only after careful research.

Podiatry Statutes or Regulations

In some states, podiatrist practice is addressed in a statute or regulation specific to podiatrists. In other states, podiatry provisions are found as sections of the medical practice act or board of medicine regulations. Like dentists, whether podiatrists may supervise nurse anesthetists in the absence of a licensed medical doctor depends on state law. Questions sometimes occur concerning the range of services a podiatrist can order a CRNA to perform. For example, podiatry statutes often restrict podiatrists from administering any type of anesthesia other than local. In such an instance, a podiatrist clearly could not personally administer regional anesthesia, but would a nurse anesthetist working with a podiatrist be precluded from administering regional anesthesia as well? This is a difficult legal question, the answer to which will depend on interpretation of a particular state's laws and regulations.

Physician Office Surgery/Anesthesia Statutes or Regulations

In contrast to regulation of hospitals and ambulatory surgical centers, as of the late 1990s less than 5 states explicitly regulated surgical and anesthesia activities in physician offices. "Physician" in this context refers to medical doctors (MDs) or doctors of osteopathic medicine (DOs), as opposed to dentists, for example, who are the subject of different statutory and regulatory provisions.

Unregulated practice in physician offices came under increasing scrutiny in the late 1990s. Reports of injury and death in office settings appeared in the media, drawing the attention of the public, as well as legislators and regulators. In response, many states have now addressed office surgery and anesthesia practice, and this trend will probably continue until most, if not every state, has provisions in place governing such practice. As

of September 2010, at least 28 states had adopted laws, regulations, guidelines, positions, or policy statements concerning office surgery and anesthesia practice.

Reasonable regulation of offices concerning requirements that are evidence-based and clearly promote patient safety, such as equipment standards, is clearly warranted. Unfortunately, however, the office surgery and anesthesia issue has often been a state battleground where anesthesiologist societies have sought adoption of provisions that would restrict CRNAs, while not improving patient safety. For example, anesthesiologist societies have sometimes sought adoption of provisions that would require surgeons who work with CRNAs in offices to have training in the particular type of anesthesia being given for the office procedure. Practically speaking, since the physicians having training in anesthesia administration tend to be anesthesiologists, such provisions, if adopted, could have the effect that all office anesthesia be administered or supervised by anesthesiologists. Such provisions would unjustifiably discriminate against CRNAs, because they would only apply when surgeons work with CRNAs, but not when surgeons work with anesthesiologists.

Pharmacy/Drug Statutes or Regulations

States usually have statutes and regulations that address various aspects of drug use including distinguishing between controlled and noncontrolled substances. In addition, states commonly have statutes governing pharmacies and regulations adopted by the board of pharmacy. State statutes and regulations governing drug use can affect nurse anesthetists, particularly if questions are raised concerning whether a nurse anesthetist is properly handling drugs or has the authority to engage in certain practices.

Attorney General Opinions

Attorney general (AG) opinions are not statutes or regulations but are mentioned here because of their relation to them. As the state's chief legal officer, an AG often provides interpretations of state laws or regulations. For example, a state administrative entity such as a BON might ask an AG to render an opinion concerning whether the agency has exceeded the scope of its statutory authority. In addition, a BON could ask an AG whether a specific activity of a nurse was permitted or prohibited by state law. An AG opinion is not binding in the manner of a court's decision but often carries significant weight. For this reason, CRNAs must carefully consider the advisability and ramifications of encouraging an administrative body to seek an AG opinion.

State Recognition of Nurse Anesthesia Practice

Few states formally recognized nurse anesthetists in statutes and regulations until the 1970s. That decade marked the beginning of an era of increased formal and specific state recognition of APRNs. Currently, all 50 states, the District of Columbia, Puerto Rico, and the US Virgin Islands mention nurse anesthetists in at least one state statute or regulation.

Although it is clear that the legitimacy of nurse anesthesia as a profession is widely accepted, the manner, type, and frequency of statutory and regulatory recognition of CRNA practice varies considerably. State statutes and regulations sometimes refer to nurse anesthetists as a type of "advanced practice registered nurse," "advanced registered nurse practitioner," or "advanced practitioner of nursing," or as nurses practicing in an "expanded role" or "specialty area." States use these categories to describe nurses such as CRNAs who have qualifications beyond those required of RNs. In some states, CRNAs are named both specifically as a discrete nursing specialty and more generally as one of several specialties that fall within a broader generic category such as "APRN." In addition, some states have general statutory or regulatory provisions that apply to all specialty nurses, and additional provisions that apply specifically to individual APRNs such as nurse anesthetists.

As Table 5.2 indicates, nurse anesthetists are specifically mentioned in all 50 states. Figures are estimates based on the AANA's review of pertinent state laws and regulations and are current as of September 2010. In many states, nurse anesthetists are

---

Table 5.2. Primary State Statutory/Regulatory Sources of Recognition[11]

Primary sources of recognition	No. of states
Nurse Practice Act only	3[a]
Board of Nursing rules or regulations only	5
Nurse Practice Act and Board of Nursing rules or regulations	41[b]
Department of Health	1

(Adapted with permission from the American Association of Nurse Anesthetists.)
[a]Plus Puerto Rico.
[b]Plus the District of Columbia and the US Virgin Islands.

mentioned in statutes and regulations other than NPAs or BON rules or regulations. The table does not attempt to categorize every statutory and regulatory reference to nurse anesthetists. The table demonstrates, however, that every state recognizes nurse anesthetists, even if there is no specific reference in the NPA or BON rules or regulations. The following is an explanation of each of the table's categories.

Nurse Practice Act Only

Three states (and Puerto Rico) explicitly mention nurse anesthetists in the NPA but not in state BON rules or regulations.

State Board of Nursing Rules or Regulations Only

Five states explicitly mention nurse anesthetists in BON rules or regulations but not in the NPA.

Nurse Practice Act and State Board of Nursing Rules or Regulations

Approximately 41 states (and the District of Columbia and the US Virgin Islands) explicitly mention nurse anesthetists in both the NPA and BON rules or regulations. This is a dramatic increase since 1993, when only 21 states mentioned nurse anesthetists in both the NPA and BON rules or regulations. Taking the preceding 3 categories together, 49 states explicitly mention nurse anesthetists in either the NPA or BON rules or regulations, or both. This is a significant increase since 1993, when 40 states explicitly mentioned nurse anesthetists in either the NPA or the BON rules or regulations. Clearly, formal state recognition of nurse anesthesia as an advanced practice nursing role is now the rule, as opposed to being the rare exception in the early 1970s.

Department of Health

One state (New York) that does not recognize nurse anesthetists in the NPA, BON rules or regulations, or MPA nevertheless explicitly mentions nurse anesthetists in state department of health facility licensing regulations.

Medical Practice Act

Although no state currently uses the medical practice act as the sole source of recognition for nurse anesthetists, a few state medical practice acts do include provisions concerning nurse anesthetists, or APRNs generally. For example, the Medical Practice Act of Texas includes provisions regarding the ordering of drugs and devices by a CRNA in a licensed hospital or ambulatory surgery center. Nurse anesthetists need to be aware that, even if their primary source of recognition is the NPA or BON rules, provisions in other statutes, such as the medical practice act, may affect nurse anesthesia practice as well.

Methods of State Regulation of Nurse Anesthesia Practice

Every state requires that RNs apply for and receive a state-issued license before practicing. Although licensure is the uniform method of state recognition of RNs, there is no such consistency concerning the way states recognize APRNs such as nurse anesthetists. It does not appear that any state deems the mere possession of a license as an RN sufficient authority to administer anesthesia. In every state, there appears to be statutory or regulatory language of some sort that enables only certain RNs to practice nurse anesthesia. States vary widely in the specific method of regulation they use to authorize nurse anesthesia practice. Some states require RNs to obtain a specialty

107

license, in addition to the RN license, before they can practice nurse anesthesia. Other states require nurse anesthetists to register, obtain a certificate, or to apply for "recognition," "authorization," or "approval" to practice. Finally, some states do not identify a specific method by which they authorize nurses to administer anesthesia. These states, however, generally state qualifications needed to practice as a nurse anesthetist.

Commentators frequently refer to licensure as the only method of state regulation that protects both a profession's practice and title, because licensure is the only method that ensures that unauthorized persons do not practice a profession. Other methods of state regulation of professions such as recognition, certification, and registration are often thought of as forms of title protection only. In other words, these methods are sometimes thought to merely prohibit individuals who do not possess certain qualifications from using a protected title, such as "CRNA." Individuals who do not use the protected title may still supposedly practice the profession. A close examination of the state statutes and regulations in which nurse anesthetists are recognized reveals the potential danger of relying on classic definitions of licensure, registration, or other methods of state regulation. There is no substitute for examining these terms as they are actually used in a particular state and evaluating their substantive effect.

In contrast to the definitions used by commentators, methods of regulation thought of as conferring only "title protection" often appear to be something more than that as they are actually used in state laws and regulations. For example, in many states in which "recognition" is the method of regulating nurse anesthesia practice, it is clear that nurses may not administer anesthetics unless they possess certain state-delineated qualifications. This is the case regardless of whether a nurse is called a nurse anesthetist or a CRNA. In these states, recognition is actually being implemented in a way that resembles licensure in the sense that both the practice and title of a profession are being protected. The practical reality is that regardless of what a state calls its particular method of regulating nurse anesthesia practice, the goal of the method is usually the same—to allow and authorize only those nurses with certain qualifications to administer anesthesia.

Table 5.3 summarizes the methods states use to authorize nurse anesthesia practice based on the AANA's review of pertinent state laws and regulations. Five states use multiple terms for the regulation process (eg, *licensure and recognition* as a CRNA). Combining all categories in the table except the last (method not specified), 45 states explicitly mention a specific process in which nurse anesthetists participate before practicing as CRNAs. These state mechanisms are described in state NPAs, or more commonly, BON rules or regulations. The mechanisms summarized in Table 5.3 are in addition to whatever state procedures nurse anesthetists must comply with to obtain their RN licenses.

Although the ostensible purpose of formal state processes for CRNA recognition is to ensure that only qualified RNs administer anesthesia, the practical importance of these state requirements is diminished by a key factor. Most hospitals require that, apart from students and new graduates, nurse anesthetists be graduates of an accredited nurse anesthesia educational program and be certified by the Council on Certification of Nurse Anesthetists (CCNA). Apart from quality of care considerations, hospitals are motivated by liability concerns.

Table 5.3. State Methods or Types of Recognition for Nurse Anesthetists[12]

Method/type of recognition	No. of states
Licensure	22
Certification	10
Authorization or approval	7
Registration or recognition	10
Notification	1
Method not specified	5

Number of States does not total to 50 because 5 states use multiple terms for the regulation process.

Regardless of whether states required CRNAs to possess certain qualifications, most nurse anesthetists would ultimately be forced to pass the CCNA's certification examination if they wished to continue to practice. The following is an explanation of each of the categories in Table 5.3; statistics are current as of September 2010.

Licensure

Twenty-two states, as of September 2010, require that nurse anesthetists obtain a state license in addition to licensure as an RN. This is an increase from 1993, when only 7 states required an additional license. The nature of the additional license varies. In some states, the additional license is as a CRNA. In others, the license is more general, such as an APRN license. States that require additional licensure do not necessarily delineate stricter qualifications for practice than states that do not require additional licensure. In no way are CRNAs who receive additional licensure better qualified than those who do not.

An example of a state using this method of recognition is Arkansas. There, RNs are granted a license as an advanced practice nurse in the category of CRNA after providing proof of completion of a nurse anesthesia educational program that meets the standards of the Council on Accreditation

of Nurse Anesthesia Educational Programs (COA) or other nationally recognized accrediting body. The applicant must also provide documentation demonstrating current certification from the CCNA or recertification from the Council on Recertification of Nurse Anesthetists (COR) or other nationally recognized certifying body.

Certification

Ten states, the District of Columbia, Puerto Rico, and the US Virgin Islands require that nurse anesthetists apply for and receive certification as a CRNA or in a particular kind of general specialty nurse category such as advanced registered nurse practitioner. The certification is not a license. Furthermore, the certification is issued by the state and should not be confused with the certification conferred by the CCNA upon passage of the council's examination. The state certification is granted after the CRNA provides evidence that he or she possesses certain qualifications.

In South Dakota, for example, an applicant for certification as a CRNA must provide written evidence to the BON that the applicant has completed an approved program of nurse anesthesia accredited by the COA. The applicant must also provide written evidence that he or she has passed a board-approved examination that has

109

been validated and scored in accordance with generally accepted testing procedures. To renew certification, the applicant must show evidence of meeting the recertification requirements of the COR.

Authorization or Approval

Seven states require that nurse anesthetists formally apply for and receive "approval" or "authorization" to practice. In Alabama, for example, CRNAs apply to the BON for approval to practice. The CRNA must submit documentation that he or she has graduated from a school of anesthesia accredited by the COA and has been certified by the CCNA or recertified by the COR. The BON then notifies the CRNA that he or she has been approved to practice by issuing the CRNA an advanced practice approval card.

Registration or Recognition

Ten states, after receipt of appropriate documentation concerning qualifications, formally recognize or register nurse anesthetists. The documentation required is typically similar to documentation required in states that approve, authorize, or certify nurse anesthetists to practice. After receiving such documentation, Nevada, for example, issues a certificate of recognition as a CRNA.

Method Not Specified

Five states do not delineate a specific method or process by which they authorize nurses to administer anesthesia. Many of these states nevertheless state qualifications needed to practice as a nurse anesthetist. In Pennsylvania, for example, the BON rules or regulations state that administration of anesthesia is a proper function of an RN who meets the requirements set forth in the BON rules or regulations. Pennsylvania, therefore, does not delineate

a specific process, such as authorization or approval, that nurse anesthetists must observe to practice. To legally practice in Pennsylvania, however, nurse anesthetists must have successfully completed a nurse anesthesia educational program accredited by the COA and be certified or recertified by the CCNA or the COR, as appropriate.

Qualifications Required for Practice

Regardless of whether a state has a specific process by which nurse anesthetists are recognized (eg, licensure, authorization, or approval), most states specify qualifications nurse anesthetists must possess to practice. These requirements are generally delineated in NPAs or BON rules or regulations; the requirements specified vary. Before practicing in a state, it is prudent for a nurse anesthetist to review the state's NPA and BON rules or regulations. These materials are commonly available online, such as at BON websites. (The National Council of State Boards of Nursing [NCSBN] website, at http://www.ncsbn.org, has links to individual BON websites). These documents are also sometimes available as paper documents from boards of nursing either at no charge or for a minimal fee. Increasingly, though, boards of nursing are no longer making paper documents available because of availability of the documents online. In addition, although requirements vary from state to state, if there are forms or applications that must be completed to practice as a nurse anesthetist, such documents are also often online. Before practicing in a particular state, however, it is wise to contact the BON directly to ensure that you have all applicable forms or applications that must be completed. Regardless of requirements (if any) that a nurse anesthetist must meet to practice in a particular state as an APRN, he or she must also comply with requirements for practice as an RN.

The most common qualifications that states specify that a nurse anesthetist must possess to practice concern education, certification, and recertification. Many states also address new graduate practice. In addition, most states delineate nurse anesthetist scope of practice in some fashion. All of the figures cited in this section are current as of September 2010.

Education

Forty-eight states require that nurse anesthetists graduate from a nurse anesthesia educational program in order to practice.[13] The other 2 states do not specifically require graduation from a nurse anesthesia educational program. Of the 48 states that require graduation, 37 states (and the District of Columbia, Puerto Rico, and the US Virgin Islands) require nurse anesthetists to have graduated from an accredited program. Approximately 11 of the 48 states require graduation from a nurse anesthesia educational program but either do not specifically refer to accreditation or have ambiguous language concerning whether the program must be accredited. In practice, the omission of a specific requirement that the nurse anesthesia educational program be "accredited" is not meaningful, because all existing programs are presently accredited.

The specific language states use to require graduation from a nurse anesthesia educational program varies. Many states require that a nurse anesthetist graduate from a program accredited by the COA. Some states do not specifically refer to the council but instead require graduation from a program that is nationally recognized or nationally accredited. These states sometimes add the caveat that the national accrediting body must be approved by the BON. Language of this sort is in effect a requirement that nurse anesthetists graduate from a program accredited by the COA, since there is no other national entity that accredits nurse anesthesia educational programs. In addition, in states that require the national accrediting body be approved by the BON, no state has failed to approve the COA as the appropriate accrediting body.

Master's Degree Requirements

In recent years, a trend toward requiring master's degrees for nurse anesthetists and other advanced practice nurses has emerged in state laws and regulations. Thirty states have enacted laws or adopted regulations that require master's degrees either currently or at a future date.[14] State requirements vary widely regarding when degree requirements will be implemented, required degree concentration, and the potential effect on CRNAs who wish to practice in states having such requirements. The COA required that, as of 1998, all programs be at the graduate level, awarding at least a master's degree.[15] Consequently, all nurse anesthetists entering nurse anesthesia educational programs in or after 1998 graduate with a minimum of a master's degree. As a result, graduates after that date should meet current state master's degree requirements.

Most states that have adopted a master's degree requirement have included a grandfather clause concerning nurse anesthetists without master's degrees. Generally, in the context of recognition or licensure of healthcare providers, a grandfather clause is a provision in a law or regulation that exempts a provider from having to comply with a new requirement that would otherwise affect prior rights or privileges. In other words, a grandfather clause allows

111

practitioners to continue to practice, even if additional restrictions imposed by a law or regulation would otherwise prohibit their practice. In the case of a master's degree requirement, a grandfather clause would allow nurse anesthetists without master's degrees who are currently recognized by a state to continue to practice with their existing educational credentials. For additional information regarding state master's degree requirements for nurse anesthetists, see Conover and Tobin[15] and the AANA website.[14]

Certification

Forty-eight states (and the District of Columbia and the US Virgin Islands) require nurse anesthetists to be certified to practice.[16] This is an increase from the approximately 40 states that required certification as of 1993. Some of these states exempt new graduates from the certification requirement for varying periods of time. Two states (and Puerto Rico) do not specifically require nurse anesthetists to be certified to practice, but nurse anesthetists must bear in mind that many individual institutions will require certification even if a particular state does not.

As with state educational requirements, the language of certification requirements varies; the manner in which certification requirements vary tends to parallel language variations in educational requirements. For example, just as numerous states require graduation from a program accredited by the COA, many states require that a nurse anesthetist be certified by the CCNA. Some states do not specifically refer to the certification council but instead require certification from a nationally recognized or national certifying body. These states sometimes also require that the national certifying body must be approved by or be acceptable to the BON. This

is in effect a requirement that one be certified by the CCNA, since there is no other national entity that certifies nurse anesthetists. In states that require that the national certifying body must be approved by the BON, no state with such a requirement has failed to approve the CCNA as the appropriate certifying body.

Recertification

Forty-five states and the District of Columbia require nurse anesthetists to be recertified at appropriate intervals.[11] This is an increase from the approximately 37 states that had such a requirement in 1993. The US Virgin Islands Board of Nurse Licensure rules are somewhat ambiguous concerning whether recertification is required, merely stating that a CRNA "shall be afforded every opportunity to maintain his/her certification status."

The comments in the preceding section of this chapter regarding variation in language used to require certification apply to recertification as well. In other words, some states specifically require that nurse anesthetists be recertified by the COR, but other states merely refer to a "nationally recognized" or "national" recertifying body. The recertifying body sometimes must be approved or accepted by the BON. In these states, the COR has uniformly been the entity approved or accepted. Again, bear in mind that regardless of state requirements, most institutions will require that nurse anesthetists be recertified.

Provisions for New Graduates

New graduates of nurse anesthesia educational programs are not certified at the time of graduation; that is, they have not yet taken and passed the national examination of the CCNA. Consequently, in states that require nurse anesthetists to be certified, the question arises as to whether new graduates are allowed to practice for a period of time following graduation before certification.

In 38 states (and the District of Columbia and Puerto Rico), there are explicit provisions in the NPA or BON rules or regulations regarding new graduate practice.[12] This is an increase from 29 states in 1993. Of the 38 states, 26 states and the District of Columbia permit new graduates to practice while they are awaiting results of the first certification examination. In these states, however, a new graduate who fails the examination must stop practicing until he or she passes the examination. Three of these 26 states permit new graduates who fail the first examination to petition the BON for an extension until they take the examination a second time. The BON grants this extension at its discretion. Eight states permit new graduates to practice for up to 1 year. Commonly, this allows graduates multiple opportunities to pass the certification examination. Finally, 2 states permit new graduates to practice for more than 1 year while awaiting results of the certification examination. Of these 2 states, 1 permits new graduates to practice for up to 18 months and 1 allows new graduates to practice for up to 2 years.

The remaining 12 states (and the US Virgin Islands) do not have explicit new graduate provisions in the NPA or BON rules or regulations. This does not necessarily mean, however, that new graduates in such states may not practice. At least 2 of the 12 states clearly do not require certification as a prerequisite to practice. In 2 states (Ohio and Utah), however, provisions in law or rule that once authorized new graduate practice have been repealed, and the boards of nursing in these states have indicated that nurse anesthetists may not practice until they are certified. In the 8 remaining states in which certification appears to be required, a state BON may or may not feel that the requirement can be interpreted to permit new graduate practice for a period of time. Questions regarding specifics of new graduate practice in any particular state should be directed to the applicable BON. There appears to be a trend, however, for states to reconsider whether to allow new graduates to practice before certification; this in part appears to be due to the evolution of computerized testing and the reality that new graduates can complete the certification process more rapidly than was the case years ago.

Scope of Practice

Although there is a lack of uniformity concerning how states regulate nurse anesthetist scope of practice, nearly every state does address or define scope of practice in some manner. Most states define it broadly, and others define it via a "laundry list" of permitted activities. Still other states say that nurse anesthetists must practice in accordance with the AANA's guidelines or standards for practice.

Every state, although not always explicitly, permits nurse anesthetists to administer local, regional, and general anesthesia. As a practical matter, nurse anesthetists are not prohibited by state law from engaging in the common anesthesia practices they were educated to perform. State law, of course, can change. Nurse anesthetists must always be alert to the possibility of proposals to change state statutes or regulations to restrict their scope of practice. While state laws and regulations are generally not an impediment to nurse anesthetists providing the full range of anesthesia services for which they are qualified, the same cannot be said for institutional policies. Institutions sometimes do not permit all functions permitted by state

113

law. Even in states with a broadly state-defined scope of practice, CRNAs must still be prepared to address scope of practice issues at the institutional level, because institutions are generally free to define scope of practice more restrictively than does the state.

Nursing Interstate Licensure Compacts

Registered Nurse/Licensed Practical Nurse Compact

The NCSBN, or National Council of State Boards of Nursing, developed the concept of an interstate compact for nursing, adopting a model compact in December 1997. The NCSBN studied a variety of regulatory models to authorize nursing practice in multiple states. Based on the recommendation of a panel of legal experts, the NCSBN Multistate Regulation Task Force decided on an "interstate compact" model for nurse licensure and regulation. The compact is modeled on the driver's license interstate compact, through which drivers are licensed in only 1 state but able to drive in all states that have entered into the compact. An interstate compact is an agreement between 2 or more states to remedy a particular problem of multistate concern. As delineated in Table 5.4, the RN/licensed practical nurse (LPN) interstate compact has been enacted into law or adopted by regulation in 24 states. The RN/LPN compact, and a list of states that have adopted the compact, are posted on the NCSBN website at www.ncsbn.org.[17]

The interstate compact significantly changes the administrative process for nurses who currently hold RN and/or LPN licenses in multiple states. If a nurse works in more than 1 state, and those states participate in the compact, the nurse must hold an RN license only in the state in which the nurse has a primary residence. The current requirements for scope of practice, disciplinary procedures, and advanced practice authorization, however, largely remain unchanged. Nurses who work in several states still have to comply with the scope of practice statutes and regulations in each state in which they practice. Under the compact, the primary state of residence is known as the "home state." "Party states" are any states that adopt the compact. A "remote state" is a party state that is not the home state.

As the NCSBN model interstate compact states, the compact "does not affect additional requirements imposed by states for advanced practice registered nursing. However, a multistate licensure privilege to practice registered nursing granted by a party state shall be recognized by other party states as a license to practice registered nursing if one is required by state law as a precondition for qualifying for advanced practice registered nurse authorization."

What does this mean? What is the effect on APRNs such as CRNAs? Suppose Joe Smith, CRNA, practices in State X and State Y, that both states are parties to the compact, and that State X is Joe's "home state," or state of residence. Joe would have to obtain an RN license only in State X, not in State Y. Assume, though, that both State X and State Y have recognition requirements in addition to an RN license that a CRNA must fulfill to practice as an APRN. Joe would still have to meet those additional application requirements and submit any necessary paperwork in both State X and State Y; the compact would only relieve Joe of the burden of obtaining a second RN license (ie, an RN license in State Y).

Table 5.4. Adoption of RN/LPN Interstate Compact[12]

State	Implementation date	State	Implementation date
Arizona	Jul 1, 2002	New Hampshire	Jan 1, 2006
Arkansas	Jul 1, 2000	New Mexico	Jan 1, 2004
Colorado	Oct 1, 2007	North Carolina	Jul 1, 2000
Delaware	Jul 1, 2000	North Dakota	Jan 1, 2004
Idaho	Jul 1, 2001	Rhode Island	Jul 1, 2008
Iowa	Jul 1, 2000	South Carolina	Feb 1, 2006
Kentucky	Jun 1, 2007	South Dakota	Jan 1, 2001
Maine	Jul 1, 2001	Tennessee	Jul 1, 2003
Maryland	Jan 1, 2000	Texas	Jan 1, 2000
Mississippi	Jul 1, 2001	Utah	Jan 1, 2000
Missouri	Jun 1, 2010	Virginia	Jan 1, 2005
Nebraska	Jan 1, 2001	Wisconsin	Jan 1, 2000

RN indicates registered nurse; LPN, licensed practical nurse.

Uniform Advanced Practice Registered Nurse Requirements

In 2000, the NCSBN developed and adopted a document titled, "Uniform Advanced Practice Registered Nurse Licensure/Authority to Practice Requirements" (hereinafter referred to as the "uniform APRN requirements"). The uniform APRN requirements are posted on the NCSBN website.[18]

The uniform APRN requirements document is not the advanced practice nursing compact. Rather, the NCSBN considers the document a "model" that boards of nursing can use as they see fit. For example, a board in a particular state could compare that state's nursing statute and rules and evaluate whether it would be desirable to revise the statute and/or rules to be consistent with the principles reflected in the uniform APRN requirements. The uniform APRN requirements concern qualifications to practice (such as having to be certified) and do not address scope of practice. The nurse anesthesia profession has already implemented the uniform requirements; none of the requirements, to the author's knowledge, would cause problems for CRNAs if the requirements were adopted by any particular state.

Advanced Practice Registered Nurse Compact

The APRN compact, adopted by the NCSBN in 2002, is similar to the RN/LPN compact. Unlike the RN/LPN compact, however, the APRN compact does not address scope of practice. The RN/LPN compact includes scope of practice elements because of the relative uniformity of RN and LPN scopes of practice across the states. The wide variation in APRN scope of practice in the states, and the controversy sometimes generated by APRN scope of practice changes, makes it difficult to include scope of practice provisions. One of the primary benefits of a licensure compact of this type is the benefit of not having to obtain multiple licenses to practice in compact states. Scope of practice elements could be very controversial and are not necessary for APRNs to achieve this licensure benefit.

115

Under the APRN compact, a state is required to meet the following premises before enacting the APRN compact: (1) adoption of the RN/LPN compact and (2) adoption of the uniform APRN requirements. As indicated above in the discussion of the uniform APRN requirements, the requirements concern qualifications to practice (eg, education and certification) and do not address scope of practice. None of the requirements, to the author's knowledge, would cause problems for CRNAs if adopted by any particular state. A list of states that have adopted the APRN compact are posted on the NCSBN website (http://www.ncsbn.org).[19] As of September 2010, Iowa, Texas, and Utah had enacted the APRN compact into law, although the implementation date for the APRN compact had not yet been determined.

Summary

Formal state regulation of the nursing profession in the United States evolved in the 20th century from the rare occurrence to the commonplace. Whereas state regulation of nursing initially focused on RNs, from the 1970s to the present, most states adopted additional statutory and regulatory provisions specific to APRNs, such as CRNAs. Institutional and employer policies may have a more immediate effect on practice than do state laws or regulations. Nevertheless, because formal state regulation of nurse anesthesia practice is widespread, the possibility always exists for adoption of state laws or regulations that could restrict or undermine nurse anesthesia practice. For this reason, it is imperative that state nurse anesthetist associations, as well as individual CRNAs, closely monitor and be involved with pertinent state statutory and regulatory developments.

References

1. Clayton JE. Licensure of health care professionals. In: Becker S, ed. *Health Care Law: A Practical Guide.* 2nd ed. New York, NY: Matthew Bender; 1999:16.1-16.56.

2. *Dent v West Virginia,* 129 US 114 (1889).

3. Bill of rights. Ratified December 15, 1791. National Archives and Records Administration website. http://www.archives.gov/exhibits/charters/bill_of_rights_transcript.html. Accessed March 9, 2010.

4. Bullough B. The current phase in the development of nurse practice acts. *St Louis University Law J.* 1984;28:365-395.

5. Greenlaw J. Definition and regulation of nursing practice: an historical survey. *Law Med Health Care.* 1985; 13(3):117-121.

6. Hadley EH. Nurses and prescriptive authority: a legal and economic analysis. *Am J Law Med.* 1989;15(2-3):245-299.

7. American Nurses Association. *Nursing Practice Act: Suggested State Legislation.* Kansas City, MO: American Nurses Association; 1990.

8. American Nurses Association. *Model Practice Act.* Washington, DC: American Nurses Association; 1996.

9. Gunn IP. Professional credentialing: tying hands while protecting the public. *CRNA Forum.* 1986;2:11-12.

10. American College of Surgeons. *Resources for Optimal Care of the Injured Patient.* Chicago, IL: American College of Surgeons; 2006:63-64.

116

11. American Association of Nurse Anesthetists. Recertification requirements. State legislative and regulatory requirements (50-state summaries). September 2010. http://www.aana.com. Accessed March 9, 2010.

12. American Association of Nurse Anesthetists. New graduate provisions. State legislative and regulatory requirements (50-state summaries). September 2010. http://www.aana.com. Accessed March 30, 2010.

13. American Association of Nurse Anesthetists. Educational requirements. State legislative and regulatory requirements (50-state summaries). September 2010. http://www.aana.com. Accessed March 9, 2010.

14. American Association of Nurse Anesthetists. Advanced education requirements. State legislative and regulatory requirements (50-state summaries). September 2010. http://www.aana.com. Accessed March 9, 2010.

15. Conover J, Tobin MH. State master's degree requirements for nurse anesthetists. *AANA J.* 1998;66(4):351-357.

16. American Association of Nurse Anesthetists. Certification requirements. State legislative and regulatory requirements (50-state summaries). September 2010. http://www.aana.com. Accessed March 9, 2010.

17. National Council of State Boards of Nursing. About nurse licensure compact (NLC). https://www.ncsbn.org/156.htm. Accessed March 30, 2010.

18. National Council of State Boards of Nursing. Uniform Advanced Practice Registered Nurse Licensure/authority to practice requirements. Aug 16, 2002. https://www.ncsbn.org. Accessed March 30, 2010.

19. National Council of State Boards of Nursing. APRN compact. https://www.ncsbn.org/917.htm. Accessed March 30, 2010.

Acknowledgment

Jana L. Conover, AANA assistant director of state government affairs, compiled the numerical summaries in the section of the chapter regarding state statutory and regulatory requirements concerning nurse anesthetists. Her input and editorial suggestions were invaluable in updating the chapter.

117

Study Questions

1. How does the definition of the practice of medicine in a state potentially affect the scope of practice of a nurse anesthetist?

2. What are common qualifications that states require nurse anesthetists to possess before they may practice?

3. How do institutional (such as hospital) policies and procedures affect nurse anesthetist practice, and are such policies and procedures similar to or different from state statutory and regulatory requirements?

4. What are the types or methods of recognition that states use for nurse anesthetists, and how are those types or methods similar or different?

5. What might be some of the implications for a nurse anesthetist who is unaware of state statutory and regulatory provisions that mention nurse anesthetists?

6. What is a statute or law, and what is a rule or regulation? If a statute and rule deal with the identical subject, which will take precedence if there are inconsistencies between them, and why?

CHAPTER 6

Professional Regulation and Credentialing of Nurse Anesthesia Practice

Karen L. Plaus, CRNA, PhD, FAAN
John C. Preston, CRNA, DNSc
Susan S. Caulk, CRNA, MA

Key Concepts

- Certification and recertification processes are developed and administered by the respective councils of the National Board of Certification and Recertification for Nurse Anesthetists (NBCRNA).

- The NBCRNA credentialing processes for nurse anesthesia practice are in accordance with external and regulatory agency requirements.

- The Councils on Certification and Recertification of Nurse Anesthetists maintain autonomous function relative to their governance, decision-making capability, and finance under the NBCRNA corporate structure.

- The councils are accredited by the National Commission for Certifying Agencies and the American Board of Nursing Specialties for their credentialing functions.

- Continuing education is a common mechanism adopted by many professional organizations through which their members can demonstrate continued competence in their specialty.

Continues on next page.

Key Concepts (continued)

- In addition, continuing education in nursing or a nursing-related specialty area is frequently identified by state boards of nursing or their regulatory equivalents as one acceptable means to maintain continued competence necessary for uninterrupted practice as an advanced practice registered nurse (eg, APRN, APN, ANP) at a state level.

- External entities involved in credentialing of nurse anesthetists include the National Council on State Boards of Nursing, state boards of medicine, and the individual state boards of nursing. These agencies recognize the councils in statute or regulation as the sole authority for regulation issues. This is often the case with regulatory issues involving Certified Registered Nurse Anesthetists by state boards of nursing.

This chapter describes the professional regulation and credentialing for Certified Registered Nurse Anesthetists (CRNAs). For this discussion, professional regulation of clinical practice will pertain to national credentialing procedures for CRNAs, including certification and recertification through mandatory continuing education (CE). The requirements for CRNA practice are congruent with standards and criteria of the National Council on State Boards of Nursing, National Commission for Certifying Agencies (NCCA), and the American Board of Nursing Specialties (ABNS). The evolution of the credentialing procedures, the role of the American Association of Nurse Anesthetists (AANA), and current trends in credentialing for nurse anesthesia also are discussed.

Paramount to continued eligibility for and recognition to practice is the concept of continued competence and the difficulty associated with demonstrating or evidencing this concept. Therefore, another purpose of this chapter will be to review CE for nurse anesthetists and to examine the unique and important symbiosis between CE, continued competency attainment, and professional credentialing for CRNAs.

Historical Perspectives

The AANA has fostered the professional growth and continued competency of CRNAs since its inception. As stated in the organizational philosophy, "The members of this professional association are dedicated to the precept that its members are committed to the advancement of educational standards and practices, which will advance the art and science of anesthesiology and thereby support and enhance quality patient care."[1] The AANA has promulgated advancement of CRNA practice through the certification and recertification processes, implementation of mandatory CE, and the publication of standards and guidelines related to clinical anesthesia.

One of the educational objectives of the AANA is to provide CE opportunities for CRNAs. This objective has been met primarily through the use of CE lectures related to nurse anesthesia practice at state and national nurse anesthesia meetings. The historical precedence for CE was established at the first AANA Annual Meeting held in 1933. Anesthesia practitioners presented clinical lectures, which included such topics as "The Induction of an Anesthetic, Intratracheal Anesthesia, Ethylene Anesthesia and Carbon Dioxide Filtration of Anesthesia."[2] At this meeting, AANA President Agatha Hodgins identified the need for continued growth of the nurse anesthesia profession: "This present meeting is the first fruit of what might be called an adventure. This spirit of adventure is then the dynamic force that keeps us constantly contrasting what we are and what we may be and supplies the necessary courage to change from static to growing conditions."[2]

Nurse anesthesia practice has continued its dynamic growth largely because of the historic leadership of the AANA and the opportunities provided by the constant evolution of technological and scientific advances by both its members and others external to nurse anesthesia. The promotion by the AANA of performance standards relating to both education and practice has subsequently served as a paradigm for other professions to pattern their own development.

In 1967 and early 1968, the AANA Board of Directors realized the increasing importance of documenting continued professional excellence. It was also recognized that CE was essential for practitioners to maintain that measure of competence. Furthermore, the growth of consumer knowledge and the demand for high-quality care required all professional associations, such as the AANA, to be accountable for the competence of their practitioners. As a result, the AANA Board of Directors charged the Education Committee to study how new requirements for CE for nurse anesthetists should evolve. The committee recommended awarding certificates to CRNAs who voluntarily attended CE meetings related to anesthesia practice. Subsequently, at the AANA Annual Meeting in 1969, a bylaw amendment was adopted providing certificates of professional excellence at 5-year intervals to members with documented completion of additional clinical and didactic experience. Participation in this optional program indicated that nurse anesthetists were highly motivated to maintain current knowledge and skills for practice. However, throughout the 1970s, the public began to require more of the health professions and their members in terms of provider competency than what volunteer efforts would be capable of sustaining.

In 1975, the AANA established the Councils on Accreditation, Certification, and Practice. This restructuring occurred partially from awareness of the 1975 proposal by the US Department of Health, Education, and Welfare (now the US Department of Health and Human Services) related to credentialing for healthcare. The final report published in July 1977 contained 2 recommendations relating to competency measurement and continued competence that were pertinent to nurse anesthesia. The recommendation on competency measurement stated:

> Certification organizations, licensure boards, and professional associations should take steps to recognize and

promote the wide spread adoption of effective competency measures to determine the qualifications of health personnel. Special attention should be given to the further development of proficiency and equivalency measures for appropriate categories of health manpower.[3]

The recommendation on continued competence stated:

> Certification organizations, licensure boards, and professional associations should adopt requirements and procedures that will assure the continued competence of health personnel. Additional studies of the best mechanisms to assure continued competence should be supported on a high-priority basis by professional associations, the proposed national certification commission, state agencies and the federal government.[3]

The reorganization of the AANA to include the formation of the councils on certification and recertification was a result of the visionary insights of the Board of Directors and the membership to further advance the profession of nurse anesthesia. The goals of restructuring are listed in Table 6.1.

At the 1976 AANA Annual Meeting, members voted to amend the bylaws to provide for mandatory CE for recertification of active practicing nurse anesthetists. The CE program, developed by the CE Committee, was adopted by the membership at the AANA Annual Meeting on August 22, 1977 and planned for implementation by August 1, 1978. As healthcare professionals, CRNAs were motivated to support and participate in this process aimed at supporting continued competency attainment and maintenance. Their support was echoed in the

> **Table 6.1. Goals of the 1975 Restructuring[4]**
>
> - Overcome questions of conjugation of membership and recertification by external agencies.
> - Allow the AANA to respond more freely to members' requests for increased activities in political and economic arenas.
> - Provide a mechanism that would separate the evaluation of professional competence from Association activities.

introductory statements of the AANA CE program:

> The rapidly changing character and increasing complexity of nurse anesthesia practice demands continuous updating of the practitioner's knowledge, understanding and skills. Any improvement in standards and expectations could not be accomplished without the ongoing involvement of knowledgeable and skillful professionals who were engaged in a lifelong growth process.[5]

Nurse anesthesia practitioners accepted responsibility for their individual actions and for participation in quality CE activities. Nurse anesthetists have always been ethically and legally responsible for the quality of their individual practices. As a profession, nurse anesthetists have accepted collective responsibility for the quality of service they offer to their communities of interest.

To facilitate implementation of the program, the AANA Board of Directors appointed an ad hoc committee on recertification. This committee drafted the initial standards, criteria, and procedures for recertification. At the 1978 AANA Annual Meeting, the members approved the formation of the Council on Recertification of Nurse Anesthetists (COR).

The AANA staff reorganization that began in 2005 resulted in the merger and separate incorporation of the Council on Certification and the Council on Recertification into the National Board of Certification and Recertification for Nurse Anesthetists (NBCRNA). The NBCRNA is a not-for-profit corporation that has the autonomous authority to carry out certification and recertification roles in the discipline of nurse anesthesia. The AANA recognizes it through separate services and recognition agreements. The NBCRNA is composed of members that include CRNAs, physicians, and public members. Table 6.2 identifies the mission, vision, and objectives of the NBCRNA.

Certification

Certification has been a requirement for nurse anesthesia practice since 1945. One of the early leaders of the profession, Gertrude Fife, identified the need to establish a National Board Examination for Nurse Anesthetists. The National Board Examination was chosen "to safeguard the surgeon's interest, the interest of the hospitals and the interest of the public."[2] The AANA Credentials Committee was organized in 1941. This committee drafted the Qualifying Examination and administered it to all eligible nurse anesthesia graduates of approved schools. In 1982, the Qualifying Examination was renamed the National Certification Examination (NCE).

Certification is defined as a process by which a professional agency or association

123

Table 6.2. The National Board of Certification and Recertification for Nurse Anesthetists: Introduction, Vision, and Mission[8]

The National Board of Certification and Recertification for Nurse Anesthetists (NBCRNA) is a not-for-profit corporation organized under the laws of the state of Illinois. The NBCRNA's two councils—the Council on Certification of Nurse Anesthetists (CCNA) and the Council on Recertification of Nurse Anesthetists (COR)—carry out the credentialing activities of the NBCRNA.

NBCRNA credentialing provides assurances to the public that certified individuals have met objective, predetermined qualifications for providing nurse anesthesia services. While state licensure provides the legal credential for the practice of professional nursing, private voluntary certification indicates compliance with the professional standards for practice in this clinical nursing specialty. The certification credential for nurse anesthetists has been institutionalized in many position descriptions as a practice requirement or as the standard for demonstrating equivalency. It has been recognized through malpractice litigation, state nurse practice acts, and state rules and regulations.

Vision
The NBCRNA is the recognized leader in nurse anesthesia credentialing.

Mission
The NBCRNA offers certification and recertification programs that are tailored to specific professional standards of nurse anesthesia practice and promote patient safety.

certifies that an individual licensed to practice a profession has met certain standards specified by that profession for specialty practice.[6] The purpose of certification is to assure the public that an individual has mastered a body of knowledge and acquired skills in a particular specialty. Licensure refers to a process by which a state government grants permission to individuals to practice their occupation as a way of ensuring that the public health, safety, and welfare will be reasonably protected. Licensure and certification are both mandated mechanisms of regulating nurse anesthesia practice; however, certification goes beyond licensure by recognizing the acquisition of additional specialized knowledge and by establishing certain professional standards.[7]

Council on Certification

The responsibilities for the development and administration of the NCE were transferred to the Council on Certification of Nurse Anesthetists (CCNA) in 1975. The council is an autonomous certifying agency under the corporate structure of the NBCRNA. The certification program has been accredited by the NCCA since 1980. The NCCA approval provides the public and other communities of interest recognition that the NBCRNA's certification program has met or exceeded the highest national voluntary standards for private certification. It indicates that the program has been reviewed by an impartial commission and deemed to have met the nationally accepted criteria and guidelines of the NCCA.

Table 6.3. Purposes of the Council on Certification of Nurse Anesthetists[8]

- Formulate and adopt requirements for eligibility for admission to the Certification Examination and for the certification of registered nurse anesthetists.
- Formulate, adopt, and administer the Certification Examination to those registered nurse anesthetists who have met all requirements for examination and have been found eligible by the council.
- Evaluate candidates' performance on the Certification Examination.
- Grant initial certification to those candidates who pass the Certification Examination and fulfill all other requirements for certification.

(Reprinted with permission from the National Board of Certification and Recertification for Nurse Anesthetists.)

The ABNS, established in 1991, is a national peer review program for specialty nursing certification bodies. The ABNS serves as the national umbrella organization for nursing specialty boards authorized and recognized to certify nurse specialists in the United States. It promotes the highest quality of specialty nursing practice through the establishment of standards of professional specialty nursing certification. The CCNA was one of the first national certification bodies to be recognized by the ABNS.

The principal purpose of the Council on Certification is related to its charge, which is to protect and serve the public by ensuring that individuals who are credentialed as CRNAs have met predetermined qualifications or standards for providing nurse anesthesia services. The additional purposes of the council are listed in Table 6.3.

The eligibility criteria for admission to write the NCE are listed in Table 6.4. In order to be eligible for certification by the council, the applicant must meet all of the eligibility requirements and successfully pass the NCE. In 2007 the CCNA implemented time-limited eligibility for certification. If applicants do not pass the NCE on their first attempt, they may retake the examination up to 4 times in a calendar

year and have up to 2 calendar years to pass the NCE following their date of nurse anesthesia program graduation. Individuals who do not pass the NCE within 2 years postgraduation, or who don't pass the examination in 8 or fewer attempts, will not be eligible to take the NCE again unless they return to and successfully complete an unabridged accredited nurse anesthesia educational program.

Content Validation Procedures for the National Certification Examination

The Council on Certification has collaborated with national testing agencies to aid in the administration of the NCE. Previous testing agencies used by the council included the Psychological Corporation (1975-1984), San Antonio, Texas; Assessment Systems, Inc (1984-1991), Bala Cynwyd, Pennsylvania; and American College Testing (1991-1996), Iowa City, Iowa. In 1995, Computer Adaptive Technologies, Inc (CAT), Evanston, Illinois, was selected to serve as the testing agency to facilitate the transition of the NCE from paper and pencil to computerized adaptive testing. Although CAT was contracted to manage item bank maintenance and test development and assembly, Prometric in

125

Table 6.4. Eligibility Requirements for Admission to the National Certification Examination (NCE)[8]

In order to be eligible to apply to take the NCE for registered nurse anesthetists and to receive a certification eligibility notification, a candidate must:

1. Comply with all state requirements for current and unrestricted licensure as a registered professional nurse;
2. Complete a nurse anesthesia educational program accredited by the Council on Accreditation of Nurse Anesthesia Educational Programs ("accredited program") within the previous two (2) calendar years;
3. Submit:
   a. A complete and accurate examination application form signed by the candidate which includes the NBCRNA *Waiver of Liability and Agreement of Authorization, Confidentiality, and Nondisclosure Statement.*
   b. An official non-handwritten notarized transcript of the candidate's record of performance in an accredited program, on a transcript form prescribed by the NBCRNA Council on Certification of Nurse Anesthetists, signed by the program director and by the candidate, which accurately documents the candidate's academic and clinical experiences, and his or her completion of the accredited program. If transcripts are submitted prior to completion of the program, a *Program Completion Verification Form* verifying that the candidate has in fact completed the program must be signed and submitted by the candidate's program director after the program has been completed;
   c. A copy of the candidate's valid license to practice as a registered professional nurse that is current on the candidate's requested examination date in at least one state. If the *state board of nursing issues a paper license* or wallet card, then a copy of that RN license must be submitted. If state law prohibits the copying of a nursing license, the candidate must submit a written statement from the state nursing board verifying current licensure and providing the license number and date of expiration. **If the state board of nursing no longer issues a paper license or wallet card, a web verification will be accepted;**
   d. Payment of the current application fee and any other applicable fees;
   e. A signed, notarized *Authentication of Applicant Identity Form* with a passport photo or digitalized photo taken within the previous six (6) months attached;
4. Make the following eligibility certifications:
   a. that his or her license has never been revoked, restricted, suspended or limited by any state, has never been surrendered, and is not the subject of a pending action or investigation;
   b. that he or she does not currently suffer from a mental or physical condition which might interfere with the practice of nurse anesthesia;
   c. that he or she does not currently suffer from drug or alcohol addiction or abuse;
   d. that he or she has not been convicted of and is not currently under indictment for any felony;
   e. that, except for incidents occurring during the nurse anesthesia educational program which were thereafter satisfactorily resolved, he or she has not been the subject of any documented allegations of misconduct, incompetent practice, or unethical behavior;

Continues on page 127.

Table 6.4. Eligibility Requirements for Admission to the National Certification Examination (NCE)[8] (continued)

    f. that he or she has never been the subject of disciplinary action, been placed on probation, suspended, or dismissed from a nurse anesthesia educational program for unethical behavior, questions of academic integrity or documented evidence of cheating. If the candidate does not so certify, he or she must provide full documentation of the reasons therefore with sufficient specificity to allow the NBCRNA to evaluate the possible impact of the problem on the candidate's current ability to take the NCE or practice nurse anesthesia and to resolve the issue to the NBCRNA's satisfaction; and

5. Sign the *Waiver of Liability and Agreement of Authorization, Confidentiality, and Nondisclosure Statement* clarifying that the individual has read, understands, and intends to be legally bound by the following statements:

    a. that he or she understands that the content of the NCE, and each of its items, is proprietary, is copyrighted and strictly confidential, and that the unauthorized retention, possession, copying, distribution, disclosure, discussion, or receipt of any NCE question, in whole or in part, by written, electronic, oral or other form of communication, including but not limited to e-mailing, copying or printing of electronic files, and reconstruction through memorization and/or dictation, before, during, or after the NCE, is strictly prohibited, and that, in addition to constituting irregular behavior subject to disciplinary action such as denial of eligibility to take the NCE now or in the future or revocation of certification, such activities violate the NBCRNA's proprietary rights, including copyrights, and may subject him or her to legal action resulting in monetary damages;

    b. that he or she understands that he or she can be disqualified from taking or continuing to sit for the NCE, or from receiving NCE scores, and may be required to retake the NCE, if the NBCRNA determines, at its discretion, through proctor observation, statistical analysis or any other means, that he or she was engaged in collaborative, disruptive, or other irregular behavior before, during the administration of, or following the NCE, or that the integrity or validity of the NCE is in question;

    c. that he or she has not been the recipient of any NCE questions, that he or she has not been involved in any disclosure, distribution or discussion of any NCE questions, and that, following this examination, he or she will not disclose, distribute, or discuss any NCE questions;

    d. that he or she will inform the NBCRNA if he or she is aware of anyone who discloses any NCE question(s) or asks them to disclose any NCE question(s); and

    e. that he or she understands that evidence of unethical or inappropriate behavior may result in revocation or permanent denial of certification.

(Reprinted with permission from the National Board of Certification and Recertification for Nurse Anesthetists.)

Baltimore, Maryland, was initially contracted for test delivery. In 2002, CAT was contracted as a single source provider for all of these services. The company has undergone a series of transitions, merging in 2002 with Assessment Systems, Inc, to create Pennsylvania-based Promissor, which was purchased in 2006 by Pearson VUE of Bloomington, Minnesota.

Representatives from the testing agencies and the council have collaborated on the procedures to build a valid, job-related examination to comply with the Uniform Guidelines on Employee Selection Procedures. These guidelines established a uniform federal position prohibiting discrimination in employment practices, particularly in the use of tests.[9] The guidelines address the importance of test validation procedures and documentation of a job analysis. Although the guidelines do not directly speak to test validation procedures for voluntary certifying organizations, there is well-established precedent in the courts that a validated test is a solid defense against allegations of discrimination.[10] The council recognized that the guidelines could apply to employers who use the certification credential for employment purposes.

In the Standards for Educational and Psychological Testing, validity is described as the appropriateness, meaningfulness, and usefulness of specific inferences made from test scores. Test validation is the process of accumulating evidence to support such inferences.[11] Credentialing examinations are validated through content, criteria, or construct validation strategies. Content validation is the most frequently used strategy for professional certification examinations. Since certification reflects the acquisition of the knowledge, skills, and abilities required for specialty practice, the content validation procedure can link the knowledge, skills, and abilities to the Certification Examination.

The content validation procedures for the NCE were documented through a job analysis in 1987 and a professional practice analysis (PPA) in 1992, 1996, 2000, and 2006. The goal of a PPA is to define performances critical to the definition of credentialed behavior and to delineate the knowledge, skills, and abilities underlying these performances.[12] Content validity refers to the degree to which the content of

the examination is representative of the area of work about which the inference is to be made.[13] In other words, a high degree of validity means that the questions on an examination accurately reflect requirements and expectations of the actual job (ie, a performance domain), and scores on the examination can be relied upon as an accurate indicator of the examinee's mastery of those requirements. Content validation studies are used to assess whether the questions on the examination adequately represent a performance domain.[13] According to national testing standards, credentialing agencies should repeat their validation studies every 3 to 5 years.

The PPA survey instruments used in 1992, 1996, 2000, and 2006 included items related to demographics, practice setting, education, and most importantly, elements of fundamental knowledge of nurse anesthesia practitioners (T. Muckle, MEd, written communication, 2007).[14-16] The knowledge areas of the survey were organized to identify the frequency and level of expertise related to patient conditions, procedures, anesthesia agents, techniques, equipment, and instrumentation and technology encountered in practice. All of the survey items were considered to have a requisite level of importance to practice. For each of the survey items, respondents were asked to indicate on a rating scale the relative importance of each of the knowledge areas, as well as the relative frequency (monthly, weekly, daily) that recall of such knowledge was necessary in the profession. Assessment of the relative importance of the responses was then used in determining appropriate emphasis weighting of the knowledge areas in the test specifications. The surveys were mailed to practitioners with a minimum of 1 year of anesthesia experience, the AANA Board of

Directors, council representatives, and committee members.

Data obtained from the PPA surveys were tabulated and analyzed by representatives from the testing agency using the Rasch rating scale model calibrations. Such an analysis generates calibrations for each survey item on a scale of relative importance. The Rasch rating scale calibrations are a log-linear transformation of the ordinal data onto a linear, equal-interval scale. The Rasch rating scale model places all of the observations on a common linear scale so that a comparison between items can be obtained (T. Muckle, PhD, written communication, 2007).[16] This measurement model facilitates the understanding, interpretation, and meaningful inferences that can be made from the PPA. The Rasch calibrations also provide the basis for making a meaningful transformation of all the responses to the items on the NCE. A positive Rasch calibration indicates a survey item of relatively high importance, whereas a negative calibration indicates an item of relatively low importance (T. Muckle, PhD, written communication, 2007).[16] The Rasch importance calibrations can be easily converted to percentage weights, which are used for content balancing of the examination.

The results using the Rasch rating scale revealed that there was agreement between respondents in most areas surveyed as indicated by high correlations obtained in each section. The results of the 1996 and 2002 survey were consistent with the frequency and level of expertise rating results from the 1992 PPA and supported the existing blueprint of the NCE. Therefore, no changes to the NCE blueprint were made through 2006. The PPA survey in 2006 marked the first electronic administration over the Internet, rather than a paper survey administered by mail. The results of the 2006 survey indicated a higher weighting on instrumentation and technology, and the test specifications were adjusted in 2007 to account for this shift in emphasis (T. Muckle, PhD, written communication, 2007).

After PPA is conducted, content validation proceeds by making explicit links between the PPA knowledge and skill statements and the test items. Using a classification scheme, every question in the item bank is tied to a specific corresponding knowledge area in the content outline. The current content outline and the percentage of the examination tested in each area are listed in Table 6.5. A conceptual overview of the relationship of each candidate's

129

Table 6.5. Content Outline of National Certification Examination[8]

Content	Percentage
1. Basic sciences	25
2. Equipment, instrumentation, technology	10
3. Basic principles of anesthesia	30
4. Advanced principles of anesthesia	30
5. Professional issues	5

For more detailed information regarding the content outline of the National Certification Examination, please consult the NBCRNA Candidate Handbook.
(Adapted with permission from the National Board of Certification and Recertification for Nurse Anesthetists.)

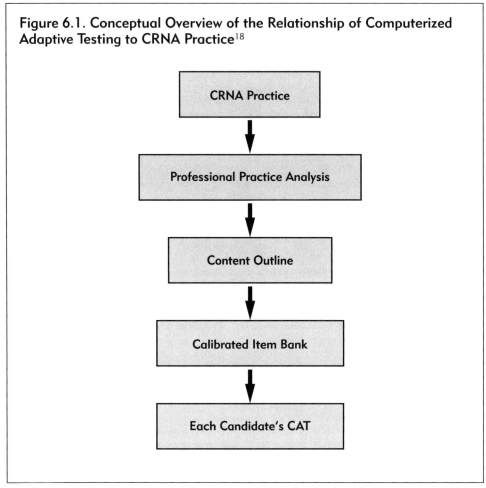

Figure 6.1. Conceptual Overview of the Relationship of Computerized Adaptive Testing to CRNA Practice[18]

CAT indicates computerized adaptive test.
(Reprinted with permission from Bergstrom.)

computerized adaptive test to CRNA practice is presented in Figure 6.1.

Questions comprising the NCE are developed by members of the NBCRNA Examination Committee, which consists of CRNA and physician representatives. This committee meets annually to write and review test questions for the approved item bank and update the item bank each year. Questions are reviewed frequently to verify the content classification. Performance statistics for questions are continuously monitored by the NBCRNA and testing agency.

Development of the Certification Examination

The NCE for nurse anesthetists was administered in paper and pencil format from 1945 to 1996 based on the standard criterion-referenced testing process. In April 1996, the CCNA implemented computerized adaptive testing procedures for their examinations.[17] This computer adaptive method of administering tests is based on the psychometric framework of item response theory. This theory uses a mathematical model to determine the difficulty of test questions and to estimate the ability of candidates.[18] With computerized adaptive testing, each candidate's test is individualized; it is assembled interactively as the candidate is tested based on his or her dynamic performance on the examination.[18] Test questions are stored in a large item bank and classified by content category and level of difficulty. After the candidate answers a question, the computer algorithm calculates an estimate of competence and selects a next question of appropriate content and difficulty. This process is repeated for each question, thus creating an examination that is tailored to each individual's knowledge and skills and also fulfills the council's test plan requirements.

The NBCRNA administers 2 computer adaptive tests: the NCE and the Self-Evaluation Examination. The purpose of the NCE is to assess the entry-level knowledge and skills required for nurse anesthesia practice. The purposes of the self-evaluation examination are to allow students to assess their knowledge of the fundamental aspects of nurse anesthesia and provide them with the opportunity to prepare for the computer adaptive Certification Examination.

The NCE is a variable-length, computerized, adaptive test of entry-level competence in the practice of nurse anesthesia. Each candidate receives a minimum of 100 questions: 70 questions representing the certification content outline and 30 unscored questions that are being assessed for validity for potential future examination use.[8] The maximum number of questions is 170 (140 scored questions, 30 unscored). Prior to 2009, the NCE consisted solely of standard, 4-option multiple choice questions. In order to enhance the ability of the NCE to assess entry-level competency in the field of nurse anesthesia, the Council on Certification of Nurse Anesthetists (CCNA) has added *alternative question formats* to the NCE. These question formats are multiple correct response, calculation, drag and drop, and hotspot questions. The purpose of introducing new question types is to assess subject matter that is important to entry-level knowledge but difficult to pose in a traditional multiple choice question format.

Examinees who perform close to the passing score are administered more questions in order to collect the most information possible regarding their performance level. Examinees who are well above (clearly passing) or well below (clearly failing) the passing score are administered fewer questions because there is little doubt of their performance with regard to the entry-level passing standard. A maximum of 3 hours is allowed for the test period.[8] Currently, the NCE is administered year-round at national testing centers.

Each test conforms to the NCE content outline, which ensures inclusion of test questions in the content areas of basic sciences, basic and advanced principles of anesthesia, equipment, instrumentation and technology, and professional aspects. The test is also administered in a way that satisfies the relative emphasis of each of these primary content areas, as determined by the PPA. All of the questions are chosen from the same item bank. The item bank contains all of the questions necessary to meet the test specifications. The same passing score is implemented for all candidates, which ensures that no candidate is at a disadvantage with regard to passing the test. All candidates have the opportunity to demonstrate their ability or competence level, because the Certification Examination will not end until a pass or fail decision is determined.[8]

131

Scoring the Certification Examination

Examinations using computerized adaptive testing are scored based on the candidate's performance relative to the difficulty of items administered. A candidate must obtain a scaled score of 450 to pass the examination. A pass/fail decision is made when one of the conditions listed in Table 6.6 has been met.

The passing score is determined using standard scoring methods of educational and psychological testing.[19] The passing standard is continually reviewed by the Board and is published on the NBCRNA website (www.nbcrna.com).

New Trends for the Certification Examination

Although the variable-length, multiple-choice, computerized adaptive testing format of the NCE has remained consistent since 1996, recent advancements in psychometric procedures and educational trends will influence the future of the NCE test development. The NCE has consisted solely of multiple-choice questions because they are relatively easy to construct and are objectively scored. The CCNA introduced innovative item formats, such as multiple correct response, supplied answer, matching, ordering formats, and video simulations for the NCE. These alternative item types are intended to assess higher-level critical thinking skills that are difficult to evaluate with traditional multiple-choice questions. The educational transition to the practice doctorate by 2025 for entry-level practitioners will play a role in the future assessment of core competencies.

Future Directions in Certification

The NBCRNA is committed to continually investigating trends related to entry-level competencies and testing procedures. These include updating the content validation process, incorporating alternative item types, and promoting research activities related to testing. Representatives from the NBCRNA participate in meetings with other agencies associated with professional certification issues. These agencies include the Institute for Credentialing Excellence (formerly the National Organization of Competency Assurance), the National Council of State Boards of Nursing, the National Specialty Nursing Certifying Organizations, the NCCA, and the ABNS.

Table 6.6. Pass/Fail Conditions for Certification Examination Scores[8]

1. The candidate has clearly demonstrated competence. This decision may be reached at any point between 100 and 170 items.
2. The candidate has clearly demonstrated incompetence. This decision may be reached at any point between 100 and 170 items.
3. The maximum number of questions (170) has been administered, and the pass/fail decision is based on whether the candidate's level of competence is above or below the pass/fail point.
4. The maximum amount of time (3 hours) is reached. A fail decision is made if the candidate has not completed more than 100 questions. If the candidate has completed more than 100 questions, the pass/fail decision is based on whether the candidate's level of competence is above or below the pass/fail point.

(Reprinted with permission from the National Board of Certification and Recertification for Nurse Anesthetists.)

Table 6.7. The Purposes of the Council on Recertification of Nurse Anesthetists[20]

- Recertify qualified CRNAs on a biennial basis.
- Formulate and adopt criteria for eligibility for recertification of CRNAs based on the current licensure, maintenance of practice skills, participation in approved CE activities, and other recognized activities conducive to professional proficiency and freedom from known mental or physical impairments that may interfere with or prevent the professional practice of nurse anesthesia. The practice of nurse anesthesia may include clinical practice and anesthesia-related administrative, educational, and research activities.
- Formulate and adopt criteria for approval of CE programs and offerings used in the recertification process.
- Develop and maintain mechanisms to provide for a hearing and appellate review for individuals seeking recertification.
- Develop and maintain a mechanism for the investigation and final resolution of charges or other allegations against individuals currently holding recertification by the council.
- Make recommendations to the Board of Directors, councils, and committees in conformity with stated purposes.

(Reprinted with permission from the National Board of Certification and Recertification for Nurse Anesthetists.)

Recertification

Following initial certification, a CRNA is eligible to apply for recertification every 2 years. Recertification is a requirement for advanced practice nursing credentialing and reimbursement. Through the recertification process, the COR seeks to advance the quality of anesthesia care provided to the public. Specifically, it endeavors to make certain that nurse anesthetists maintain their skills and keep current with scientific and technological developments. It also strives to ensure that appropriate limitations are placed on those who are known to have developed conditions that might adversely affect their ability to practice anesthesia.[20]

Recertification, of course, is not and cannot be a guarantee of competence to perform all anesthesia procedures. Full recertification is, however, an indication that the CRNA has maintained a current license to practice, has been substantially engaged in nurse anesthesia practice, has participated in approved CE activities, and is not known to have developed any impairment that could interfere with the administration of anesthesia.[20] The NBCRNA has set forth established guidelines and criteria for recertification with input from the AANA membership. The purposes of the Council on Recertification of Nurse Anesthetists are listed in Table 6.7.

Categories of Recertification

Two categories of recertification have been established by the council: full recertification and interim recertification. The criteria for full recertification are listed in Table 6.8. The process of recertification includes meeting all of the criteria and completing the application procedures.

A CRNA applying for recertification needs to submit the following information to the NBCRNA by the July 31 deadline: the completed application and fee, documentation of current nursing and advanced practice nursing licensure, proof of completion of 40 hours of approved CE, and documentation of substantial engagement in

133

Table 6.8. Criteria for Full Recertification[20]

In order to receive Full Recertification, an applicant must comply with all of the following requirements:

1. Initial Certification
   Receipt of initial certification by the Council on Certification of Nurse Anesthetists or its predecessor.
2. Licensure
   a. Documentation of compliance with all state requirements for licensure as a registered nurse performing nurse anesthesia, including a current unrestricted license to practice as a registered nurse, with authority to practice nurse anesthesia if such authority is granted, in at least one state and in all states in which the applicant currently practices. For those individuals employed by the United States government, "state requirements" refer to the requirements of any state or territory of the United States; and
   b. Certification by the applicant that his or her license has never been revoked, restricted, suspended or limited by any state, has never been surrendered, and is not the subject of a pending action or investigation, except for those actions or pending actions that previously were reported to the Council in writing. If the applicant does not so certify, he or she must provide full documentation of the reasons therefore so that the Council may evaluate whether any revocation, restriction, suspension, limitation, surrender, or any pending action impacts on the applicant's current ability to practice nurse anesthesia.
3. Continuing Education
   Documentation of completion of 40 hours of approved continuing education, as set forth in the Continuing Education Program of the AANA, within the two-year period prior to the applicant's upcoming August 1 recertification date or, if the applicant's recertification period is shorter than two years, within such shortened period prior to the applicant's upcoming August 1 recertification date.
4. Practice
   Certification by the applicant that he or she has been or will have been substantially engaged in the practice of nurse anesthesia during the two-year period prior to the applicant's upcoming August 1 recertification date. It is recommended that substantial engagement in the practice of nurse anesthesia generally should consist of a minimum of 850 hours of practice over the two-year recertification period. Because individual practice experiences vary, it is the responsibility of the applicant to assess whether his or her practice experience constitutes substantial engagement and to so certify.

   The practice of nurse anesthesia may include clinical practice, nurse anesthesia-related administrative, educational or research activities, or a combination of two or more of such areas of practice. To be nurse anesthesia-related, activities must have as their primary objective and be directly related to the delivery of anesthesia care to patients or the improvement of delivery of anesthesia care to patients.

   Where there is an inconsistency between the applicant's practice certification and his or her record of practice, or other information received by the Council, the decision as to whether an applicant has satisfied the practice requirement is at the discretion of the Council.

Continues on page 135.

Table 6.8. Criteria for Full Recertification[20] (continued)

5. Certifications by Applicant that he or she:
   a. does not currently suffer from a mental or physical condition which might interfere with the practice of nurse anesthesia;
   b. does not currently suffer from drug or alcohol addiction or abuse;
   c. has not been convicted of, and is not currently under indictment for, any felony; and
   d. has not been the subject of any documented allegations of misconduct, incompetent practice or unethical behavior.

   If the applicant does not so certify, he or she must state the reasons therefore with sufficient specificity to allow the Council to evaluate the possible impact of the problem on the applicant's current ability to practice nurse anesthesia and to resolve the issue to the Council's satisfaction.

(Reprinted with permission from the National Board of Certification and Recertification for Nurse Anesthetists.)

practice. The recertification period is effective for a 2-year period from August 1 through July 31. Individuals who do not meet the July 31 deadline suffer a lapse in their recertification and loss of all privileges that accompany recertification. Individuals suffering a lapse in status are recertified on the date all materials are received and processed. The recertification status is renewed every 2 years and expires automatically at the end of the recertification period unless renewed.

The category of interim recertification includes provisional recertification and conditional recertification. Provisional recertification may be granted for any of 5 reasons: pending review of an application, pending fulfillment of the practice requirements, pending completion of a treatment or rehabilitation program, pending completion of probation, and pending the outcome of an investigation or disciplinary or legal action. The council will grant a CRNA provisional status while reviewing an application if questions arise as to the fulfillment of the established criteria. After completion of the investigation, the council may grant or deny recertification.[21]

For a CRNA who is currently able to practice nurse anesthesia but who has not been substantially engaged in practice during the 2-year period before recertification, provisional recertification may be granted. A CRNA who is participating in a drug, alcohol, or other type of substance abuse treatment or rehabilitation program may be assigned provisional recertification if all of the other recertification criteria are met. After completion of the rehabilitation or treatment program, the CRNA may receive full recertification.[20]

Conditional recertification is granted to those CRNAs who meet the recertification criteria but have restrictions placed on their professional nursing license. The conditional recertification will reflect any conditions imposed by the appropriate state licensure authority. Examples of a restricted license include a license to practice only under supervision and a license to practice provided the individual remains in a drug, alcohol, or other type of treatment program for a stated period. The status may be changed to full recertification when the restrictions are removed from the license.[20]

135

The NBCRNA has the authority and the ability to revoke or modify the recertification status of an anesthesia practitioner with cause. Reasons for automatic revocation of recertification include the failure to maintain licensure as a registered nurse, adjudication by a court that the individual is mentally incompetent, and conviction of or pleading no contest to a felony that is, in the view of the council, related to the practice of nursing or nurse anesthesia.

Discretionary revocation of recertification is used for the following reasons:

- Failure of the individual to maintain licensure as a registered nurse, with authority to practice nurse anesthesia if such authority is granted in all states in which the individual practices.
- Conviction of or pleading no contest to a felony.[20]

The recertification status of a CRNA may be modified at any time to reflect applicable information that comes to the attention of the NBCRNA. The NBCRNA has established procedures for reconsideration of any modification in the recertification status of a CRNA. The NBCRNA strives to maintain the integrity of the nurse anesthesia profession and to protect the welfare of the public in its decisions about the recertification status of CRNAs.[20]

Refresher Program

The NBCRNA, in concert with AANA CE, set forth and agree on the requirements and guidelines for the Refresher Program. The Refresher Program is designed for CRNAs who have not been substantially engaged in the practice of nurse anesthesia for more than 3 years and must update their skills and knowledge of current clinical practice and theoretical practice in anesthesia in order to meet the prevailing standards of practice and to apply for recertification.

The objectives of the Refresher Program are twofold: (1) to foster acquisition of the current knowledge, attitudes, and skills necessary for safe nurse anesthesia practice and (2) to establish minimum requirements for CE and clinical anesthesia experience needed to enable the nurse anesthetist who is not currently engaged in the practice of nurse anesthesia to become recertified.[21]

The Refresher Program consists of a CE component and a clinical component, both of which must be completed within a 24-month period. There are specific requirements for the CE and clinical components depending on the number of years a nurse anesthetist has not been substantially engaged in the practice of anesthesia (Table 6.9). In addition, if the nurse anesthetist has not been substantially engaged in the practice of anesthesia for 5 or more years, he or she must retake and pass the NCE.[21]

The NBCRNA continuously evaluates the recertification requirements based on education trends, scope of and authority for practice, and regulatory oversight. In response to these areas, the NBCRNA has conducted a recertification practice analysis (RPA) and a national benchmarking study. The RPA was developed and conducted in 2008 in collaboration with Castle Worldwide Inc, Research Triangle Park, North Carolina. The purpose of the RPA was to determine the knowledge and skill that reasonably experienced nurse anesthetists must have to provide competent service, especially in contrast with entry-level expectations as defined for initial certification. As part of this work, the 3 domains identified that are essential for nurse anesthesia include: (1) clinical practice, (2) practice evaluation and improvement, and (3) professional responsibility.

Table 6.9. Refresher Program Requirements

A certified registered nurse anesthetist must fulfill the following Refresher Program requirements to become eligible for full recertification.

A. **Not substantially engaged in clinical anesthesia practice for more than 3 years but less than 5 years.** Certified registered nurse anesthetists who have not been engaged in nurse anesthesia practice for *3 years but have practiced substantially within the last 5 years* must meet the following criteria:

1. Documentation of **100 CE credits** which have been prior approved by a recognized approval organization:

   40 CE credits: Scientific foundations to include Patho-physiology and Pharmacology.

   40 CE credits: Advanced Principles of Anesthesia Practice to include Specialty Case Management, Pediatrics, Obstetrics, Geriatrics, and Regional anesthesia.

   10 CE credits: Professional Standards and Safety.

   10 CE credits: Anesthesia Equipment, Instrumentation and Technology.

2. Documentation of **250 hours** of clinical anesthesia time on the *Transcript for Completion of the Clinical Anesthesia Refresher Component.*

3. Documentation of completion of the number of required clinical anesthesia experiences which include a broad range of general anesthesia, monitored anesthesia care, and the management or administration of regional anesthesia. The required cases are listed on the *Transcript for Completion of the Clinical Anesthesia Refresher Component.*

4. Documentation of current ACLS, PALS, and NRP provider certification.

B. **Not substantially engaged in clinical anesthesia practice for more than 5 years but less than 7 years.** Certified registered nurse anesthetists who have not been engaged in nurse anesthesia practice for *5 years but who have practiced substantially within the last 7 years* must meet the following criteria.

1. Documentation of **200 CE credits** which have been prior approved by a recognized approval organization:

   80 CE credits: Scientific foundations to include Patho-physiology and Pharmacology.

   80 CE credits: Advanced Principles of Anesthesia Practice to include Specialty Case Management, Pediatrics, Obstetrics, Geriatrics, and Regional anesthesia.

   20 CE credits: Professional Standards and Safety.

   20 CE credits: Anesthesia Equipment, Instrumentation and Technology.

2. Documentation of **300 hours** of clinical experience on the *Transcript for Completion of the Clinical Anesthesia Refresher Component.*

3. Documentation of completion of the number of the required clinical anesthesia experiences which include a broad range of general anesthesia, monitored anesthesia care, and the management or administration of regional anesthesia. The required cases are listed on the *Transcript for Completion of the Clinical Anesthesia Refresher Component.*

4. Documentation of current ACLS, PALS, and NRP provider certification.

5. Documentation of successful completion of the NCE. The examination may be attempted up to four (4) times within one year from the date of official notification that the didactic and clinical requirements of the Refresher Program have been completed. The nurse anesthetist must successfully pass the exam within that time frame.

Continues on page 138.

Table 6.9. Refresher Program Requirements (continued)

C. **Not substantially engaged in clinical anesthesia practice for more than 7 years.** Certified registered nurse anesthetists who have not been substantially engaged in nurse anesthesia practice for *more than 7 years* must meet the following criteria.

1. Documentation of **300 CE credits** or class hours which have been prior approved by a recognized approval organization:

   120 CE credits: Scientific foundations to include Patho-physiology and Pharmacology.

   120 CE credits: Advanced Principles of Anesthesia Practice to include Specialty Case Management, Pediatrics, Obstetrics, Geriatrics, and Regional anesthesia.

   30 CE credits: Professional Standards and Safety.

   30 CE credits: Anesthesia Equipment, Instrumentation and Technology.

2. Documentation of **400 hours** of clinical anesthesia time on the *Transcript for Completion of the Clinical Refresher Component.*

3. Documentation of completion of the number of required clinical anesthesia experiences which include a broad range of general anesthesia, monitored anesthesia care, and the management or administration of regional anesthesia. The required cases are listed on the *Transcript for Completion of the Clinical Anesthesia Refresher Component.*

4. Documentation of current ACLS, PALS, and NRP provider certification.

5. Documentation of successful completion of the NCE. The examination may be attempted up to four (4) times within one year from the date of official notification that the didactic and clinical requirements of the Refresher Program have been completed. The nurse anesthetist must successfully pass the exam within that time frame.

138

(Reprinted with permission from the National Board of Certification and Recertification for Nurse Anesthetists.)
ACLS indicates Advanced Cardiac Life Support; PALS, Pediatric Advanced Life Support; NRP, Neonatal Resuscitation Program; and NCE, National Certification Examination.

The National Recertification Benchmarking Study was conducted in collaboration with Castle Worldwide and the Institute for Credentialing Excellence. The goal of this study was to identify current practices in recertification throughout the certification community, specifically to investigate views on CE requirements and the assessment of competence. These documents will assist the NBCRNA in determination of any future changes in recertification.

Future Directions in Recertification

The NBCRNA is dedicated to consistently evaluating and updating the criteria and procedures related to recertification. Through the established recertification process, the NBCRNA seeks to ensure that nurse anesthesia practitioners maintain the high level of knowledge and skill required for practice. It also aims to ensure that appropriate limitations are placed on CRNAs who are known to have developed conditions that might adversely affect their ability to practice. The NBCRNA will continue to explore strategies to meet its goals and the needs of the profession. The future requirements for recertification and the possibility of specialty credentialing for subspecialty areas (pain management, pediatric, cardiac, and other clinical specialties) are under consideration.

Continuing Education

Continuing education for CRNAs has been a requirement for recertification since 1978. The AANA believes that nursing, and therefore, nurse anesthesia, is accountable to the public for promulgating standards of nursing practice that improve the delivery of services and promote high-quality patient care. As the national professional association for nurses specializing in anesthesia, the AANA holds itself responsible for providing CE activities that help CRNAs excel in practice. It further meets this commitment to society and the profession by establishing and maintaining standards that foster high-quality CE activities offered by other providers, but approved by the AANA.

Nurse anesthesia professional development is the lifelong process of active participation in learning activities that assist in developing and maintaining continuing competence, enhancing professional practice, and supporting achievement of anesthesia career goals. Nurse anesthesia professional development begins within the basic nurse anesthesia educational program, continues throughout the career of the nurse anesthetist, and encompasses the educational concepts of CE staff development (SD) and academic education. Staff development consists of employer-provider orientation, in-services, and continuing education. Continuing education is an organized and evaluative process that promotes the enrichment of knowledge toward the goal of maintaining anesthesia expertise.

The CE program for nurse anesthesia seeks to enhance the professional competence of healthcare providers in the specialty of nurse anesthesia and thereby ensure a higher quality of anesthesia healthcare service. The AANA's CE program includes standards and criteria for the review, approval, and recognition of CE activities for nurse anesthetists for purposes of recertification. The AANA CE program provides a structure and framework for this educational content review, approval and recognition and the departmental organization is prepared to assist each AANA member in achieving the goal of professional competence enhancement.

Specifically, the goals of the CE program facilitate the promotion of quality CE for nurse anesthetists.[11] The goals are to:

1. Examine the CE approval process and recommend needed changes.
2. Utilize environmental scanning process to identify directions for the CE program.
3. Continue to support and guide state associations and applicants in complying with CE program requirements.
4. Support CE staff and process
5. Coordinate CE goals and strategies with those of the AANA Board of Directors and the NBCRNA.

The AANA's CE Committee, in conjunction with the AANA CE Department, oversees the Association's CE program and continually monitors the process to ensure that the standards and criteria are met. The purpose of the AANA CE approval process is to ensure that CE for nurse anesthetists is appropriate and acceptable for recertification. The AANA has also established standards and criteria for the CE program to ensure the quality of educational programs for nurse anesthetists. Continuing education credits are required for recertification. Therefore, certain criteria have been defined in a manner that recognizes those non-AANA CE programs whose content is relevant to the practice of anesthesia or that contribute to the improvement of the nurse anesthetist's practice in 1 or more of 4 specific areas:

139

education, administration, research, or clinical practice.

The AANA has developed specific pa rameters on which to base its CE approvals, and these parameters are directly linked to the recertification process. This structure enables the professional Association to carry out its responsibilities to the public with respect to ensuring that the CE process is meaningful for the purposes of credentialing in the field of nurse anesthesia. An equally important purpose of the CE process is to support continued competence to promote the delivery of the highest quality patient care and patient safety.

These standards and criteria are used to evaluate applications for approval of CE credits both internal to the Association as well as external to the Association and are listed in Table 6.10. All applicants must adhere to these standards and criteria in order to have their content receive AANA approval.

Each CRNA is required to obtain a minimum of 40 CE credits every 2 years as part of the recertification criteria. One CE credit is equal to 60 minutes or 1 contact hour. Individual CRNAs must first perform a self-assessment to identify the areas and types of CE activity that correspond to their need in professional practice. Then CRNAs elect to participate in the CE activity that provides the most benefit to them in terms of content, location, and cost. Table 6.11 lists the types of educational activities available to CRNAs for CE credit.

Generally, the provider of any CE activity is responsible for securing approval for the educational opportunity. Accommodations are designed to allow recipients to make application for content not processed by a provider. Therefore, the AANA CE program has 2 types of approval for CE activities: prior approval and nonprior approval. The criteria for each of the standards provide further clarification of their meaning. The AANA CE Committee may withdraw approval status of a CE activity if the provider fails to comply with the established standards and criteria. Educational activities that are not congruent with the AANA CE program philosophy may be denied approval. An appeal mechanism exists for providers or individuals who are not satisfied with a committee decision.

Continuing Education Committee

The CE Committee is a standing committee of the AANA. Members are appointed by the president-elect with approval from the Board of Directors. According to AANA By-laws, the committee shall formulate CE criteria for eligibility for use toward recertification. Such criteria shall be submitted to the NBCRNA for evaluation and adoption. The committee shall also supervise CE projects conducted by the Association, evaluate applications for program approval, and approve refresher courses based on established criteria that are required before transference to active recertified membership.

The CE Committee believes that CE activities are most effective when the learning needs of participants are considered and when the principles of adult education are applied to the creation and delivery of the educational content. The committee supports these beliefs by developing and upholding the AANA standards of CE that include those basic concepts. The CE Committee also monitors and appraises the CE activities of other providers to ensure that they adhere to established standards that promote quality CE for nurse anesthetists.[5]

The CE Committee is primarily responsible for providing opportunities for

Table 6.10. Standards and Criteria for Continuing Education Programs[5]

These standards and criteria are used to evaluate applications for approval of CE credits. The CE Committee and the CE Department work together to approve programs that are appropriate for the continuing education and recertification of nurse anesthetists. All applicants must adhere to the following standards and criteria.

Standard I: Official Application
Providers of CE for nurse anesthetists who request approval from the AANA must submit an appropriate application to the AANA's CE Department.
Criteria:
A. Applications for prior approval must include the following: application fee; date and location of CE activity; CE credits (contact hours) requested; purpose/goal(s); planning; needs assessment/target audience; learner objectives; content; teaching methods; faculty; physical facilities/resources; recordkeeping, certificate of attendance and evaluation.
B. Applications for nonprior approval must include all required documentation, as specified on the form.
C. CE activities must be appropriate for nurse anesthetists and their recertification process.

Standard II: Purpose/Goals
Eligible CE activities support and promote quality CE for nurse anesthetists. The program's statement of purpose must include information to substantiate this standard. The purpose/goal(s) is a statement of the "what" and the "why" of the activity.
Criteria:
A. The overall intent for whom, what and why of the CE activity must be described.
B. The statement of purpose must describe how the CE activity will enhance the quality of care provided by nurse anesthetists.

Standard III: Planning
A planning process for developing, implementing, and evaluating the CE activity must be in place.
Criteria:
A. The program coordinator responsible for planning and implementing the CE activity must be identified. It is recommended that the program coordinator be a nurse anesthetist or a registered nurse.
B. The resumes of the program coordinator and members of the planning committee must be available upon request.
C. The provider must comply with the requirements published in the CE Program.

Standard IV: Needs Assessment/Target Audience
The CE activity must have been developed on the basis of a documented need of the potential target audience.
Criteria:
A. The target audience for the CE activity must be identified.
B. The method by which the need for the CE activity was assessed and validated must be described.

Continues on page 142.

141

Table 6.10. Standards and Criteria for Continuing Education Programs[5] (continued)

Standard V: Learner Objectives

Learner objectives for the CE activity must be stated in behavioral terms.

Criteria:

A. Objectives must flow from the purpose/goal and be consistent with the identified needs of the target audience.

B. Objectives must clearly define expected outcomes for the learner.

C. Objectives must be stated in behavioral terms that are measurable, so that the learner can readily assess the achievement of each objective.

Standard VI: Content

The content provides knowledge, skills, and abilities, beyond the basic level for preparation of nurse anesthetists, while being mindful of the need to periodically relearn, refresh, or update those basic competencies or to adapt them to new practice situations or settings.

Criteria:

A. The content must not only meet the needs of the participants but also support current practice for nurse anesthetists in education, administration, research, or clinical practice.

B. The content must flow from learner objectives.

C. The content must be described in outline form, and an hourly schedule of the content must be set forth to include presentations, meals, breaks, etc. The provider must submit sufficient content to adequately appraise its relevance and value to nurse anesthetists.

D. The time allotted for the CE activity must be consistent with the learner objectives and appropriate to the content being presented.

Standard VII: Teaching Methods

Teaching methods must be consistent with the content and learner objectives and reflect the use of adult principles of learning.

Criteria:

A. Teaching methods must facilitate learning and maximize the achievement of identified objectives.

B. The program coordinator must explain how adult principles of learning are reflected in the teaching methods.

Standard VIII: Faculty

The faculty members for the CE activity must deliver content in an area in which they have knowledge and expertise and must take an active part in planning their presentations.

Criteria:

A. The program coordinator must describe how the faculty members participate in planning their presentations.

B. The program coordinator must submit the name, title, and credentials that identify the educational/academic preparation and professional qualifications of each faculty member; short resumes must be provided upon request.

C. Curriculum vitae information must validate faculty members' content expertise and experience in the subject matter.

Continues on page 143.

142

Table 6.10. Standards and Criteria for Continuing Education Programs[5] (continued)

Standard IX: Physical Facilities/Resources

The site for the CE activity must be suitable in terms of teaching methods, environmental comfort, and target audience accessibility. Resources allocated for the CE activity must be adequate to provide for a quality CE effort.

Criteria:

A. The program coordinator must describe the physical facility and its suitability.

B. The program coordinator must describe the human, financial, and material resources that will be used to implement a quality CE activity.

Standard X: Recordkeeping

Criteria:

A. The provider must maintain the following information: needs assessment; target audience; purpose; planning committee; learner objectives; content; faculty; teaching and evaluation methods; title, date, and site of activity; name of the person responsible for coordinating and implementing the activity (program coordinator); participant roster, with names, AANA ID numbers, and addresses of participants; summary of participant evaluations; the number of CE credits (contact hours) awarded to each participant; verification of attendance process and a copy of the certificate awarded; marketing materials; co-provider/sponsor agreement (if applicable); and documentation, if commercially supported, of how program integrity is maintained and proof of disclaimers or declarations regarding vested interest by each presenter.

B. This information must be stored securely and be retrievable for at least 60 months.

Standard XI: Verification of Attendance

All participants must receive a certificate of attendance that verifies their participation in or attendance at the CE activity.

Criteria:

A. The certificate of attendance must include the following information: name of participant; AANA membership or recertification; APRN number and/or RN license number; title of CE activity; date of activity; city and state for location of CE activity; AANA code number and expiration date; number of CE credits (contact hours) awarded to the individual; name, city and state of provider; and signature of provider to verify attendance.

B. Following the program, the program coordinator must submit the attendance record in alphabetical order.

Standard XII: Evaluation

There must be a clearly defined method of evaluating the CE activity.

Criteria:

A. The program coordinator must submit an evaluation instrument that includes an appraisal of the following: the learner's achievement of each objective; the teaching effectiveness of each program faculty member/presenter; the relevance of content to objectives; the effectiveness of teaching methods; the appropriateness of physical facilities; and the achievement of personal objectives by the learner.

B. The program coordinator must state how planners and learners participated in the evaluation and how the results will be used.

143

CE indicates continuing education; ID, identification; APRN, advanced practice registered nurse; and RN, registered nurse. (Reprinted with permission from the American Association of Nurse Anesthetists.)

Table 6.11. Types of Continuing Education Activities

- Attendance at local, state, national, and international nurse anesthesia meetings
- Participation in hospital or anesthesia department in-services
- Participation in research activities
- Attendance at college and university courses relevant to anesthesia practice
- Publication of original manuscripts
- New clinical anesthesia experiences beyond the requirements of basic preparation
- Audiovisual media programs such as videos, audiotapes, and computerized instruction
- Simulation activities

---

continued learning by individuals and groups of nurse anesthetists. It believes that lifelong learning is essential for the continued acquisition of knowledge and skills required to maintain competence. The committee maintains that nurses, by entering the field of anesthesia, hold themselves accountable and responsible for seeking out learning experiences that will improve and advance the practice of anesthesia and the quality of care they provide.[5]

Prior-Approved Continuing Education Activities

Prior approval is the process used to review applications and award CE credit based on predetermined criteria. Prior approval by the AANA designates that a CE activity has met or exceeded specific published standards and has been awarded CE credit before its actual presentation. In addition, this status obliges providers of educational program activities to assume responsibilities for specific published and publically available requirements related to record keeping and recording attendance. Additionally, program content must be consistent with the overall purpose and goals of the AANA's CE program. The types of activities that are eligible for prior approval include educational programs sponsored by associations and organizations at the local, state, regional, national, or international level; in-service programs; provider-directed independent study; and simulation.

To obtain prior approval, the provider must submit the completed application form with all required supporting documentation to the AANA CE Department in advance of the proposed CE activity. Additional materials required include the application fee, evaluation form, and an event-specific certificate of attendance. Notification of approval is furnished in writing within 30 days of receipt of the application and all other required materials. If additional information is required for prior approval, the provider must submit it before the presentation of the CE activity, or approval will not be granted. A unique identification code number is assigned to the CE activity and must appear on promotional activities, certificates of attendance, attendance records, and correspondence sent to the CE Department, which are associated with the specific program. The record-keeping process involves submission of an official AANA attendance record with the participants' names, AANA numbers, and CE credits for each participant within 30 days after completion of the program. The provider must issue a certificate of attendance to all participants.[5] Currently, all necessary forms required to complete the prior approval process are available on the AANA's website. These forms are prepared in an interactive format and can be electronically transmitted directly to the AANA CE Department.

Nonprior-Approved Continuing Education Activities

The nonprior approval process is used to award CE credit to individuals for attendance at or participation in learning activities that have not received prior approval by the AANA, but which were approved by a recognized approval or accrediting organization before their presentation. This approval mechanism is initiated by the individual who submits the application. Continuing education credit is not considered until an application and all required documentation have been submitted.

Applications for nonprior approval should be submitted within 60 days following the conclusion of the CE activity. Examples of activities that are eligible for nonprior approval include programs that have received approval or accreditation for CE credit from another recognized professional organization. Also eligible for credit are graduate-level college or university courses, life support courses, publication of an original manuscript, new clinical anesthesia experiences, and research in anesthesia-related fields. The individual or group requesting the CE credit must complete the appropriate application and provide the required documentation.

Written notification of approval or denial of CE credit is sent after review of the application. The committee ensures that the nonprior-approved program meets the standards and criteria for the AANA CE program.[5] Currently, all necessary forms required to complete the nonprior approval process are available on the AANA's website. These forms are prepared in an interactive format and can be electronically transmitted directly to the AANA CE Department.

Record Keeping

The AANA CE Department maintains records of CE credits earned by its members. In addition, nonmembers can contract with the AANA for this service. At the end of the recertification period, CE documentation is forwarded to the NBCRNA for both members and nonmembers with record-keeping contracts. The CE credits are recorded during each year from August 1 through July 31 to coincide with the recertification period. Members of the AANA can use the AANA website as well as nonmembers who pay for an AANA record-keeping contract to access their transcript of CE credits 24 hours a day. In addition, they may also access and print a transcript of their CE activities for any time period of interest via the AANA website.

Summary

The professional regulation (credentialing) of CRNAs comprises the certification and recertification processes through mandatory CE and compliance with external accreditation agency requirements. This chapter has described the development and implementation of these regulatory procedures. The AANA's leadership and members have supported and maintained sound regulatory practices for CRNAs, which have long been noted among other provider organizations as some of the strongest and most effective standards and programs ever developed. Each individual CRNA, as a member of the specialty profession of nurse anesthesia, must remain committed to maintaining the quality of anesthesia care through CE and demonstration of contemporary practice patterns of the highest standard.

References

1. Philosophy. In: Bylaws and Standing Rules of the American Association of Nurse Anesthetists. Park Ridge, IL: American Association of Nurse Anesthetists; 2008:2.

2. Bankert M. *Watchful Care: A History of America's Nurse Anesthetists*. New York, NY: Continuum Publishing; 1989:80-81.

3. *Credentialing Health Manpower*. Washington, DC: US Dept of Health, Education, and Welfare; 1977:16-17.

4. Proposed AANA restructuring detailed at Assembly of States. *AANA NewsBull*. May 1978:1,5,7.

5. Continuing Education Program of the American Association of Nurse Anesthetists. Park Ridge, IL: American Association of Nurse Anesthetists; 2008:2-30.

6. American Nurses Association. The Study of Credentialing in Nursing: A New Approach. Washington, DC: American Nurses Association; 1979. A Report of the Committee; vol 1.

7. Scofield R. Certification: what does it mean? *Curr Concepts Nurs*. 1988;2(1): 6-10.

8. Council on Certification of Nurse Anesthetists. *2010 Candidate Handbook*. Park Ridge, IL: American Association of Nurse Anesthetists. http://www. nbcrna.com/downloads/CCNA/NBCR NA_2010_Candidate_Handbook.pdf. Accessed March 2, 2010.

9. Civil Service Commission. Uniform Guidelines on Employee Selection Procedures. *Fed Regist*. 1978;43:166.

10. Bryant SK. Voluntary certification and the uniform guidelines on selection procedures: a potential problem for personnel managers. *Health Policy Educ*. 1981;2(2):135-152.

11. American Psychological Association. *Standards for Educational and Psychological Testing*. Washington, DC: American Psychological Association; 1985:1-92.

12. Wolgemuth RR, Samph T. *A Summary Task Analysis Report*. American Association of State Social Work Boards. 1983;1:1-12.

13. Henderson JB. Job analysis. In: Browning AH, Bugbee AC, Mullins MA, eds. *Certification: A NOCA Handbook*. Washington, DC: National Organization of Competency Assurance; 1996:41-65.

14. Zaglaniczny KL. Council on Certification Professional Practice Analysis. *AANA J*. 1993;61(3):241-255.

15. Zaglaniczny KL, Healey T. A report on the Council on Certification 1996 Professional Practice Analysis. *AANA J*. 1998;66(1):43-62.

16. McShane F, Fagerlund KA. A report on the Council on Certification of Nurse Anesthetists 2001 Professional Practice Analysis. *AANA J*. 2004;72(1):31-52.

17. Zaglaniczny KL. The transition of the National Certification Examination from paper and pencil to computer adaptive testing. *AANA J*. 1996;64(1): 9-14.

18. Bergstrom BA. Computer adaptive testing for the National Certification Examination. *AANA J*. 1996;64(2): 119-124.

19. Schoon CG, Smith IL. Standard setting. In: Browning AH, Bugbee AC, Mullins MA, eds. *Certification: A NOCA Handbook*. Washington, DC: National Organization of Competency Assurance; 1996:149-189.

20. Council on Recertification of Nurse Anesthetists. Criteria for Recertification. Park Ridge, IL: American Association of Nurse Anesthetists. 2008:2-19. http://www.nbcrna.com/downloads/COR/Recert/NBCRNA_Recertification_Criteria.pdf.

21. Refresher program. In: *Criteria for Recertification*. Park Ridge, IL: American Association of Nurse Anesthetists; 2008:1-6. http://www.nbcrna.com/downloads/COR/Refresher/NBCRNA_Refresher_Program_Book.pdf.

147

Study Questions

1. What are the key factors that were instrumental in the development of continuing education for CRNAs?

2. What is the difference in the criteria for certification and recertification of CRNAs?

3. What is the role of the NBCRNA and each of the councils that are incorporated in it?

4. What are the processes and procedures to obtain prior approval for a continuing education program?

5. What is the responsibility of each CRNA in maintaining continued competence?

CHAPTER 7
Standards of Care in Anesthesia Practice

Sandra K. Tunajek, CRNA, DNP

Key Concepts

- Standards of practice contribute to professional autonomy, accountability, and high-quality clinical practice.

- Evidence-based practice standards enable the delivery of high-quality anesthesia care.

- Applications of research to education and practice can greatly influence the quality and delivery of nurse anesthesia care.

- Professional organizations have a key role in clinical research and the promulgation of standards and practice.

- Standards and guidelines are effective benchmarks for professional competency and accountability.

- New and evolving standards and guidelines must be effectively disseminated.

The existence of professions depends on a social contract, a tacit agreement in which society confers privileges in exchange for obligations. In most countries, the legislative or regulatory process provides a framework for the identification and the extent of the legal authority delegated to the specified profession. The legal authority, usually in the form of government regulation, implies social responsibility and public accountability. Therefore, a profession acquires further recognition, relevance, and meaning through mechanisms to ensure both accountability and responsibility.

In our society, certain professions and occupations perform work of such a nature that, if it is undertaken in a negligent or fraudulent way, it can be dangerous or contrary to the public interest. As a result, it has been the accepted practice to regulate the activities of groups such as doctors, nurses, engineers, and lawyers.

Self-governing professions exhibit 3 essential characteristics: (1) a unique combination of knowledge and skills, (2) a commitment to duty above self-interest or personal gain, and (3) self-governance and freedom from external interference. Two additional key points are clear: (1) Self-regulation is granted in order to serve the public interest, and (2) Self-regulation is a privilege.

The principal stakeholders having an interest in the fairness and appropriateness of professional regulation include the public, the profession, and the members of the profession. The public has an interest in seeing that only competent, accountable professionals are allowed to provide potentially dangerous healthcare services. The profession has a stake in regulation to ensure that the reputation of the profession and its practitioners is credible, and people will have sufficient confidence in the practitioners. Members of the profession have a stake in regulation not only as a legitimate need to earn a living at a profession for which they have devoted much time and energy in preparation but also as a model of work that can be a value and a source of motivation and personal satisfaction.

Nursing and medicine have enjoyed positions of honor based on their social contract with the public they serve.

Self-regulating professions possess a collective knowledge that implies proprietorship. Although possession of this knowledge is a social asset and provides the underpinning for professional organization, ownership also compels stewardship and responsibility for advancing the profession. Professional knowledge also encompasses certain behaviors and attitudes, as well as a spirit of courtesy, generosity, and cooperation.

The profession as an institution serves as a normative reference group for individual practitioners, and through a code of ethics clarifies for both its members and outsiders the norms that ought to govern professional behavior. To enter a profession is to assume a certain kind of social identity as a person of valuable knowledge and skill, a recognized contributor to valuable public services but also as a trustee of the knowledge and skill that defines the professional domain.

Professionalism embraces a continuum of behaviors guided by personally held principles, beliefs, and values. Measuring professionalism is an elusive endeavor. Barondess[1] noted that professional values are standards that are accepted by the practitioner and professional group and that provide a framework for evaluating beliefs and attitudes that influence behavior. Initiation to the socialization process begins within the various training programs and contributes to the molding of and internalization of both personal and professional values specific to that particular discipline. Studies suggest this socialization provides the basis for self-regulation and continues throughout one's career, further influencing commitment to evolving ethical requirements and increasing demands for competency assessment, as well as compulsory maintenance of skills, professional development, and regulatory mandates for updates to practice.[2,3]

Studies show that a fundamental characteristic of a profession is self-regulation.[4,5] Accountability and public interest, both of which are inherent and necessary in professionalism and self-regulation, are maintained by individual members through adherence to standards, competence, and ethical conduct. Society has always valued and continues to value the importance of professionalism and self-regulation.

Self-Regulation

Self-regulation is the inherent privilege of any occupation that holds a specialized body of knowledge with implied public accountability. Responsibility and accountability is made more specific through the establishment of a professional definition and a code of ethics. The profession is further expected to foster research and to develop, disseminate, implement, and enforce various standards for education and practice. The profession may also set rules for ethics, credentials for entry into practice, accreditation standards, and mechanisms for monitoring compliance.

Professional practitioners distinguish themselves from other occupations by the special character of the knowledge required to perform their tasks. Expert knowledge, cognitive thinking, clinical skill, and

legal scope of practice are critical for professional identity and accountability. The principles of self-regulation acknowledge the professions' authority to determine and evaluate the technical knowledge used in its work. The profession then is responsible for the expertise, skill, and judgment that best regulates a continuing commitment to professional conduct and competence. The scope of professional practice includes the roles, functions, and accountabilities for which members of the profession are educated and authorized to perform. By a profession's adherence to these principles, the public trust and confidence are sustained and quality of performance is ensured.[4]

Self-regulation among professions can also be described as how individuals or groups monitor their own behavior and how that behavior is judged in relation to personal and social standards. Furthermore, the professions encourage mechanisms or self-reactive incentives to moderate the individual or group behavior. This integrated self-regulating system involving beliefs, systems, and structures provides professional self-satisfaction and a sense of self-worth.[5] The members of the profession acknowledge an obligation to maintain competence, integrity, ethical practice, altruism, and the promotion of the public good. These commitments form the basis of the social contract between a profession and society, which in return grants the profession the right to autonomy in practice and the privilege of self-regulation. Additionally, the contract between professions and society grants a proprietary use of an expert body of knowledge, a considerable degree of autonomy, prestige, and financial rewards.[4]

Greater autonomy and control translate into the independence of individual members of a profession, allowing an authority to practice with less or no supervision. Furthermore, it allows the ability of the profession to set entry requirements and standards for practice instead of having government or another profession impose requirements on the profession. In addition, the profession has a means of gaining access to regulatory entities, which allows it to express its point of view and even negotiate for additional authority.

Society has accorded the profession of nursing and its specialty practice the right to regulate its own practice. This responsibility is reflected in professional policies and standards for education and practice that encompass accountability, integrity, competence, and commitment to patient advocacy, safety, and access to high-quality care.

Self-regulation has been inherent to the nurse anesthesia profession since 1931 when the National Association of Nurse Anesthetists, now the American Association of Nurse Anesthetists (AANA), set the objective "to develop educational standards and techniques in the administration of anesthetic drugs."[6] This and other self-regulatory parameters that are grounded in knowledge of and adherence to the current standards of care are central to professional recognition of nurse anesthesia. Standards promulgated by a profession are representative models that delineate contemporary principles of practice; reflect the theory, evidence, philosophic values, and clinical priorities of the profession; and provide a foundation by which clinical practice can be evaluated and measured.[7,8] Furthermore, the standards are the fundamental principles for ensuring that its members act in the public interest by adhering to processes of professional and legal regulation.

The dictionary definition of a standard refers to "something set up and established by authority, custom, or general consent as a model, example or rule for the measure of quantity, weight, extent, value, or quality."[9] A standard is also defined as a criterion, gauge, or yardstick by which judgments or decisions may be made. The word *standard* also refers to both the model and the example of criteria for determining how well one's performance approximates the designed model. Thus, a standard is both a goal (what should be done) and a measure of progress toward that goal (how well it was done).

Standards then may be described as the benchmark for expected behaviors, which are based on a desired level of excellence. A standard may be mandatory (required by law), voluntary (established by professional organizations), or de facto (generally accepted by custom or practice). Standards may be formulated by professional and specialty organizations, state boards of nursing, federal organizations, and regulatory bodies at both the federal and state levels. Furthermore, standards can be measured and enforced in a wide variety of ways.[8,10,11]

Evidence-Based Practice

Although many aspects of nursing and medical practice have been based on tradition and clinical experiences, the healthcare professions have consistently valued the scientific foundations of practice. Educators and clinicians have traditionally linked anecdotal practice information with theory and available research. However, in the past decade, there has been a movement toward evidence-based practice (EBP) that articulates interventions based on methods of researched, evidence-based, clinical outcomes that are important for practice and patient care.

Evidence-based practice began in England in the 1990s as a way to ensure that decisions regarding the provision of clinical services were driven by evidence that clinical care was effective as well as cost-efficient. Sackett et al[12] described evidence-based medicine or evidence-based nursing as the integration of the best research with clinical expertise and patient values. The integration of the best research tells us that evidence-based nursing and medicine is not just research utilization of isolated studies but a rigorous method by which all the research data for a particular problem or issue are analyzed together, synthesized, and put into an integrative review. The work of Sackett and colleagues[12] underlines the importance of practitioner experience and recognizes the expertise of the clinician.

Evidence-based practice has increasingly influenced decision making in health policy. Major factors in the movement toward EBP focused on improving care and saving money for health delivery systems. The driving forces for the development of EBP include the high cost of care, variability in delivery systems, and increased demands for practitioner accountability. Reviews in the nursing and medical literature further highlighted the problems, emphasizing the gap between best evidence and practice.

Evidence-based practice approaches are assuming prominence in many healthcare specialties and are a paradigm shift from traditional clinical practice. The Agency for Healthcare Research and Quality created Evidence-based Practice Centers in 1997 to synthesize existing scientific literature about important healthcare topics and promote EBP and evidence-based decision making. The expertise of the evidence-based practice center is now also used for comparative effectiveness reviews or research reviews. These reviews use a research method that systematically and critically appraises existing research to synthesize knowledge on a particular topic and to communicate the effectiveness and complexities that surround it; in other words, to inform healthcare-related decisions.

Although Wilensky[13] and others discuss comparative effectiveness in various policy papers and analysis, no standard definition of comparative effectiveness has emerged. However, discussion on comparative effectiveness generally incorporates the work of Chalkidou, Tunis, and coworkers[14] and uses the following definition: "a set of analytic tools that allow for the comparison of one treatment—drug, device, or procedure—to another treatment on the basis of risks, benefits, and potentially, cost." Furthermore, the discussions suggest a focus on the research setting as real-world healthcare interactions, rather than randomized controlled trials. A caveat: although comparative effectiveness can be a valuable tool to inform the decision making of the clinician, the patient, and policy makers, it cannot provide a simple template or one-size-fits-all answer. Finally, another important aspect of the comparative effectiveness reviews is the identification of research gaps, as well as recommendations for studies and approaches to fill the gaps between research and clinical practice.[15]

In 2009, additional funding for evidence-based comparative effectiveness research was created by the American Recovery and Reinvestment Act, an initial, potentially important move toward modernizing the US healthcare system.[16]

In 2001, the Institute of Medicine (IOM)[17] highlighted quality issues in healthcare delivery and recommended a redesign of the system to better administer and improve quality. A major feature of the IOM report called for evidence-based decision making

153

and a healthcare environment characterized by the application of evidence, improved outcomes, and technology to monitor and deliver care. Furthermore, the report suggested that healthcare professionals must gain, assess, apply, and integrate new knowledge in order to adapt to changing environments and improved outcomes in patient care. Additionally, payment systems were to be realigned with improvements in recommended areas, resulting in the evolution of the pay-for-performance initiatives launched by the Centers for Medicare & Medicaid Services (CMS) programs.

Although the IOM report recognized the technological advances and improvements in anesthesia safety and quality, much of anesthesia research has focused on laboratory investigations or those that build on evidence-based techniques that are confirmed by careful clinical observation and expert consensus opinion.

Evidence-based practice is a clinical decision-making approach critical to promoting best patient outcomes. The definition of EBP has evolved over time and is the integration of the best available research with clinical expertise in the context of patient characteristics, culture, and preferences. This definition closely parallels the definition of EBP that the IOM adapted from Sackett and colleagues.[18] Review studies of current anesthetic interventions in routine practice indicate that many are supported by evidence in the literature.[19,20] Both the AANA and the American Society of Anesthesiologists (ASA) support safe and relevant best practices and continually utilize research-based clinical standards, practice parameters, and consensus guidelines in both education and practice.

Translating research into practice is not a simple task. Often, many years pass before information acquired from research studies is applied in the clinical setting. It is a complex process, and successful integration of research into practice requires critical appraisal of study methods and results and most importantly, consideration of the applicability of the evidence to the particular clinical setting. The assessment of applicability is imperative before evidence can be incorporated into professional recommendations. Qualitative considerations, such as patient preferences, must also be assessed before the evidence can be determined to be applicable. Because of their role, education, and the respect they have earned, Certified Registered Nurse Anesthetists (CRNAs) and other advanced-practice nurses are in an ideal position for leading EBP changes in the clinical arena.

The AANA recognizes that evidence derived from clinical experiences, reasoning, or judgment is relevant to translating evidence into practice. Therefore, the AANA Board of Directors has adopted a definition for nurse anesthesia EBP that incorporates the elements that emphasize the need for balance between expertise and evidence (Table 7.1). Additionally, the AANA Practice Committee is focusing efforts toward incorporating key steps into the review of existing practice recommendations and the development of new standards. These include processes to (1) ask a clinically important question; (2) search the literature, including conducting a meta-analysis; (3) evaluate the published evidence and applicability of the results to clinical practice; and (4) form consensus opinion.

Evidence-based anesthesia practice is strongly rooted in consensus formation based on use of consensus expertise that acknowledges clinical and scientific training, theoretical understanding, experience, self-reflection, knowledge of current research,

154

Table 7.1. AANA Definition of Evidence-Based Nurse Anesthesia Practice[18]

Evidence-based nurse anesthesia practice is defined as the "integration and synthesis of the best research evidence with clinical expertise and patient values" in order to optimize the care of patients receiving anesthesia services. Best research evidence is "clinically relevant data, information and research (often taken from the basic sciences of medicine and nursing) including patient-centered research into the accuracy and precision of diagnostic tests (including clinical examinations), utilizing the power of prognostic markers, and the efficacy and safety of therapeutic, rehabilitative and preventive regimens" (Sackett et al., 2000). Patient values are "unique preferences, concerns and expectations each patient brings to a clinical encounter and which must be integrated into clinical decisions in order to serve the patient" (Sackett et al., 2000). Clinical expertise is "the ability to use our clinical skills and past experience to rapidly identify each patient's unique health state and diagnosis, their individual risks and benefits of potential interventions, and their personal values and expectations" (Sackett et al., 2000). Anesthesia services are those activities within the scope of practice of a certified registered nurse anesthetist.

Adopted AANA Board of Directors January 2009.

(Reprinted with permission from the AANA.)

and continuing education and training.[21,22] This type of proactive approach is particularly useful because it accelerates the acceptance and application of these documents throughout the practicing community.

The systematic merging of evidence from these sources can offer anesthesia providers scientifically supportable findings that are flexible enough to deal with clinically complex problems. This process also addresses issues of dissemination, implementation, and sustainability of effective interventions. Furthermore, the process recognizes that clinical decisions should be made in collaboration with the patient based on the best available and relevant clinical evidence and with consideration for the probable costs, outcome benefits, accessible resources, and alternative options.

Healthcare workers are increasingly accountable to patients and institutions for demonstration that they are maintaining currency and competence. In a rapidly changing healthcare environment, an essential factor in professional development is a lifelong commitment to learning and improving practice. Efforts to define and develop competency frameworks, as well as mechanisms to identify and measure characteristics that are supported by evidence, are among the emerging challenges for professions.

Although dissemination of standards and guideline recommendations may be readily achieved, studies suggest that the use or application of research knowledge is not always transferred to practice. Additionally, the introduction of new evidence or tools in practice involves major changes in thinking of both individual and institutional behavior. Although knowledge transfer facilitates the dissemination of research to practitioners and the public, unless it is consistent with practitioner cultural beliefs and norms, it is unlikely to be successful.[22,23]

The barriers identified to changing clinical practice include individual and organizational

155

cultural resistance, ineffectual continuing education programs, poor access to information technology, lack of evidence in many clinical situations, and practitioner lack of skill sets. The latter includes computer skills, information searching, and interpreting statistical information, and methods to evaluate effective implementation and positive patient outcomes. One of the most commonly cited barriers is misperceptions or negative attitudes about research and evidence-based care.[15,22,24-25] Clearly, practitioners must understand the new practices and their utility before they can be expected to adopt them.

Evidence-based medicine is not an entirely new concept but aims to highlight a solid and conscientious scientific basis of clinical decision making. A growing body of evidence demonstrates that evidence-based interventions do benefit patients. Although evidence-based comparative effectiveness research does not contain recommendations or instruct clinicians as to what to do, these initiatives have created considerable controversy. The greatest concerns focus on the potential loss of personalized care, the issues related to rationing of services, and the economic implications of any measure that reduces spending growth and income for the healthcare industry. The healthcare industry argues that judgment, reasoning, and consideration of values of relevant stakeholders (patients, clinicians, policy makers, and society) must also play a role in developing strategies for reforming the system.

The concept of evidence-based research is relatively well supported. However, a cautionary concern noted by detractors lies in translating research into new clinical interventions. It is time-consuming, and the acceptance by practitioners is often slow or nonexistent.[22,24-25]

Currently, thousands of studies are being conducted on dissemination of innovation and implementation of health and mental health services. Both federal and state initiatives are being implemented and assessed for the effective integration of objective and observational evidence, clinical expertise, the needs and expectations of patients, and cost-efficiencies.[26,27]

Certainly, savings from health information technology, prevention, pay-for-performance, and comparative effectiveness research are attractive strategies for improving quality of care and reducing costs. Evidence-based practice initiatives are intended to enhance a transition of new discoveries into safe and high-quality healthcare for patients.[27]

Effective EBP strategies may serve as procedural processes to help clarify the best course of action in clinical decision making and improving the provision of care to patients. Furthermore, they may guarantee a more rapid transfer of knowledge from outcomes-related research to clinical patient care, and they may encourage continued engagement in research.

More detailed information about EBP as it relates to the nurse anesthetist appears in Chapter 9.

Professional and Public Accountability

Professional attitudes and behaviors are critical to the survival and enhancement of professions. Accountability for quality of patient care is a social practice in which the conduct of a healthcare professional is reviewed in light of public policy and professional standards of conduct.

Quality of care is most often defined as that activity involving patient and provider behavior and communication that is based on solidly defined standards of practice.

Practice standards are the highest mandate for individual judgment and clinical behavior. Standards and other practice guidelines furnish practitioners and the judiciary with confirmation of what constitutes the standard knowledge and skills that a healthcare practitioner should apply in the daily care of patients.[11,28,29]

A standard represents a performance behavior that allows for little variation and is consistently exercised by a prudent nurse anesthetist or other practitioner in similar circumstances. Nurse anesthetists must be accountable to the public for adhering to all published standards, including comprehensive documentation that supports compliance with expected behaviors and professional conduct.[28]

The AANA has maintained responsibility to the public by promulgating standards and defining the acceptable level of anesthesia care that is provided by nurse anesthetists. Although it was not until 1974 that the AANA codified what had been generally accepted practice into formal written guidelines for the rendering of optimal anesthesia care,[30] the Association has fostered growth and continued competency from its inception. The initial guidelines clarified the scope of nurse anesthesia practice to the public and provided a structural framework for accountability of the practitioner. Those traditional common practice standards are acknowledged as the original source of the nurse anesthetists' standard of care that further evolved into consensus standards and policies adopted by the professional organization.

The standards and guidelines promulgated by the AANA are intended to provide professionals and healthcare policy makers with a basic framework of conduct and practice that illustrates the expected professionalism and technical skills befitting those who hold licenses to practice as nurse anesthetists. Standards of care are continually updated and revised as the changing body of knowledge, clinical evidence, and technology occur. Promulgated practice guidance documents are further influenced by such factors such as malpractice insurance claims, accrediting agency recommendations, equipment manufacturer requirements, the judiciary, and government policies.[28,29]

As a specialty association dedicated to meeting the highest standards of competence and ethical conduct, the AANA is a recognized leader in anesthesia safety and quality. The AANA Board of Directors first adopted standards of practice in 1980 with the publication of the *Guidelines for Nurse Anesthesia Practice*. Subsequent revisions followed in 1983, 1989, 1992, 1996, and 1999. Currently, the AANA *Professional Practice Manual for the Certified Registered Nurse Anesthetist*, first published in 1989, is a compendium of documents that reflect self-regulation, professional accountability, educational integrity, and continual performance improvement. Inherent to the discipline of nurse anesthesia practice, the Scope and Standards of Nurse Anesthesia Practice and other document definitions of the collection of integrated resources are highlighted in Tables 7.2 and 7.3 and are printed in the *Professional Practice Manual for the Certified Registered Nurse Anesthetist*,[31] which is available through the AANA website and bookstore.

Standards of Practice

Standards are rules or minimum requirements that describe specific responsibilities and principles of patient care and define the expectations against which professional performance can be measured.

Table 7.2. Scope and Standards for Nurse Anesthesia Practice[31]

The AANA Scope and Standards for Nurse Anesthesia Practice offer guidance for Certified Registered Nurse Anesthetists (CRNAs) and healthcare institutions regarding the scope of nurse anesthesia practice. The scope of practice of the Certified Registered Nurse Anesthetist addresses the responsibilities associated with anesthesia practice and is performed in collaboration with other qualified healthcare providers. Collaboration is a process which involves two or more parties working together, each contributing his or her respective area of expertise. CRNAs are responsible for the quality of services they render.

Scope of Practice
The practice of anesthesia is a recognized specialty in both nursing and medicine. Anesthesiology is the art and science of rendering a patient insensible to pain by the administration of anesthetic agents and related drugs and procedures. Anesthesia and anesthesia-related care represents those services which anesthesia professionals provide upon request, assignment, and referral by the patient's physician or other healthcare provider authorized by law, most often to facilitate diagnostic, therapeutic and surgical procedures. In other instances, the referral or request for consultation or assistance may be for management of pain associated with obstetrical labor and delivery, management of acute and chronic ventilatory problems, or the management of acute and chronic pain through the performance of selected diagnostic and therapeutic blocks or other forms of pain management. Education, practice and research within the specialty of nurse anesthesia promote competent anesthesia care encompassing the diversity of patient populations, age, ethnicity and gender. CRNAs practice according to their expertise, state statutes and regulations, and institutional policy.

CRNA scope of practice includes, but is not limited to the following:
1. Performing and documenting a pre-anesthetic assessment and evaluation of the patient, including requesting consultations and diagnostic studies; selecting, obtaining, ordering, and administering pre-anesthetic medications and fluids; and obtaining informed consent for anesthesia.
2. Developing and implementing an anesthetic plan.
3. Initiating the anesthetic technique which may include: general, regional, local, and sedation.
4. Selecting, applying, and inserting appropriate non-invasive and invasive monitoring modalities for continuous evaluation of the patient's physical status.
5. Selecting, obtaining, and administering the anesthetics, adjuvant and accessory drugs, and fluids necessary to manage the anesthetic.
6. Managing a patient's airway and pulmonary status using current practice modalities.
7. Facilitating emergence and recovery from anesthesia by selecting, obtaining, ordering and administering medications, fluids, and ventilatory support.
8. Discharging the patient from a post-anesthesia care area and providing post-anesthesia follow-up evaluation and care.
9. Implementing acute and chronic pain management modalities.
10. Responding to emergency situations by providing airway management, administration of emergency fluids and drugs, and using basic or advanced cardiac life support techniques.

Continues on page 159.

Table 7.2. Scope and Standards for Nurse Anesthesia Practice[31] **(continued)**

Additional nurse anesthesia responsibilities which are within the expertise of the individual CRNA include:

1. Administration/management: scheduling, material and supply management, supervision of staff, students or ancillary personnel, development of policies and procedures, fiscal management, performance evaluations, preventative maintenance, billing and data management.

2. Quality assessment: data collection, reporting mechanism, trending, compliance, committee meetings, departmental review, problem focused studies, problem solving, interventions, documents and process oversight.

3. Educational: clinical and didactic teaching, BCLS/ACLS instruction, inservice commitment, EMT training, supervision of residents, and facility continuing education.

4. Research: conducting and participating in departmental, hospital-wide, and university-sponsored research projects.

5. Committee appointments: assignment to committees, committee responsibilities, and coordination of committee activities.

6. Interdepartmental liaison: interface with other departments such as nursing, surgery, obstetrics, post-anesthesia care units (PACU), outpatient surgery, admissions, administration, laboratory, pharmacy, etc.

7. Clinical/administrative oversight of other departments: respiratory therapy, PACU, operating room, surgical intensive care unit (SICU), pain clinics, etc.

The functions listed above are a summary of CRNA clinical practice and are not intended to be all-inclusive. A more specific list of CRNA functions and practice parameters is detailed in the *AANA Guidelines for Core Clinical Privileges.*

CRNAs strive for professional excellence by demonstrating competence and commitment to the clinical, educational, consultative, research, and administrative practice in the specialty of anesthesia. CRNAs should actively participate in the development of departmental policies and guidelines, performance appraisals and peer reviews, clinical and administrative conferences, and serve on healthcare facility committees. In addition to these activities, CRNAs should assume a leadership role in the evaluation of the quality of anesthesia care provided throughout the facility and the community.

The scope of practice of the CRNA is also the scope of practice of nurse anesthetists who have graduated within the past 24 months from a nurse anesthesia educational program, accredited by the Council on Accreditation of Nurse Anesthesia Educational Programs, but have not yet passed their initial certification examination. Students enrolled in nurse anesthesia educational programs accredited by the Council on Accreditation of Nurse Anesthesia Educational Programs practice pursuant to the Council's Standards and Guidelines.

Continues on page 160.

159

Table 7.2. Scope and Standards for Nurse Anesthesia Practice[31] **(continued)**

Standards for Nurse Anesthesia Practice

Introduction

These standards are intended to:

1. Assist the profession in evaluating the quality of care provided by its practitioners.
2. Provide a common base for practitioners to use in their development of a quality practice.
3. Assist the public in understanding what to expect from the practitioner.
4. Support and preserve the basic rights of the patient.

These standards apply to all anesthetizing locations. While the standards are intended to encourage high quality patient care, they cannot assure specific outcomes.

Standard I

Perform a thorough and complete preanesthesia assessment.

Interpretation

The responsibility for the care of the patient begins with the pre-anesthetic assessment. Except in emergency situations, the CRNA has an obligation to complete a thorough evaluation and determine that relevant tests have been obtained and reviewed.

Standard II

Obtain informed consent for the planned anesthetic intervention from the patient or legal guardian.

Interpretation

The CRNA shall obtain or verify that an informed consent has been obtained by a qualified provider. Discuss anesthetic options and risks with the patient and/or legal guardian in language the patient and/or legal guardian can understand. Document in the patient's medical record that informed consent was obtained.

Standard III

Formulate a patient-specific plan for anesthesia care.

Interpretation

The plan of care developed by the CRNA is based upon comprehensive patient assessment, problem analysis, anticipated surgical or therapeutic procedure, patient and surgeon preferences, and current anesthesia principles.

Standard IV

Implement and adjust the anesthesia care plan based on the patient's physiological response.

Interpretation

The CRNA shall induce and maintain anesthesia at required levels. The CRNA shall continuously assess the patient's response to the anesthetic and/or surgical intervention and intervene as required to maintain the patient in a satisfactory physiologic condition.

Continues on page 161.

Table 7.2. Scope and Standards for Nurse Anesthesia Practice[31] (continued)

Standard V
Monitor the patient's physiologic condition as appropriate for the type of anesthesia and specific patient needs.

    A. **Monitor ventilation continuously.** Verify intubation of the trachea by auscultation, chest excursion, and confirmation of carbon dioxide in the expired gas. Continuously monitor end-tidal carbon dioxide during controlled or assisted ventilation including any anesthesia or sedation technique requiring artificial airway support. Use spirometry and ventilatory pressure monitors as indicated.

    B. **Monitor oxygenation continuously** by clinical observation, pulse oximetry, and if indicated, arterial blood gas analysis.

    C. **Monitor cardiovascular status continuously** via electrocardiogram and heart sounds. Record blood pressure and heart rate at least every five minutes.

    D. **Monitor body temperature continuously** on all pediatric patients receiving general anesthesia and when indicated, on all other patients.

    E. **Monitor neuromuscular function and status** when neuromuscular blocking agents are administered.

    F. **Monitor and assess the patient positioning** and protective measures except for those aspects that are performed exclusively by one or more other providers.

Interpretation
Continuous clinical observation and vigilance are the basis of safe anesthesia care. The standard applies to all patients receiving anesthesia care and may be exceeded at any time at the discretion of the CRNA. Unless otherwise stipulated in the standards a means to monitor and evaluate the patient's status shall be immediately available for all patients. When any physiological monitoring device is utilized, variable pitch and low threshold alarms should be turned on and audible in most circumstances. The omission of any monitoring standards shall be documented and the reason stated on the patient's anesthesia record. As new patient safety technologies evolve, integration into the current anesthesia practice shall be considered. The CRNA shall be in constant attendance of the patient until the responsibility for care has been accepted by another qualified healthcare provider.

161

Standard VI
There shall be complete, accurate, and timely documentation of pertinent information on the patient's medical record.
Interpretation
Document all anesthetic interventions and patient responses. Accurate documentation facilitates comprehensive patient care, provides information for retrospective review and research data, and establishes a medical-legal record.

Standard VII
Transfer the responsibility for care of the patient to other qualified providers in a manner which assures continuity of care and patient safety.
Interpretation
The CRNA shall assess the patient's status and determine when it is safe to transfer the responsibility of care to other qualified providers. The CRNA shall accurately report the patient's condition and all essential information to the provider assuming responsibility for the patient.

Continues on page 162.

Table 7.2. Scope and Standards for Nurse Anesthesia Practice[31] (continued)

Standard VIII

Adhere to appropriate safety precautions, as established within the institution, to minimize the risks of fire, explosion, electrical shock and equipment malfunction. Document on the patient's medical record that the anesthesia machine and equipment were checked.

Interpretation

Prior to use, the CRNA shall inspect the anesthesia machine and monitors according to established guidelines. The CRNA shall check the readiness, availability, cleanliness, and working condition of all equipment to be utilized in the administration of the anesthesia care. When the patient is ventilated by an automatic mechanical ventilator, monitor the integrity of the breathing system with a device capable of detecting a disconnection by emitting an audible alarm. Monitor oxygen concentration continuously with an oxygen analyzer with a low concentration audible alarm turned on and in use.

Standard IX

Precautions shall be taken to minimize the risk of infection to the patient, the CRNA, and other healthcare providers.

Interpretation

Written policies and procedures in infection control shall be developed for personnel and equipment.

Standard X

Anesthesia care shall be assessed to assure its quality and contribution to positive patient outcomes.

Interpretation

The CRNA shall participate in the ongoing review and evaluation of the quality and appropriateness of anesthesia care. Evaluation shall be performed based upon appropriate outcome criteria and reviewed on an ongoing basis. The CRNA shall participate in a continual process of self evaluation and strive to incorporate new techniques and knowledge into practice.

Standard XI

The CRNA shall respect and maintain the basic rights of patients.

Interpretation

The CRNA shall support and preserve the rights of patients to personal dignity and ethical norms of practice.

The "Standards for Nurse Anesthesia Practice" were adopted in 1974 and subsequently revised in 1981, 1989, 1992, 1996, 2002, and 2005. In 1983, the "Standards for Nurse Anesthesia Practice" and the "Scope of Practice" statement were included together in the *American Association of Nurse Anesthetists Guidelines for the Practice of the Certified Registered Nurse Anesthetist* document. That document subsequently has had the following name changes: *Guidelines for Nurse Anesthesia Practice* (1989); *Guidelines and Standards for Nurse Anesthesia Practice* (1992); and *Scope and Standards for Nurse Anesthesia Practice* (1996). In addition, the "Scope of Practice" statement was first published in 1980 as one part of the *American Association of Nurse Anesthetists Guidelines for the Practice of the Certified Registered Nurse Anesthetist* document.

(Reprinted with permission from the AANA.)

Table 7.3. AANA Document Definitions[31]

AANA Document Definitions: These definitions are intended to assist nurse anesthetists and other entities in distinguishing the different types of documents developed by the American Association of Nurse Anesthetists.

Code of Ethics

Principles of conduct and professional integrity that guide decision making and behavior of nurse anesthetists.

Practice Standards

Authoritative statements that describe the minimum rules and responsibilities for which nurse anesthetists are accountable. Represents expected behaviors that must be demonstrated by a nurse anesthetist's professional practice.

Practice Guidelines

Systematically developed statements to assist practitioners in clinical decision making that are commonly accepted within the discipline of the anesthesia profession.

Position Statements

Articulate the AANA official position or belief about certain nurse anesthesia practice related topics. May define the knowledge and abilities necessary to fulfill the professional functions and role of the nurse anesthetist.

Advisory Opinions

Statement that provides general recommendations reflecting consensus of the anesthesia profession. Describes appropriate role/behavior/decision making for specific situations.

Protocols

Evidenced-based statements of appropriate process of care and effective management for individual patient needs or specific clinical conditions.

Algorithms

Clinical recommendations prepared in flow-chart form describing processes and decisions involved in addressing specific conditions.

Considerations for Policy Development

Informational advisory documents intended to assist external entities in the development of policies that impact nurse anesthesia practice.

Joint Statements

Consensus statements promulgated by the AANA and other professional organizations.

White Paper

A complete description of a particular concept, position or solution to a problem, from overview to detailed facts, created to promote professionalism and advocacy. Intended to guide decision-makers on policy development.

163

(Reprinted with permission from the AANA.)

Standards evolve through consideration of existing research evidence and consensus opinion. Standards have been used to evaluate nurse anesthesia care in a number of ways. They serve to provide direction and a framework for the evaluation of practice, to describe the profession's accountability to the public, and to set benchmarks for a nurse anesthetist's performance outcomes. Standards also establish an expected level of patient care and enable the measurement of a nurse anesthetist's competency. Standards have been used to evaluate and ensure quality and to manage individual and institutional risk.[8,28]

Standards are classified as regulatory, voluntary, and involuntary. Regulatory standards are usually based on government mandates. Voluntary standards cover a wide range of services and products and serve an important role to ensure quality and safety. They are often developed by consensus with input from important stakeholders. Those developed by healthcare practitioners are often the work of the professional organization or accrediting entities. Voluntary standards may have the weight of regulatory standards because the government often relies on voluntary standards and individuals chosen to participate in and adhere to these standards as a means of standardized approaches to patient care.

Involuntary standards are those requirements defined by an obligatory participation and adherence in order to achieve or receive a benefit. Professional liability carriers are an example. Standards may also be categorized according to the scope of influence such as national, state, local, or institutional.

Standards are designed to provide guidance, but in the event of a lawsuit, such standards may be relied on to define the standard of care. Practitioners and students should note that there is a single standard for the provision of anesthesia care in this country. The nurse anesthesia profession has established standards of care that are not different from those of anesthesiologists. As Blumenreich[29] has indicated, "there is a rather uniform quality of care between nurse anesthetists and anesthesiologists, and that is further evidence that the 'standard of care' is the same." With the emergence of national consensus standards, new technology and evidence-based measures, and the ability to rapidly disseminate such knowledge, there is a trend for healthcare practitioners to be held to a single national standard of care. Professional standards, developed by specialty organizations, may also be contained in federal legislative or regulatory language. Therefore, local policy development must be scrutinized to reflect national standards.[8]

Previous authors have discussed the use of the comparative practice documents and information as it relates to the establishment of quality anesthesia care, including clinical practice standards, clinical practice guidelines, and position statements that support nurse anesthesia practice. Although each is distinctly different, they are often used interchangeably, with each providing a necessary component in determining quality of care.[8] Furthermore, the documents also serve as a valuable guide to hospitals, boards of nursing, accrediting organizations, CRNA managers, and government and private payers as a comprehensive resource for CRNA services in a constantly changing healthcare environment.

As the healthcare professions continue to move toward evidenced-based benchmarks to ensure professional competence and accountability, professional standards and guideline documents serve as the cornerstone for individual performance measures.

Performance Measures

The importance of collecting and reporting data about the performance of healthcare institutions as well as practitioners who are providing services and care has increased dramatically in the last 10 years. The importance of performance measures has emerged somewhat predictably, largely because of concerns about healthcare quality and costs, patient safety, access to care, and disparities in care. Diverse programs have been initiated to address these issues including the imbalance between cost and quality outcomes.

Taking the lead is the National Quality Forum (NQF), a private organization representing every sector of the healthcare system: consumer organizations; public and private purchasers; physicians, nurses, hospitals, and other healthcare providers; accrediting and certifying bodies supporting industries, and healthcare research and quality improvement organizations.[26] The NQF serves as a neutral evaluator of performance measures developed by others. It does not develop performance measures.

Endorsement by the NQF, which involves rigorous, evidence-based review and a formal consensus development process, has become the benchmark for comparative effectiveness and healthcare performance measures.

Practice Documents

Standards for professional practice have been used to evaluate nurse anesthesia care in a number of ways. They serve as a framework for measurement of a nurse anesthetist's practice by establishing the expected level of expertise, clinical care and performance outcomes, and management of individual and institutional risk for CRNA services. The standards are authoritative statements designed to describe the specific principles and responsibilities for which nurse anesthetists are held accountable. As mentioned earlier, there is a single standard of care for the provision of anesthesia services in the United States. Standards do not vary according to type of anesthesia provider or locality of the service.[8,29]

Practice guidelines are recommendations for patient care designed to assist the provider in critical decision making; they are based on the best evidence available and commonly accepted practices within the anesthesia profession. Practice guidelines are not mandated recommendations but may be tied to performance initiatives.

Position statements have less forceful criteria than either practice guidelines or standards. They usually represent an official position on emerging trends or consultant findings, or they discuss procedural policies, both clinical and nonclinical. Frequently, they evolve as the result of an identified clinical practice issue or concerns related to patient safety. Either practice guidelines or position statements may ultimately evolve into standards, given time, appropriate testing, discussion, and review.

For example, in response to a perceived lack of oversight for patient care in the office outpatient setting, the AANA Board of Directors and the Practice Committee initiated data collection on this emerging practice trend in June 1997. Subsequently, the AANA first introduced a position statement, then guidelines, and finally, adopted in February 1999 the office-based standards. The standards are intended to assist anesthesia practitioners seeking guidance for patient safety in this setting and are based on the concept that the standard of care is the same regardless of the practice setting. The AANA is the first organization to adopt such stringent recommendations for

165

this setting, further supporting the role of the profession as advocates for patient safety.

In response to public and private concerns relating to patient care, practice guidelines and standards have received renewed attention. Healthcare practitioners are being asked to further define, justify, improve, and document their quality of care. In short, the public, government agencies, business, and industry are demanding accountability from healthcare providers, accountability that requires entities to publicly disseminate, continually review and update, and impose appropriate standards of care.

It is the inherent responsibility of a professional association to develop, disseminate, and assist in the implementation of practice guidelines and standards of practice. Additionally, the profession must hold members accountable for using the standards and must protect the public from practitioners who have not acquired sufficient expertise or have chosen not to follow professional standards. The professional organization must also educate the public and regulatory agencies relative to the standards and must be responsible for disseminating new standards to the public and to practitioners.

The AANA has accepted and maintained this responsibility to the public by promulgating standards and defining the accepted level of anesthesia care that its members provide. The development of professional standards is largely the responsibility of the AANA Practice Committee, which, with the input of the membership and the Board of Directors, tracks emerging trends and issues, seeks consultation and research for best practices, and develops recommendations for adoption and implementation.

More recently, the emerging trend of research-based evidence and a more systematic approach to the development of standards and guidelines has led to emphasis on specific objectives and clinical outcomes and cost-benefit analysis for the intended objectives. Processes for developing guidelines and standards evolve from scientific evidence, expert opinions, and clinical experience. Expert opinion is vital to the process to assist in the collection of evidence, but more importantly, input from practitioners must be solicited to ensure that the guidelines are functional in clinical settings.[18,25]

As the growing demand for objective, comparative information about practitioner performance and patient care outcomes increases, outcome measures are rapidly becoming the benchmarking tool for healthcare institutions. Furthermore, providers of care, including nurse anesthetists, are being assessed with competencies documented and linked to overall institutional patient care results.[32,33]

Most healthcare professions acknowledge that the contract with the public now includes insurers, purchasers, other healthcare providers, patients, and consumers in general. Rigorous selection and training of nurse anesthetists and their dedication to responsible patient care may not automatically result in the trust, control, and autonomy that such professionalism once ensured. Practitioners are now required to constantly prove competence and professional behavior, and that behavior is being monitored closely by those outside the profession.[32]

Epstein and Hundert[33] and others[34] have defined competence as the habitual and judicious use of communication, knowledge, technical skills, clinical reasoning, emotions, values, and reflection in daily practice for the benefit of the individual and the communities of interest being served.

Current assessment and evaluations of basic skills are no longer the norm and may underemphasize some important domains of professional practice, including interpersonal skills, lifelong learning, professionalism, and integration of core knowledge into clinical practice. The ongoing challenge and implementation of new formats that reflect reliability and validity are areas of much discussion and debate among the professions.

Deliberations such as these are essential to the maintenance of professional independence, because society grants the privilege of self-regulation, conditional on the responsible assurance that nurse anesthetists possess the knowledge, training, and skills necessary to properly serve the public.[11]

The use of performance data based on the standard of care as a measure of competency is an emerging approach for competency assessment. Developing any program intended to ensure that health professionals continue to practice in a safe and effective manner is challenging.[32-34] The design and implementation is difficult, and valid assessment has been elusive. Although, further research is needed to gain a better understanding of the varied source and nature of determinants of quality practice, institutional and regulatory efforts to use performance measures to assess quality of care continue to expand.[35]

Performance measurement standards may be divided into 2 types: process and outcome. Process standards refer to a particular behavior or the mechanism by which a specific task is performed. Process standards mandate a clinical conduct. Outcome measures tell whether the changes being made are leading to improvement— that is, helping to achieve the aim (eg, decreasing waiting time in the emergency department, increasing the number of continuing education seminars for providers). Process measures tell whether a specific process change is having the intended effect (eg, percentage of telemetry patients not meeting criteria for telemetry utilization, practitioners who cannot demonstrate a skill). In determining whether these measures are relevant and practical, it is critical to address valid mechanisms for data collection.[36,37] Consequently, it is imperative that the individual CRNA, as well as the professional organization, be involved in the collection and interpretation of outcomes data that accurately reflect the high quality of care provided to patients.

Practice Guidelines

Practice guidelines are official policy statements of a professional association that are developed to assist the nurse anesthesia practitioner to understand the indications for and the methods to perform clinical procedures (eg, administration of anesthesia to the obstetrical patient). They also may depict basic clinical management options for complications of a disease process, such as the treatment of a malignant hyperthermia crisis. Practice guidelines not only are useful in guiding practice but also have relevance in education, research, and the development of continuous quality improvement processes. Practice guidelines assist in the instruction of the student registered nurse anesthetist in the administration of anesthesia for specific surgical procedures, guide the researcher in the identification and development of methods to investigate a specific clinical problem, and serve as a benchmark to measure and improve practice. Although they do not carry the influence of standards, practice guidelines can be and have been used in malpractice litigation.[8]

Practice guidelines are systematically developed recommendations supported by analysis of current literature and by a synthesis of expert opinion, clinical feasibility data, and consensus surveys. The development of EBP guidelines is an endeavor that looks at the literature available, evaluates it on the basis of scientific merits, evaluates the results, and makes recommendations as to the best options for patient care.

Although based on validated research, guidelines are not intended to be standards or absolute requirements. Practice guidelines, to be understood and implemented, should be accompanied with statements that interpret or explain the intent of the guideline. Although clinical practice guidelines may be described in many different terms (including practice parameters, practice guidelines, patient care protocols, clinical pathways, and care maps), the intent of each evidence-based guideline is to encourage practitioners to improve patient care services. Practice guidelines also examine the quality of care provided and serve as a reminder to practitioners to practice in an acceptable, prudent, and cost-effective manner.

The wording of the guideline is intentionally structured to allow for flexibility and individual patient needs. They are advisory and recommend behaviors that most commonly lead to positive outcomes. Guidelines are subject to change as new technology and procedures become available or are developed. As new information is communicated or specific issues and trends require an official position from a professional association, the AANA will develop new guidelines and modify the existing ones.

Position Statements

Position statements represent an official recommendation by a professional entity, such as the AANA Board of Directors, developed to address professional or generic issues affecting nurse anesthesia. Position statements related to clinical anesthesia practice are not published as standards by a professional organization, but may refer to a specific practice that is accepted and commonplace within the anesthesia profession. Accordingly, position statements, like practice guidelines, may form a functional standard. As a functional standard, the statement would reflect the care that a reasonable and prudent anesthetist would provide to his or her patient in similar circumstances.

The position statements may assist the CRNA in the development of institutional and departmental policies regarding insertion of central venous, pulmonary artery, and arterial monitoring catheters, as well as the provision of pain management services.

Anesthesia practitioners are often required to participate in policy development and interpretation. The AANA documents that relate to considerations for policy development arose from clinical practice questions and are designed to assist CRNAs and professional practitioners.

Advisory statements, or practice parameters, are intended to assist in decision making in areas of patient care where scientific evidence is insufficient. Advisories are a synthesis of expert opinion, clinical feasibility, and consensus surveys. They are not intended to be standards of practice and may be accepted as is, modified, or rejected according to clinical needs and constraints. Parameters are intended to promote beneficial or desirable outcomes but cannot guarantee any specific outcome. Variances in practice may be acceptable based on the judgment of the practitioner.

Sources of Professional Standards

Standards relevant to anesthesia also originate from a number of ancillary sources. Additionally, individual practitioners often develop personal standards based on clinical habits (eg, the use of a pericardial stethoscope or an anesthesia machine checkout list) that are repeated daily and become incorporated into the practice for that practitioner or a department of anesthesia.

When evidence is ambiguous or conflicting, or where scientific data are lacking, the clinical experiences of involved practitioners are used to guide the development of consensus-based recommendations. For example, anesthesia department policies address such issues as "nothing by mouth" policies that are formulated from clinical experience and scientific support of the morbidity associated with aspiration. Such policies outline the anesthesia care of the patient who is considered at risk of aspiration. The departmental policy is derived from the consensus of the department members who recognize that a rapid-sequence induction would be the standard of care for the induction of general anesthesia to this patient. Additionally, the policy identifies a specified provision of care to patients and the expected practitioner behavior.

Nonprofessional sources such as insurance companies often introduce standards that have an impact on the administration of anesthesia. Medical malpractice insurance companies can and do mandate specific clinical behaviors, such as the use of specific monitoring devices, as requirements for insurance. Citing the minimum monitoring recommendations from Harvard Medical School, malpractice insurers began to advise anesthesia providers to use pulse oximetry during each anesthesia procedure and encouraged the use of capnography.[38]

Currently, failure to monitor patients with pulse oximetry and capnography is considered a breach of the standard of care. Any insurance company strongly influences the development and use of standards by refusing to insure those who do not adhere to specific monitoring modalities and standards of care.

Federal agencies such as the CMS continue to have an impact on the development and use of standards. The CMS has proposed broad, sweeping revisions to the hospital and ambulatory care standards, including performance measures, credentialing criteria, and stronger enforcement of compliance requirements. Furthermore, heightened attention focused on medical errors has sparked growing interest in the use of healthcare practices that reduce the risk of harm resulting from the processes, systems, or environments of care. According to the NQF, "never events" are errors in medical care that are clearly identifiable, preventable, and serious in their consequences for patients, and that indicate a real problem in the safety and credibility of a healthcare facility or provider competence.[39]

Through the Medicare Prescription Drug, Improvement, and Modernization Act of 2003,[40] the US government has agreed to honor any standards that are set through a voluntary consensus process. As such, the Medicare program has initiated processes that tie the standards to performance outcomes for both institutions and providers. More importantly, the CMS is proposing payment incentives as a means of ensuring compliance.[38] Voluntary agencies for accreditation, such as the Joint Commission, and more recently, accreditation agencies for the office ambulatory care setting, have expanded the capacity for the establishment of guidelines and standards of practice. For example, accreditation

169

standards specify that a comprehensive preoperative and postoperative anesthesia assessment (a process standard) must be performed. The Joint Commission is an independent, nonprofit organization established nearly 60 years ago that sets the standards by which healthcare quality is measured in America and around the world. The Joint Commission requires accredited healthcare providers to collect and submit performance data on a full set of core quality-of-care standards. It surveys hospitals regularly to evaluate their performance against these standards and publishes the information to the public.

Equipment manufacturers and product standard organizations publish voluntary standards that assist practitioners in the operation, maintenance, or purchase of anesthesia-related equipment. An example is the Z-79 Committee of the American National Standards Institute. The Z-79 Committee is responsible for the development of standards for anesthesia machine construction as well as the construction and testing of endotracheal tubes, anesthesia ventilators, and oxygen analyzers. The US Food and Drug Administration (FDA) is a federal agency that is responsible for published standards on anesthesia equipment. The FDA Anesthesia Apparatus Checkout Recommendations resulted in the development of preanesthesia checklists, which have evolved into an expected behavior for practitioners in the clinical setting.

The judiciary may also determine the standard of care. As previously stated, the standard of care is expected to be the same in all settings, and anesthesia providers are generally required to meet such a standard of care. When a judge or jury, based on testimony by an expert witness, determines a standard would have prevented a mishap or error, the standard is reaffirmed. Therefore, it is critical that any testimony convey factual information relative to the case being litigated. The opinions of these experts, if accepted by the judge or jury, assist in the reinforcement of existing standards or the establishment of new ones.

Personal standards are acknowledged as an original source of promulgated professional standards and may further evolve into consensus policies and procedures that are subsequently adopted.[8] A defining characteristic of a professional organization is the formulation of a code or system of standards that prescribes acceptable professional behaviors for the members of that group. The establishment of a code of ethics signifies the maturation of a profession and results from the evolution of a collective professional identity within the organization.[4,41]

Summary

Members of the profession are responsible for interpreting, sharing, and applying practice standards and guidelines in their own institutions and individual practices. Research has shown there is greater acceptance if the standards and guidelines are reasonable, define expected performance clearly, and do not demand radical change.

Standards and other practice parameters provide practitioners and the judiciary with a consistent benchmark and confirmation of the knowledge and skills that constitute the expected level of care and quality patient outcomes. Professional standards of performance in general practice may be an essential component of measures for quality assurance. They render practitioners' performance transparent to the "outside world" and provide support for general practitioners themselves.

Members of the profession are responsible for personal and professional development by seeking new knowledge and skills to enhance performance. Therefore, the prudent professional association should contribute to efforts that focus on the development of standards that are tailored to the individual clinician and professional values.

The organization must continue its efforts to support research and develop evidence-based standards and guidelines of practice that provide effective care. The profession must examine how standards and practice guidelines can be rapidly disseminated and used more effectively to enhance and promote the quality of clinical practice. The future clearly indicates increasing reliance on practice standards and guidelines, with far-reaching implications for the profession's ability to maintain practice rights, reimbursement authority, and statutory and legal recognition.

In the future, CRNAs can anticipate multiple changes in the nurse anesthesia specialty. The profession will come under increasing pressure to deliver value-based care and to demonstrate the worth and quality of the care delivered. To best serve the public and the nurse anesthesia profession, it is imperative that all CRNAs be aware of the practice standards, guidelines, and position statements of the professional organization. Each is a measure for the evaluation of the nurse anesthetist and a method to validate professional practice.

Professionals are expected to master new knowledge, to incorporate it continually into practice, and to inform the discipline. The standard of care provides guidance in practice and encourages positive outcomes. Nurse anesthetists must use their own knowledge and expertise to guide their clinical practice and adherence to existing standards. Furthermore, nurse anesthetists have the challenging responsibility to engage in self-monitoring to maintain competence. Practitioners must continually review any changes in existing standards or the introduction of new standards and successfully transfer those recommendations into practice.

Professionalism is a behavior that defines the nurse anesthetist's relationship with physicians, other healthcare providers, and society. The standards define, support, and enhance professional self-regulation. Self-regulation is a privilege, not a right, and maintaining the public trust is essential to sustaining professional longevity. The standards set a framework that underscores the collective sense of professional responsibility, accountability, integrity, and competence of the individual nurse anesthetist as well as the profession's commitment to ensuring high-quality patient care and the public confidence and trust.

171

References

1. Barondess JA. Medicine and professionalism. *Arch Intern Med.* 2003; 163(2):145-149.

2. Waugaman WR, Lohrer DJ. From nurse to nurse anesthetist: the influence of age and gender on professional socialization and career commitment of advanced practice nurses. *J Prof Nurs.* 2000;16(1):45-56.

3. Weidman J, Twale D, Stein E. Socialization of graduate students in higher education. *ASHE-ERIC Higher Educ Rep.* 2001;28(3):34-39.

4. Bayles M. Professional power and self-regulation. *Business Prof Ethics J.* 1988;5(2):26-43.

5. Bandura A. Social cognitive theory of self-regulation. *Organ Behav Hum Decis Processes.* 1991;50:248-287.

6. Bankert M. *Watchful Care: A History of American's Nurse Anesthetists.* New York, NY: Continuum; 1989:76.

7. Klein R. Competence, professional self regulation and the public interest. *BMJ.* 1998;316(7146):1740-1742.

8. Tunajek S. Standards of care in anesthesia practice. In Foster S, Faut-Callahan M, eds. *A Professional Study and Resource Guide for the CRNA.* Park Ridge, IL: American Association of Nurse Anesthetists; 2001:256-285.

9. *American Heritage Dictionary of the English Language.* 4th ed. Boston, MA: Houghton Mifflin; 2000.

10. Mantha S, Roizen MF, Fleischer LA, Thisted R, Foss J. Comparing methods of clinical measurement: reporting standards for Bland and Altman analysis. *Anesth Analg.* 2000;90(3):593-602.

11. Stobo J, Blank L. *Project Professionalism: Staying Ahead of the Wave.* Philadelphia, PA: American Board of Internal Medicine; 1998:1-3.

12. Sackett DL, Rosenberg WM, Gray JA, Haynes RB, Richardson WS. Evidence based medicine: what it is and what it isn't. *BMJ.* 1996;312(7023):71-72.

13. Wilensky GR. Developing a center for comparative effectiveness information. *Health Aff.* 2006;25(6):w572-w585.

14. Chalkidou K, Tunis S, Lopert R, et al. Comparative effectiveness research and evidence-based health policy: experience from four countries. *Milbank Q.* 2009;87(2):339-367.

15. Naik AD, Petersen LA. The neglected purpose of comparative-effectiveness research. *N Engl J Med.* 2009;360(19):1929-1931.

16. American Recovery and Reinvestment Act of 2009 (ARRA) Pub L 111-5.

17. Institute of Medicine Committee on Quality of Health Care in America. *Crossing the Quality Chasm: A New Health System for the 21st Century.* Washington, DC: National Academies Press; 2001.

18. Sackett DL, Straus SE, Richardson WS, Rosenberg W, Hayes RB. *Evidence-based Medicine: How to Practice and Teach EBM.* 2nd ed. London, UK: Churchill Livingstone; 2000.

19. Myles PS, Bain DL, Johnson F, McMahon R. Is anaesthesia evidence-based? A survey of anaesthetic practice. *Br J Anaesth.* 1999;82(4):591-595.

20. Pronovost PJ, Berenholtz SM, Dorman T, Merritt WT, Martinez EA, Guyatt GH. Evidence-based medicine in anesthesiology. *Anesth Analg.* 2001;92(3):787-794.

21. Tramer MR. *Evidence-Based Resource in Anaesthesia and Analgesia.* London, UK: BMJ Books; 2000.

22. Grol R, Grimshaw J. From best evidence to best practice: effective implementation of change in patient's care. *Lancet.* 2003;362(9391):1225-1230.

23. Leape LL, Rogers G, Hanna D, et al. Developing and implementing new safe practices: voluntary adoption through statewide collaboratives. *Qual Saf Health Care.* 2006; 15(4):289-295.

24. Haynes B, Haines A. Barriers and bridges to evidence-based clinical practice. *BMJ.* 1998;317(7153):273-276.

25. Retsas A. Barriers to using research evidence in nursing practice. *J Adv Nurs.* 2000;31(3):599-606.

172

26. National Quality Forum. *Safe Practices for Better Healthcare: Summary: A Consensus Report.* Rockville, MD: Agency for Healthcare Research and Quality; 2006. http://www.ahrq.gov/qual/nqfpract.htm. Accessed May 8, 2009.

27. Clancy CM, Slutsky JR. Advancing excellence in health care: getting to effectiveness. *J Invest Med.* 2005; 53(2):65-66.

28. Tunajek SK. Professional standards and public accountability. *AANA J.* 2006;74(1):25-27.

29. Blumenreich GA. The standard of care. *AANA J.* 1991;59(4):302-304.

30. Editorial. *AANA J.* 1974;42(2):95,154.

31. American Association of Nurse Anesthetists. *Professional Practice Manual for the Certified Registered Nurse Anesthetist.* Park Ridge, IL: AANA; 2007.

32. Pawlson LG, O'Kane ME. Professionalism, regulation and the market: impact on accountability for quality of care. *Health Aff.* 2002;21(3):200-207.

33. Epstein RM, Hundert EM. Defining and assessing professional competence. *JAMA.* 2002;287(2):226-235.

34. van der Vleuten CP, Schuwirth LW. Assessing professional competence: from methods to programmes. *Med Educ.* 2005;39(3):309-317.

35. Corrigan JM, Burstin H. Measuring quality of performance: where is it headed, and who is making the decisions? *J Fam Pract.* 2007;56(10 suppl A):4A-7A.

36. Timmermans S, Mauck A. The promises and pitfalls of evidence-based medicine. *Health Aff.* 2008;24(1):18-28.

37. Mant J. Process versus outcome indicators in the assessment of quality of health care. *Int J Qual Health Care.* 2001;13(6):475-481.

38. Eichhorn J, Cooper J, Cullen D, Maier W, Philip J, Seeman R. Standards for patient monitoring during anesthesia at Harvard Medical School. *JAMA.* 1986;256(8):1017-1020.

39. Serious Reportable Events in Healthcare: A Consensus Report. The National Forum for Healthcare Quality Measurement and Reporting. 2002. http://www.qualityforum.org/pdf/news/prSeriousReportableEvents10-15-06.pdf. Accessed April 15, 2010.

40. Medicare Prescription Drug, Improvement, and Modernization Act (MMA) of 2003. Pub L No. 108-173, 117 Stat 2066.

41. Sox HC. The ethical foundations of professionalism: a sociologic history. *Chest.* 2007;131(5):1532-1540.

173

Study Questions

1. Healthcare policy discussions are moving toward evidence-based comparative effectiveness. Discuss professional responsibility for the development of standards of care, including reasons why professions will most likely continue to develop standards.

2. Evidence-based practice has increasingly influenced decision making in patient care. Describe the implications for dissemination of new standards to the nurse anesthesia professionals.

3. Evidence-based outcomes support documentation of practitioner competency. Describe mechanisms for measurement of competency currently incorporated into practice.

4. Practice standards and guidelines best serve the public health and the nursing profession when developed by clinicians in the discipline of nursing. Why?

5. Clinical practice guidelines appear to be effective tools, in part, to ensure quality of care. Outline the main components of a clinical practice guideline. How is it different from standards?

6. Evidence-based standard development and adoption is focused on implementation mechanisms. What are the primary strategies for implementation?

CHAPTER 8

Credentialing and Privileging in Clinical Practice

Jeanne Learman, CRNA, MS

Key Concepts

- Credentialing and privileging of Certified Registered Nurse Anesthetists (CRNAs) and others who provide healthcare with a high level of autonomy help assure the public that there is a process of self-regulation to promote safe patient care.

- Credentialing includes verifying that the applicant meets initial educational requirements for licensing and the profession, checking current licenses and certifications for the states of practice, and assessing current clinical competencies.

- CRNA credentialing may be accomplished through 2 different pathways: through human resources (usually used for employees) or through the medical staff office as an allied health provider (usually used for contracted CRNAs).

- The awarding of specific clinical privileges for CRNAs is typically part of credentialing as allied health providers. As a patient protection, clinical privileges should accurately reflect current competencies. For the CRNA, similar to medical staff, clinical privileges may be considered a "property right."

- All CRNAs should maintain their own credentialing file.

Continues on next page.

Key Concepts (continued)

- Healthcare entities must query the National Practitioner Data Bank (NPDB) when granting and renewing privileges. The NPDB receives reports about payments made for medical malpractice, and these reports may have an impact on a healthcare facility's recredentialing decisions.

- The credentialing process may help the profession by promoting order, consistency, and control in the practice of nurse anesthesia.

Purposes of the credentialing and privileging process include assuring the public that there is self-regulation of the medical staff and other individuals who provide healthcare with a high level of autonomy, and bringing "order, consistency, and control"[1] to the profession. The credentialing process should look at education, experience, and skill. Hravnak,[2] points out that professionally imposed regulations can increase the validity of practice through peer review, ensure public safety, and limit practice by unqualified individuals.

Inherent in the concept of awarding privileges, but difficult to quantify, is an expectation of professionalism. Practitioners are expected to demonstrate behaviors that reflect a commitment to continual professional development, ethical practice, an understanding and sensitivity to diversity, and a responsible attitude toward their patients, their profession, and society.

Before 1975, hospital leaders, attorneys, third-party payers, the medical-legal environment, and regulatory agencies such as the Joint Commission were barely concerned with the issue of medical staff credentialing. In fact, physicians were generally given lifetime privileges. In contrast, today's hospital medical staffs find themselves involved in increasing numbers of interdepartmental credentialing issues for a number of reasons: the medical-legal environment has become far more invasive; the Joint Commission has featured the issue of hospital credentialing prominently in the results of its surveys; and the National Committee for Quality Assurance, which accredits HMOs, has required an active credentialing process as a prerequisite of accreditation. In addition, examples of improper or ineffectual credentialing are often discussed in professional circles and sensationalized in the lay media.

As a result of these changes, hospital leaders are challenged to establish corporate policies and procedures that ensure objectivity, consistency, and clinical competence throughout the appointment, privileges delineation, and reappointment process. Hospitals generally accomplish this through medical staff bylaws, governing board bylaws, and/or departmental rules and regulations.

Clinical privileges are the procedures the clinician is qualified and permitted to perform within a healthcare facility. Historically, CRNAs were employed with their responsibilities outlined in a job description or, in many small hospitals, were included as part of the regular medical staff. It was rare to have individual clinical privileges delineated. During the 1980s and 1990s, other mid-level practitioners such as certified nurse practitioners, nurse midwives, and physician assistants have increased in numbers, and most hospitals now have medical staff bylaws that define a category for allied health professionals, which typically includes clinical psychologists, podiatrists, advanced practice nurses, physician assistants, and others whom the medical staff believes are necessary to offer specialized services at their institution. Inherent in the concept of awarding privileges, but more difficult to quantify, is an expectation of professionalism: "Practitioners are expected to demonstrate behaviors that reflect a commitment to continuous professional development, ethical practice, an understanding and sensitivity to diversity, and a responsible attitude toward their patients, their profession, and society."[3]

This increased availability of allied health providers creates many political, legal, and practical questions. Which allied health professionals may have access to the facility? Will there be a different process for

177

employed providers and contracted providers? What is the process for initial credentialing and the process for ongoing monitoring or renewal of privileges? The governing body must approve the categories of allied health providers who are permitted access to the facility and must define the method of evaluating current competency. Whether an allied health provider has access to a hospital or other healthcare facility depends on 2 factors: state law, including the state's licensing act, and the facility's governing body bylaws, rules, and regulations.

Hospital or healthcare facility bylaws may define whether mid-level practitioners will provide services independently to hospital clients or whether they will collaborate with a member of the medical staff. The CRNA may be considered a "licensed independent practitioner" if state regulations (including the nurse practice act and hospital licensing regulations) do not require physician supervision. In reality, attempting to divide practitioners into 2 camps in which some function independently and others must be under supervision obscures the fact that the level of independence of individuals who deliver care, diagnostics, and supportive healthcare services is a continuum. Allied health providers (AHPs) are typically individuals with advanced degrees or training and, although technically unable to function totally independently by law in some states, they practice with independent judgment and decision making, and in reality, the degree of control or supervision exerted by others may be quite limited.

Implications for CRNAs

Currently, a multiplicity of approaches to credentialing CRNAs exists. When CRNAs are hospital employees, their initial verification of credentials and experiences is documented by human resources and the anesthesia department manager. When CRNAs are contracted by the hospital to provide services, they will most likely be required to apply and be credentialed as an AHP, usually through regular medical staff credentialing channels. Individual clinical privileges should be delineated regardless of the contractual or employment relationship that exists within the practice setting. Privileges are granted for a period not to exceed 2 years.

Temporary privileges may be granted for a limited period of time under certain circumstances.[3] The 2 circumstances in which temporary privileges may be granted are: 1) to meet an important patient care need for a specified time period, and 2) for new applicants awaiting review and approval by the organized medical staff. The temporary privileges must be granted by the chief executive officer or designee on the recommendation of the medical staff president or designee and may be granted for no more than 120 days. Before receiving temporary privileges, new applicants must have the following information already submitted: a complete application, current licensure, relevant training or experience, current competence to perform the privileges requested, a query of the National Practitioner Data Bank (NPDB), and no previous limitation or termination of privileges or licensure.

Nurse anesthetists are responsible for seeking clinical privileges that reflect their educational preparation, clinical experience, and level of professional competence. To establish credentials for employees, the hospital should establish an appropriate interface between the credentialing office and human resources. In the absence of a specific privileging process, CRNAs practice according to departmental policy. In some clinical settings, CRNAs' privileges change

---

Table 8.1. Key Points Regarding Level of Autonomy

CRNAs should seek practice settings that offer the desired level of autonomy.

CRNAs should have the educational preparation and the clinical experience to perform the privileges they have requested.

CRNAs should be familiar with the level of autonomy that their practice settings allow, as defined by job descriptions or clinical privileges.

---

on a case-by-case basis according to decisions made by the anesthesiologist providing medical direction. This situation creates confusion for CRNAs, surgeons, and operating room staff and should be avoided if possible. The patient's best interests are served when the CRNA is privileged according to education and experience, not according to departmental control issues.

Nurse anesthetists practice with various levels of autonomy in different practice settings (Table 8.1). For example, in most office settings and small hospital settings, CRNAs autonomously manage the anesthesia care from preanesthesia evaluation through discharge in collaboration with the surgeon. Hospitals do not have to permit CRNAs to do everything they are permitted to do by state statutes,[4] and some hospitals do limit CRNAs' scope of practice. Faut-Callahan[5] states: "It should be noted that no states have nursing rules or regulations that require that nurse anesthetists be supervised by anesthesiologists." Some nurse practice acts or state laws governing healthcare do have statements that indicate that a nurse anesthetist practices under physician supervision or direction. As Blumenreich[6] explains in the article, "The Nature of Supervision" from the *AANA Journal,* it is a term that can have many interpretations, and for CRNAs practicing with surgeons, it is typically a collaborative practice with each bringing their respective skills together for the care of the patient.

In the past, when the CRNA was an employee of a physician group or contracted through a locum tenens agency, many facilities would count on the physician group or locums tenens agency to do the initial credentialing and required only evidence of current licenses, certification, and professional liability to be given to the hospital. The Joint Commission standards regarding primary source verification and hospital liability concerns have changed this approach, and now each hospital does its own credentialing. Traditionally, hospitals were not held accountable for the errors and omissions of credentialed members of the medical staff. Instead, staff members were viewed as independent contractors to patients, using the hospital premises. This assumption has changed as courts have recognized how much authority healthcare entities exert in the selection and retention of members of the medical staff. Thus, liability has been imposed in situations in which a healthcare entity knew or should have known that a clinician was likely to cause injury to patients. Benda and Rozovsky[7] state that "This direct corporate liability for the selection and credentialing of medical staff/allied health providers is likely to force the undeniable conclusion that AHPs must be credentialed." To protect themselves from claims of corporate negligence, hospitals and healthcare facilities may increase their oversight of hiring, credentialing, monitoring, and supervising of AHPs. This is now true whether the AHP is employed by the healthcare facility, contracted, or employed through a physician's group.

The goals of credentialing are laudable, but as Blumenreich[8] points out, "the power to determine in what areas a practitioner may practice and from which areas the practitioner will be excluded *can* be used to benefit *others* besides society and patients." The power to credential can be used to benefit the person granting privileges—usually by limiting the privileges of certain providers. This can be done for purposes of controlling the financial flow of dollars to certain practitioners or simply to remove a competitor.

A healthcare facility must also decide how to provide due process if AHPs are denied access to the hospital or are subjected to disciplinary action. The Joint Commission requires hearing and appeal mechanisms for termination of privileges for licensed independent practitioners defined as "any individual permitted by law and by the hospital to provide patient care services without direction or supervision, within the scope of the individual's license and consistent with individually granted clinical privileges." As Blumenreich[9] explains, "Hospital privileges have been interpreted as establishing that the practitioner has a property right. Ideally, this property right cannot be taken away without due process."

When a hospital or healthcare entity denies privileges or revokes already granted privileges, it becomes a serious issue for CRNAs, because an almost universally asked question on CRNA applications is "Have your privileges ever been denied or revoked?" This can create problems because sometimes the nurse anesthetist may not even be able to find out why his or her privileges were denied.

Blumenreich,[8] legal counsel for the American Association of Nurse Anesthetists, suggests language to use when requesting the hospital to provide a reason for any denial and provide the nurse anesthetist applicant with a chance to present evidence. This may meet with limited success because most hospitals do not extend the same protections to AHP as those required by the Joint Commission 2007 Standards for medical staff. In fact, the Joint Commission Official Handbook[3] states, "The Fair Hearing and Appeal Process for Adverse Privileging Decisions may differ for members and non-members of the medical staff." Medical staff are traditionally given the right to hearings, the right to present evidence, correct accusations, and appeal decisions of the credentialing committee.

Initial Credentialing

The credentialing process (Figure 8.1), while striving to meet the same goals of ensuring competent providers for patient safety, may differ from one facility to another. In fact, key points in Joint Commission recommendations for credentialing state: "The organization establishes hospital specific mechanisms for appointment of medical staff/allied medical staff members, and for granting and renewing or revising specific clinical privileges. These mechanisms may differ for medical staff members and other individuals."[3] For the hospital-employed CRNA, the human resources department and anesthesia department determine that initial requirements for education, licensing, certification, and experience have been met. The anesthesia department director assesses whether the CRNA has the required competencies to meet the needs of the anesthesia department.

The procedures for credentialing CRNAs may follow the procedures for medical

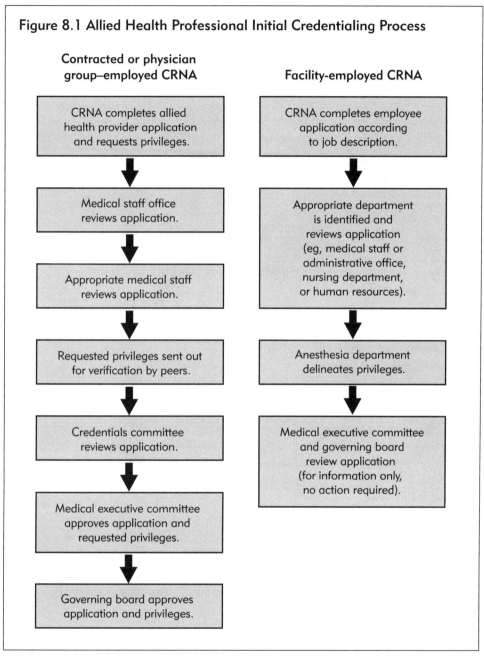

Figure 8.1 Allied Health Professional Initial Credentialing Process

Contracted or physician group–employed CRNA

CRNA completes allied health provider application and requests privileges.

↓

Medical staff office reviews application.

↓

Appropriate medical staff reviews application.

↓

Requested privileges sent out for verification by peers.

↓

Credentials committee reviews application.

↓

Medical executive committee approves application and requested privileges.

↓

Governing board approves application and privileges.

Facility-employed CRNA

CRNA completes employee application according to job description.

↓

Appropriate department is identified and reviews application (eg, medical staff or administrative office, nursing department, or human resources).

↓

Anesthesia department delineates privileges.

↓

Medical executive committee and governing board review application (for information only, no action required).

CRNAs must adhere to specific credentialing/verification process as outlined in the governing board or medical staff bylaws, rules and regulations, or policies and procedures, or use the procedures above.

181

staff membership or reappointment. Ideally, the process includes an application specifically tailored to reflect the qualifications of a CRNA and the privileges applicable to their practice (Figure 8.2); however, some hospitals prefer to use a uniform credentialing application for all medical and allied health staff.

Figure 8.2. Sample Letter for Credentialing or Recredentialing a CRNA

Hospital Address:_____

The following CRNA has applied for allied medical staff privileges:_____
Please complete the following questionnaire:

Do you have direct knowledge of this applicant's current level of skill and knowledge?
_____ yes _____ no

1. If so, for how long? from _____ to _____
    Please comment: _____
    Dates of affiliation with _____Hospital:_____ to _____

2. In your opinion, is the applicant's current and overall competence:
    _____ less than adequate _____ competent _____ above average
    If less than adequate, please explain: _____

3. Would you be willing to have this applicant participate in the clinical care and
    management of yourself or your family? _____ yes _____ no

4. Does the applicant have the ability to work cooperatively in a setting with all members
    of the interdisciplinary team? _____ yes _____ no

5. Are the applicant's ethical standards in conformance with the ethical standards
    maintained by the other members of your professional staff? _____ yes _____ no

6. If the answer to questions 3, 4, or 5 was no, please explain:

    _____

    _____

7. Does the applicant have any mental or physical problems or disabilities that, to your
    knowledge, would prevent him or her from adequately performing clinical duties?
    _____ yes _____ no

8. Has the applicant ever been the subject of any disciplinary action to your knowledge?
    _____ no _____ yes

9. Has the applicant, to your knowledge, ever had his or her membership, status, and/or
    clinical privileges revoked, suspended, reduced, or not renewed in any facility?
    _____ yes _____ no

10. To your knowledge, has this applicant's license and/or certification to practice in any
    jurisdiction ever been suspended or terminated? _____ no _____ yes

11. If the answer to question 7, 8, 9, or 10 was yes, please explain:_____

    _____

Additional Comments:

_____

                                              Signature:_____
                                                  Title:_____
                                              Address:_____

Clinical Privileges

The American Association of Nurse Anesthetists (AANA) has developed a document titled Guidelines for Core Clinical Privileges. This document is a valuable guide to hospitals establishing allied medical staff privileges for CRNAs because it includes a CRNA-specific application form and a listing of anesthesia privileges. It is included in the *Professional Practice Manual for the Certified Registered Nurse Anesthetist.*[10] Nurse anesthetists are most knowledgeable of the educational requirements and clinical practices of their profession and should take a leadership role in developing the experience requirements and definitions of privileges for their profession.

Privileges should be appropriate to the scope and complexity of care provided by CRNAs and should not be overly specific or restrictive (Table 8.2). Clinical privileging should be so defined as to permit CRNAs to provide selected procedures under specific conditions with or without supervision. The clinical privileging process includes checking the qualifications of the provider; confirming current licenses, education, and competence; reviewing the actual practice privileges requested and granted; determining the conditions or limits of practice; and establishing the process for evaluation and renewal of privileges.

Sample Grouping of Privileges for CRNAs

Hospitals have used many different formats to award privileges to CRNAs. I have found it useful to use the following distinctions in our community hospital:

Core Privileges include the skills that are mandatory for a CRNA to practice appropriately in a specific clinical setting. For example, in our hospital, spinal anesthesia is a part of core privileges.

Special Privileges include skills that may be appropriate for some CRNAs based on experience but not for other CRNAs. Some examples include thoracic epidural, continuous femoral pain block, and placement of central or arterial lines.

Emergency Privileges recognize that occasionally circumstances may occur that require the use of skills that are not a regular part of a CRNA's practice. The following is a sample statement for emergency privileges, which CRNAs may be given as part of the privilege application:

> I also understand that it is not necessary to request emergency clinical privileges. An emergency is deemed to exist whenever serious permanent harm or aggravation of injury or disease is imminent, the life of a patient is in immediate danger, or any delay in administering treatment could add to that danger. In such an emergency, I am authorized and will assist to do everything possible to save the patient's life or to save the patient from serious harm, to the degree permitted by my license, but regardless of department affiliation, staff category or level of privileges. If I provide services to a patient in an emergency, I am obligated to utilize appropriate consultative assistance when available and arrange for appropriate follow-up care as soon as possible.

The preceding paragraph was crafted based on The Joint Commission Standard MS.4.100, Temporary Privileges, which states "Medical staff bylaws or other documents may stipulate that in an emergency, any medical staff member with clinical privileges is permitted to provide any type of patient care, treatment, and services necessary as a life-saving measure or to prevent serious

Table 8.2. Guidelines for Core Clinical Privileges[10]

CRNA privileges and responsibilities must be consistent with law and may, without limitation, include the following:

Preanesthetic Preparation and Evaluation
- Obtaining an appropriate health history.
- Conducting an appropriate physical screening assessment.
- Recommending or requesting and evaluating pertinent diagnostic studies.
- Selecting, obtaining, ordering, and administering pre-anesthetic medications.
- Documenting the pre-anesthetic evaluation and obtaining informed consent for anesthesia, anesthesia induction, maintenance, and emergence.

Intraoperative Care
- Obtaining, preparing, and using all equipment, monitors, supplies and drugs used for the administration of anesthesia, performing and ordering safety checks as needed.
- Selecting, obtaining or administering the anesthetics, adjuvant drugs, accessory drugs, fluids and blood products necessary to manage the anesthetic.
- Performing all aspects of airway management, including fiberoptic intubation.
- Performing and managing regional anesthetic techniques including, but not limited to: subarachnoid, epidural and caudal blocks; plexus, major and peripheral nerve blocks; intravenous regional anesthesia; transtracheal, topical and local infiltration blocks; intracapsular, intercostal and ocular blocks.
- Providing appropriate invasive and non-invasive monitoring modalities utilizing current standards and techniques.
- Recognizing abnormal patient response during anesthesia, selecting and implementing corrective action and requesting consultation whenever necessary.
- Evaluating patient response during emergence from anesthesia and instituting pharmacological or supportive treatment to insure patient stability during transfer.

Postanesthesia Care
- Providing postanesthesia follow-up and evaluation of the patient's response to anesthesia and surgical experience, taking appropriate corrective actions and requesting consultation when indicated.
- Initiating and administering respiratory support to insure adequate ventilation and oxygenation in the postanesthesia period.
- Initiating and administering pharmacological or fluid support of the cardiovascular system during the postanesthesia period to prevent morbidity and mortality.
- Initiating acute postanesthesia pain management techniques.
- Discharging patients from a postanesthesia care area. according to facility policy.

Continues on page 185.

harm—regardless of his or her medical staff status or clinical privileges—provided that the care, treatment and services provided are within the scope of the individual's license"[11]

Nonclinical responsibilities may also be included in the privileges list but are most often part of a job description or part of a contract. These may include responsibilities related to administration, management,

---

Table 8.2. Guidelines for Core Clinical Privileges[10] (continued)

Clinical Support Functions
- Inserting peripheral and central intravenous catheters.
- Inserting pulmonary artery catheters.
- Inserting arterial catheters and performing arterial puncture to obtain arterial blood samples.
- Managing emergency situations, including initiating or participating in cardiopulmonary resuscitation.
- Providing consultation and implementation of respiratory and ventilatory care.
- Management of interventional pain therapy utilizing drugs, regional anesthetic techniques or other accepted pain relief modalities.
- Using consultation when appropriate, selecting, obtaining, ordering and/or administering medications or treatments related to the care of the patient.
- Accepting additional responsibilities which are within the expertise of the individual CRNA and appropriate to the practice setting.

(Reprinted with permission from the AANA.)

scheduling, policy development, quality assessment, problem solving, committee meetings, educational activities for students and operating room staff, research projects, and interdepartmental liaisons.

Primary Source Verification

The medical staff credentialing and privileging path is more complex and includes requirements that are not in the human resources path. An example is that the medical staff standards require primary source verification of education and training:[3] "Current licensure and/or certification verified with the primary source" and "The applicants' specific relevant training, verified with the primary source." This requirement for primary source verification was instituted by the Joint Commission in 1988 and eliminated the physician or AHP as the intermediary to transmit the credentials, documents, or experience. The purpose of primary source verification is to reduce the possibility of forgery or falsification of credentials. Hospitals cannot accept material in the possession of medical staff applicants as sufficient evidence of credentials. Thus,

credentials committees will require original letters of reference, request transcripts directly from colleges, and call the state board of nursing instead of accepting photocopies. Hospitals may still request photocopies of documents such as licenses and diplomas in the credentialing verification process. Credentialing verifications are now available online through the American Association of Nurse Anesthetists website. The following information may be verified for CRNAs: 1) date of initial certification, 2) name of the nurse anesthesia educational program completed, and 3) recertification dates. This information is updated each night at midnight by the Council on Certification of Nurse Anesthetists and the Council on Recertification of Nurse Anesthetists.[12] In an effort to establish that they have used due diligence to verify an applicant's experience, many hospitals contact all past employers and/or practice settings for the previous 3 to 5 years. Because of this need for primary source verification, there are a number of things applicants can do to help the credentialing process go more quickly and smoothly (Table 8.3). With the

185

Table 8.3. Suggestions for Facilitation of the Credentialing Process

- Provide complete addresses for all educational institutions and practice sites.
- List a key contact person for each practice site (department manager or former colleague).
- If your work at the hospital was through an agency, provide the agency name, address, and phone number.
- Contact the colleagues you list as references and let them know a timely response will be appreciated.
- If the facility will allow you to assist in getting references, sending a structured reference letter (See Figure 8.2) may encourage a more rapid reply. Enclose a stamped envelope, preaddressed to the medical staff coordinator at the facility where you are applying for privileges.
- When selecting references, choose people who are familiar with your skills and patient outcomes, such as CRNAs, anesthesiologists, surgeons, and administrators.

---

recent attention to credentialing and increased numbers of HMOs and hospital mergers, requirements of the credentialing process have put additional strain on medical staff coordinators and the physicians and allied health providers who must provide ever more information (Table 8.4). A cooperative attitude is essential. Efforts in making the credentialing process go smoothly for the medical staff coordinator will most likely be rewarded by return cooperation when assistance is needed with policy changes or educational endeavors.

Occasionally it is not possible to contact primary sources, such as when the anesthesia program has closed. In this situation, the Joint Commission has allowed that reliable secondary sources may be used.[11]

National Practitioner Data Bank

Hospitals and other credentialing bodies must query the National Practitioner Data Bank (NPDB) when granting and renewing privileges. Reports are made to, and obtained from, the NPDB regarding claims of medical malpractice against healthcare practitioners. Congress voted the NPDB into existence with the federal Health Care Quality Improvement Act of 1986[13] with the purpose of restricting the ability of incompetent physicians and other healthcare providers to move from state to state without disclosure or discovery of the practitioners' previous damaging or incompetent performance. The NPDB receives information about 5 different types of actions taken against practitioners: 1) malpractice payments made for the benefit of physicians, dentists, and other healthcare practitioners, 2) licensure actions taken by state medical boards and state boards of dentistry against physicians and dentists, 3) professional review actions primarily taken against physicians and dentists by hospitals and other healthcare entities including HMOs, group practices, and professional societies, 4) actions taken by the Drug Enforcement Administration (DEA), and 5) Medicare/Medicaid Exclusions.

In 2005, the NPDB received 17,298 medical malpractice payment reports and 6,302 adverse action reports.[14] As Kremer and Faut-Callahan[15] note, "A limitation of NPDB information is that malpractice payments recorded in the NPDB do not necessarily constitute a comprehensive and definitive reflection of actual health

---

Table 8.4. What CRNAs Should Maintain in Their Own Credentials File

- Nursing and anesthesia program addresses, transcripts, and diplomas

- Resume or curriculum vitae

- Practice sites with *dates*—regularly updated

- Registered nurse licenses

- Certification and recertification certificates

- Specialty certification (if applicable in your state)

- Basic cardiac life support and advanced cardiac life support documentation

- Letters of reference from colleagues who practice with you

- Transcript of continuing education hours

- Immunization status documentation for hepatitis B virus

- Tuberculin test results

- Professional liability insurance policy documentation

- List of appropriate clinical privileges

---

care incompetence." As discussed by Metter, Granville, and Kussman,[16] the NPDB practice of using claims payment as an indicator of substandard care results in significant inaccuracies, because about 30% of claims with substandard care are not paid and will not be reported to the NPDB. The Data Bank cannot alter a report once it has been entered, but the subject of the report may review it and add a clarifying statement. After a practitioner's statement is added to the NPDB file, it will be sent to all hospitals or other healthcare entities who query the NPDB. There is also a process to follow if the subject of a report wishes to dispute the factual accuracy of the report. CRNAs should be aware of the reporting requirements of the NPDB, its potential impact on their ability to be credentialed, and their right to enter an explanation regarding a claim.

Assessment of Continued Competency/Recredentialing

Periodic reevaluation is necessary to satisfy the Joint Commission and requirements for institutional licensing. The recredentialing decision is based partly on updating qualifications, but should be primarily on information about performance.

Written evidence of continued competency (Figure 8.3) for the employed CRNA will generally be summarized in an annual review completed by a hospital-employed

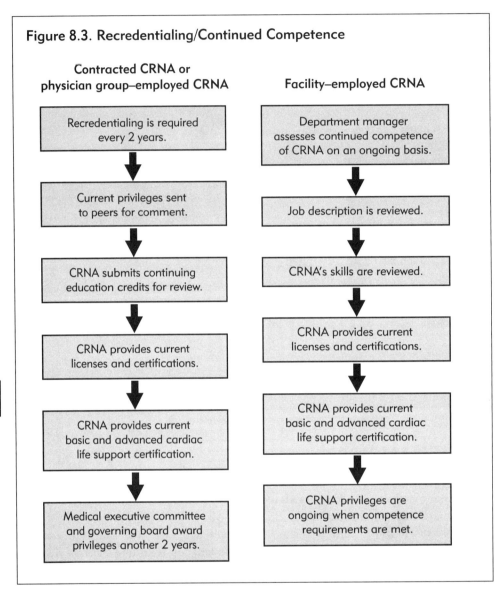

Figure 8.3. Recredentialing/Continued Competence

Contracted CRNA or physician group–employed CRNA

- Recredentialing is required every 2 years.
- Current privileges sent to peers for comment.
- CRNA submits continuing education credits for review.
- CRNA provides current licenses and certifications.
- CRNA provides current basic and advanced cardiac life support certification.
- Medical executive committee and governing board award privileges another 2 years.

Facility–employed CRNA

- Department manager assesses continued competence of CRNA on an ongoing basis.
- Job description is reviewed.
- CRNA's skills are reviewed.
- CRNA provides current licenses and certifications.
- CRNA provides current basic and advanced cardiac life support certification.
- CRNA privileges are ongoing when competence requirements are met.

manager or, for the physician group–employed CRNA, by physicians in the group. A determination of current competencies may include demonstrations of knowledge of cardiorespiratory resuscitation and other emergency procedures, use of anesthesia and emergency equipment, and review of specific skills, (eg, arterial line placement). Requests for renewal of specific anesthesia privileges should be based on the CRNA's education, training, experience, demonstrated ability, and judgment. Requests for new privileges may be awarded after documentation of education and observed skills (Figure 8.4). Results of quality improvement studies should be considered. Patient satisfaction surveys can help in the recredentialing process but should not be the sole resource of measuring quality patient care.

For the contracted CRNA or physician group–employed CRNA with allied health

Figure 8.4. Application for Clinical Privileges Form

APPLICATION FOR CLINICAL PRIVILEGES

CLINICAL PRIVILEGES DELINEATION FORM

Type of Request: ☐ Initial   ☐ Renewal

Category: Certified Registered Nurse Anesthetist

Soc. Sec. # _____

Please check the procedures for which you are making application:

☐ Preanesthetic assessment
☐ Requesting laboratory/diagnostic studies
☐ Preanesthetic medication
☐ General anesthesia and adjuvant drugs
☐ Regional anesthesia techniques
    ☐ Subarachnoid
    ☐ Epidural
    ☐ Caudal
    ☐ Upper extremity
    ☐ Lower extremity
    ☐ Diagnostic and therapeutic nerve blocks
    ☐ Local Infiltration
    ☐ Topical
    ☐ Periocular block
    ☐ Transtracheal
    ☐ Intracapsular
    ☐ Intercostal
    ☐ Other _____

☐ Cardiopulmonary resuscitation management
☐ Perianesthetic invasive and noninvasive monitoring
☐ Tracheal intubation/extubation
☐ Mechanical ventilation/oxygen therapy
☐ Fluid, electrolyte, acid-base management
☐ Blood, blood products, plasma expanders
☐ Peripheral intravenous/arterial catheter placement
☐ Central venous catheter placement
☐ Pulmonary artery catheter placement
☐ Acute and chronic pain therapy
☐ Post anesthesia care/discharge
☐ Conscious and deep sedation techniques
☐ Perianesthesia management of patient using accessory drugs or fluids.
☐ Other _____

I am mentally and physically capable of performing the privileges which I have requested:

Signature_____ Date _____

Name (Please print) _____

The above nurse anesthetist is granted the full privileges which he/she has requested with the following exceptions, and/or limitations (if none, so state).

Decision: ☐ Approval   ☐ Disapproval

Signature, Chief Nurse Anesthetist _____

Signature, Medical Director _____

Signature, Director, Medical/Professional Staff Office_____

Date Practitioner Notified:_____

These privileges are granted initially for one calendar year following approval and must be renewed on a biennial basis. The applicant may request to have privileges changed as required during this period.

(Reprinted with permission from the AANA.)

189

provider status at the hospital, written evidence of continued competency will usually be assessed every 2 years. This privilege reappointment process may ask 2 or 3 colleagues familiar with the CRNA's work to verify the CRNA's continued qualifications for a specific list of privileges and attest to the CRNA's continued competence by completing a letter of reference similar to that in Figure 8.5. The Joint Commission standards recommend quality improvement and risk management data be considered as part of the reappointment process. Responsibility

for the assessment and improvement of clinical processes and patient outcomes are characteristics of professional work, and CRNA involvement in these activities will be scrutinized. The documentation of unusual or unexpected anesthesia events on all anesthetics is one way to assess continued competency. This approach allows for the identification of providers who are having the same problems (eg, difficult airway management or hypotension) and allows for an evaluation of management and outcome of the anesthesia event. It is possible

---

Figure 8.5. New Anesthesia Clinical Privileges Form

Anesthesia Provider: _____

New Privilege Requested: _____

Didactic review: (articles, lectures, and audio or video tapes)

_____

_____

Clinical experience: Date: Observed By:

_____   _____   _____

_____   _____   _____

_____   _____   _____

_____   _____   _____

Approved by: _____   Date: _____

Director of Anesthesia

---

that in the future, a more active recredentialing will be required, such as skills verification by simulator testing.

Some hospitals require a 50% or 60% attendance rate at medical staff meetings for active medical staff. This requirement rarely extends to the AHPs, but CRNAs will find time spent attending medical staff meetings to be insightful in understanding the concerns of medical staff relative to the anesthesia services. Your presence means you will help develop policies for anesthesia delivery and be able to educate the medical staff about CRNA practice. Committees (eg, cardiopulmonary rescuscitation, infection control, conscious sedation, and obstetrics) will develop policies that have an impact on CRNA practice. Nurse anesthetists serving on these committees have found them an important way to influence hospital policy, provide education to nursing staff, and create positive relationships for CRNAs throughout the hospital.

It is beyond the minimum requirements for credentialing and a mark of excellence to take an active part in identifying and maintaining the qualifications and competencies necessary to provide anesthesia care for your patient group. For example, if the hospital adds trauma care, open heart surgery, pain management, or a labor epidural service, the professional CRNA should take an active role in establishing reliable competencies. In addition to patient care, the recredentialing process typically includes an assessment of the CRNA's documentation, teamwork, and personal accountability.

Nonmedical Issues in Credentialing

Practitioners should be evaluated on criteria that are directly related to patient care and the practitioner's ability to perform the requested privileges. If practitioners are disciplined, it will usually be because of problems that directly affect the quality of care provided.

However, as Lansberg[19] points out, both state and federal courts have upheld decisions by healthcare entities to exclude or discipline a physician for reasons not directly related to patient care. These include:

1. Giving incomplete or false information on the application form
2. Unfavorable reports or references from other facilities including those related to attitude and personality problems
3. Violation of bylaws or rules, such as refusing, even after warning, to follow hospital criteria for performing a particular procedure or refusing to accept every third indigent OB/GYN patient who comes to the hospital
4. Disruptive behavior or inability to work with others, for example, dealing with hospital staff in a volatile, hostile, and uncooperative manner
5. Refusal to execute a release for a transfer of information from another hospital
6. Physician's termination for alcohol abuse
7. Criminal conduct, for example, a conviction of driving while intoxicated, second offense
8. Economic criteria such as termination of a radiologist's privileges based on his or her refusal to sign employment contracts with the physician who was awarded an exclusive contract
9. Noncompliance with bylaws provisions such as those that specify the conditions under which a medical staff member or allied healthcare provider may request a leave of absence and detail the procedure for a reinstatement of privileges

Credentials Verification Organizations

Although hospitals cannot accept evidence of credentials carried by applicants, they may rely on other organizations to conduct primary source verification. Credentials verification organizations (CVOs) acting as agents have started up all over the country, many of them managed by hospital and physician associations. For example, the Michigan Professional Credential Verification Services, Inc, was started as a joint venture of the Michigan Hospital Association and the Michigan State Medical Society. Managed care organizations have contributed to the growth of CVOs because a typical managed care organization will enroll several hundred practitioners and the burden of credentialing could be enormous. Once a CVO checks a practitioner's credentials, it does not need to check them again when another hospital requests credentialing (within a reasonable time frame). This reduces the cost and time required for credentialing and reduces the number of inquiries that agencies issuing the credentials must handle.

In 2008, an example of CVO fees were $100 per physician or allied health provider for credentialing and $55 for recredentialing. In an effort to reduce their costs for credentialing, some health systems are establishing an area-wide approach to credentialing with a uniform application package that, when completed, may be mailed to each healthcare facility at which a practitioner is requesting initial or renewal privileges. The National Committee for Quality Assurance certifies some CVOs. This reduces the oversight required by the healthcare facility using the CVO.

Trends

Using the services of AHPs can maximize the opportunities for hospitals, healthcare systems, and physician group practices to maintain quality of care and patient satisfaction while increasing the level of service and reducing costs. Market forces continue to change our healthcare delivery systems, including *where* care is delivered (outpatient clinics and offices), and *who* is providing the care. Many observers of evolving healthcare market forces believe that AHPs will play an ever-increasing and important role in healthcare. AHPs can help accomplish the goals of the new healthcare environment, which are to deliver health services differently using fewer resources yet maintaining quality outcome and customer satisfaction. "You can be a victor over change or a victim of change. Set up a training program in your mind and make sure your top employee (you!) is updating his or her skills."[18]

Summary

The public expects (and increasingly demands through litigation) that hospitals and healthcare entities have mechanisms in place to screen the providers who care for them. The Joint Commission, as an external regulatory agency, presents itself to the public as the group that will assess whether hospitals have appropriate mechanisms to review the credentials of physicians, AHPs, and employees. Approximately 15,000 healthcare organizations and programs report to their local communities that they are accountable to the public because they have met Joint Commission recommendations assessed during an on-site visit.[19] Hospitals are increasingly using CVOs to provide primary source verification of data required to credential medical and allied health providers. One factor spurring this change is the merger of many large hospitals and managed care systems, which has necessitated the processing of large numbers of new medical staff simultaneously.

Although The Joint Commission requires physician members of the medical staff to be credentialed and privileged, hospitals may choose to verify the CRNA credentials through 1 of 2 mechanisms: the human resources department, or AHPs' credentialing. Employed CRNAs' qualifications are processed by human resources. In addition, employees may go through allied medical staff credentialing.

The process to award specific clinical privileges is always part of AHPs' credentialing and may or may not be implemented for employed CRNAs. The credentialing and privileging process should provide an objective mechanism for initial application and renewal of clinical privileges based on education, experience, legal qualifications, and a practitioner's competence and ability to render quality care. There is substantial evidence that many CRNAs' privileges are restricted not by initial training or experience, but by medical staff bylaws or by the employing or supervising physician anesthesiologist group.

Healthcare attorneys and risk managers are encouraging hospitals to use the allied health providers' credentials verification process to credential all mid-level providers, (eg, advanced practice nurses, physician assistants, physical therapists, psychologists, podiatrists, and chiropractors). They recommend that hospitals may gain some legal protection by regular recredentialing of providers who exercise a high level of independent decision making in the provision of patient care and providing similar due process rights as are customarily afforded medical staff.

All CRNAs should be prepared for the potential changes to the AHPs credentialing and clinical privileges process by maintaining their own credential file. Credentialing verifications are now available on the American Association of Nurse Anesthetists website. The following information can be verified: date of initial certification, name of the nurse anesthesia educational program completed, and recertification dates.

References

1. Affara F. The fundamentals of professional regulation. *Int Nurs Rev.* 39 (4):113-116.

2. Hravnak M. Credentialing and privileging: insight into the process for acute-care nurse practitioners. *AACN Clin Issues.* 8(1):108-115.

3. *Comprehensive Accreditation Manual for Hospitals: The Official Handbook.* Oakbrook Terrace, IL: Joint Commission. 2007: CAMH Update 1, March 2007:MS-16.

4. Blackmond B. Risk management and allied health professionals. *NAMSS Overview.* 1997:21-24.

5. Faut-Callahan M. Credentialing of CRNAs. *Adv Pract Nurs Q.* 1998:54-62.

6. Blumenreich G. The nature of supervision. *AANA J.* 1997;165(3):208-211.

7. Benda GC, Rozovsky FA. *Managed Care and the Law: Liability and Risk Management.* Boston, MA: Little, Brown and Company; 1996.

8. Blumenreich G. Fairness in credentialing and the Certified Registered Nurse Anesthetist. *AANA J.* 2002; 70(5):347-351.

9. Blumenreich G. Hospital privileges. *AANA J.* 1990;58(1):66-68.

193

10. American Association of Nurse Anesthetists. Guidelines for Core Clinical Privileges. *The Professional Practice Manual for the Certified Registered Nurse Anesthetist.* Park Ridge, IL: American Association of Nurse Anesthetists:1-4.

11. *Comprehensive Accreditation Manual for Hospitals.* Oakbrook Terrace, IL: Joint Commission; 2007:MS-27

12. National Board of Certification and Recertification for Nurse Anesthetists website. http:www.nbcrna.com. Accessed August 4, 2008.

13. Health Care Quality Improvement Act of 1986. 42 USC §11101.

14. National Practitioner Databank. Healthcare Integrity and Protection Databank. http://www.npdb-hipdb.hrsa.gov/annualrpt.html. Accessed May 8, 2008.

15. Kremer M, Faut-Callahan M. The national practitioner data bank: implications for nurse anesthetists. *CRNA.* 1998;9(4):157-162.

16. Metter EJ, Granville RL, Kussman MJ. The effect of threshold amounts for reporting malpractice payments to the National Practitioners Data Bank: analysis using the closed claims data of the office of the assistant secretary of defense (health affairs). *Mil Med.* 1997;162(4):257-261.

17. Landsberg B. Physician integrity and other non-medical issues in credentialing. Lecture presented at the national health lawyers' association conference. March 12-14, 1997.

18. Waitley D. Personal coach. *Priorities.* 1999;3(5):30-32.

19. Facts About the Joint Commission. http://www.jointcommission.org/AboutUs/Fact_Sheets/joint_commission_facts.htm. Accessed February 18, 2010.

Key References

1. Health Resources Services Administration. US Department of Health and Human Services. National Practitioner Data Bank Guidebook.

2. Learman J, Loppnow N. Credentialing of CRNAs: time for a new look. *AANA J.* 1997;65(3):228-234.

194

Study Questions

1. Define credentialing and privileging and describe the typical process CRNAs follow in securing both as requirements for practice.

2. Discuss the reasons why credentialing and privileging are increasingly important both to the facilities that employ CRNAs as well as to a CRNA's scope of practice.

3. Discuss the intended purpose of the National Practitioner Data Bank and how CRNAs are affected by it.

4. Describe why it is important for CRNAs to maintain their own credentialing file and what should become a part of the file.

195

CHAPTER 9
Evidence-Based Practice and the CRNA

Michael J. Kremer, CRNA, PhD, FAAN

Key Concepts

- Certified Registered Nurse Anesthetists (CRNAs) are adopting the principles of evidence-based practice advocated by the Institute of Medicine.

- Nurse anesthesia education and practice reflects patient-centric care, delivered by an interdisciplinary team.

- Nurse anesthetists use the best evidence when planning and implementing anesthesia care.

- Nurse anesthetists are committed to quality improvement and use of data to improve practice and education.

- Anesthesia practice involves competencies in technology and informatics. CRNAs use information systems to support and improve patient care. Nurse anesthetists critically evaluate clinical and research databases used as clinical decision support resources.

New clinical information develops more quickly than its rate of assimilation by trainees and practicing clinicians. Certified Registered Nurse Anesthetists (CRNAs), students, and faculty need the most current information regarding healthcare and anesthetic interventions. This information need is pressing for student registered nurse anesthetists because they are rapidly learning complex specialty-related concepts and must be able to objectively justify clinical decisions to their faculty.[1] Using evidence-based medicine methods helps balance the demand for current information with the burgeoning supply of general and specialty-related research findings.

Evidence-based practice (EBP) has been described as "the integration of individual clinical expertise with the best available external clinical evidence from systematic research."[2] Healthcare professionals may believe that their practices have always reflected EBP, but performance assessments indicate this is not the case.[3] Current literature advocates for increased adoption of EBP, but EBP implementation is inconsistent.

The Institute of Medicine Committee (IOM) on the Health Professions Education Summit suggested a paradigm shift for health professions education. The primary goal of this process is that "all health professionals will be educated to deliver patient-centric care as members of an interdisciplinary team, emphasizing evidence-based practice, quality improvement approaches and informatics."[4] Included in this paradigm shift is movement of healthcare delivery away from the traditional physician-dominated practice toward the concept of the physician as team leader seeking the best evidence for patient care. Ideally, such physicians and teams will have the ability and expectation to continually learn and change, through use of evidence-based clinical decision support, informatics, and clinical data repositories. The potential scope of this initiative clearly includes all health professionals.[5]

The impact of EBP on medical education and practice will be reviewed briefly in the following section. A discussion of EBP influence on nursing and advanced practice nursing education and practice will follow, with an emphasis on implications for nurse anesthesia.

Evidence-Based Practice and Physicians

Evidence-based practice concepts first appeared in the medical literature in the early 1990s.[6] As integrated into medical education, EBP training provides physicians with critical search and appraisal skills to review medical literature, describes continual quality assessment, and provides the basis for lifelong learning that is linked to patient care. One generational aspect of learning EBP is the near universal facility of current students with information technology. Evidence of increased familiarity with EBP in the first 3 years following medical school graduation is beginning to be reported, but there are few reports describing EBP use in posttraining clinical practice.[7]

Challenges have been described in fostering increased EBP use by practicing physicians. Physicians are a diverse group, with a wide range of time from completion of medical training. For example, 18% of practicing physicians are between 55 and 64 years old and completed medical school an average of 30 to 40 years ago. Similarly, the average nurse anesthetist is 48 years old and may have been away from an academic environment for many years. The duration of time away from clinical training correlates with lower adherence to EBP and greater use of tests and therapies without proven benefit.[8]

Access to and comfort with computers and information technology can be highly variable among medical practitioners.[9-11] Remaining current with recent evidence to provide optimal care requires easy access to internet-based knowledge repositories. Multiple computer-based clinical decision support systems have demonstrated improved clinical performance and patient outcomes.[12,13] The optimal integration of informatics with clinical decision making has been studied by CRNA investigators,[14] but routine fusion of these information sources and widespread clinical application of EBP is slowly evolving.

Nursing and Evidence-Based Practice

Nurses have used EBP since the era of Florence Nightingale. The challenges of responding to the IOM imperatives for clinical education in the health professions will drive nursing to find effective mechanisms to bridge the gap between research and clinical practice. Clearly, translational clinical research is a major imperative in health professions research.[15]

Nurses are the largest group of healthcare providers, with 2.7 million in the United States[16] and some 40,000 CRNAs.[17] There is a significant nursing workforce shortage with an 8.5% national registered nurse vacancy rate[18] and a 12.5% CRNA vacancy rate.[19] Fostering EBP in the registered nurse and advanced practice nurse workforces, given these data, is a daunting challenge.

A survey of 3,000 US licensed nurses demonstrated that almost half of the respondents were unfamiliar with the term "evidence-based medicine." More than half of these survey respondents had not identified a clinical problem that required research, and 43% "sometimes, rarely or never" read nursing journals or texts.[20] Given the workforce needs for nurses and advanced practice nurses coupled with the need to optimally develop skills related to EBP, there are major challenges to fully operationalize this paradigm. Nurse anesthesia educators and practitioners can be leaders in nursing with respect to implementing EBP from entry-level education to daily clinical practice.[1]

Substantial information literacy and access to adequate technology is necessary to implement EBP with tools such as best-practice databases, clinical practice guidelines, electronic medical records, and computerized physician order entry. Nurses report that access to evidence-based information can be "extremely difficult." Fewer than 50% of respondents to the survey by Pravikoff et al[20] reported available workstation access to the Internet. Attitudes toward evidence-based medicine are complex, with a majority of nurses identifying a colleague or supervisor as their primary source for information, versus any independent literature source.

Given these baseline dynamics, integrating EBP into nursing education and practice will require a multifaceted approach that includes changes in attitudes toward the value of EBP and widespread education in information literacy, computer skills, and access to the necessary information technology.

The Future of Evidence-Based Practice in Nursing Education

Nursing education programs must prepare students at all academic levels to understand and value the importance of maintaining practice based on incoming knowledge rather than a mix of tradition, intuition, and experience. Evidence-based clinical practice has been a nursing education goal since the 1980s when a meta-analysis of patient outcomes indicated better outcomes were attained when nursing interventions were based on scientific evidence instead of traditional practices.[21] Trends in nursing education will be reflected in the graduates who seek to enter nurse anesthesia programs. Knowledge and skills inculcated in these nurses about EBP at the level of best practices will be refined and enhanced in graduate nurse anesthesia programs and in continuing education content for practicing CRNAs.

Traditional nursing research education sought to prepare a subset of students to generate research in addition to the broader goal of preparing all students to use research in clinical decision making. A recent National League for Nursing survey of nursing educators showed that, on average, 70% of faculty reported implementation of evidence-based courses and curricular innovation in their teaching.[22] However, this trend was more pronounced in baccalaureate, master's degree, and doctoral programs. Similar to medical faculty, nursing faculty must be fluent in methods to access research along with integration of related findings into practice to model the use of evidence in practice.

Nursing education at the baccalaureate and master's degree levels has focused on preparing graduates to generate research rather than to critique and use research, translating research findings into practice to improve care. However, the American Association of Colleges of Nursing contends that nursing education should prepare students to "use scientific knowledge in their practice."[23]

Research in academic programs often has been taught in isolation from other courses. Students may not connect research to clinical practice.[24] The sometimes tedious instructional methods related to research content and perceived lack of relevancy to actual clinical situations have contributed to pervasive negative attitudes toward research among practicing nurses along with the misperception that EBP is not realistic in today's healthcare environment.[24]

To prepare nursing graduates as evidence-based practitioners, faculty must have in-depth knowledge and skills to teach and model EBP. In a survey of 79 nurse practitioner educators from the National Organization of Nurse Practitioner Faculties and the Association of Faculties of Pediatric Nurse Practitioners, the self-reported knowledge of participants about EBP was high, and they believed in the benefits of EBP and the need to integrate EBP into academic curricula. At the same time, faculty survey responses showed a knowledge gap in teaching EBP strategies. Few of the programs with which respondents were affiliated had foundational courses in EBP. Survey respondents believed that EBP improved clinical care and would advance the profession and described the extent to which EBP clinical competencies were incorporated into clinical specialty courses.[25]

Findings from a recent literature review showed that classroom teaching of EBP was useful, but clinically integrated teaching improved EBP skills, attitudes, and behaviors. Consistent integration and skills building in EBP through an interdisciplinary approach to learning (including health information technology) throughout education programs is needed to prepare clinicians who will deliver evidence-based care when entering the clinical workforce.[25]

Curricular integration of EBP requires establishment of EBP as a core competency throughout all levels of nursing curricula.

Related competencies should include formation of PICOT questions, the mnemonic for patient population, intervention or area of interest, comparison intervention or comparison group, outcome, and timeframe. Students need to be able to search for the best evidence, specifically pre-appraised evidence, and evidence-based clinical practice guidelines and integrate the best evidence with their clinical expertise and patient preferences related to clinical decisions. Students also need to be able to assess outcomes based on EBP changes and participate in team EBP projects. At the graduate level, students should be competent in all components of EBP. They should also demonstrate facility with synthesis of a body of evidence to initiate and evaluate practice changes to improve the health of individuals, lead practice changes based on the best evidence for populations of patients, generate evidence through outcomes management, and mentor others in EBP.[5]

A recent position statement from the National League for Nursing calls for new models of nursing education that will address demands for competencies in EBP.[22] In a related vein, the AANA Doctoral Task Force identified competencies for CRNAs educated at the practice doctoral level.[26]

Nurse Anesthesia Competencies and Curricular Models

Organizations seek to identify the core capabilities, or competencies, that have sustainable value and wide applicability to the customers whom they serve. Professional nursing organizations, which serve the interests of patients, generally identify role-related competencies that describe their vision of the skills and abilities the individual nurse must possess.[27] For example, in the *AANA Code of Ethics for the Certified*

Registered Nurse Anesthetist,[28] competencies include engaging in lifelong professional educational activities, participating in continual quality improvement activities, and maintaining licensure according to statutory and regulatory requirements and recertification.

In education, the AANA has adopted master's degree level educational competencies required of the CRNA for entry into practice. These are the acquired knowledge, skills, and competencies in patient safety, perianesthetic management, critical thinking, communication, and the professional role identified by the Council on Accreditation of Nurse Anesthesia Educational Programs Standards for Accreditation of Nurse Anesthesia Educational Programs (effective January, 2010) Standard III: Program of Study, Criterion 2129 listed in Table 9.1. EBP is reflected in subcriterion C, which describes providing nurse anesthesia care based on sound principles and research evidence.

The *Competencies for the CRNA Practitioner at the Clinical Doctorate Level*[26] (Table 9.2) may serve as the framework upon which the curricula of practice-focused doctoral education programs in nurse anesthesia will be based. The *Competencies for the CRNA Practitioner at the Clinical Doctorate Level* complement the *Practice Doctorate Nurse Practitioner Entry-Level Competencies 2006* developed by the National Organization of Nurse Practitioner Faculties.[30] A commitment to EBP is demonstrated in these competencies, eg, "uses a systematic outcomes analysis approach in the translation of research evidence . . . to demonstrate they will have the expected effects on nurse anesthesia practice; uses evidence-based practice to inform clinical decision making."

201

Table 9.1. Standards for Accreditation of Nurse Anesthesia Educational Programs, Standard III: Program of Study, Criterion 21[29]

C 21. The program demonstrates that graduates have acquired knowledge, skills and competencies in patient safety, perianesthetic management, critical thinking, communication and the professional role.

a. Patient safety is demonstrated by the ability of the graduate to:
   1. Be vigilant in the delivery of patient care.
   2. Protect patients from iatrogenic complications.
   3. Participate in the positioning of patients to prevent injury.
   4. Accomplish a comprehensive and appropriate equipment check.
   5. Utilize standard precautions and appropriate infection control measures.

b. Individualized perianesthetic management is demonstrated by the ability of the graduate to:
   1. Provide care throughout the perianesthetic continuum.
   2. Use a variety of current anesthesia techniques, agents, adjunctive drugs and equipment when providing anesthesia conditions for a variety of surgical and medically related procedures.
   3. Administer general anesthesia to patients of all ages and physical conditions for a variety of surgical and medically related procedures.
   4. Provide anesthesia services to all patients, including trauma and emergency cases.
   5. Administer and manage a variety of regional anesthetics.
   6. Function as a resource person for airway and ventilatory management of patients.
   7. Possess current advanced cardiac life support (ACLS) and pediatric advanced life support (PALS) recognition.
   8. Deliver culturally competent perianesthetic care throughout the anesthesia experience.

c. Critical thinking is demonstrated by the graduate's ability to:
   1. Apply theory to practice in decision-making and problem solving.
   2. Provide nurse anesthesia care based on sound principles and research evidence.
   3. Perform a preanesthetic assessment and formulate an anesthesia care plan for patients to whom they are assigned to administer anesthesia.
   4. Identify and take appropriate action when confronted with anesthetic equipment-related malfunctions.
   5. Interpret and utilize data obtained from noninvasive and invasive monitoring modalities.
   6. Calculate, initiate and manage fluid and blood component therapy.
   7. Recognize and appropriately respond to anesthetic complications that occur during the perianesthetic period.
   8. Pass the Council on Certification of Nurse Anesthetists' certification examination in accordance with the council's policies and procedures.

d. Communication skills are demonstrated by the graduate's ability to:
   1. Effectively communicate with all individuals influencing patient care.
   2. Utilize appropriate verbal, nonverbal and written communication in the delivery of perianesthetic care.

Continues on page 203.

Table 9.1. Standards for Accreditation of Nurse Anesthesia Educational Programs, Standard III: Program of Study, Criterion 21 (continued)[29]

e. Professional responsibility is demonstrated by the graduate's ability to:
  1. Participate in activities that improve anesthesia care.
  2. Function within appropriate legal requirements as a registered professional nurse, accepting responsibility and accountability for his or her practice.
  3. Interact on a professional level with integrity.
  4. Teach others.
  5. Participate in continuing education activities to acquire new knowledge and improve his or her practice.

(Reprinted with permission from the Council on Accreditation of Nurse Anesthesia Educational Programs.)

Table 9.2. Competencies for the CRNA Practitioner at the Clinical Doctorate Level[26]

Competency Area: Biological Systems, Homeostasis and Pathogenesis
  • Develops best-practice models for nurse anesthesia patient care management through integration of knowledge acquired from arts and sciences within the context of the nurse anesthesia philosophical and scientific framework.
  • Uses a systematic outcomes analysis approach in the translation of research evidence and data in the arts and sciences to demonstrate they will have the expected effects on nurse anesthesia practice.

Competency Area: Professional Role
  • Demonstrates increased ability to undertake complex leadership roles in nurse anesthesia.
  • Demonstrates ability to provide leadership that facilitates intraprofessional and interprofessional collaboration.
  • Integrates critical and reflective thinking in leadership style.
  • Demonstrates ability to utilize a variety of leadership principles in situational management.

Competency Area: Healthcare Improvement
  • Uses evidence based practice to inform clinical decision-making in nurse anesthesia.
  • Evaluates how complex organizations, public policy processes and world markets impact the financing, delivery and quality of anesthesia and healthcare.
  • Develops, implements and assesses strategies to improve patient outcomes and quality of care.

Continues on page 204.

203

Table 9.2. Competencies for the CRNA Practitioner at the Clinical Doctorate Level[26] (continued)

Competency Area: Practice Inquiry
- Demonstrates the ability to assess and evaluate health outcomes in a variety of populations, clinical settings and systems.
- Demonstrates ability to disseminate research evidence to diverse audiences through a variety of methods.

Competency Area: Technology, and Informatics
- Uses information systems/technology to support and improve patient care and health-care systems.
- Designs, selects and uses information systems/technology to evaluate programs of care and care systems.
- Critically evaluates clinical and research databases used as clinical decision support resources.

Competency Area: Public and Social Policy
- Advocates for health policy change based on an intent to achieve excellence, and to do so within an ethical context, upholding cultural mores and values.
- Influences the statutory and regulatory aspects of health policy in relation to nurse anesthesia care.
- Evaluates the impact of local and global political change on the globalization of health-care policy development.

Competency Area: Health Systems Management
- Demonstrates the ability to analyze the structure, function and outcomes of integrated delivery systems and complex organization.
- Negotiates, implements and assesses business plans in a collaborative organization.
- Develops and implements an integrated risk management plan based on information systems and technology to promote outcome improvement for the patient, organization and global populations.

Competency Area: Ethics
- Applies ethically sound decision making for complex issues.
- Informs the public of the role and practice of the doctorally prepared CRNA and represents themselves in accordance with the *Code of Ethics for CRNAs*.
- Fulfills the obligation as a doctorally-educated professional to uphold the *Code of Ethics for CRNAs*.

(Reprinted with permission from the Council on Accreditation of Nurse Anesthesia Educational Programs.)

Integration of Evidence-Based Practice Into Nurse Anesthesia Education

Pellegrini[1] noted that as nurse anesthesia education and practice evolve, instructional methods will need to reflect EBP, elements of which are captured in the competencies above. The paradigm of using clinical judgment and expertise as the basis for clinical decision making will shift to a paradigm that uses the best available evidence to formulate clinical decisions along with clinical experience and expertise. Implementation of EBP principles into nurse anesthesia education will yield a well-informed student and ensure that students and faculty remain at the forefront of the latest evidence available in the literature.[1] When presented with a clinical question, student registered nurse anesthetists and practitioners can use the steps in Table 9.3 to do an EBP evidence analysis. Table 9.4 describes a tool by Pellegrini[1] for evaluating evidence, and Figure 9.1 illustrates the Pyramid of Evidence.

Evidence-Based Practice Resources

It is a difficult task for practitioners and trainees to remain current with the relevant evidence in their field of interest. The major bibliographic databases cover less than half of the world's literature and are biased toward English language publications. Textbooks, editorials, and reviews that have not been prepared systematically may be unreliable. Much evidence is unpublished, but the findings may be significant for clinical practice or future research. More easily accessible research reports may exaggerate the benefits of the interventions described.

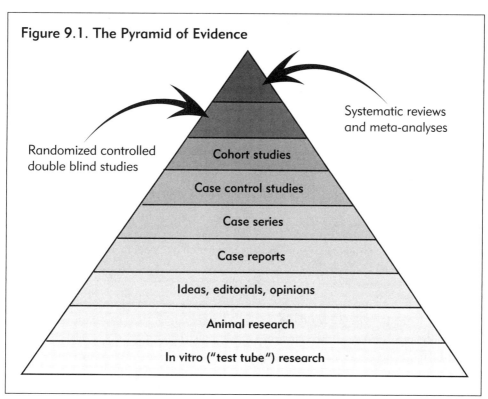

Figure 9.1. The Pyramid of Evidence

Systematic reviews and meta-analyses

Randomized controlled double blind studies

Cohort studies

Case control studies

Case series

Case reports

Ideas, editorials, opinions

Animal research

In vitro ("test tube") research

Table 9.3. Steps for Evidence-Based Practice Evidence Analysis

1. Define the problem or question in terms of the patient or problem, the intervention or comparison interventions used to answer the question, and the findings of the research reviewed.
2. Outline the current steps in one's clinical practice to address the problem.
3. Use a ranking system to determine the quality of evidence available in the literature. This hierarchy, in descending order, consists of findings from systematic review of well-designed clinical studies (meta-analyses); results of one or more appropriately designed studies (randomized trials, cohort studies); results of large case series and case reports; editorials and opinion pieces; animal research, and in vitro research.
4. Identify the resources available to implement any proposed changes to practice to differentiate which evidence is applicable to the current clinical setting.
5. Assess the validity of the research presented with a consistent rubric to review clinical trials that includes these questions:
    a. Did the clinical trials studied include elements such as randomization of subjects, adequate sample size, and appropriate statistical analysis?
    b. Were the results relevant to clinical practice?
    c. Were the therapeutic interventions reported feasible for clinical practice?
    d. Were all research subjects accounted for at the end of the study?

Table 9.4. Elements of Evidence Evaluation[1]

Title, author(s), journal and date, volume number, pages
Research questions/hypotheses
Research methods and design, including setting and sample
Independent and dependent study variables
Instruments used for measurement including reported validity and reliability
Data collection methods
Results reported
Strengths of the study
Decision/reservations
Level of evidence and overall grade:
   A: Strongly recommended; good evidence
   B: Recommended; fair evidence
   C: Not recommended; balance of benefits and harm too close to justify recommendation.
   D: Recommend against; fair evidence of ineffectiveness or harm outweighs risk.
   F: Insufficient evidence; evidence is lacking or research is of poor quality.

(Reprinted with permission from Pellegrini.[1])

The Cochrane Library is a regularly updated collection of evidence-based medicine databases, including The Cochrane Database of Systematic Reviews. This database includes systematic reviews of healthcare interventions that are produced and distributed by the Cochrane Collaboration. *The Cochrane Library* is published quarterly and is available on CD-ROM and the Internet. The review abstracts are available to browse

---

Table 9.5. Structure of a Cochrane Collaboration Review

1. Plain language summary: a short statement summarizing the review, specifically aimed at lay people.
2. Structured abstract: a structured summary of the review, subdivided into sections similar to the main review. This may be published independently from the review and appears in the medical bibliographic database MEDLINE.
3. Background: this gives an introduction to the question considered, including details on causes and incidences of a given problem, the possible mechanism of action of a proposed treatment, uncertainties about management options, etc.
4. Objectives: short statement of the aim of the review.
5. Selection criteria: brief description of the main elements of the question under consideration. This is subdivided into:
   a. Types of studies, eg, randomized controlled trials.
   b. Types of participants: the population of interest. This section may include details of diagnostic criteria, if desired or appropriate.
   c. Types of interventions: the main intervention under consideration and any comparison treatments.
   d. Types of outcome measures: any outcome measures/endpoints, eg, reduction in symptoms, that are considered important by the reviewer, defined in advance. Not only outcome measures used in trials.
6. Search strategy for identification of studies: details of how an exhaustive identification of relevant information was attempted, including details of searches of electronic databases, searches for unpublished information, hand searching of journals or conference proceedings, searching of reference lists of relevant articles, etc.
7. Methods of the review: description of how studies eligible for inclusion in the review were selected, how their quality was assessed, how data were extracted from the studies, how data were analyzed, whether any subgroups were studied or whether any sensitivity analyses were carried out, etc.
8. Description of studies: how many studies were found, what were their inclusion criteria, how big were they, etc.
9. Methodological quality of included studies: were there any reasons to doubt the conclusions of any studies because of concerns about the study quality?
10. Results: what do the data show? The results section may be accompanied by a graph to show a meta-analysis, if this was carried out.
11. Discussion: interpretation and assessment of results.
12. Authors' conclusions: subdivided into implications for practice and implications for research.

(Reprinted with permission from The Cochrane Collaboration.)

---

and search without charge on this website: http://www.cochrane.org/reviews/revstruc.htm.31 The structure of a Cochrane Review is detailed in Table 9.5.

Use of Evidence-Based Practice Findings in Practice

Outcomes research findings that use EBP methods are becoming evident in anesthesia and critical care. As noted earlier, EBP approaches to care integrate the expertise of the clinician with data from systematic research findings. EBP originated with internal medicine, which, unlike anesthesia, involves treatment and diagnosis. However, EBP is applicable to nontherapeutic specialties such as anesthesia and critical care.[32] Some examples of EBP anesthesia literature follow.

The reported frequency of anesthesia awareness is 0.1% to 0.2% in adults who undergo general anesthesia. Clinical predictors of potential intraoperative awareness have been identified.[33] Monitoring technology is available that may decrease the incidence of intraoperative awareness, but the American Association of Nurse Anesthetists and the American Society of Anesthesiologists have not mandated use of these monitors.

An AANA Position Statement, Unintended Awareness Under General Anesthesia,[33] addresses intraoperative brain function monitors. These monitors can be used by anesthesia providers to assess the level of consciousness with a number based on signal processing algorithms of the patient's electroencephalogram. A variety of brain function monitors are available. These devices are based on the cortical electroencephalogram and measure the relative hypnotic effect of the anesthetic rather than anesthetic depth. This position statement recommends using brain function monitors as adjuncts to other patient monitoring modalities.[33] The evidence-based nature of this position statement is reinforced by a Cochrane review.

The Cochrane review on bispectral index (BIS) investigated whether BIS incorporated as a standard monitor reduced anesthetic consumption, recovery time, incidence of recall awareness during surgery, and total cost of anesthetic management. The strategy was to search published studies from MEDLINE, Embase, and the Cochrane Central Register of Controlled Trails. The authors selected all randomized controlled trials in which BIS was used during anesthesia, and the level of consciousness in control groups was determined by use of traditional clinical criteria. Two reviewers independently collected data for anesthetic consumption, recovery time, duration of time in the recovery room, time to discharge, incidence of intraoperative awareness, and the cost of anesthesia management. Searching these databases revealed 17 applicable studies. A total of 719 patients from 9 studies with data met the inclusion criteria for this review.[34]

The BIS monitor was used to determine the dose of propofol needed (2 studies), or required concentrations of sevoflurane (4 studies), desflurane (2 studies), and isoflurane (1 study). Reviewers assessed adequate heterogeneity across the studies with respect to the type of anesthetics, methods of administration, and clinical criteria. Decreased propofol consumption in the BIS group was consistently reported in 2 studies. However, the amount of volatile anesthetic used varied across the study. There were consistent reports of prompter recovery times in the BIS group throughout the studies. Reported duration of recovery room stay was inconsistent throughout studies. In outpatient settings (4 studies, 210 patients), there was no difference in discharge time with or without the BIS monitor. There were no reports of intraopertive recall in either group. The total anesthesia drug cost was only calculated in 1 study and was lower in the BIS group.[34]

Reviewers concluded that, with the clinical heterogeneity throughout the studies reviewed, BIS values could improve immediate recovery time when used to guide anesthetic dosing. More controlled trials with protocols for anesthesia delivery were advocated to determine the effects of BIS monitoring on quality of care, effectiveness, and efficiency.[34]

Another area of interest to anesthesia providers is fasting guidelines, which have evolved. A systematic review of the evidence behind modern fasting guidelines reviewed the development of evidence-based practice in this area.

A Cochrane review studied the effects of various preoperative fasting practices related to the duration of nothing-by-mouth time and type and volume of intake allowed on perioperative complications and patient well-being. Only a few trials reported the incidence of aspiration, regurgitation, or related morbidity, but relied on indirect measures of patient safety such as intraoperative gastric volume and pH. Of interest, there was no evidence to suggest fluid intake up to 2 hours preoperatively had an impact on the gastric volume or pH of patients studied. Fluid intake up to 90 minutes preoperatively also had no impact on gastric contents, but the sample sizes from which these conclusions were derived were smaller. Investigators noted that permitting preoperative water consumption resulted in significantly lower gastric volumes. The authors suggested that clinicians should evaluate this evidence and potentially adjust existing fasting policies.[35]

These studies demonstrate the applicability of EBP to clinical practice, which will become second nature when processes and standards in education, accreditation, and licensure fully incorporate EBP principles.

Incorporation of Evidence-Based Practice in Education, Accreditation, and Licensure

Findings from a recent literature review showed that classroom teaching of EBP improved the knowledge of students and that clinically integrated teaching improved EBP skills, attitudes, and behaviors. Consistent integration of EBP into clinical and didactic curricula through an interdisciplinary approach to learning, including incorporation of health information technology, will help prepare clinicians who will deliver evidence-based care when they enter practice and throughout their careers.[22]

As noted earlier, research in educational programs has often been taught separately from other courses and students often fail to see the application to clinical practice.[24] The sometimes tedious teaching methods for research and seeming lack of application to clinical practice contribute to pervasive negative attitudes toward research in practicing nurses and the belief that EBP is not feasible given the demands of today's clinical environment.

In addition to the previous master's degree level and doctoral-level competencies discussed, research-intensive doctoral programs should foster competency in the skills required at the master's degree level, knowledge generation related to the science of best translating efficacious interventions into clinical practice, and the generation of external evidence through appropriate research methods to answer important clinical questions where evidence does not exist. EBP competencies will need to be established throughout all academic curricula and leveled appropriately.[36] Clinical and academic faculty will need to model EBP. Interdisciplinary collaborative approaches involving clinicians, academicians, academic institutions, and healthcare systems will need to become partners to rapidly translate evidence into clinical practice.

EBP may affect entry to nursing practice through curricular mandates at the level of the National Council of State Boards of Nursing, which is responsible for regulating nursing practice at the state level through its 60 member boards. These boards of nursing are governmental agencies that approve

209

nursing programs and promulgate rules and regulations that address entry to practice standards that nursing programs are mandated to meet. If the programs do not meet regulatory standards, the boards can sanction these programs.[5]

National nursing accreditation is a voluntary process accomplished via either the National League for Nursing Accrediting Commission or the Commission on Collegiate Nursing Education. Specialty accreditation, in some cases including institutional accreditation, is provided for nurse anesthesia educational programs by the Council on Accreditation of Nurse Anesthesia Education Programs. Accreditation addresses quality through a voluntary nongovernmental peer review process.[5]

A proposed initiative related to EBP for these agencies is for the National Council of State Boards of Nursing, National League for Nursing Accrediting Commission, and Commission on Collegiate Nursing Education to develop mandatory standards for curricular content in EBP as part of the licensing, relicensing, and accreditation processes for nursing schools. This could include explicit EBP wording, expectations, and criteria in the review of nursing education programs.[5] It is possible that the National Council of State Boards of Nursing Examination Committee and national certification bodies for advanced practice nursing, such as the Council on Certification of Nurse Anesthetists, may at some point include assessment of EBP competencies, such as knowledge, process, outcomes, and application, as an essential component of licensing and certification examinations.[5] The implications for the nurse anesthesia accreditation, certification, and recertification processes are substantial. The respective communities of interest and councils would need to communicate regarding possible inclusion of EBP into the requirements for nurse anesthesia education, certification, and recertification.

Creating and Sustaining an EBP Culture in Healthcare Systems

As clinicians and educators acquire the knowledge, skills, and abilities to implement EBP, it will be essential to have a culture that supports EBP. Leaders in healthcare organizations, with input from interdisciplinary healthcare professionals, need to create a shared vision and strategic plan for EBP.[37] The strategic plan must be clearly communicated to all healthcare professionals. The expectations related to EBP should be established and integrated throughout the philosophy and performance standards of the healthcare system, with staff having accountability and incentives for meeting those standards.

Research findings demonstrate that the following factors facilitate EBP use in healthcare systems:

- Knowledge and skills of healthcare providers in EBP
- Belief of healthcare providers that EBP improves care and outcomes
- Belief of healthcare providers in their ability to implement EBP
- EBP mentors who are skilled in EBP as well as organizational change
- Administrative and organizational support
- Journal clubs and EBP fellowship programs[37,38]

Findings from recent survey research demonstrate that healthcare professionals who rate themselves higher on knowledge and beliefs about EBP are more likely to teach it to others.[39] To advance EBP, healthcare systems will need to implement educational and fellowship programs to enhance EBP knowledge, beliefs, and skills of its staff; provide EBP mentors who can work with staff on the implementation of EBP initiatives such as journal clubs and EBP implementation and outcomes management projects; and provide the necessary administrative support and resources at the point of care.

Existing models to guide EBP implementation provide process frameworks for EBP use by individual practitioners. These include:

- Stetler's model[40]
- DiCenso, Cullum, Ciliska, and Guyatt's model[41]
- The Clinical Scholar Model[42]

There are also models focused on system-wide EBP implementation, including:

- The Iowa Model.[43]
- Rosswurm and Larrabee's Model[44]
- The Advancing Research and Clinical Practice Through Close Collaboration Model[39]

Evidence has not yet been generated in the form of model testing or full-scale randomized clinical trials to support the majority of these models. There is a major need for studies of this nature.

As integration of EBP into education and practice continues, 3 broad areas will need to be addressed:

1. Establishment of a vision, clear expectations, and interdisciplinary strategic planning for the use of EBP in education and practice
2. Implementation of strategies for creating and sustaining a culture of EBP in healthcare systems
3. Measurement of EBP outcomes and generation of future research[5]

Conclusions

Nurse anesthetists have a long history of leadership in their specialty and in healthcare. As leaders, we must understand the characteristics and realities of creating an evidence-based specialty. In that process, we must comprehend and apply sound leadership and management of the related infrastructure, processes, and behaviors that incorporate evidence in every aspect of clinical practice. Evidence-driven practice is no longer optional and is now an expectation in all clinical settings.[45]

The dedication to EBP demonstrated by Florence Nightingale and nurse anesthesia leaders such as Alice Magaw, Agatha Hodgins, Helen Lamb, and others will be continued by current and future generations of nurse anesthetists. The commitment to clinical excellence and organizational strength historically demonstrated by nurse anesthetists will be reinforced by dedication to full integration and use of EBP in CRNA education and practice.

References

1. Pellegrini JE. Using evidence-based practice in nurse anesthesia programs. *AANA J.* 2006;74(4):269-273.

2. Sackett DL. Evidence-based medicine [editorial]. *Spine.* 1998;23(10):1085-1086.

3. McGlynn EA, Asch SM, Adams J, et al. The quality of health care delivered to adults in the United States. *N Engl J Med.* 2003;348(26):2635-45.

4. Grenier AC, Knebel E. *Health Professions Education: A Bridge to Quality.* Washington, DC: The National Academies Press; 2003:1-18

211

5. Institute of Medicine. IOM round-table on evidence-based medicine, health professions sector statement. http://www.iom.edu/Reports/2003/Health-Professions-Education-A-Bridge-to-Quality.aspx. Accessed May 7, 2010.

6. Medical School Objective Project Writing Group. Learning objectives for medical student education—guidelines for medical schools: report I of the Medical School Objectives Project. *Acad Med* 1999;74(1):13-18.

7. Dorsch J, Aiyer MK, Gumidyala K, Meyer LE. Retention of EGM competencies. *Med Ref Serv Q.* 2006;25(3): 45-57.

8. Conway PH, Edwards S, Stucky ER, Chiang VW, Ottolini MC, Landrigan CP. Variations in management of common inpatient pediatric illnesses: hospitalists and community pediatricians. *Pediatrics.* 2006;118(2):441-447.

9. Jha AK, Ferris TG, Donelan K, et al. How common are electronic medical records in the United States? a summary of the evidence. *Health Aff.* 2006;25(6):w496-w507.

10. Gans D, Kralewski J, Hammons T, Dowd B. Medical groups' adoption of electronic health records and information systems. *Health Aff.* 2005;24 (5):1323-1333.

11. Garritty C, El Emam K. Who's using PDAs? estimates on PDA use by health providers: a systematic review of surveys. *J Med Internet Res.* 2006;8(2):e7.

12. Hunt DL, Haynes RB, Hanna SE, Smith K. Effects of computer-based clinical decision support systems of physician performance and patient outcomes: a systematic review. *JAMA.* 1998;280(15):1339-1346.

13. Kuperman GJ, Teich JM, Bates DW, et al. Detecting alerts, notifying the physician, and offering action items: a comprehensive alerting system. *J Am Med Inform Assoc.* 1996;3(suppl): 704-708.

14. Coopmans V, Biddle C. CRNA performance using a handheld, computerized, decision-making aid during critical events in a simulated environment: a methodologic inquiry. *AANA J.* 2008;76(1):29-35.

15. McDonald, L. Florence Nightingale and the early origins of evidence-based nursing. *Evid Based Nurs.* 2001;4(3):68-69.

16. Spratley E. The registered nurse population March 2000: findings from the National Sample Survey of Registered Nurses. Rockville, MD: US Department of Health and Human Services; 2006.

17. AANA. Who we are. http://www.aana.com. Accessed October 11, 2009.

18. American Hospitals Association. The state of America's hospitals—taking the pulse. Findings from the 2006 AHA Survey of Hospital Leaders. http://www.aha.org/aha/research-and-trends/health-and-hospital-trends/2006.html. Accessed September 30, 2010.

19. Merwin E, Stern S, Jordan L. Executive summary of the AANA Foundation faculty workforce study. Park Ridge, IL: AANA Foundation: 2007.

20. Pravikoff DS, Tanner AB, Pierce ST. Readiness of US nurses for evidence-based practice. *Am J Nurs.* 2005;105 (9):40-51.

21. Heater BS, Becker AM, Olson RK. Nursing interventions and patient outcomes: a meta-analysis of studies. *Nurs Res.* 1988;37(5):303-307.

22. National League for Nursing Board of Governors. Transforming nursing education: position statement. http://www.nln.org/aboutnln/Position Statements/index.htm. Accessed May 7, 2010.

23. American Association of Colleges of Nursing. AACN position statement on nursing research. http://www.aacn. nche.edu/Publications/positions/NsgRes.htm. Accessed May 28, 2008.

24. Burke LE, Schlenk EA, Sereika SM, Cohen SM, Happ MB, Dorman JS. Developing research competence to support evidence-based practice. *J Profess Nurs.* 2005;21(6):358-363.

25. Melnyk B, Fineout-Overholt E, Feinstein N, Sadler L, Green-Hernandez C. Nurse practitioner educators' perceived knowledge, beliefs, and teaching strategies regarding evidence-based practice: implications for accelerating the integration of evidence-based practice into graduate programs. *J Profess Nurs.* 2008;24(1):7-13.

26. American Association of Nurse Anesthetists. Report of the Taskforce on Doctoral Education for CRNAs. Park Ridge, IL: AANA Publishing; 2008.

27. Callahan L. Competence models: from theory to practical applications. *AANA J.* 1988;56(5):387-389.

28. AANA Code of Ethics for the Certified Registered Nurse Anesthetist. www.aana.com. Accessed March 2, 2011.

29. Standards for Accreditation of Nurse Anesthesia Educational Programs. Park Ridge, IL: Council on Accreditation of Nurse Anesthesia Educational Programs; 2006.

30. National Organization of Nurse Practitioner Faculties Domains and Core Competencies of Nurse Practitioner Practice. http://www.nonpf.org/associations/10789/files/DomainsandCoreComps2006.pdf. Accessed January 8, 2008.

31. The Cochrane Collaboration. http://www.cochrane.org/reviews/revstruc.htm. Accessed July 14, 2008.

32. Schulman CS. Strategies for starting a successful evidence-based practice program. *AACN Adv Crit Care.* 2008; 19(3):301-311.

33. AANA. Position Statement 2.12. Unintended awareness under general anesthesia. http://www.aana.com. Accessed September 30, 2010.

34. Punjasawadwong Y, Bunchungmongkol N, Pongchiewboon A. Bispectral index for improving anaesthetic delivery and postoperative recovery. The Cochrane Collaboration. http://www.cochrane.org/colloquia/abstracts/ottawa/P-118.htm. Accessed. June 8, 2008.

35. Stuart P. The evidence base behind modern fasting guidelines. *Best Pract Res Clin Anaesthesiol.* 2006;20(3): 457-469.

36. Stevens K. *Essential Competencies for Evidence-Based Practice in Nursing.* San Antonio, TX: The University of Texas Health Sciences Center School of Nursing at San Antonio Academic Center for Evidence-Based Practice; 2006.

37. Melnyk B, Fineout-Overholt E. *Evidence-Based Practice in Nursing and Healthcare: A Guide to Best Practice.* Philadelphia, PA: Lippincott, Williams & Wilkins; 2005:15-21.

213

38. Pagoto SL, Spring B, Coups EJ, Mulvaney S, Coutu MF, Ozakinci G. Barriers and facilitators of evidence-based practice perceived by behavioral science health professionals. *J Clin Psychol.* 2007;63(7):695-705.

39. Melnyk BM, Fineout-Overholt E, Fischbeck Feinstein N, et al. Nurses' perceived knowledge, beliefs, skills, and needs regarding evidence-based practice: implications for accelerating the paradigm shift. *Worldviews Evid Based Nurs.* 2004;1(3):185-193.

40. Stetler C. Updating the Stetler model of research utilization to facilitate evidence-based practice. *Nurs Outlook.* 2001;49(6):272-278.

41. DiCenso A, Ciliska D, Guyatt G. Introduction to evidence-based nursing. In: DiCenso A, Guyatt G, Ciliska D. eds. *Evidence-Based Nursing: A Guide to Clinical Practice.* Philadelphia, PA: Elsevier; 2005:105-110.

42. Fineout-Overholt E, Melnyk BM, Schultz A. Transforming health care from the inside out: advancing evidence-based practice in the 21st century. *J Prof Nurs.* 2005;21(6):335-344.

43. Titler M. Use of research in practice. In: LoBiondo G, Haber J, eds. *Nursing Research Methods: Critical Appraisal and Utilization.* 5th ed. St Louis, MO: Mosby; 2003:75-80.

44. Rosswurm MA, Larrabee JH. A model for change to evidence-based practice. *Image J Nurs Sch.* 1999;31(4):317-322.

45. Porter-O'Grady T, Malloch K. Beyond the myth and magic: the future of evidence-based leadership. *Nurs Admin Q.* 2008;32(3):176-187.

214

The Healthcare Environment

CHAPTER 10
Healthcare Delivery in the United States

Scot D. Foster, CRNA, PhD, FAAN
Ira P. Gunn, CRNA, MLN, FAAN

Key Concepts

- The US healthcare system is unique in the world because (1) the United States spends far more on health services than any other industrialized country, (2) segments of the US health system serve as corporate, for-profit centers, and (3) there is no universal coverage for all citizens.

- The current delivery system is based on social values of autonomy, choice, free enterprise, market demand, and domination by the medical community. This was achieved through restrictive licensing, credentialing, and legislative protections. Since the advent of managed care, medical domination within the system has waned as control from managed care companies and insurance providers increases.

- The healthcare system is composed of 5 basic elements or sectors: health providers (individuals and institutions or agencies), health payers (health insurers—public and private, industry, individuals), health regulators (public and private), health manufacturers (eg, equipment, pharmaceuticals), and health clients.

- The current delivery system is highly fragmented and characterized by uneven levels of quality, service, and reimbursement; lack of system access; and emphasis on cure rather than prevention. These issues have all contributed to the astronomical increase in medical costs from 9.1% of the gross domestic product in 1980 to 16% in 2005, resulting in profoundly negative effects on business and individuals.

Continues on next page.

Key Concepts (continued)

- Wholesale reform of the national healthcare system is again being fiercely debated, posited largely on disparate views of the federal government's role in providing and regulating services. Although a few states have adopted systems of "universal access" with arguable success, change will come only when required by popular mandate or a major economic threat to the nation's economic growth and stability.

The healthcare system in the United States differs substantially from those in other developed countries. As such, many of its problems and features are unique. Although touted as providing the best and most comprehensive care in the world, it does so only for a privileged class of people or at extraordinary cost for others. Expenditures clearly exceed that of any industrialized nation in the world. Further indictment of the system is revealed by low rankings in patient outcomes areas such as infant mortality, life expectancy, obesity, diabetes, cardiovascular disease, and cancer. The World Health Organization reported in 2000 that the United States ranked 37th in the world in the quality and function of its healthcare delivery system.[1] Structurally, the US system of care delivery is highly fragmented and plagued by for-profit sectors of control, as opposed to European countries in which a central authority, such as a minister of health, oversees and tightly manages service distribution, quality, and financing of services.

By most estimates, nearly 45 million US citizens are uninsured or underinsured. This situation portends huge financial costs in terms of increased and untreated illness, not to mention the moral dimension of effectively withholding care for those not positioned to pay for services. For those who can afford care, the experience of illness, recovery, and health maintenance is often characterized by delivery systems that are overextended, too costly, egregiously slow, and that fail to emphasize preventative care and don't document quality improvement efforts well. It is clear that the system remains in crisis because of its failure to contain costs, protect its users from potentially catastrophic financial loss for lack of coverage, or serve the basic, preventative healthcare needs of all citizens.

Nearly every US president since the turn of the century has attempted to influence the healthcare system to make it more available and responsive to the needs of ordinary citizens. Although there have been many notable and successful efforts at reform, such as legislating Medicare and Medicaid programs, most progress has come incrementally in the form of insurance portability, changes in reimbursement mechanisms, and more inclusive access for at-risk populations. Unfortunately, substantive progress toward a more systemized mode of delivery has been elusive, culminating in the failed attempt by the Clinton administration to implement wholesale revision of the system via the 1994 Health Security Act.

The debate has become increasingly vigorous as a result of the recession that began in late 2007, often referred to as the worst economic downturn of the US economy since the Great Depression. Largely because of nearly doubling and in some cases, tripling unemployment rates, massive home foreclosures, and bank and business failures, the Obama administration determined that recovery should be based on cost control of major sectors of the economy, chief among them, healthcare.

Recent debates and attempts at reform have largely been focused on the role of the federal government, specifically on the extent to which governments should provide care through a single-payer system, reliance solely on private enterprise to manage the system of service and delivery or options for a functional merger of both. For some advocates there is the traditional fear that government will eliminate choice in the form of a single-payer system or public option, akin to an expansion of the current Medicare system, and estrange patients from their doctors. Most within this group maintain that although reform is needed, the means to

219

achieve it should protect the traditional pre-rogatives of private control, minimal regulation, promotion of market forces, and tax reductions or credits for financing. Opposing advocates maintain that the system has proven to be nonfunctional, with increasing costs by lack of regulation and lack of competition, universal access, and cost control. They advocate more central authority of system management, increasing government subsidy, increased access to care and control of risk pool vagaries. In sum, the arguments center on traditional values of choice and private control vs public regulation, entrepreneurial models, and the moral question regarding whether healthcare is a right or a privilege.

The predominant delivery system in the future will likely continue to rely on the tenets of managed care (either public or private), although it is increasingly obvious after several decades of this structure's dominance, that even this paradigm is not the panacea once imagined. The public has become increasingly vocal in its concerns that managed care organizations more frequently cater to the interest of corporate profit than public good, fail to offer promised services by denial of service, and ignore meaningful work that emphasizes quality of care and transparency in making those results public, although the relatively recent proliferation of public and private "watchdog" groups has made substantial inroads into requiring public disclosure of patient outcomes.

Institutions themselves are finding that the mega-mergers of the 1990s too often failed to save money by streamlining services, that teamwork with physicians was increasingly costly and difficult, and that governmental regulations appeared to increase in direct proportion to the decreases in third-party reimbursements. Providers also became disenchanted with erosion of their traditional decision-making authority and practice autonomy, not to mention the continuing squeeze by the government on reimbursement schedules.

Philosophical arguments aside, it is important for Certified Registered Nurse Anesthetists (CRNAs) to appreciate the historical role and pervasive influence of organized medicine on the design and maintenance of our system, because CRNA work and opportunity is inextricably bound to the medical community of providers and the byzantine delivery structure in which we work.

Historical Overview

The configuration of the healthcare delivery system in the United States is a product of this country's founding economic tenets and the medical profession's influence on its design, as described in Paul Starr's book, *The Social Transformation of American Medicine.*[2] Since the late 1800s, state and federal governments legislatively codified much of the structural design of the healthcare system promulgated by organized medicine. Because of these early and effective attempts at control of the system, it has taken substantial effort to make any statutory or regulatory revision that would enhance system flexibility or accommodate social need. Since those times of physician dominance, however, other entities have been increasingly effective at exerting controls and bringing about change, including equipment suppliers, pharmaceutical houses, insurance companies, hospital and professional organizations, and citizen advocacy groups. However, the increasing clatter of voices too often yields little in the way of patient benefit.

Although there were a variety of types of physicians in the United States in the late

1800s, the allopathic physicians ultimately won control of the healthcare delivery system. The early design of the system made physicians gatekeepers to healthcare and ensured that persons seeking care would initially have to be seen by a physician. This was accomplished largely by passage of medical practice acts that mandated the licensing of physicians in each of the states, beginning in 1873. Although some practice acts were enacted in the late 17th and 18th centuries, most were repealed by 1850 because of the chaotic state of medical education and wide variations in the quality of physician providers.

Some of the early practice acts were aimed at setting reimbursement rates for physicians based on their varying levels of competence and education. Although some physicians were university educated, others had been trained in apprenticeship programs. It was another quarter of a century before the medical education system was sufficiently stable to allow physicians to publicly endorse a monopoly over the whole of healthcare. Bullough,[3] Safreit,[4] and Hadley[5] state that physicians claimed the whole of healthcare for themselves because no other health providers were licensed at the time, including nurses. In the intervening decades, nonphysician health providers have had to work diligently to reclaim their areas of practice through the legislative process. Early versions of the South Carolina Medical Practice Act provided an apt example of the pervasiveness of this controlling influence by medicine, stating:

> Medical Practice includes any person who shall diagnose, cure, relieve in any degree or profess or attempt to diagnose, cure or relieve any human disease, ailment, defect, abnormality, or complaint, whether of a physical or mental origin, by attendance or advice, by prescribing, using or furnishing any drug, appliance, manipulation, adjustment or [other] method or by any therapeutic agent whatsoever.[6]

Licensing acts not only placed the physician in a position to control the care provided to patients but essentially extended that control over other healthcare providers. Consequently, their economic control of the healthcare dollar was ensured. Certainly, physicians had more education than other healthcare workers at the time, so it was not difficult for them to achieve dominance. Furthermore, they were organized to achieve that purpose, but organization of other health providers came much later; however, neither the economic stature nor economic rewards for physicians at the turn of the century compare with what they are today. The US population was mostly rural, and the distance between patients and their doctors meant that a significant portion of a doctor's time was spent traveling. Consequently, the number of patients treated was much smaller than is common today. Pay took the form of a dozen eggs, a couple of chickens, and in some instances, money.

There were only a few services that early physicians could provide because medical knowledge was still ill-defined and poorly understood. Many of those responsibilities today fall within the nature and practice of nursing. Few rural areas had hospitals, and therefore patients were cared for in their homes. Thus, physicians did not rely extensively on nurses or other health professionals. In fact, except for nurses and pharmacists, many allied health professions and technicians did not exist. The physicians' greatest competitors at the turn of the century were the so-called nostrum makers, that is, makers and sellers of

221

patented medicines. It was not until the passage of the Federal Pure Food and Drug Act in 1906 that the American Medical Association began to gain some control over pharmaceuticals and prescription by declaring it within the rightful and exclusive domain of medicine.[2]

Although nursing, or nurturing, existed even in prehistoric times, as did elements of medicine, formalized nursing in the United States did not appear until physicians were well into the process of seeking licensure. In 1873, there were 3 schools of nursing. By 1900, there were 432. Many of these schools were established as a cheap source of labor for the developing hospital industry. Florence Nightingale, whose nursing philosophies and traditions influenced early American nursing, did not believe in state licensing, but felt that educational programs should be of such quality as to make graduation the sole requisite for professional credibility and recognition. However, the proliferation of nursing programs in the United States indicated that there was such variation in quality that nursing leaders eventually sought state licensure.

Unfortunately, early legislation adopted the practice of registration, wherein the title was protected, but not the practice. That is, the scope of nursing practice was not defined within a registration model as would have been the case under a licensure model. The first state to enact legislation was North Carolina. Also important and unlike other professional education disciplines in the United States, state boards of nursing were given responsibility for approving nursing education programs, in addition to registering nurses.[7] In 1938, the National League for Nursing Education began a private sector accreditation program for nursing education. Subsequently, its name was changed to the National League for Nursing.

The urbanization of the United States began in earnest with the industrial revolution. In the early 1900s, physicians, church groups, and others began building hospitals for the care of the sick, predominantly in cities. By this time, the germ theory had been enunciated and principles of disinfection and sterilization were employed, which stimulated the growth of hospitals, allowing large numbers of patients to be confined in one institution without fear of patient-to-patient contamination. Furthermore, because of urbanization and industrialization, few families were well equipped at home to take care of family members during serious illnesses. Through efforts of nurses and social workers, the Henry Street Settlement in New York City pioneered the public health movement and the visiting nurse concept for care of the indigent. Congress passed the Sheppard-Towner Act of 1921 to help finance public health nurses, and state laws were passed to register births and license midwives. Soon statistics documented lower maternal and infant mortality and at lower cost. Predictably, opposition by organized medicine arose because these programs were not under physician control or direction. This led inevitably to the discontinuation of the Sheppard-Towner Act.[8,9]

Major expansion of community-based hospitals, particularly in rural areas, awaited the passage of the Hill-Burton Act by Congress in 1946. In its first 20 years, 4,678 projects were undertaken, almost half directed to communities with populations under 10,000.[10] Provider discrimination became a popular mechanism in many early hospitals in awarding staff membership and clinical privileges. Most often, privileges were restricted to white, male physicians.

Early female physicians had to build their own hospitals if they were to benefit from this mode of practice, as did black physicians. Often a qualification for hospital staff privileges was membership in the medical society. At that time, women and blacks were not readily admitted to these societies and were essentially forced to establish their own professional organizations.[7-9] This, of course, was a reflection of the social mores of the nation, at least until the civil rights legislation of the 1960s.

The Advent of Health Insurance

National interest in adopting a model of health insurance had begun in the United States by 1910. The idea put forth was for universal coverage for which payment for insurance was divided between state governments, employers, and employees. In spite of early and vehement opposition by the American Medical Association, many physicians believed its emergence was inevitable, and most eventually abandoned their traditional opposition and endorsed early initiatives. However, World War I intervened, and compulsory insurance began to be viewed as un-American. It was often termed a "Prussianization of America." Many in the medical profession were relieved that the issue of insurance was temporarily, at least, "off the table," because it was viewed by some as a potential threat to the doctor-patient relationship, not to mention traditional methods of reimbursement.

Commercial insurance companies; physicians in New York; and a labor leader, Samuel Gompers, who preferred higher wages to fringe benefits, began to oppose universal health insurance.[11] In 1925, the New York State Medical Society reported that "health insurance is a dead issue in the United States. . . . It is not conceivable that

any serious effort will again be made to subsidize medicine as the handmaiden of the public."[11] A medical historian stated that physicians of the time did not reckon with the Great Depression that was soon to come, which would threaten the financial security of both physicians and hospitals and have the effect of reopening the debate on the advisability of health insurance.

In 1929, voluntary health insurance got its start in Dallas, Texas, when teachers agreed to pay Baylor University Hospital 50 cents a month for hospital insurance. This insurance afforded each teacher 21 days of hospitalization per year. The concept was the forerunner of Blue Cross, a private, non-profit hospital insurance corporation. Blue Shield, the other part of the "Blues" which covers physician payments, was not formalized until 1946. The major impetus for the acceptance and spread of private health insurance came from the labor movement shortly after World War II, when the Supreme Court ruled that labor unions could appropriately negotiate and strike over healthcare benefits for their members. As more and more American industries offered health benefits to employees, it became almost unthinkable that major employers would someday not offer health insurance as a paid benefit. However, this benefit is now perceived by many business leaders as one central reason for their declining competitiveness in a global economy. Consequently, continued provision of health benefits is undergoing substantial review and change. For example, retirees are now being eliminated from plans promised for life, coverage is being reduced or is unavailable, and beneficiaries are paying larger deductibles and copayments. This may presage the inevitability of employee-paid health insurance for the future, although that potential would likely require federal mandate of individual coverage, an unpopular notion with the public.

Essentially, as an outgrowth of American medicine's design, the healthcare delivery system became physician-controlled, acute care–centered, and hospital-based. The payment system was designed to permit physicians to be reimbursed directly by patients on a fee-for-service basis. Thus, medicine had gained through its state licensing acts exclusive privileges and a monopoly as gatekeeper to the delivery of health services in the United States. In more recent years, traditional fee-for-service is becoming more rare, replaced by heavily discounted reimbursements for services, capitated rates, and increasingly decremented reimbursements by public payers. In fact, the current healthcare reform debate centers around substantial shifts of funding out of Medicare to pay for portions of newly proposed reform packages. There are numerous reports that many physicians may likely opt out of the Medicare program if this happens because current reimbursement rates could not cover costs of service. Clearly, the potential of decreased Medicare funding is of grave importance to CRNAs, whether they are medically directed or not.

Medicine, as a state-endorsed monopoly, has been traditionally protected from restrictive practices that in the business world would have made individuals, groups, or companies subject to federal and state antitrust laws. It was not until 1976 that the US Supreme Court ruled that the nation's antitrust laws also applied to the professions.[12] Thus, monopolization of markets, conspiring to restrain trade, and price fixing, wherein the profession did not have an exclusive legal prerogative, made physicians vulnerable to actions under both federal and state antitrust laws. A variety of antitrust allegations have been made against groups of physicians or professional societies with varying results; however, the cost of such litigation and the length of time required to finalize court decisions have reduced the number of actions taken under these laws. In some instances, either the state or federal government's antitrust operatives may seek consent decrees from persons charged with antitrust violations to correct situations in which restrictive practices and/or price fixing were alleged.

Insurance companies offering healthcare coverage have maintained exemption from original antitrust legislation through the McCarran-Furgeson Act since 1944. Attendant to the current healthcare reform debate is increasing support to repeal that act, and thus, make insurers susceptible to competition borne of the widespread view that these companies may be actively involved in collusion, rate setting, and denying claims. Whether or not insurance companies are actually involved in such activities, threats of repeal clearly are attempts to force the industry to accept reforms that they view as not in their best financial interest.

Although many of the arguments the medical profession made for designing the system were based on quality concerns, there can be little question that the profession was equally concerned about its economic status. Physicians and hospitals have usually been allowed to determine the value of their own services and been given authority to charge what they believed the market would bear. Such practice is usually consistent with a capitalistic system based on the supply and demand theory of a market economy. Unfortunately, the demand for healthcare services is often influenced by the principal suppliers of that system: hospitals and physicians. Some health policy analysts view the healthcare system as a traditional market, when it is really an aberration of this model, a view that constitutes a major factor in the current cost crisis in healthcare.[13]

Today's Healthcare System

There are 5 health services program sectors that compose US healthcare: 1) principal government health authorities; 2) other government agencies; 3) private healthcare sectors; 4) nonhealth commercial sectors; and 5) voluntary sectors.[14] Within each of these program sectors are the operational components of the system, that is, the groups of individuals or organizations that, within each program sector, actually produce health services. These operating components are 1) healthcare facilities; 2) workforce production (providers); 3) health manufacturers (equipment and pharmaceuticals); 4) financers (public or private payers); and 5) healthcare clients (patients). All operating components function within each of the program sectors. The complexity of the system becomes apparent when it is viewed that each component is guided by separate, unaligned missions, incentives, goals, and base of power. Too often, this delicate balance is not coincident with the overall goal of benefitting the patient alone.

As is often the case, the relative power or influence of each operating component is in constant flux. For instance, physicians' power can be strengthened by refusing to accept Medicare patients when reimbursements are inadequate. At the other extreme, doctors may be victims of decreased influence when insurance companies refuse to authorize services to their patients for cost considerations. In the case of insurance companies, their power to increase premium rates may be offset by increasing government sponsorship of payment services that threaten direct competition. For clients,

power can potentially be increased in direct proportion to their legislative influence or attenuated by unregulated or monopolistic practices by insurers, as is too often the case. These tensions can and do cause patient harm, if not properly balanced. The rest of this chapter will be given to a discussion of the role and function of primary program sections and the operating components referred to previously.

Health Services Program Sectors

Principal Federal Government Healthcare Authorities

Governments, at national, state, and local levels, assume primary and fundamental roles in healthcare when measured by the percentage of healthcare dollars and services transacted annually. Federal and state governments are both authorized by the federal constitution to offer services, described by most as an uneasy alliance. The federal government derives its authority from the constitutional authority to tax and spend, provide for the general welfare, and regulate interstate and foreign commerce.[15] The states derive their power through the 10th amendment of the constitution, which essentially reserves power to states, not otherwise delegated to the federal government.

The largest of 3 health management divisions of the federal government is the Department of Health and Human Services, followed by the Department of Veterans Affairs and the Department of Defense. The Department of Health and Human Services operates more than 300 distinct programs under 11 subdivisions, chief among them, the Public Health Service, the Centers for Medicare & Medicaid Services, the Agency for Healthcare Research and Quality, the

225

Health Resources and Services Administration, the Centers for Disease Control and Prevention, the Food and Drug Administration, and the National Institutes of Health.[16] The Public Health Service remains a functional entity that comprises several of the aforementioned divisions. All of these divisions are the ones that most directly affect or influence CRNA practice through policy and regulation. The specific function of each is widely described in a variety of Internet sources.

Principal State Government Agencies

States provide a range of services within a variety of organizational structures, primarily through a department of health services. Primary services usually include mental illness treatment, licensing authority for care providers, vocational rehabilitation, occupational health, environmental protection, collection and analysis of vital and health statistics, and, most importantly, administration of Medicaid. Medicaid affords health services for the indigent, with the federal government and state governments jointly funding the program and the states operating it. Thus, eligibility for Medicaid is determined by each state, as are any restrictions on health services and reimbursement rates for providers. Unless reimbursement to selected providers is mandated by federal law, the state determines who will be directly reimbursed for covered services.

States are also authorized to empower local health service agencies, generally focused on public health efforts and services for the poor and more parochial issues involving clean water supplies, sanitary sewage, and solid waste disposal. Other common services may include maternal and child health, venereal disease control, home care, family planning, and health code enforcement. It is generally agreed that these services provide the foundational elements of public health services.

Federal and State Services Financing

Although the federal government has been a provider of healthcare services since the Revolutionary War, its role as a major financier of health services came with the enactment of Medicare and Medicaid legislation in 1965. Medicare was conceived as an earned entitlement health insurance program for the elderly paid for by Social Security taxes. The program initially afforded insurance for physician services and hospitalization. Over the years, other healthcare providers, including CRNAs, gained direct reimbursement from Medicare for services. Many outpatient services are now covered, particularly after the enactment of the Prospective Payment System in 1983, which was devised to contain hospital costs. Because patients are now being discharged earlier as a cost-containment measure, coverage for selected home health services was added because many patients required extended or rehabilitation care.

Medicare payment is administered through 4 means:

- Part A: hospital payment, hospice, and home health care,
- Part B: provider payment (including CRNAs),
- Part C: Medicare beneficiary enrollment in managed care organizations, and
- Part D: drug prescription coverage.

Funding for payment for all of these programs is derived from Social Security taxes, general revenues, and enrollee premium payments and administered by the Centers for Medicare & Medicaid Services. The

Centers for Medicare & Medicaid Services (formerly the Healthcare Financing Administration) is the major payer for the federal government, using the private insurance industry as its intermediary for reimbursing health services associated with the Medicare program. The Centers for Medicare & Medicaid Services is also responsible for providing the federal portion of funding to the states for their Medicaid programs. Medicaid is usually operated by the state department of health, using a private insurer as intermediary.

The federal government also assumes major responsibility in funding basic and applied biomedical research associated with disease, injury, treatment modalities, and delivery systems. In addition to establishing and funding the National Institutes of Health, including the Center for Nursing Research, many university and private research groups derive funding from government or private foundations that support healthcare services and a plethora of health education programs.

Finally, the government plays a major role in providing educational funding for a variety of health professionals, thus directly affecting the available supply of health manpower. The federal government maintains a Health Manpower Division and a Division of Nursing within the US Department of Health and Human Services to monitor health and human resources and to oversee disbursement of federal funds related to education. Unfortunately, their effectiveness depends in part on annual congressional appropriations. Consequently, manpower issues too often become a function of the political and legislative process rather than one dependent on fact-based data demonstrating bona fide manpower shortages. At present, advanced practice registered nurses (Certified Registered Nurse Anesthetists, nurse practitioners, certified nurse midwives, and clinical nurse specialists) receive only 1% of the nearly $9 billion expended annually by the federal government for expanding the healthcare workforce. Well over half of that amount is reserved for physician training.[17]

Health payers, both governmental and private, determine directly or indirectly how healthcare will be delivered, where it will be delivered, how often, and to whom it will be delivered. Nonphysician health professionals seeking more autonomy in practice and the ability to be reimbursed for services ignore at their peril the influence healthcare funding and reimbursement have on practice. The skills and capability to influence legislation and regulation are as important in configuring the environment for nurse anesthesia practice as the skills to perform intubations are to the administration of anesthesia. Table 10.1 provides an overview of the healthcare roles of federal, state, and local governments.

Private or Voluntary Healthcare Sector

Private sector functions in healthcare assume a wide variety of roles and can be nonprofit or for-profit. Their roles and functions are expansive and include direct delivery of patient care (nursing homes, employee health services, general hospitals, managed care companies), education and advocacy (professional organizations, such as the AANA), financing (insurance companies), research and manufacturing (pharmaceutical houses, devices), and regulation (credentialing, quality watch-dog groups). Other groups such as the American Heart Association, the Red Cross, and the Visiting Nurse Association, among many other groups, are considered voluntary agencies that perform services according to their own

227

Table 10.1. Major Healthcare Roles of Federal, State, and Local Governments

	Financing	Delivery	Regulation
Federal	Plays a large role through Medicare, Medicaid, and other government-sponsored programs; subsidizes selected health professional educational programs; subsidizes much health-related research and other studies.	Operates healthcare clinics and hospitals for care of military, veterans, American Indians, and research subjects at the National Institutes of Health; formerly provided services at public health hospitals and clinics for seamen and patients with infectious diseases.	Regulates health programs it finances by setting conditions for participation as well as qualifications, conditions, and rates for reimbursement; approves drugs and devices for use in healthcare; regulates controlled substances distribution; prohibits provider discrimination in care provisions; enforces laws applicable to healthcare delivery.
State	Funds Medicaid with help of the federal government, including some long-term care and mental health services; provides some public health services; subsidizes health professional and occupational education.	Operates mental health and mental retardation hospitals, health departments, academic health centers, prison medical facilities.	Regulates health and liability insurance; licenses or otherwise credentials health institutions and personnel; defines scopes of practice; establishes health codes and standards; enforces standards.
Local	Subsidizes public and teaching hospitals; funds local public health departments and clinics; subsidizes some indigent care in the absence of a municipal hospital.	Operates clinics and municipal hospitals; operates public health departments.	Establishes and enforces local health codes.

mission or as adjunct services at the behest of or to support gaps in the federal government services. Table 10.2 summarizes the roles of private and voluntary providers or organizations, which in many cases are fundamental to the provision of comprehensive healthcare services.

These groups by no means take a back seat to the larger governmental function of providing healthcare. Private sector groups maintain a highly visible and authoritative advocacy role for their constituents, members, and clients alike. Among the most vocal in the healthcare debate are health provider associations, consumer health groups, insurance and managed care companies, and community activist organizations. In addition to providing direct services, these activist groups monitor healthcare quality, identify needs and solutions requiring public and private support, and educate the public on health matters. These groups may be national or local in scope; may be defined along racial, age, economic status, or other lines; and may, in most instances, have substantial power to local, state, and federal governments. Most importantly, many of these groups promote the underlying value that services emanating from the private sector are vastly preferential to government-based services.

Health Services Operating Components

Workforce

Although many health professionals engage in private practice either as individuals or as groups, the healthcare delivery system today is one of the major and most stable employers in the United States. In 2004, almost 13.8 million people, about 9.9% of all persons employed in the United States, were working in the healthcare industry. Of workers throughout the United States, 41%

were employed in hospitals, 13% in nursing and personal care facilities, and more than 14% in physicians' offices. Today there are more than 700 categories of skilled health occupations, including 2.3 million nurses and over 750,000 allopathic and osteopathic physicians.[15] Pharmacists, dentists, optometrists, and podiatrists account for another 400,000 professionals. It is estimated that it requires 15 other healthcare workers to support each physician. Although physicians remain a dominant force in healthcare, their traditional influences are waning as managed care bureaucrats make inroads into practice autonomy and nonphysicians expand their traditional scope of practice into areas once considered exclusive to physicians.

Financing

National healthcare spending is expected to reach $2.5 trillion in 2009, accounting for 17.6% of the gross domestic product. By 2018, national healthcare expenditures are expected to reach $4.4 trillion—more than double 2007 spending.[18] Historically, healthcare costs have exceeded general inflation by at least double; however, that number is expected to increase if healthcare reform measures are not adopted.

Jonas et al[14] summarize the financing or transfer of monies (services payment) from the public via 3 primary mechanisms: government (federal and state); insurance or managed care companies; or private pay, commonly know as "out of pocket." Nearly half of all payment for services is from government sources, including the services it operates directly or for which it pays independent providers. Regardless of the mechanism of payment, the source of payment is always the same—the patient.

The primary issue involving the financing of health services centers around skewed incentives and issues of affordability. Examples

229

Table 10.2. Summary of Private Sector Roles in Healthcare

	Financing	Delivery	Credentialing/regulations
Business/industry	Often provides health insurance for employees; may provide health coverage using HMOs or PPOs; pays for workers' compensation insurance; provides coverage for selected addiction rehabilitation.	Operates occupational health clinics; may provide some health maintenance services.	May regulate smoking and areas to smoke.
Credentialing bodies	Affect costs of care	Affect delivery of healthcare services; configure institutional delivery mechanisms, available resources, etc.	Accredit institutional or agency providers; accredit educational programs for preparing health professionals; and certify health personnel.
Health insurance	For a price, pays for health services; reimburses health professionals and institutions; performs utilization reviews and billing audits.	Affects delivery systems based on inherent incentives in insurance policies, providers and services reimbursed, conditions, and levels of reimbursement.	Determines qualifications for insurance coverage.
Health personnel		Provide direct health services, paid salary, or pay on the basis of charge or allowable fees.	
Health institutions*	May have a financing function.	Provide health services through an organized delivery system; reimbursed by insurance or health client for most services rendered as an institution.	Often provide institutional credentialing for physicians and in some instances for other nonphysician health professionals in independent practice.

Continued on page 231.

The Healthcare Environment

Table 10.2. Summary of Private Sector Roles in Healthcare (continued)

	Financing	Delivery	Credentialing/ regulations
Professional organizations		Recruit new members in the profession to ensure adequacy of personnel resources for healthcare delivery; promote change and innovation in professional practice and healthcare delivery.	Set education and practice standards for the profession and its members; may participate in or provide quality assurance, risk management programs, or continuing education programs; may publish ethical code for members.
Liability insurers/ product liability insurers	For a price, underwrite costs of malpractice and product-liability claims, defense costs, and/or payments or judgments.		Determine conditions for acquiring liability insurance and liability limits available; malpractice insurance may be required to obtain institutional clinical privileges.

*Health institutions include hospitals, ambulatory health centers, diagnostic or treatment centers, hospices, long-term care facilities, etc.

of misaligned incentives are plentiful and commonly occur in the failure of plans to closely monitor pharmaceutical costs by substituting generic medications, payment for acute care procedures at the expense of preventative care, and failure to base payments on best practices, or known quality indicators, or performance measures. Affordability is a problem shared by the individual (insurance premiums), businesses (costs for employer-based health benefits), and even governments (state and federal) related to their ability to sustain cost increases in operating Medicare, Medicaid, veterans facilities, and myriad other ancillary health service programs, especially those involving healthcare for children.

The picture for healthcare financing is bleak under the current system of delivery. It is estimated that the average employer-sponsored premium for a family of 4 costs close to $13,400 a year and the employee pays about 27% of this cost,[19] which equates to about 10% of a median family salary in the United States of $40,000. Public programs fare no better. The Medicare Hospital Insurance Trust Fund is expected to pay out more in hospital benefits this year than it receives in taxes. Small business suffers also; it is estimated that nearly $1 trillion in profits this decade will be lost to paying healthcare costs. This has the effect of increasing job losses, stifling production, and hampering consumer purchasing power, a recipe for disastrous effects on the US economy.

Facilities

Acute care hospitals remain the predominant institutions supplying inpatient care. In 2008, there were about 5,815 acute care hospitals—including federal and state government-owned, private nonprofit, and private for-profit—loosely classified by service category as general, special, rehabilitation and chronic disease, and psychiatric. Approximately one-third of the US healthcare dollar is spent on inpatient hospital care, making hospital care the single most expensive component of the healthcare system.[15]

Hospitals continue to endure major financial stresses as government and other payers try to constrain the cost of care. Paltry profit margins, hospitals claim, stem largely from the 1997 Balanced Budget Act, which substantially reduced hospital payments, coupled with the failure of merged institutions to save costs from duplicate expenditures and increases in operating and personnel costs. Furthermore, the chronic cost cuts in Medicare reimbursements have highlighted the stark reality that payer mix is perhaps the single most critical factor in maintaining financial margins and quality. Historically, congressional implementation of the Prospective Payment System as the vehicle for Medicare reimbursement of hospitals has led to shortened hospital stays and lower bed occupancy, prompting the closure or merger of many hospitals. Closures were hastened by the advent of freestanding ambulatory health clinics and surgicenters that took many of the profit-making services away from hospitals.

Hospitals in the United States affect the delivery of health services in several ways.

Hospital ownership reflects the pluralism of American society itself. They are owned by the government and by private groups, usually held by various religious, racial, ethnic, and organizational groups. They may be community supported at local levels or supported by municipalities, the state, or the federal government. Historically, hospitals have served to define social class and race, including the poor, the wealthy, and ethnic groups. Although civil rights laws eliminated overt hospital segregation of races, public and private hospitals still often segregate the poor from the wealthy in more discreet and subtle ways.

Obviously, most hospitals focus on acute care. They are often characterized as procedure based, that is, oriented to providing services that yield high revenue, such as surgery, scans, access to specialists, interventional procedures, and high-tech treatment modalities. Although many have incorporated a greater outpatient focus, the fact that the highest percentage of the healthcare dollar goes to these institutions clearly offsets any comparable revenue for preventative services in a nonacute setting. Although many hospitals have, during the last decade, begun to sponsor aggressive wellness initiatives to both patients and employees with benefits, there is still much to be done to integrate a broad range of services that meet the needs of the acutely ill yet maintain incentives to keep patients well and out of the hospital.

All CRNAs should be aware of the symbiotic relationship that exists between hospitals and physicians—the physician needs hospitals in which to admit patients, and the hospital needs physicians to fill beds and pay for its operation. Doctors are "privileged" to work in hospitals and to admit patients, and they exert a privileging control via medical staff policies to keep other providers out who might afford competition. Physician influence dominates the hospital environment, especially in policy making, often to the detriment of other health providers, including nurses, therapists, and technicians. At the practical level, this power-sharing arrangement between the institution and physicians requires that CRNAs be ever vigilant to policy issues that would have a deleterious effect on their scope of practice borne of bias, inappropriate use of power, or decisions made absent of fact or rationale, especially those related to clinical best practices, sound business practice, and regulatory issues.

Summary

The US healthcare system is not easy to explain or understand. Its structure is unique among world delivery systems and in many specialties and services, provides the best care available in the world—at least for those who can access and afford it. The system is maintained through a delicate balance of historical prerogatives, political interests, capitalistic incentives, powerful advocacy groups, and skewed incentives, that by most measures ill fit the health needs of the ordinary US citizen. Reform is required and will eventually happen by choice or economic and political peril.

References

1. The World Health Organization's ranking of the world's health systems. World Health Organization website. http://www.photius.com/rankings/healthranks.html. Accessed November 11, 2009.

2. Starr P. *The Social Transformation of American Medicine*. New York, NY: Basic Books; 1983:102-112.

3. Bullough B. Introduction to nursing practice law. In: Bullough B, Bullough V, Soukup M, eds. *Nursing Issues and Nursing Strategies of the Eighties*. New York, NY: Springer Publishing; 1983:279-291.

4. Safreit BJ. Healthcare dollars and regulatory sense: the role of advanced practice nursing. *Yale J Reg.* 1991;9(2):417.

5. Hadley EH. Nurses and prescriptive authority: a legal and economic analysis. *Am J Law Med.* 1989;15(2-3):245.

6. Code of Laws of South Carolina; Medical Practice Act. 1976.

7. Waddle F. Licensure: achievements and limitations. In: *The Study of Credentialing in Nursing: A New Approach*. Kansas City, MO: American Nurses' Association; 1979:126-132.

8. Melosh B. *The Physician's Hand: Work Culture and Conflict in American Nursing*. Philadelphia, PA: Temple University Press; 1982:113-158.

9. Diers D. Nurse-midwives and nurse anesthetists: the cutting edge in specialist practice. In: Aiken LH, Fagin CM, eds. *Charting Nursing's Future: Agenda for the 1990s*. Philadelphia, PA: JB Lippincott; 1992:159-180.

10. Stevens R. *In Sickness and in Wealth: American Hospitals in the Twentieth Century*. New York, NY: Basic Books; 1989:200-227.

11. Numbers RL. The third party: health insurance in America. In: Lee PR, Estes DL, Ramsay NB, eds. *The Nation's Health*. 2nd ed. San Francisco, CA: Boyd and Fraser; 1984:196-204.

12. Wing KR. *The Law and the Public's Health*. Ann Arbor, MI: Health Administration Press; 1985:177-195.

233

13. Ribicoff A, Danaceau P. *The American Medical Machine.* New York, NY: Harrow Books, Harper & Row; 1972:135-167.

14. Jonas S, Goldsteen R, Goldsteen K. *An Introduction to the US Healthcare System.* 6th ed. New York, NY: Springer Publishing; 2007:1-30.

15. Grad FP. *The Public Health Law Manual.* 3rd ed. Washington, DC: American Public Health Association; 2005: 9-23.

16. US Department of Health and Human Services Organizational Chart. http://www.hhs.gov/about/orgchart/index.html. Accessed November 11, 2009.

17. American Association of Colleges of Nursing. Support Medicare Graduate Nursing Education: Increase Access to Quality Health Care. www.aacn.nche.edu/Government/pdf/GNEFactsheet.pdf. Accessed October 17, 2009.

18. Sisko A, Truffer C, Smith S, et al. Health spending projections through 2018: recession effects add uncertainty to the outlook. *Health Aff.* 2009; 28(2):346-357.

19. Jensen E, McKinsey and Company. Will Health Benefit Costs Eclipse Profits? National Coalition of Healthcare Forum and National Healthcare Reform and Its Potential Impacts on New York, May 27, 2009.

Key References

1. Jonas S. *An Introduction to the US Healthcare System.* 4th ed. New York, NY: Springer Publishing. 1998:1-26.

2. Safreit BJ. Healthcare dollars and regulatory sense: the role of advanced practice nursing. *Yale J Reg.* 1991;9(2):417.

3. Starr P. *The Social Transformation of American Medicine.* New York, NY: Basic Books; 1982.

Study Questions

1. From a historical context, discuss the ways that physicians came to exert control over healthcare delivery and services in the United States.

2. What are the characteristics of the healthcare system that have developed from the social tenets of the United States?

3. Early nursing leaders failed to secure nursing practice through licensure, which had substantial ramifications for practice in years to come. What are the characteristics of licensure (as opposed to recognition, registration, or certification) that would have made practice for CRNAs more secure?

4. Identify the basic elements of the healthcare system and describe how each is interrelated. Specifically, describe the relationship between the health service program sectors and its operational components.

5. Describe the functional intent of the 4 major sections of the Medicare Program relating to reimbursement of qualified entities.

6. What are some of the primary failures of today's healthcare delivery system? What do you feel the priorities for change are and why? What, if any role, do CRNAs play in those changes?

CHAPTER 11
Managed Care and Healthcare Reform

Scot D. Foster, CRNA, PhD, FAAN*

Key Concepts

- Managed care is based on the principles of cost control through reduced provider payment, resource management, controlled patient access through "gatekeeping," limited panels of provider staff, and use of information and data that reduces redundancy and unjustified care.

- Although the basic constructs of managed care will likely characterize any healthcare delivery system of the future, the last decade witnessed many system changes, spawned by consumer demand, to bring choice and flexibility to the system that better balance provider choice with cost. These changes, if not carefully monitored, may threaten financial viability of the system by increasing costs.

- Evolved managed care systems of the future will most likely be based on collaborative models in which risk is shared and will, perhaps, include emphasis on new, direct relationships between providers and payers.

- Certified Registered Nurse Anesthetists working in a managed care environment must be increasingly aware of managing cost, documenting quality of care provided, and purposefully improving patient outcomes.

- Healthcare reform measures Congress passed in March 2010 ostensibly reduce cost and broaden opportunity for coverage of the noninsured population. Many of the bill's controversial system changes will require another decade of testing to demonstrate the capacity to deliver intended outcomes.

* Author note: Historical sections of this chapter, which appeared in the first edition of this text, were the work of Jeffrey C. Bauer, PhD, partner in the management consulting practice of ACS Healthcare Solutions, Dearborn, Michigan.

Managed care was a defining feature of the US health system for the last third of the 20th century, and its importance grew continually throughout this period. Few concepts appeared more frequently in a keyword search of the era's popular press and professional literature on American medicine. Managed care attracted so much attention because it played a major role in controlling access, determining quality, redistributing income, and otherwise changing the delivery of healthcare services.

Yet, managed care continues to be viewed simultaneously as the solution to and the cause of problems within the healthcare delivery system. Its proponents have become its opponents within just a few years, and sometimes vice versa. Providers who profited greatly from managed care one year could be bankrupted by it in the next. Consumer satisfaction with managed care was often very high; at the same time, most people seemed to be clamoring for major health plan reform. Many politicians reversed their positions on managed care from one election to the next just to get re-elected. Intense divisions on managed care issues could be found in the 2 major parties by the end of the 1990s.

If you are a bit confused by these contradictions, you are beginning to understand managed care. Managed care has never had a coherent or consistent meaning, despite its increasingly powerful presence over several decades. Indeed, the situation is aptly summarized by the popular quip, "If you've seen one managed care plan, you've seen one managed care plan." You certainly haven't seen them all because plans could be substantially different from market to market at the same time, or they could change substantially in the same market from year to year.

This chapter would ideally start with a definition of managed care, but a consistent and enduring definition does not exist. As will be shown in the next section, managed care effectively encompasses several forms of reimbursement that are not traditional fee-for-service. Managed care plans generally incorporate 1 or more limitations (eg, access control via a "gatekeeper," an approved drug formulary, a limited provider panel) not normally found in indemnity plans that historically allowed providers to bill without restrictions other than their own clinical judgment. However, the differences between managed care plans can be just as great as the differences between managed care and fee-for-service. A standardized definition is inherently imprecise, potentially misleading, and probably outdated soon after it appears in print.

So what's a practitioner to do in the face of such ambiguity and uncertainty? To help answer this important question, this chapter begins with a brief review of the history of managed care and then provides an analysis of its status at the end of the 20th century. Next, some thoughts are presented about its evolution as reflected in the 2010 Patient Protection and Affordable Care Act, which will likely have broad ramifications for the functionality of managed care terms of service. The context for these changes is unique because this act is built on a new philosophical premise that US citizens have a moral right to care; that is, healthcare services are now considered a fundamental right and not a privilege accorded to those who can afford it. Furthermore, the potential for sustaining major reforms as proposed in this legislation must be viewed in the context of a fragile world economy, contemporary political ideology, and thoughtful analysis of the congruence of the act's provisions in the context of personal interpretations of basic democratic values.

A Conceptual Definition

As previously stated, a strict definition of managed care is likely not possible because there are major variations on the theme. However, a listing of characteristics that underlie the concept may be of benefit. Managed care can best be viewed as a continuum of plan types that, to a varying extent, incorporate limited provider networks, primary care gatekeeping of access to specialty services, medical necessity authorization, and negotiated payments including provider risk sharing to aggressively control health care costs.[1] Often the key to successful managed care organizations (MCOs) relies on growing plan membership to gain leverage in provider negotiations and resultant economies of scale.[1] In all cases, the variation among plan types depends on the extent to which the plan does or does not provide strict control of these basic characteristics. Wagner and Kongstvedt[2] provide a visual representation of the continuum of predominant managed care models (Figure 11.1). The left arrow represents looser

controls on choice (with associated increased cost) with progressively stricter controls as one moves to the right of the figure, characterized by the closed-panel HMO. This type of plan would theoretically impose less cost, less choice, and stricter quality controls. Accompanying this figure is a table that briefly describes the characteristics of these models (Table 11.1).[2]

A Brief History of Managed Care

The creation of the prepaid group practice (PPGP) delivery model in the 1920s is generally identified as the beginning of the movement that ultimately became managed care. PPGPs represented a substantial change from the traditional form of reimbursement—fee-for-service—because they charged members a fixed monthly fee for a defined set of benefits. This practice was called capitation because the monthly charge was assessed per capita, that is, per head. The "cap" rate is also commonly designated as the premium per member per month.

Although offering health benefits for a fixed monthly charge was not an entirely new idea at the time, the revolutionary

239

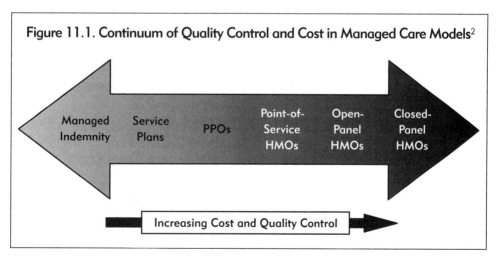

Figure 11.1. Continuum of Quality Control and Cost in Managed Care Models[2]

Managed Indemnity — Service Plans — PPOs — Point-of-Service HMOs — Open-Panel HMOs — Closed-Panel HMOs

Increasing Cost and Quality Control

HMO indicates health maintenance organization; PPO, preferred provider organization.
(Kongstvedt PR. Managed Care: *What It Is and How It Works.* Sudbury, MA: Jones & Bartlett; 2009. jblearning.com. Reprinted with permission.)

Table 11.1. Predominant Models of Managed Care[2]

Model nomenclature	Descriptive characteristics
Indemnity with precertification, mandatory second opinion, and case management	• Traditional insurance with specific schedule of benefits. • Members not restricted in choice of providers. • Providers paid based on usual, customary, and reasonable fee. • Benefits subject to deductible and coinsurance to patient (average 20%). • Market penetration decreasing because of high cost of product.
Service plan with precertification, mandatory second opinion, and case management	• Plan reimburses providers directly and providers agree to plan's fee schedule. • Balance billing other than deductible and coinsurance prohibited. • Provider fees discounted from usual, customary, and reasonable fee and may be based on diagnosis-related groups. • Heavy hospital discounts from large volume and other cost saving factors.
Preferred provider organization (PPO)	• Similar to service plans but cost savings from reduced and approved panel of providers. • Pricing to PPO cannot exceed that provided to other competitors. Balance billing prohibited. • Failure to comply with pricing results in financial penalty to provider. • Benefits reduced if member seeks care outside PPO network. • Most popular managed care organization option.
Point-of-service (POS) plan	• Developed in response to conflict between cost control and freedom of choice of provider. • Member chooses compliance with strict HMO authorization systems (in network), or pays higher fees when for self-referral (out of network). • Decreasing popularity because costs not competitive with HMO or PPO.
"Open-access" HMO	• Members may access any provider in HMO through self-referral. • Benefits substantially lower with high cost sharing for specialist care. • Works only when primary care physician can provide most services without specialists.

Continues on page 241.

Table 11.1. Predominant Models of Managed Care[2] (continued)

Model nomenclature	Descriptive characteristics
Open-panel HMO	• HMO contracts providers as independent contractors under contracted or capitated rates. • Members choose primary care physician for authorization, but have access to wider range of providers. • Provider at risk if cost of care exceeds capitation. • HMO can contract with independent practice organization or directly with provider, which is the most popular method.
Network model	• HMO contracts with several large multispecialty medical groups, usually paid under capitated rates. • Groups pay physicians under a variety of mechanisms. • Network models popular in California where managed care organization penetration is highest in the US.
Closed-panel HMO	• Physicians provide services in HMO facilites to HMO members only. Types include staff and group models. • For staff model, providers are employess of HMO, which pays salary and incentive plan. • Group model more common. Autonomously governed physicians contract with HMO to provide services per capitation. Group pays provider salary and incentives. Group at risk if cost exceeds capitation, but HMO generally provides stop-loss reinsurance • Kaiser Permanente best known group model.

HMO indicates health maintenance organization; PPO, preferred provider organization.
(Kongstvedt PR. Managed Care: *What It Is and How It Works*. Sudbury, MA: Jones & Bartlett; 2009. jblearning.com. Reprinted with permission.)

241

aspect of the PPGP movement was putting providers at risk. Under the traditional fee-for-service arrangement, doctors theoretically got paid for all the care they provided. Under a capitated PPGP plan, however, doctors were obligated to provide care in accordance with the terms of the contract. Providers lost money if the costs of patient care exceeded the premium per member per month. The only way to make a net profit from the arrangement was to have other patients whose care cost proportionally less.

PPGPs had a financial incentive to avoid providing medical services that did not keep the patient healthy according to the terms of the contract.

Health Maintenance Organizations

Perhaps the best known PPGP was the plan organized in the late 1920s by Henry Kaiser, a very successful and socially concerned industrialist in Oakland, California. The Kaiser Plan identified itself as a health maintenance organization (HMO) to emphasize the proposition that keeping people healthy was a win-win situation. Preventive care, such as screening to identify diseases in early stages when treatment was less expensive, presumably maintained members' health and allowed the plan to make a fair profit. The HMOs' presumed orientation to preventive care became the key distinguishing feature of their reputation for at least 50 years, even though the research literature offers scant evidence that the theory was commonly put into practice. Organized medicine staunchly opposed the PPGP-HMO movement from the beginning on grounds that capitation gave doctors an incentive to undertreat (ie, to withhold care that was medically necessary). Indeed, medical associations argued that fixed reimbursement forced doctors to consider their remuneration when determining the course of treatment—a clear violation of the Hippocratic dictum that money should not influence a doctor's decisions. Due to the overall political strength of organized medicine, the early stages of managed care were effectively confined to California and a few Midwestern states for 4 decades.

As indemnity health insurance matured under the control of organized medicine, the highly politicized fight against capitation diverted public attention from the countervailing proposition that fee-for-service reimbursement promoted overtreatment.[3] Excessive care received almost no attention until the costs of Medicare and Medicaid began to skyrocket far beyond projected levels in the late 1960s and the early 1970s. As luck would have it, the president of the United States believed strongly in capitation and PPGP. President Richard M. Nixon successfully led the fight to base the nation's first federal health reform program on HMOs. The Health Maintenance Organization Act of

1973 gave special status to capitated health plans, legitimizing "managed care" in the process. HMOs suddenly attracted attention because they were presumably less expensive than traditional health insurance products.

The meaning of managed care became muddled almost immediately. Academic researchers and policy analysts touted HMOs for their presumed emphasis on prevention, but employers were more interested in the potential price advantage of the new alternatives to fee-for-service, or AHPs, for most of the 1970s, when managed care was not yet a common term. Preferred provider organizations (PPO) entered the market as another alternative. PPOs reduced employers' costs of health insurance by securing discounts from medical groups and hospitals and listing them on the panel of providers authorized by the health plan. PPOs were based almost entirely on fee-for-service arrangements and seldom put providers at risk, but like HMOs, they attracted attention because they were an alternative to traditional insurance. The use of gatekeepers, health plan employees (often nurses) charged with the task of denying coverage for "unnecessary" services, was the only major feature shared by HMOs and PPOs. Nevertheless, with almost nothing else in common, both were lumped together under the rubric of managed care beginning in the early 1980s. By the end of the decade, managed care was firmly established as the challenger to fee-for-service health plans, even though the term itself encompassed 2 very different alternatives that still relied predominantly on fee-for-service arrangements below the surface.

Managed Care in the 1990s

The scope of managed care expanded even further in the early 1990s. Employee provider organizations, point-of-sale options, and other variations on the general theme added to the "alphabet soup" of managed care. Indeed, managed care's power was so strong that it became the cornerstone of President Clinton's intense but failed effort at national health reform in 1993 and 1994. The healthcare marketplace of Minneapolis-St. Paul was used widely as the model for national reform because it reportedly had the nation's lowest rate of health plan inflation and highest concentration of HMOs and PPOs. As a sign of the quick ebb and flow of managed care, the Twin Cities had some of the nation's highest premium increases and most troubled health plans just 5 years later. Managed care did not deliver as promised by the politicians, pundits, and policy wonks.

Managed care attracted a remarkable amount of attention over the past several decades, but did not develop a coherent definition or consistent form. The closest thing to a common trait in the evolving versions of managed care is probably the use of restrictions to prevent practitioners from making decisions free of economic constraints. The best that might be said of managed care so far is that it is an antidote for some serious problems of fee-for-service medical care. However, it has not yet proven to be a cure for the underlying economic disease of increased healthcare costs and associated ills of disparate access, sometimes dubious health outcomes, and uneven quality of care.

Managed Care at the Turn of the Century

By the end of the century, almost 80 million Americans, approximately 30% of the US population, were enrolled in HMOs, the predominant form of managed care. Tens of millions more were covered by PPOs. Despite their huge rise in popularity in the last 3 decades, as well as some success in holding down care costs, managed care systems were not viewed as entirely successful. Premiums were climbing, medical care inflation was re-emerging, and its expansion slowed, especially among HMOs. Many MCOs were losing money and experienced myriad complaints from the public about their quality, efficiency, and patient-centeredness at the expense of corporate shareholder profit. Many viewed managed care as providing only a modicum of benefit when compared with the clearly flawed fee-for-service system. In such circumstances, defining the practice environment of the early 21st century was difficult. Far from being models of competition and cost management, most of the large HMOs and insurers in the nation simply wanted to reverse their recent losses. Health plans shifted their focus from growth to profitability in the late 1990s, and their provider and customer relations deteriorated at about the same time. As a result, many industry observers wrote articles predicting the imminent failure of managed care.[4,5] The reasons for these predictions were varied and included:

- Inability to control medical loss ratio (percentage of premium paid to medical services) due in part to high administrative expenses
- Rise of pharmaceutical costs by 11% to 12% yearly
- Increasing resistance from organized providers to HMO discounts
- Limited application of disease management programs, prevention, screening, or wellness
- Lack of sophisticated computer systems that could facilitate a competent administrative infrastructure

243

- The advent of rapidly developing medical technology and genomics
- Greater consumer demand including an exploding aging population with greater life expectancy
- Cost of complying with governmental regulation

The first decade of the 21st century brought other changes to managed care, the most important of which was a significant drop in HMO enrollment in preference to the PPO, where choice and flexibility were more characteristic. Nationwide, between 1996 and 2003, HMO market share dropped from 31% to 24% of covered workers while PPOs rose from 28% to 54% of covered workers.[6] In 2009, managed care enrollment totaled nearly 130 million people, evenly split between HMOs and PPOs. The HMO penetration rate was 24% nationwide, and nearly 71% of the Medicaid population was enrolled in managed care with about half that number in the Medicare population.[7] Reasons for this shift were largely in reaction to new consumer protection legislation, disgruntled consumers regarding access to and quality of care, limited consumer choice, and provider angst over the corporatization of healthcare decision making.

In response, there was general loosening of the tightly managed application of traditional managed care practices. These loosened restrictions varied substantially among plans; however, all MCOs employed a variety of strategies to stem the tide of decreased HMO enrollment, including elimination of the gatekeeper approval for access to specialists, shifting risk away from providers (capitation or risk pools), and decreasing utilization management as well as reducing mandated prior authorizations. Most importantly, many plans were offering less restrictive products and greater

choice. In sum, HMOs and PPOs became markedly less differentiated.

Managed Medicare and Medicaid

Currently there are nearly 100 million enrollees in Medicare and Medicaid,[8] most in managed care arrangements. The efforts of the healthcare reform act will likely have profound influence on total enrollment in these public programs given the massive infusion of enrollees into Medicaid expected as a means for individuals and businesses to access healthcare services. On the other hand, there may be tremendous effects on Part C of Medicare (Advantage programs—from substantial decrements to reimbursements that are scheduled). Specifically, $110 billion in cuts are part of the proposed Medicare savings from across-the-board "productivity adjustments" to fund broader access via Medicaid. These cuts would affect payments to both hospitals and providers. In short, the act will have profound and yet unknown effects. These unknown effects could come in the form of several issues and assumptions:

- Will the penalties for not buying mandated insurance plans provide sufficient incentive to prompt the younger population to move into plans that would counterbalance higher cost, older patients?
- Congress currently struggles with the dilemma of how to maintain reasonable reimbursement that would give providers incentives to continue to participate in these public programs. Congress keeps overriding the anticipated 21% provider payment cuts, but only for temporary periods. A sustainable solution is not in sight, and the health reform act anticipates nearly $330 billion of the $1 trillion total reform cost to be

generated from these cuts as well as those anticipated from cutting reimbursements for imaging services, rehabilitation, and long-term care hospitals and from reducing the prescription drug benefit to drug makers.

- What will the insurance exchanges look like? What are their operational details? Specifically, what constitutes minimum benefit packages and regulatory costs required to ensure compliance with benefit standards? Regulatory specifics were not available as of this writing.

- Several state attorneys general introduced lawsuits that test the constitutionality of the individual mandate. They contend that Congress lacks the authority under the interstate commerce clause to require individuals to buy health insurance. If successful and the individual mandate is found unconstitutional, a large portion of income anticipated to pay for reform from individuals will not be forthcoming, thus stifling the reform attempt. If unsuccessful, insurers may be forced to cover additional unhealthy customers without the benefit of new, healthy customers to offset costs.

There is much yet unknown about the future of Medicare and Medicaid and its ultimate effects on provider practice, including CRNAs. However, these entitlement programs have become enormously popular with the citizenry, who will likely not tolerate draconian change. On the other side of that equation, providers remain wary because excessive austerity measures that decrease provider reimbursement will likely cause them to abandon service provision in greater numbers, because many now claim that reimbursement rates do not sufficiently cover cost, much less afford reasonable profit.

Although initial attempts at reform legislation included proposals for Medicare Part B reimbursement reform, many if not all of those attempts were abandoned at least temporarily when legislators began to understand that comprehensive payment reform could not be implemented for hospitals or physicians in a timely manner and without major system disruption. Currently, reform efforts do not affect private insurance payment for CRNA services, and rates for CRNA services under state-based exchanges have not been set. It is not until 2014 that individual insurance mandates will become effective that may, in part, offset anticipated cuts in other areas. Still, much of the work of the AANA on its members' behalf will necessarily be focused on maintaining access to and fair reimbursement from both public and private managed care plans.

The Future of Managed Care

It is unlikely that the healthcare delivery system will shift dramatically away from a basic paradigm of managed care or managed competition in favor of a single-payer system prevalent in many European countries. Given the current political climate in which fears abound (founded or not) that increasing governmental intrusion or takeover of large segments of the economy ultimately threaten private business by promoting socialistic public policy, managed care will likely continue in its present form, experimenting with new strategies that balance cost and choice. Unless or until rampant medical inflation emerges or the public refuses to assume greater cost-sharing responsibilities, the system is unlikely to change, without expanded enrollments and reduced benefits. Although recent health reform measures will likely affect the configuration of managed care, there is a general lack of clarity on the end results (positive or negative) of new iterations of managed care.

In the past 5 years, increasing attention has been paid to the concept of *consumerism* as a viable, new model of managed care. Under this concept, there is a general move away from provider-centric to consumer-centric plans that emphasize substantial patient cost sharing and financial incentives for patients to make better choices in plans based on service quality. Succinctly stated, "providers (physicians, hospitals and other suppliers of health care) would compete for consumers who would be armed with the quality and cost information needed to make informed choices and motivated to do so by paying a larger share of the cost of their health care."[9] The goal of this new paradigm was to stimulate competition among providers that would drive quality improvement and contain costs more effectively than the managed care tools used by HMOs and other health plans in the past, for example, limited provider networks, primary care gatekeeping of access to specialty services, medical necessity authorization, and provider risk sharing.[1]

Robinson[10] provides a similar perspective on the consumer model. "Consumerism and managed competition share the market paradigm that social resources, including medical care, should be allocated based on individual rather than collective decisions. Informed and price-conscious individual choices represent the values and preferences of the patient better than the choices of even the most benevolent third party. The performance of the delivery system is enhanced by consumer and provider incentives that align the pursuit of individual self-interest and the social interest in promoting a high-quality, cost effective

system of care." This author summarizes his concept by describing it as a market-oriented system that combines the best elements of the demand side of consumerism with the supply-side approach characteristic of traditional managed care organizations. Table 11.2 describes divergent perspectives between consumerism and managed competition relative to market and factors influencing healthcare and insurance coverage. Factors characterizing the operational view attendant to this new model include:

- *Consumer-driven care and decision making:* Consumerism is built around the concept that individual choice, as opposed to provider/MCO choice, is preferred to ensure that cost is controlled, and service is more likely to be aligned with patient need. Therefore, in this new, hybrid system, there are greater amounts of data to which the consumer has access relating to the type of quality of service provided, and the consumer is always in the best position to make an informed and accurate decision about care alternatives and service providers. In essence, the consumer will, in trade for choice, assume greater financial risk.

- *Health benefit designs:* From the consumer perspective, the desirable benefit package comes with high-deductible, indemnity-type coverage, supported by a health savings account, from which the consumer pays for noncatastrophic medical expenses.[9] These consumer-directed health plans and health savings accounts have met with mixed success in the market, predicated largely on the demographic of the employee, such as wage range, length of employment, and whether or not they have union representation.

Table 11.2. Contrasting Views of Consumerism and Managed Competition on the Markets for Healthcare and Health[10]

Market for healthcare	Consumerism	Managed competition
Physician-patient interaction	Price-conscious consumer choice generates appropriate provider behavior.	Practice variations, quality shortfalls result from weak consumer choices.
Large physician and hospital organizations	Often bureaucratic, monopolistic	Source of coordination, incentive alignment
Preferred practice setting	Small physician practices, single specialty hospitals	Multispecialty medical groups, integrated delivery systems
Preferred provider payment method	Fee-for-service, episode-of-illness pricing	Capitation for provider organizations, salary for individual physicians
Preferred method of performance measurement	Performance measures of individual physicians and clinical services	Performance measures of physician organizations and the spectrum of services
Role of economic incentives at time of seeking care	Central: With substantial cost sharing, consumer faces strong incentive to consider cost as well as quality.	Peripheral: With limited cost sharing, consumer focuses on quality rather than cost.

Market for health insurance coverage	Consumerism	Managed competition
Health insurance plans	Skeptical: Insurance is needed to spread risk, but it fosters price-unconscious demand.	Positive: Support consumer choice and provider coordination, as well as spreading risk.
Preferred benefit design	Extensive consumer cost sharing: High deductible with health savings account	Limited consumer cost sharing: Comprehensive coverage with modest copayments
Preferred network design	Broad PPO network with competing, nonintegrated providers	Integrated HMO network, ideally centered on physician group practices

Continues on page 248.

247

Table 11.2. Contrasting Views of Consumerism and Managed Competition on the Markets for Healthcare and Health[10] (continued)

Market for health insurance coverage	Consumerism	Managed competition
Role of employer and governmental sponsors as active purchasers of insurance coverage	Skeptical: Third parties distort consumer incentives; ideal is individual insurance market with tax subsidies.	Positive: Sponsors need to play active role in comparing quality, offsetting risk selection, and not merely subsidizing coverage.
Role of economic incentives at time of choosing insurance coverage	Peripheral: Health plans should offer similar, overlapping provider networks; consumer has choice focused on benefit design, not network design.	Central: Health plans should offer distinct, competing provider networks; consumer choice focused on network design, not benefit design.

- *Hospital consolidation:* It is an accepted assumption that hospitals will continue to consolidate for a variety of reasons, including higher likelihood of accessing capital for building and service expansion and a greater and more efficient use of expensive information technologies required to track performance and financial economies of scale.

- *Health and wellness and case management programs:* These programs are enjoying increased popularity among both consumers and MCOs on the precept that they provide postacute services, enhance routine management of health issues (eg, obesity, smoking, fitness), and keep a hand in managing cost in patients with higher-risk disease processes. Most programs are not as tightly controlled as traditional "utilization" panels, and many employers have incorporated wellness programming into benefit plans by means of aggressive incentives to participate, and thus keep employees out of the hospital and decrease cost. Again, success is spotty relative to the newness of these programs and the fact that cost sharing among some may provide less incentive to the consumer.

- *Quality performance and price transparency:* Any emerging iteration of managed care, including a new emphasis on consumerism models, will necessarily incorporate more attention to service price transparency and consistency of price throughout service sectors. This price transparency will enhance CRNA desirability as preferred providers when the public shops for high-quality, low-cost providers. Furthermore, it is increasingly likely that, commensurate with pay-for-performance programs, somewhat common in medicine, other providers will be subject to the same programs that directly link pay with outcomes, including patient satisfaction, resulting financial efficiencies, and productivity profiles.

Practical Advice for Practitioners

Skills required by a select group of independent CRNAs for forging managed care contracts will not be addressed specifically in this narrative. Suffice it to say that legal advice is highly recommended to ensure clear delineation of rights and responsibilities of both parties. Alternatively, professional advice from other billing and contracting professionals is a desirable first step to ensure a strong business structure and adequate profit margin.

For those CRNAs practicing in the healthcare team model, there is practical advice of another nature, not directly related to contract acquisition and management. These factors include the need for CRNAs to be aware of their need to not only provide, but also to document the quality of their work according to professional industry standards. A CRNA's ability to acquire and maintain liability coverage will depend on it, as will a hospital's reporting of patient outcomes to state and federal authorities and a variety of accrediting or institutional certification or regulatory agencies. Other requisite activities for CRNAs to keep at the forefront of daily practice include a keen sensitivity to and vigilant monitoring of equipment cost and supplies, especially pharmaceutical agents. CRNAs can also be effective at keeping costs in line by organizing their time such that productivity standards are met and exceeded, as well as patient expectations of clinical performance. Above all, an employed CRNA should never become indifferent to the need to help

the institutions for which they work meet the underlying tenets of managed care. Remember, it is you, the provider, who exerts substantial influence over the expense side of the ledger, regardless of whether you are self-employed or employed by a group or hospital. It is not enough to be clinically excellent; you must be work-smart.

Perhaps the most important concern of CRNA employers is to hire and retain CRNAs with optimum clinical flexibility in order to meet clinical productivity requirements. The greatest threat to a CRNA's continued employment is his or her unwillingness or inability to maintain a comprehensive and diverse clinical skill set, in other words, to maintain a full scope of practice. Too often, CRNAs become "comfortable" in their jobs and start demanding fewer hours and limitations to cases managed (eg, obstetrics, regional blocks, trauma). Other CRNAs may refuse to work in particular surgical environments, such as inpatient areas, preferring outpatient or surgical centers, or they may refuse remote site surgeries such as interventional radiology, to the comfort of well-supervised, inpatient surgical suites. Some CRNAs will refuse to serve other anesthesia settings in the network of contracted service areas to accommodate their own need for the security of routine. In all these cases, it is important to realize that such behaviors contribute to an increasing lack of value of the CRNA to the employer. In times of full employment of CRNAs, this will and should lead to dismissal. CRNAs must be ever mindful that experience and clinical skill alone will not suffice to achieve the perceived status of desirable employee. Your employer, in most cases, is contracted to provide service to a diverse array of surgical need in diverse environments. Flexibility is a key component of an employee's work ethic. Given the high

249

range of salaries currently enjoyed by most CRNAs, it is an unreasonable expectation that those levels of compensation can accommodate a recalcitrant attitude or self-imposed restrictions on scope of practice.

One final thought: All CRNAs must realize that as the market in healthcare becomes more managed and scrutinized for factors that make services efficient and of high quality, the same concepts regarding plan evaluation will apply to CRNAs, demanding that they become more competitive with other provider groups. Although about 80% of CRNAs work in a team setting, this work arrangement in no way precludes the need for CRNAs to practice independently in terms of decision making. It is not beyond the realm of possibility that, as federal reimbursement schema changes, so will the competitive nature of employment. That is, regardless of work environment, CRNAs should not consider themselves a protected class by an employer or believe that they are somehow magically removed from competitive forces. With high salaries and high demand come high competition to demonstrate value unique to the professional service provided by CRNAs alone and not defined by support mechanisms from other providers. In every case, CRNAs should be valued by employers because they are capable of independent thought and practice. That is the only way in which an employer can exploit (in the positive connotation of the term) the vast skills and resources the employee brings to patient care.

The concept of managed care is dynamic and evolving. Nevertheless, there are certain principles that underlie the process about which CRNAs need to be attentive. Notions of cost efficiency, control of resources, meaningful quality measures, and evidence-based outcomes remain paramount, regardless of the iteration of managed care structure. Some of the best and most productive networks to increase understanding of these concepts are personal contacts with other experienced CRNAs via attendance at state and national professional meetings.

Healthcare Reform

On March 23, 2010, President Barack Obama signed a comprehensive healthcare reform bill into law, titled the Patient Protection and Affordable Care Act. This historic legislation, pursued in some form by virtually every president since Franklin D. Roosevelt, has both its ardent supporters and opponents, but nonetheless portends substantial, and hopefully, positive change. Most analysts agree that it will take at least a decade to make any competent analysis of its effects and long-term potential to improve healthcare accessibility, quality, and affordability for millions of Americans. In broad terms, the health reform package provides government subsidies to low- and middle-income families buying health insurance on their own, expands eligibility rules for Medicaid, and provides coverage for a majority of uninsured Americans. It would also establish a number of insurance reforms.[11] The Congressional Budget Office determined that the new bill would provide coverage to 32 million people in the United States previously not covered (bringing the total covered to 94% of the US population). The cost of the coverage components of the new law are estimated by the Congressional Budget Office to be $938 billion over 10 years, financed through a combination of savings from Medicare and Medicaid and new taxes and fees, including an excise tax on high cost insurance.[12] They also expect that the healthcare reform law will reduce the deficit by $124 billion over 10 years. The balance of this chapter will highlight the bill's major features and issues of specific importance to

CRNAs. Clearly, provisions of this act will have ramifications for current managed care services and available products. It is likely, however, that those changes will continue to exist within the context of the delicate balance between cost and choice, and of course, the public's taste for additional taxes, potential threats to entitlement programs such as Medicare, and perceptions of excessive federal authority over individuals.

Features of the New Law

Approach and Design
This law requires that most US citizens and legal residents have health insurance that can be obtained in several ways. First is by individual mandate to obtain insurance or pay an annual financial penalty. Second is the expansion of Medicaid coverage for all individuals under age 65 with incomes up to 133% of the federal poverty level. For people with incomes more than 133% of the poverty level, there will be 2 types of state health insurance exchanges established, one for individuals to afford coverage through a variety of premium and cost-sharing subsidies and one for small businesses, which are afforded a variety of tax incentives to offer affordable health insurance to employees. All plans in the exchanges would be required to offer benefits that meet a minimum standard. Under this new law, funding levels for the Children's Health Insurance Program (CHIP) would extend through 2015, and there will be increased payments to primary care doctors who participate in Medicaid.

Changes to Private Insurance
There are important new requirements in the law that will codify a substantial number of new insurance reforms, a few of which are highlighted here. Insurance regulations will prevent insurers from denying coverage to people for any reason, including health status or from charging more based on health status and gender. Insurance companies will be required to establish a temporary national high-risk pool to provide health coverage to individuals with preexisting medical conditions. New health plans must provide comprehensive coverage that includes minimum service, caps on annual out-of-pocket spending, and limits annual or lifetime limits of coverage. Furthermore, insurers will be prohibited from rescinding coverage unless fraud is proven. Increases in health plan premiums will be subject to review before they are implemented, and employers who impose a waiting period for coverage greater than 60 days will be fined. The new law also will provide dependent coverage for adult children up to age 26 for individual and group policies. Importantly, the law requires health plans to report the proportion of premium dollars spent on clinical services that will, it is hoped, close the gap most apparent when comparing public and private plans.

Improvements to Medicare
Many advocates of this legislation believe that the new law contains provisions that will improve the sustainability and administrative efficiency of Medicare, close benefit gaps, and improve care for Medicare beneficiaries. Some claim that cost savings borne of these changes may add a decade of solvency of the Medicare Hospital Insurance Trust Fund; however, at this point, such assumptions are largely theoretical. For example, Congress has yet to solve issues that relate to stabilizing Medicare Part B provider reimbursement. Congress has repeatedly extended, on a temporary basis, long-term relief from threats of huge Medicare payment cuts to providers, and

251

more than half of the total cost of healthcare reform is scheduled to come from this new Medicare restructure. Much of the detail regarding the practical effects on providers is unknown (as of this writing) for lack of regulatory specificity. To further illustrate this point, during legislative debate on the bill's merits, much was made of "bending the cost curve" by putting downward pressure on health spending, closing unintended tax loopholes, and promoting tax compliance. Exactly how and to what extent there will be success in achieving those 3 goals and on whom downward pressure on spending and taxation will apply provide ample justification for doubt about the law's ultimate value or benefit.

Cost Containment

Cost containment strategies in this statute are as varied as they are controversial, because projected cost constraints are based on assumptions not shared by all engaged in the debate. The most important component of this category is the establishment of an Independent Payment Advisory Board whose role is to submit proposals containing recommendations to Congress to reduce the per-capita rate of growth in Medicare spending if spending exceeds a target growth rate. The board cannot submit proposals that ration care, increase revenues, or change benefits or eligibility or Medicare beneficiary cost sharing. The AANA remains concerned, as it would be with most national advisory boards of this sort, that CRNAs, ARNPs, or RNs be represented on the 15-member board and that the Independent Payment Advisory Board establish a means of appeal or recourse if their decisions impair patient access to care from nonphysician provider groups.

Improving Public Health, System Performance, and Quality

These statutory provisions involve the implementation of new programs that focus on promoting quality through the better use of research, integrating care services, increasing funding for community health centers (including nurse-managed clinics), increasing national emergency and trauma center capacity, promoting wellness programs and standards, and promoting research and care practices that are firmly based on demonstrated patient health outcomes. In addition, the law requires that consumers be provided with information about physician ownership of hospitals and medical equipment companies, nursing homes, and other business entities. Knowledge of potential conflicts of interest may result in better patient choices regarding sources of care.

Most notable is the establishment of a nonprofit, patient-centered outcomes research institute to compare the clinical effectiveness of medical treatments. These efforts may eventually lead to congressional actions that result in revised reimbursement schema, actions by insurance providers to make justifiable decisions to accept or deny coverage or by purchasers to combat denied claims or negotiate coverage on the basis of treatment effectiveness. However, these research findings cannot currently be construed as mandates for change; rather, they lay the foundation for legislative action in the future. Finally, renewed efforts will be made to establish compliance programs and data sets that justify systemic change to eliminate waste, fraud, and abuse in all public programs.

Healthcare Workforce

There are a number of workforce initiatives in the new healthcare reform law. They

252

include establishing a Workforce Advisory Committee to develop a national workforce strategy; making key investments in training doctors, nurses, and other healthcare providers; and establishing scholarship and loan repayment programs. The focus of statutory provisions in this legislation is on expanding the workforce, especially in primary care and care in rural areas.

AANA Contributions to Health Reform

The AANA helped to secure several provisions in the comprehensive health reform legislation important to the patients, practice, and the profession of nurse anesthesia. These include provider nondiscrimination in healthcare, nurse workforce and development provisions, graduate nursing education initiatives, and the pain care policy act. Tables 11.3 to 11.6 contain the language of these provisions developed by the AANA.[13]

A Call for Critical Analysis

It is imperative that all CRNAs and students carefully examine the myriad provisions of this new statute to decide for themselves both the ultimate value it brings to the public and the effects the provisions will have on individual clinical practitioners. It should be no surprise that the CRNA electorate reflects the same philosophical polarities of the general public, so given the historical and profound change this statute imposes, its provisions should be analyzed in the context of our time, including the current national political scene, economic conditions, effects on social structure, and personal interpretations of democratic values that each citizen brings to the evaluation process.

This type of critical analysis is the basis on which our professional organization must build its own philosophical and political agendas to serve both our patients and ourselves. It should be apparent to all informed CRNAs that a statute of this magnitude will have high value for some and unintended consequence for others. As with any other historic statute of this sort, it will and should remain a dynamic framework upon which positive change can be based.

253

Table 11.3 Provider Nondiscrimination Language[13]

SEC. 2706. NON-DISCRIMINATION IN HEALTH CARE.

(a) PROVIDERS.—A group health plan and a health insurance issuer offering group or individual health insurance coverage shall not discriminate with respect to participation under the plan or coverage against any health care provider who is acting within the scope of that provider's license or certification under applicable State law. This section shall not require that a group health plan or health insurance issuer contract with any health care provider willing to abide by the terms and conditions for participation established by the plan or issuer. Nothing in this section shall be construed as preventing a group health plan, a health insurance issuer, or the Secretary from establishing varying reimbursement rates based on quality or performance measures.

This language of the bill addressing the long-standing issue of provider nondiscrimination will help protect and advance patient access to healthcare services provided by CRNAs. Implementation date for this provision is 2014.
(Reprinted with permission from the American Association of Nurse Anesthetists.)

Table 11.4 Nurse Workforce Development Provisions[13]

With the support and involvement of the nursing community, the legislation includes language reauthorizing Title 8 nurse workforce development programs (Secs. 5308 – 5312) identical to what the nursing community requested with the AANA's involvement, and which would also establish a National Health Care Workforce Commission (Sec. 5101). The legislation also includes an AANA-sought provision removing a statutory cap that previously limited certain traineeship funds so that only 10% or less could be allocated to doctoral-level education.

(Reprinted with permission from the American Association of Nurse Anesthetists.)

Table 11.5. Graduate Nursing Education Initiative[13]

Legislation includes a Graduate Nursing Education (GNE) demonstration project (Sec. 5509) to support the expanded development of advanced practice registered nurses (APRNs). This four-year, $200 million initiative takes effect beginning FY 2012. However, concerns with the GNE provision relate to it being limited to only five hospitals. The AANA, AARP and the nursing community are working to address this situation with Congress and appropriate federal agencies.

(Reprinted with permission from the American Association of Nurse Anesthetists.)

254

Table 11.6 Pain Care Policy Act[13]

The legislation authorizes but does not fund an initiative called the National Pain Care Policy Act (Sec. 4305). It authorizes the Secretary of Health and Human Services to convene a conference on pain management to increase the recognition of pain as a significant public health problem, and directs the Secretary to report to Congress her findings no later than June 30, 2011. It also authorizes a Pain Consortium at the National Institutes of Health to enhance and coordinate clinical research on pain causes and treatments. Finally, not later than one year after enactment there shall be established an Interagency Pain Research Coordinating Committee to coordinate efforts among federal agencies that relate to pain research. The AANA will be working throughout the implementation process to ensure CRNA viewpoints are taken into account.

(Reprinted with permission from the American Association of Nurse Anesthetists.)

References

1. Draper DA, Hurley RE, Lesser CS, Strunk BC. The changing face of managed care. *Health Aff.* 2002;21(1):11-23.

2. Wagner ER, Kongstvedt PR. Types of managed health care plans and integrated healthcare delivery systems. In: Kongstvedt PR, ed. *Managed Health Care: What It Is and How It Works.* 3rd ed. Sudbury, MA: Jones and Bartlett Publishers; 2009.

3. Bauer JC. *Not What the Doctor Ordered: How to End the Medical Monopoly in Pursuit of Managed Care.* New York, NY: McGraw-Hill; 1998.

4. Robinson JC. The end of managed care. *JAMA.* 2001;285(20):2622-2626.

5. Swartz K. The death of managed care as we know it. *J Health Polit Policy Law.* 1999;24(5):1201-1205.

6. Gabel J, Claxton G, Holre E, et al. Health benefits in 2003: premiums reach thirteen-year high as employers adopt new forms of cost sharing. *Health Aff.* 2003;22(5):117-126.

7. Kaiser Family State Health Facts.org. State HMO Penetration Rate: July 2008. http://www.statehealthfacts. org/comparemaptable.jsp?ind=349&cat=7. Accessed May 27, 2010.

8. Managed Care Online. http://www. mcareol.com/factshts/factnati.htm. Accessed August 23, 2010.

9. Christianson JB, Ginsburg PB, Draper DA. The transition from managed care to consumerism: a community–level status report. *Health Aff.* 2008;27(5):1362.

10. Robinson JC. Managed consumerism in health care. *Health Aff.* 2005;24 (6):1479.

11. Sahadi J. Health reform: the $$$ story. CNNMoney.com website. http://money. cnn.com/2010/03/20/news/economy/ cbo_reconciliation/index.htm. Accessed March 7, 2011.

12. Kaiser Family Foundation website. www.kff.org. Publication 8061. Summary of New Health Reform Law: Last Modified: March 26, 2010. Associated source: www.democratic leader.house.gov/. Accessed March 7, 2011.

13. Walker JR. Letter from the AANA President to Speaker Nancy Pelosi and Leader John Boehner. March 17, 2010. www.aana.com/healthreform. aspx. Accessed March 7, 2011.

255

Key References

Kongstvedt PR. *Managed Care: What It Is and How It Works.* 3rd ed. Sudbury, MA: Jones and Bartlett Publishers; 2009.

Study Questions

1. What are the primary characteristics of managed care and how do they affect care delivery and consumer satisfaction and choice?

2. Managed care has failed to universally control healthcare costs. What are some reasons that may be contributing to this continuing problem?

3. How can practicing CRNAs contribute to their employers' need to manage the cost of care? Devise a project in your own surgical environment that addresses (and yields results) in decreasing the cost curve.

4. How can the healthcare reform statute contribute positively to better healthcare? What are some of the primary pitfalls of the new legislation? Make certain your analysis is not based on assumption, but fact.

5. What are the primary mechanisms used by state and national leadership within the AANA to influence healthcare policy, such as healthcare reform?

CHAPTER 12

Reimbursement for Anesthesia Services

James R. Walker, CRNA, DNP
Lee S. Broadston, ABA, COBS

Key Concepts

- Reimbursement is one of the most complex aspects of anesthesia practice. Several case-specific components must be evaluated individually to maximize Certified Registered Nurse Anesthetist (CRNA) professional fees.

- Healthcare consumers desire anesthesia services that reflect safety, efficiency, and economic responsibility.

- Medicare Part A provides pass-through funding to eligible rural or critical access hospitals for CRNA services. CRNAs cannot receive direct reimbursement from Medicare Part A.

- Medicare Part B provides direct reimbursement to CRNAs for anesthesia services. There are important differences between the reimbursement models including medical direction, medical supervision, and nonmedical direction.

- Many third-party payers including state Medicaid, private insurers, and others use reimbursement mechanisms similar to those used by Medicare.

Continues on next page.

Key Concepts (continued)

- Teaching CRNAs and teaching anesthesiologists have specific reimbursement considerations that influence the education of future anesthesia providers.

- Reimbursement from governmental and nongovernmental payers for chronic and acute pain management services and other nonanesthesia services is different from the reimbursement for anesthesia services. Understanding these differences is key to a successful chronic and acute pain practice.

- Reimbursement for anesthesia services requires understanding of how anesthesia services are valued (eg, relative value scale, relative value guide, resource-based relative value scale) and the associated conversion factors.

- CRNAs must understand the reimbursement process including the importance of National Provider Identifier numbers as well as accurate diagnosis and procedural coding on all submitted claims.

Certified Registered Nurse Anesthetists (CRNAs) in all practice environments must recognize that fair reimbursement for services is vital to the success of their practices and of the nurse anesthesia profession. Today's competitive healthcare marketplace and complex practice environments demand not only advanced clinical skills, but also practice management knowledge and skills. These skills will advance a CRNA's ability to excel both clinically and financially. Each of the elements that contribute to successful reimbursement must be identified and monitored by daily procedures throughout the life of the practice in order to achieve and maintain success.

Medicare Reimbursement

Medicare is a health insurance program provided by the United States government. Medicare is available to those who are 65 years of age or older, those under 65 years of age with certain disabilities, or any age with end-stage renal disease.[1] The Medicare program provides insurance to eligible beneficiaries for hospital insurance (Part A), medical insurance (Part B), optional managed care plans (Part C), and prescription drug insurance (Part D). Before January 1989, Medicare Part B directly reimbursed only anesthesiologists for anesthesia services. Because CRNAs were not eligible for direct reimbursement from Medicare Part B, hospitals were reimbursed for CRNA services under Medicare Part A. Through federal legislative efforts, CRNAs became eligible for direct Medicare reimbursement through the enactment of the Omnibus Reconciliation Act (ORA) of 1987.[2] Effective January 1, 1989, CRNAs became eligible for direct reimbursement for anesthesia services through Medicare Part B.[2] This change was budget neutral for the Medicare program because the reimbursement for CRNA services was shifted from Medicare Part A to Medicare Part B. Because Medicare recognizes CRNA services, most private health insurers and state public health plans also provide separate reimbursement for CRNA services. These changes in reimbursement policy have brought greater parity for reimbursement for CRNA services, as compared with anesthesiologist services. The implementation of these reimbursement policies introduced complexity and often confusion to the healthcare reimbursement arena. Today's healthcare spending is highly scrutinized. Reimbursement opportunities cannot be left untapped, including those for CRNA services. It is crucial that CRNAs understand not only the reimbursement systems, but also the other forces influencing the healthcare market. These understandings will equip CRNAs with an improved ability to understand their cost-effectiveness and to educate decision makers and the public regarding the value of CRNA services.

Medicare Part A

Medicare Part A is an insurance plan that provides reimbursement to inpatient hospitals, including critical access hospitals (CAHs), for the care they provide to Medicare beneficiaries.[3] In order for hospitals to be reimbursed by Medicare, they must remain compliant with the conditions of participation published by the Centers for Medicare & Medicaid Services (CMS) in title 42 of the Code of Federal Regulations. There are conditions of participation for hospitals[4] and CAHs[5] as well as conditions of coverage for ambulatory surgery centers.[6] In each of these rules, hospitals are required to ensure that anesthesia services provided by a CRNA are supervised by the operating physician or an anesthesiologist unless the state's governor

259

has opted out of the supervision requirement. Medicare Part A does not provide any reimbursement to the operating physician or an anesthesiologist who provides supervision in order for the facility to be compliant with Medicare Part A conditions for participation/coverage. As of December 2010, 16 states have opted out of the CRNA supervision requirement[7] (Table 12.1), allowing maximal flexibility to healthcare facilities using CRNA services in those states.

Pass-Through Funding

In 1983, the Medicare program implemented the prospective payment system that provided a lump sum payment from Medicare Part A to hospitals based on diagnosis-related groups (DRGs) for services provided to a Medicare beneficiary.[2] This policy change assumed that the cost for CRNA services would come out of the DRG payment, but anesthesiologists would continue to bill Medicare directly and receive a separate payment from Medicare Part B. This created a disincentive to the use of CRNA services. Hospitals could replace CRNA staff with anesthesiologists, who could seek direct reimbursement from

Medicare Part B thereby allowing the hospital to retain the full DRG payments from Medicare Part A.

The Congressional response to this issue was the creation of the pass-through funding process. This process allowed eligible hospitals to be reimbursed for CRNA expenses from the Medicare program over and above the DRG payment of the prospective payment system, restoring reimbursement equity for anesthesiologists and CRNAs.

Because CRNAs are now eligible for direct reimbursement from Medicare Part B pursuant to the Omnibus Budget Reconciliation Act of 1986, the pass-through process is available only to smaller healthcare facilities that meet specific criteria. Generally, if a designated rural hospital does not employ or contract with more than 1 full-time CRNA, does not employ or contract with any anesthesiologists, and performs fewer than 800 surgical procedures per year, the facility may qualify for the pass-through process. If this process is selected, the CRNA and the facility agree not to bill Medicare Part B for CRNA anesthesia services but rather include the costs of the services provided to Medicare patients in the annual Medicare Cost Report. Medicare will

Table 12.1. Medicare Part A Supervision Requirement Opt-Out States[7]

State	Opt-out year	State	Opt-out year
Iowa	2001	Washington	2003
Nebraska	2002	Alaska	2003
Idaho	2002	Oregon	2003
Minnesota	2002	Montana	2004
New Hampshire	2002	South Dakota	2005
New Mexico	2002	Wisconsin	2005
Kansas	2003	California	2009
North Dakota	2003	Colorado	2010

then return a portion of these CRNA expenses to the facility during the next calendar year. Rural healthcare facilities are not automatically included in the pass-through process; rather they must elect it and prove eligibility each year.

In a facility that participates in the pass-through process, CRNAs are allowed to bill third-party payers directly but must not submit charges directly to Medicare Part B. CRNAs in this practice situation must seek reimbursement for services performed for Medicare patients from the facility. Submitting charges to Medicare Part B would be a violation of the pass-through regulations and could result in government sanctions against both the CRNA and the facility. CRNAs are free to negotiate for adequate compensation with pass-through facilities. These negotiations are not required to use the fee schedules established by Medicare.

Critical Access Hospitals

A facility must meet certain CMS criteria (Table 12.2) to be designated as a CAH.[8] CRNAs providing services in a designated CAH can be reimbursed through Medicare Part B. Alternatively, the CAH may elect to bill for the services of its contracted or employed CRNAs using the Method II billing option. This option allows the CAH to submit all CRNA charges for services provided to Medicare beneficiaries on the

---

Table 12.2. CMS Criteria for Designation as a Critical Access Hospital[8]

- Is located in a State that has established with CMS a Medicare rural hospital flexibility program; *and*

- Has been designated by the State as a CAH; *and*

- Is currently participating in Medicare as a rural public, non-profit or for-profit hospital; or was a participating hospital that ceased operation during the 10-year period from November 29, 1989 to November 29, 1999; or is a health clinic or health center that was downsized from a hospital; *and*

- Is located in a rural area or is treated as rural; *and*

- Is located more than a 35-mile drive from any other hospital or CAH (in mountainous terrain or in areas with only secondary roads available, the mileage criterion is 15 miles); *and*

- Maintains no more than 25 inpatient beds; *and*

- Maintains an annual average length of stay of 96 hours per patient for acute inpatient care; *and*

- Complies with all CAH Conditions of Participation, including the requirement to make available 24-hour emergency care services 7 days per week.

CAH indicates critical access hospital.
(Reprinted from the Centers for Medicare & Medicaid Services Critical Access Hospital Fact Sheet.)

261

facility's UB-04 institutional billing document and receive 115% of 80% of the applicable Medicare fee schedule for CRNA services. This provision is not to be confused with other CAH billing methods available for other nonphysician services (eg, nurse practitioners, clinical nurse specialists, or physician assistants) for which these providers are paid 115% of 85% of the allowable Medicare fee schedule. Only the facility can adopt Billing Method II; a CRNA billing Medicare Part B directly cannot.

Medicare Part B

Medicare Part B provides medical insurance to beneficiaries to help cover the costs of care from physicians, eligible nonphysicians, outpatient care, and medically necessary supplies. Eligible nonphysicians include, but

are not limited to CRNAs, nurse practitioners, physical therapists, and occupational therapists.[9] It is common for CRNAs to assign their billing rights to their employer or practice group. By doing so, CRNAs give permission to that entity to bill third-party payers for the services they provide. Assigning billing rights to another entity does not relieve the CRNA of the responsibility to ensure that billing practices are legally consistent. The Medicare Part B reimbursement to anesthesiologists and CRNAs can occur in a variety of anesthesia delivery models[10] (Table 12.3). These are reimbursement models and not standards of care. These Medicare-defined delivery models were developed to provide different levels of reimbursement to CRNAs and anesthesiologists practicing in these various models. It is important to understand

Table 12.3. Medicare Part B Anesthesia Reimbursement Models[10]

Billing modifier	Delivery characteristics	Anesthesiologist reimbursement
Care delivered by anesthesiologist		
AA	Personally performed by anesthesiologist	100%
AD	Medical supervision by anesthesiologist (> 4 concurrent cases)	50% of 3 or 4 units
QK	Medical direction by anesthesiologist (2-4 concurrent cases)	50%
QY	Medical direction by anesthesiologist (1 case only)	50%
Care delivered by CRNA		**CRNA reimbursement**
QX	CRNA being medically directed by anesthesiologist	50%
QZ	CRNA without medical direction	100%
Other modifiers (informational only—no effect on reimbursement)		
QS	Monitored anesthesia care (MAC)	—
G8	MAC for deep complex, complicated, or markedly invasive surgical procedure	—
G9	MAC for patient who has history of severe cardiopulmonary condition	—
GC	Certification modifier for physician resident	—

(Reprinted from the Centers for Medicare and Medicaid Services Medicare Claims Processing Manual.)

The Healthcare Environment

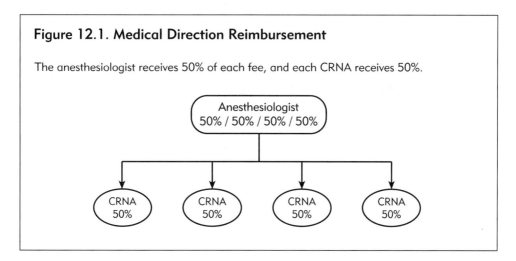

Figure 12.1. Medical Direction Reimbursement

The anesthesiologist receives 50% of each fee, and each CRNA receives 50%.

the terminology associated with these various reimbursement models.

Personally performed anesthesia services describes anesthesia care that is personally provided by an anesthesiologist in a single case. The anesthesiologist would seek reimbursement for 100% of the anesthesia fee provided for the anesthesia service using the AA billing modifier[10] (See Table 12.3).

Medical direction describes care provided by an anesthesiologist in 1 to 4 concurrent cases, each involving a primary anesthetist who is a CRNA (Figure 12.1). Medicare requires anesthesiologists to meet 7 service criteria in order to be reimbursed for medical direction[11] (Table 12.4). Operating physicians cannot be reimbursed for medical direction. In the medical direction model, the anesthesiologist and CRNA split the anesthesia fee for the service provided, each receiving 50%. The CRNA would use the QX billing modifier, and the anesthesiologist would use the QY or QK billing modifier[10] (See Table 12.3). Anesthesiologists may also seek reimbursement for medical direction of 1 to 2 concurrent cases, each involving a student registered nurse anesthetist as the primary anesthetist. Although student registered nurse anesthetists are not eligible to receive

Medicare reimbursement, the anesthesiologist providing medical direction to the student can be reimbursed for 50% of the anesthesia fee for the service provided using the AA billing modifier.

Medical supervision describes care provided by an anesthesiologist to more than 4 concurrent cases, each involving a CRNA (Figure 12.2). Under the medical supervision model, the CRNA may be reimbursed for 50% of the anesthesia fee for the service. The anesthesiologist can be reimbursed for 3 billing units for each case, and may seek a fourth unit if he or she is present for induction of anesthesia. Billing units will be covered in the next section. The CRNA would use the QX billing modifier, and the anesthesiologist would use the AD billing modifier[10] (See Table 12.3). Operating physicians cannot be reimbursed for medical supervision. This reimbursement model is rarely employed because it provides the least amount of reimbursement for anesthesiologists.

Nonmedically directed CRNA describes care personally provided by a CRNA in a single case. The CRNA would seek reimbursement for 100% of the anesthesia fee provided for the anesthesia service using the QZ billing modifier[10] (See Table 12.3).

263

Table 12.4. Conditions for Payment: Medically Directed Anesthesia Services[11]

The anesthesiologist must perform and document the following activities:

1. Performs a pre-anesthetic examination and evaluation;

2. Prescribes the anesthesia plan;

3. Personally participates in the most demanding aspects of the anesthesia plan including, if applicable, induction and emergence;

4. Ensures that any procedures in the anesthesia plan that he or she does not perform are performed by a qualified individual as defined in operating instructions;

5. Monitors the course of anesthesia administration at frequent intervals;

6. Remains physically present and available for immediate diagnosis and treatment of emergencies; and

7. Provides indicated post-anesthesia care.

The anesthesiologist is deemed to have met the Medicare requirements to be reimbursed for directing a CRNA if he or she performs and documents all 7 criteria.

(Reprinted from the Centers for Medicare & Medicaid Services Conditions for Payment.)

Figure 12.2. Medical Supervision Reimbursement

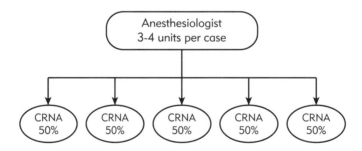

The CRNA receives 50% of the fee for each case, and the anesthesiologist receives 3 or 4 units per case.

This model does not allow for any reimbursement to an anesthesiologist. It is typically is used in settings where there are no anesthesiologists, where CRNAs practice independently from anesthesiologists, or where anesthesiologists do not meet the required criteria to bill for medical direction or medical supervision.

Figure 12.3. Teaching Anesthesiologist Reimbursement

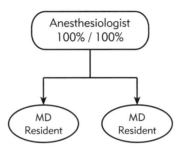

The teaching anesthesiologist receives 100% of the fee for 2 cases with anesthesiology residents.

Figure 12.4. Nonmedically Directed Teaching CRNA Reimbursement

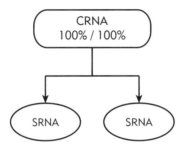

The nonmedically directed teaching CRNA receives 100% of the fee for 2 simultaneous cases with student nurse anesthetists.
CRNA indicates Certified Registered Nurse Anesthetist.

265

Teaching anesthesiologist describes an anesthesiologist providing care in 1 or 2 concurrent cases, each involving a physician resident (Figure 12.3). The anesthesiologist is required to meet the medical direction criteria for each case[11] (See Table 12.4). The anesthesiologist may seek 100% reimbursement for each case using the AA and GC billing modifiers (See Table 12.3).

Nonmedically directed teaching CRNA describes a CRNA providing care in 1 or 2 concurrent cases, each involving a student registered nurse anesthetist (Figure 12.4).

The CRNA would seek reimbursement for 100% of the anesthesia fee provided for each case using the QZ billing modifier[10] (See Table 12.3). There is no billing modifier for students. This reimbursement model is only available to nonmedically directed teaching CRNAs. The CRNA must devote full time to only those cases and be present for care provided both preanesthesia and postanesthesia for each case.

Medically directed teaching CRNA describes a CRNA being medically directed in 1 or 2 concurrent cases, each involving a

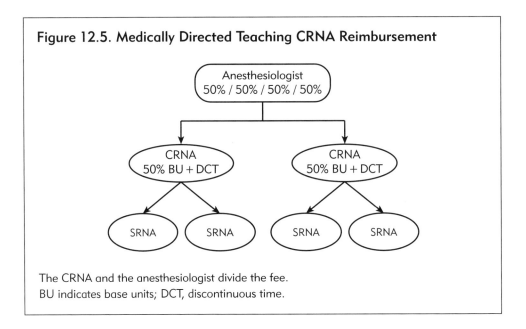

Figure 12.5. Medically Directed Teaching CRNA Reimbursement

The CRNA and the anesthesiologist divide the fee.
BU indicates base units; DCT, discontinuous time.

266

student registered nurse anesthetist (Figure 12.5). If the CRNA is involved in a single case with a student, the medical direction reimbursement method applies and the CRNA would receive only 50% of the anesthesia fee provided. If the medically directed teaching CRNA is involved in 2 concurrent cases, each involving a student registered nurse anesthetist, the CRNA would be eligible to receive only 50% of the base units and discontinuous time spent in each case (ie, sum of the face-to-face time in each case).

The Relative Value Scale

The terms relative value scale (RVS) and relative value guide (RVG)[12] refer to methods of establishing a measurement of intensity for a particular anesthesia service. The Medicare program has adopted a modified version of the RVS developed by the American Society of Anesthesiologists (ASA) known as the ASA RVG.

Measurement of Intensity

The RVS is the most accurate method available to quantify the intensity of the provision of anesthesia services for specific surgical and diagnostic procedures. The Medicare RVS assigns weights of measurement, or base units, to anatomical groups that correspond to the codes in the anesthesia section of the American Medical Association publication, *Current Procedural Terminology*(CPT).[13] The RVS also includes the element of time. One time unit is equal to 15 minutes of anesthesia service. Combining the base units and the time units results in a total number of units for the administration of a particular anesthetic. The RVS is a measurement of only the intensity of an anesthesia service and is not a pricing method for professional services. Only after a conversion factor, or dollar amount per unit, is applied to the total number of procedure units does the RVS become a basis for a professional anesthesia charge.

For example, an appendectomy with an anesthesia service duration of 1 hour would equate to 10 procedure units. This includes 6 base units according to the CPT code 00840, "Anesthesia Services for Intraperitoneal Procedures" and 4 time units (ie, 60 minutes divided by 15 equals 4 time units. The base units and time units are summed resulting in 10 total procedure units. The 10 RVS units are then multiplied by a conversion factor to arrive at the actual charge for anesthesia services provided. Although a particular third-party payer may require the reporting of the duration of service in a specific way, it is extremely important that the anesthesia practice use the same method to measure time units for all services regardless of the payer involved.

Obstetrical Anesthesia Services

In December 2009, CMS published a revision to the *Hospital Anesthesia Services Interpretive Guidelines – State Operations Manual (SOM) Appendix A*.[14] It stated, "During labor and delivery, the provision of acute analgesia (ie, relief of pain, via an epidural or spinal route) is not considered anesthesia, and a CRNA administering these forms of anesthesia services does not require supervision by the operating practitioner or anesthesiologist. However, if the operating practitioner decides that an anesthesia effect (loss of voluntary and involuntary movement and total relief of pain) is necessary for a safe operative delivery of the infant, then the CRNA supervision requirement would apply."[14] This increased the flexibility for hospitals offering obstetric services to provide safe and effective labor analgesia.

The duration of anesthesia services for labor and delivery is defined as the time when the anesthesia provider is face-to-face with the patient. This face-to-face time must be adequately documented in the patient's medical record.

The customary obstetrical pain relief services include interventions such as continuous epidural infusion and intrathecal narcotic injection. Labor analgesia is reimbursed in various ways, including flat fee reimbursement (no time units considered) and traditional RVS units including base and time units. If cesarean delivery is required, additional anesthesia care is required regardless of the reimbursement method. For example, CPT code 1967 provides 5 base units for neuraxial labor analgesia for planned vaginal delivery. If the parturient required additional anesthesia care for cesarean delivery, CPT code 1968 provides 2 additional base units for cesarean delivery following neuraxial labor analgesia. Time units would also be added for the duration of the anesthesia service for the cesarean delivery. The sum of base units and time units would provide the RVS for the overall anesthesia care provided.

Healthcare facilities nationwide continue to broaden and enhance all aspects of obstetrical care and comprehensive pain relief. CRNAs are integral in providing access to high-quality anesthesia services, including pain management during childbirth and other conditions. CRNAs should be fully versed in all aspects of obstetrical and pain management services.

Pain Management Services

Anesthesiologists and CRNAs often provide chronic and acute pain management services that may include single and continuous epidural injections or infusions, intrathecal injections, peripheral nerve blocks, and other interventional techniques. Third-party payers view these as medical services, not anesthesia services. The RVS systems set forth in the ASA RVG do not reflect the reimbursement system established in the marketplace for these services. The Medicare program and most nongovernmental payers recognize pain management as medical services and not anesthesia

267

services. Therefore, a different type of intensity measurement known as the resource-based relative value scale (RBRVS) is employed.

The RBRVS is based on methods similar to the RVS.[15] The RBRVS has been developed to place an intensity measurement on all aspects of medical services provided to patients. Pain management services are based on a fixed weight or value. The time spent providing care is not considered separately, nor is it a factor in developing a pain management service charge. The fixed weight is multiplied by an RBRVS conversion factor to calculate the RBRVS.

The conversion factor used in the RBRVS calculation should not be confused with the conversion factor used in RVS computations. These are 2 separate conversion factors. For example, the Medicare fee schedule may calculate an anesthesia conversion factor of $21 per RVS unit, but for medical services, the conversion factor may be $35 per RBRVS unit of measure.

When nongovernmental payers establish reimbursement rates for these services, they will use the RBRVS method multiplied by a conversion factor that is a percentage of the Medicare RBRVS conversion factor. For example, the RBRVS weight for an epidural steroid injection (CPT code 62311) is 5.42. This weight multiplied by the RBRVS Medicare conversion factor of $35 equates to an allowable amount of $189.70. A commercial payer may offer a CRNA a pain services fee schedule that is a percentage of the Medicare RBRVS conversion factor such as 125% of $35 or, for the epidural example, a reimbursement of 5.42 (35 x 1.25) or $237.13. Commercial payers often have clauses in their agreements that slowly reduce this percentage of the Medicare RBRVS conversion factor over time, such as 125% for the first year, 100% the second year, 95%

the third year, etc. Because these reimbursement methods are integrated into the Medicare RBRVS, any changes that are made to Medicare RBRVS—weights or conversion factors—automatically affect these non-Medicare reimbursement contracts. This can be particularly troubling as well as financially damaging.

Therefore, it would be prudent for any pain management service providers to design their charge basis for chronic and acute pain management services around the RBRVS. The values assigned to all medical procedures by the Medicare program are available from many private organizations and from the Medicare program. A pain management practice should not adopt the RBRVS conversion factor or dollar amount per RBRVS unit, but rather only the weights or measurements of intensity by procedure. These weights must be updated annually because the RBRVS values are evaluated and revised each year. The conversion factor is established by the group of providers based on the local market conditions.

Conversion Factors for Anesthesia Services

A conversion factor is a dollar amount per unit used to convert the RVS intensity measurement into an actual charge for services. Medicare publishes conversion factors for anesthesia services, adjusted by geographic location, on an annual basis.[16] Medicare considers 3 separate variables when establishing conversion factors: 1) the *work effort* of the individual physician or CRNA providing the service; 2) *practice expense* including overhead costs such as supplies, equipment, and labor; and 3) the estimated cost of professional *liability insurance* for a single procedure. Similar considerations are required when an anesthesia group establishes its conversion factor. An anesthesia practice must establish a conversion factor that is competitive within the geographic area. If the factor and the resulting gross charges are too high, it may reflect negatively on the practice. A reasonably well-priced practice should not exceed the locally identified conversion factors by more than 10% to 12%. Typically, the conversion factor will be 3 to 4 times the Medicare conversion factor.

The gross charge for the services provided is determined by multiplying the total procedure units by the conversion factor. To maintain compliance within your charge structure, this chosen conversion factor must remain the same for all patients treated, despite their source of healthcare funding (eg, Medicare, Medicaid, health insurance company, private pay).

National Provider Identifier

The Health Insurance Portability and Accountability Act (HIPAA) regulations require that all healthcare providers, including CRNAs, obtain a National Provider Identifier (NPI).[17] The online NPI application process is relatively easy, with an NPI usually being assigned within 24 hours via email. A CRNA can only have one NPI, no matter how many employers he or she may have. If a group entity bills for services directly, the group entity must also obtain an NPI. All providers, including CRNAs, must use the NPI on all anesthesia claim data submitted to any payer for reimbursement.

Applicants are required to create a user name and password when applying for an NPI. On occasion, it will be necessary to update a provider's NPI file so that claims for services can be properly processed and paid. Therefore, CRNAs will either need to provide their NPI user name and password to

a trusted practice manager or assume the responsibility of updating their NPI files so that the practices are allowed to bill and receive payment.

The Payer Credentialing Process

Third-party payers typically require each provider of service to be identified following a detailed application and credentialing process. This process is a requirement by the Medicare Part B program and all state Medicaid plans. To sidestep this requirement with any nongovernmental payer will result in nonpayment or reduced payment for services. In today's marketplace, all anesthesia practices must evaluate and identify the third party payers that require these credentialing and contracting processes in order to succeed both financially and politically.

Generally, it will take approximately 60 to 90 days to complete the credentialing process with each payer. Once the credentialing process is completed, the payer will assign a participating effective date. This date is extremely important to the success of an anesthesia practice. Medicare and a few nongovernmental plans will allow a participating effective date to be retroactive, but most payers will not allow a retroactive participating date. Therefore, CRNAs must be credentialed with all the possible payers they may encounter before treating patients or risk denial of payment for the services provided.

Periodic recredentialing is required by third-party payers. The Medicare program will determine if a full credentialing process is due when a CRNA or his or her employer makes any change to the CRNA's Medicare enrollment file. Medicare will tie the requested change to the reenrollment/credentialing requirement and will refuse to

269

make the change until the CRNA's enrollment file is updated.

The Billing Process for Anesthesia and Chronic or Acute Pain Management Services

The payers for today's healthcare services are broad and numerous. Third-party payers include the Medicare program, the state Medicaid systems, private health maintenance organizations, preferred provider organizations, commercial and indemnity payers, and the US military healthcare system known as TRICARE.[18] TRICARE is the new name for the Civilian Health and Medical Program of the Uniformed Services (CHAMPUS) following its rebirth under a managed care structure. The healthcare reimbursement process involves charges for healthcare services that are divided into facilities/hospital charges and professional charges. Charges for facilities/hospitals are submitted using the UB-04 form,[19] created by the Uniform Billing Act of 1982, which was revised in 1992 and 2004. The UB-04 form is also known as the CMS-1450 form. Professional charges are submitted using the CMS-1500 form,[20] created by the CMS. Both governmental and nongovernmental payers use the CMS-1500 form to process professional reimbursement claims.

In compliance with the Administrative Simplification Compliance Act (ASCA),[21] all Medicare providers are required to submit their claim data electronically to the Medicare payer. There are a few exceptions to this ruling. For example, providers with fewer than 25 full-time employees in their practice may qualify for exemption. It is difficult to qualify a group that meets the exception criteria. Internal Revenue Service documents such as quarterly payroll tax returns must be filed as proof. Some Medicare

carriers do not acknowledge that these exception rules exist, while others do grant exceptions. If granted, the ruling states that this exception qualification must be proven once per year.

Since 2006, providers are required to execute an electronic funds transfer (EFT) document at the time they submit a CMS 855B to update their Medicare Group Enrollment file or submit a new Medicare group application. This allows all Medicare payments to be made electronically. The EFT document must include a valid bank account. If this information is missing, the forms will be returned and the provider will not be allowed to submit claims until the forms are satisfactorily completed.

International Classification of Diseases, 9th Revision, Clinical Modification (ICD-9-CM) Coding System

A product of the World Health Organization (WHO), ICD-9 is a specific alpha-numeric coding scheme developed to identify nearly every known medical condition and disease. This coding document is referred to as the International Classification of Diseases, 9th Revision, Clinical Modification (ICD-9-CM).[22] Because of its highly technical nature, the ICD-9-CM coding process should only be performed by certified coding individuals who have completed an educational and certification program. Every CMS-1500 form requires ICD-9-CM codes, without which the claim would be rejected. The coding process is critical to correct processing and reimbursement maximization.

The actual ICD-9-CM code itself can be numeric or alpha-numeric, with up to 5 digits, including a 2-place decimal. For example, 650 and 789.06 are both valid ICD-9-CM codes. More digits equate to higher specificity. Most payers require 5-digit ICD-9-CM coding to ensure complete and accurate claim data. Codes that are too general are often returned for more information regarding the condition of the patient and the services provided. The ICD-9-CM is updated annually. If a diagnosis needs to be coded from a previous year, only valid ICD-9-CM codes for that year should be used. Although ICD-9-CM coding should be left to those who are properly trained and certified, CRNAs should be aware of ICD-9-CM codes and their relationship to reimbursement.

The ICD-10-International Classification of Diseases and Related Health Problems, is the replacement system for the aging ICD-9 system. The ICD-10 is not only a coding system for health conditions and diseases, but also addresses signs, symptoms, abnormal findings and complaints, social circumstances, and external causes of injury or diseases, as classified by the WHO. Developed in 1999, the ICD-10 is now operational outside the United States. The US implementation date for ICD-10-CM is October 1, 2013.

The Current Procedural Terminology (CPT) Coding System

The CPT coding system,[13] developed by the American Medical Association, is the nationally recognized method of identifying professional medical services provided to patients. Payers nationwide require that at least 1 CPT code appear on the CMS-1500 form in order for payment processing to be completed. As noted earlier, CPT is divided into various anatomical and specialty sections such as anesthesia, surgery, medicine, and radiology. In the area of anesthesia practice management, the primary section of CPT that is used is the anesthesia section

CPT codes 00100-01999. The CPT codes are 5-digit numeric codes with no digits to the right of the decimal place. As with ICD-9-CM, only certified coding specialists should perform CPT coding. The CPT is updated annually, resulting in some codes being changed or deleted. If a procedure needs to be coded from a previous year, only valid CPT codes for the previous year should be used. CPT coding should be left to those who are properly certified, however, every provider should be aware of CPT and its relationship to reimbursement.

Anesthesia Practice Environments

Anesthesia services are provided in a variety of practice environments. These environments have significant impact on not only salaries of the anesthesia providers, but also on the profit margin for the anesthesia group. With a challenging world economy and the resultant decline in third-party reimbursement for healthcare services, it is very important to structure the practice environment to optimize the financial bottom line. The cost-effectiveness of CRNA practice has been thoroughly studied. The most cost-effective anesthesia delivery model is the CRNA-only model, where all care is delivered by nonmedically directed CRNAs. Many institutions use an anesthesia delivery model that includes both anesthesiologists and CRNAs who practice as an anesthesia care team (ACT). ACT models typically use the medical direction reimbursement methodology. The most cost-effective ACT model is one in which there is 1 anesthesiologist medically directing 4 CRNAs. As the ratio of CRNAs to anesthesiologist decreases, so does the cost-effectiveness of the ACT. The least cost-effective models are those involving anesthesiologist-only care, medical super-

271

vision, and medical direction in a 1:1 ratio of anesthesiologist to CRNA.[23] There is considerable market pressure to improve the financial bottom line for healthcare systems, which will likely lead to more cost-effective delivery models for anesthesia services in the near future.

Summary

Understanding the complexities of reimbursement is critical to achieving and maintaining a successful anesthesia practice. Each of the contributing elements must not only be initially identified, but also continually monitored throughout the life of the practice in order to maintain success. The impact of a correctly developed and supported charge structure for all anesthesia and related services is critical for practice survival and maximization of available reimbursement. The practice can be damaged financially and politically if the CRNA fails to properly identify and negotiate with the practice's third-party payers or selects incorrect procedure and/or diagnosis codes that further delay reimbursement.

The services provided by CRNAs are in high demand and are key components in clinical anesthesia and pain management services. As reimbursement pressures continue, more light will continue to be shed on the critical role of CRNAs as full-service anesthesia providers. The proper management of this economic pressure determines the success or failure of an anesthesia practice. CRNAs must remain knowledgeable, vigilant, and facile in order to maximize reimbursement and remain competitive in today's healthcare marketplace.

References

1. Centers for Medicare & Medicaid Services. Medicare Program General Information. http://www.cms.gov. Accessed November 23, 2010.

2. American Association of Nurse Anesthetists. Medicare Reimbursement. http://www.aana.com. Accessed November 24, 2010.

3. Centers for Medicare & Medicaid Services. Medicare Part A. http://www.cms.gov. Accessed November 24, 2010.

4. Centers for Medicare & Medicaid Services. Conditions of Participation: Hospitals. Accessed November 24, 2010.

5. Centers for Medicare & Medicaid Services. Conditions of Participation: Critical Access Hospitals. http://edocket.access.gpo.gov/cfr_2009/octqtr/42cfr485.639.htm. Accessed November 24, 2010.

6. Centers for Medicare & Medicaid Services. Conditions for Coverage: Ambulatory Surgical Services. http://edocket.access.gpo.gov/cfr_2009/octqtr/42cfr416.42.htm. Accessed November 24, 2010.

7. Fact Sheet Concerning State Opt-Outs and November 13, 2001 CMS Rule. http://www.aana.com. Accessed November 23, 2010.

8. Centers for Medicare & Medicaid Services. Critical Access Hospital Fact Sheet. https://www.cms.gov. Accessed November 23, 2010.

9. Centers for Medicare & Medicaid Services. Medicare Part B. https://www.cms.gov. Accessed November 24, 2010.

10. Centers for Medicare & Medicaid Services. Medicare Claims Processing Manual, Chapter 12, Physicians/Nonphysician Practitioners. https://www.cms.gov. Accessed November 24, 2010.

11. Centers for Medicare & Medicaid Services. Conditions for payment: Medically directed anesthesia services. http://edocket.access.gpo.gov/cfr_2009/octqtr/42cfr415.110.htm. Accessed November 24, 2010.

12. Dexter F, Thompson E. Relative value guide basic units in operating room scheduling to ensure compliance with anesthesia group policies for surgical procedures performed at each anesthetizing location. *AANA J.* 2001;69(2):120-123.

13. American Medical Association. *Current Procedural Terminology.* http://www.ama-assn.org. Accessed November 24, 2010.

14. Centers for Medicare & Medicaid Services. Revised Hospital Anesthesia Interpretive Guidelines – State Operations Manual Appendix A. https://www.cms.gov. Accessed November 24, 2010.

15. American Medical Association. Resource Based Relative Value Scale. https://www.ama-assn.org. Accessed November 24, 2010.

16. Centers for Medicare & Medicaid Services. Anesthesia Conversion Factors. https://www.cms.gov. Accessed November 24, 2010.

17. Centers for Medicare & Medicaid Services. National Provider Identifier Standard. http://www.cms.gov/. Accessed November 24, 2010.

18. TRICARE. http://www.tricare.mil/mybenefit/NewToTricare.jsp. Accessed November 24, 2010.

19. Independence Blue Cross. UB-04 Claim Form and Instructions. http://www.ibx.com. Accessed November 24, 2010.

20. Centers for Medicare & Medicaid Services. Professional Paper Claim Form (CMS-1500). https://www.cms.gov. Accessed November 24, 2010.

21. Centers for Medicare & Medicaid Services. Administrative Simplification Compliance Act. https://www.cms.gov. Accessed November 24, 2010.

22. Centers for Disease Control and Prevention. International Classification of Diseases Functioning, and Disability 9th Revision, Clinical Modification. http://www.cdc.gov. Accessed November 24, 2010.

23. Hogan PF, Seifert RF, Moore CS, Simonson BE. Cost effectiveness analysis of anesthesia providers. *Nurs Econ.* 2010;28(3):159-169.

273

Study Questions

1. What is the difference between Medicare Part A and Medicare Part B? How are anesthesia services reimbursed under each?

2. What advantages or disadvantages did the shift from Medicare Part A to Medicare Part B for CRNA reimbursement create?

3. Describe the characteristics of a critical access hospital. What is rural pass-through funding, and how does it relate to CRNA reimbursement?

4. Define and contrast Medicare Part B reimbursement models to include medical direction, medical supervision, and nonmedical direction.

5. Outline the differences in reimbursement for teaching anesthesiologists and teaching CRNAs. What are the implications for nurse anesthesia education?

6. Considering the cost-effectiveness analysis of CRNAs, discuss the economic advantages and disadvantages of the various practice models.

7. What methods are used to quantify the intensity of anesthesia services, and how do they relate to CRNA reimbursement?

8. How does reimbursement for obstetric analgesia differ from other anesthesia services?

9. Explain the differences in reimbursement when comparing anesthesia services and pain management services.

10. What is a conversion factor, and how is it used for reimbursement purposes? What variables are considered when establishing a conversion factor?

11. What is the primary purpose of the ICD-9-CM and CPT coding systems, and how does each relate to anesthesia reimbursement?

12. Explain the significance and purpose of the NPI.

CHAPTER 13

Improving Quality in the 21st Century

Sandra K. Tunajek, CRNA, DNP

Key Concepts

- Quality assurance is a process-driven approach to improving patient safety by means of specific steps that help define and attain outcome goals. Outcomes are determined through application of patient care standards and evaluation of performance indicators.

- The value of healthcare is linked to the capacity to improve health outcomes, satisfaction with services, and management of costs to individuals and populations.

- Improving quality in healthcare must be a continuous process comprising components that can be measured, evaluated, and improved.

- Quality assessment requires implementation of multifaceted strategies to create sustained change within complex healthcare systems and processes of care.

- There are several quality improvement methodologies in current use that have spurred immediate improvement in healthcare delivery and performance. They include the Plan-Do-Study-Act cycles, Root-Cause Analysis, Six Sigma System, Failure Modes and Effects Analysis, and Situation-Background-Assessment-Recommendation.

- The American Association of Nurse Anesthetists has an extensive history of leadership in assessment of quality care and patient safety activities.

The US healthcare system is complex, costly, and often inefficient. This unfortunate circumstance is further complicated by recent reports of egregious medical errors, waste, and patient treatments only loosely related to best clinical practices. In addition to skyrocketing healthcare insurance premium costs and lack of access for patients, these issues are often cited as among the most substantial threats to overall patient safety and well-being.

Quality and safety concerns are not new. Hospitals, large healthcare purchasers, including employers and public programs and providers, and other health system stakeholders have experimented with wide-ranging efforts to reduce costs, increase safety, and improve patient care outcomes. Within the last several decades, incentive programs for reducing costs while improving patient care have fostered widespread development and adoption of evidence-based quality programming.

Issues involving mandates for quality standards and monitoring have reached a fever pitch of public and industry interest. How did this happen in the relatively short period of several decades? The most frequently cited etiologies include the following:

- Escalating healthcare costs have led the public to view the system as losing value when compared to cost. For millions of people, loss of value translates, in the extreme, as complete loss of access to the system because services are neither available nor affordable.
- Business and industry have, in the recent past, recognized that escalating healthcare costs are making them less globally competitive as larger segments of revenue are shunted to healthcare benefits for employees. This has resulted in business assuming a pivotal position in managing cost through strict application of quality control mechanisms.
- Today's healthcare system of organization and deployment is highly complex, composed of multiple subsystems interacting with each other, resulting in an extraordinarily fragmented healthcare delivery system.[1] This reality exacerbates system waste, fraud, overregulation, redundancy, duplication, and error, all of which contribute to escalating cost.
- Healthcare technologies have exploded that entail higher costs as well as the need to confront ethical issues of access, technology use, and potential rationing of services.

Perspectives on the Quality Movement

The conceptual foundation of the quality movement in the United States is based largely on the work of W. E. Deming. His organizational theory offered 14 key principles for transforming business effectiveness, addressing problem-solving techniques and productivity development, increasing market share, and supporting growth in the face of competition. Deming concluded that quality can be improved only if top management is part of the solution and participates appropriately and actively in the quality program.[2,3]

As policymakers, researchers, and healthcare leaders began to recognize and document deficiencies in the quality of care, Deming's principles were used as quality assessment constructs to guide improvement efforts. In addition, the work of Avedis Donabedian, MD, MPH, suggested the concept of quality of care could be defined and measured against a standard and that subsequent adjustments could be made and quality ensured or improved.[3] Donabedian's classic model for assessing quality had 3 components: (1) structure, (2) process, and (3) outcomes (first assessed by Florence Nightingale in 1855). Donabedian also believed quality was the product of 2 factors, (1) the science and technology of healthcare and, (2) the application of that science and technology into actual practice. Furthermore, he emphasized that the components of acceptable quality and the activities of professionals must be monitored in order to identify instances in which the quality of care falls beneath the expected or desired level.[3] Evidence of his teachings is at work in many current strategies, including Medicare's quality improvement efforts.

Early work to ensure quality in hospitals emerged from an accreditation process developed by the Joint Commission on Accreditation of Hospitals, later known as the Joint Commission on Accreditation of Healthcare Organizations and more recently, the Joint Commission. The Joint Commission establishes standards or measures for ensuring quality in hospitals voluntarily accredited by them. These standards for quality assurance (QA) are viewed to constitute adequate, acceptable, or excellent care. Meeting established standards is important from a quality perspective and for reimbursement purposes. Hospitals and other healthcare institutions that seek Medicare reimbursement must meet certain predetermined conditions of participation established by the Social Security Amendments of 1965, Public Law 98-97.[4] Meeting the Joint Commission standards satisfies Medicare conditions of participation. Furthermore, Medicare relies on accreditation as an indicator of quality in participating hospitals.[2,5]

Subsequent legislation, the Tax Equity and Fiscal Responsibility Act of 1982 (TEFRA, PL 97-248),[6] created peer review organizations whose responsibility was to review the appropriateness and quality of care provided to Medicare beneficiaries. In addition to review and monitoring functions, these entities may invoke sanctions, penalties, or other corrective actions for noncompliance with organization standards. The peer review organization review was more focused on utilization of care rather than quality of care. In 2002, Medicare expanded the program with a new emphasis on broader community projects to improve healthcare, and peer review organizations were renamed quality improvement organizations.[6]

Quality improvement organizations are private contractors that work under the auspices of the US Centers for Medicare & Medicaid Services (CMS). In 2005, the quality improvement organizations introduced the theme of *transformational change* to be achieved through accelerating the rate of quality improvement, raising the bar for performance, and incorporating information technologies. One example of their work is the national coordination and support of the Surgical Care Improvement Project (SCIP), a hospital-based quality improvement initiative led by CMS that focuses on reducing the rate of adverse outcomes of common surgical procedures. The initiative, supported by multiple professional entities, including the American Association of Nurse Anesthetists (AANA), was focused on a 25% reduction of surgical mortality by 2010.[6,7] That goal was successful, incorporating a larger SCIP measure set and module for prevention of infection. Implementation was required for all hospitals in fiscal year 2007.

In 1998, the Joint Commission issued standards for hospitals related to reporting of errors, known as sentinel events. A *sentinel event* is an unexpected occurrence involving

277

death or serious physical or psychological injury or the risk thereof. Serious injury specifically includes loss of limb or function. Such events are called "sentinel" because they signal the need for immediate investigation and response.[8] The first sentinel event report coincided with the release of the Institute of Medicine report[9] noting an alarming number of patient safety concerns. The 2 reports resulted in accelerated efforts to educate professionals and consumers on patient safety. Quality improvement became a targeted objective for policymakers, consumer protection groups, insurers, and practitioners.

Of great concern is wrong-site surgery, which encompasses surgery performed on the wrong side or site of the body, wrong surgical procedure performed, and surgery performed on the wrong patient. In 2003, the Joint Commission convened a summit specifically designed to bring healthcare professionals and others together to address and develop strategies to lessen or eliminate wrong-site surgery. Despite endorsements from multiple professional organizations for the document Universal Protocol for Preventing Wrong Site, Wrong Procedure, Wrong Person Surgery and related changes in operating room policy, the Joint Commission reported 867 incidents of wrong-side surgery between 2003 and September 30, 2009.[8] Organizations have adopted the Joint Commission's accrediting standards as models of monitoring and evaluating appropriateness and quality of care. Hospitals incorporated methodologies using QA, usually involving initiatives identified by regulatory or accrediting agencies. Initially, the QA process emphasized review of patient records to monitor variances in care and obvious problems involving delivery processes or safety. As QA mechanisms evolved, indicators were developed to use in measurement tools to assess performance and outcomes. Typical indicators employed in most hospitals were derived from case analyses, often including patient death, medical complications, unexpected events, and complaints about services. Unfortunately, process variance identification, correction, and remediation were perceived as punitive by many providers. Administrators viewed the process as an additional responsibility that did little to decrease the overall cost of doing business or improving quality.[1,10]

As healthcare services expanded to multiple settings, networks of hospital systems emerged, technology advances improved transfer of information, and patient care increasingly moved toward outpatient delivery of services. Largely in response to these changes in the environment, regulatory and accrediting bodies developed new standards and recommendations for monitoring and evaluating quality of care. The focus on quality improvement shifted toward evaluation of the organization as a system by using total quality management and continuous quality improvement methods for planning and accomplishing quality initiatives.[1] Objectives for these activities have a cause-and-effect relationship that emphasizes direction (Did care improve or decrease?); indicators of performance (eg, quality, customer satisfaction); target value (eg, cost, occupancy); and time limit.

In 2000, the Institute of Medicine (IOM) Committee on Quality Health Care in America launched its initiatives on healthcare quality. Established in 1970, the IOM works outside the framework of the US federal government and provides independent guidance and analysis by a volunteer workforce of scientists and other experts. Operating under a rigorous, formal, peer-review system, the Institute provides unbiased,

278

evidence-based, and authoritative information and advice concerning health and science policy to policy makers, professionals, leaders in every sector of society, and the public at large.[9]

In recent years, a series of groundbreaking IOM quality reports identified gaps in overall quality of healthcare in such areas as patient safety, medication errors, disparities, access, work environments, information communication errors, and variable or ineffective delivery of services. Their recommendations shifted the focus of quality improvement programming to identifying faulty systems and inefficient processes and bringing about general improvements in patient safety and overall quality. The identification by IOM of specific system and provider performance deficiencies has come to serve as a primary locus of debate that is guiding the redesign of the American healthcare system. All student registered nurse anesthetists should avail themselves to the study of these reports, because many have direct application to anesthesia practice and provide startling reminders of how critical quality endeavors are to the practice of clinical anesthesia.

The Quality Framework

There has been a proliferation of both private and public initiatives undertaken by organizations and agencies at the local, state, and national levels to address the quality issue. Although slow, progress has been made in stimulating improvement and accountability in many sectors of healthcare. Several key organizations have spearheaded the search for solutions with an eye toward measuring, developing evidence, public reporting, and linking payment with quantifiable performance.

The Agency for Healthcare Research and Quality

The Agency for Healthcare Research and Quality (AHRQ) is the lead federal agency charged with improving the quality, safety, efficiency, and effectiveness of healthcare for all Americans. The AHRQ quality indicators (QIs) were developed with an extensive process that included interviews from organizations that represented users, literature reviews identifying potential quality measures, evaluation of several risk-adjustment methods for use with the potential measures, empirical analysis, and validation. Originally designed as an internal quality improvement tool to assist hospitals in identifying and targeting areas of intervention, the process can be divided into 2 phases: (1) identifying measures or indicators, and (2) analyzing viable measures or indicators. Hospitals specifically use QIs to initiate case finding, root-cause analyses, and cluster identification, as well as to monitor performance over time.[11,12]

The AHRQ also develops Patient Safety Indicators (PSIs), a set of quality measures that use hospital inpatient discharge data to provide additional perspectives on patient safety. Specifically, the PSIs identify problems that patients experience within the health-care system that could be prevented by implementing system level changes. The problems identified are referred to as complications or adverse events. The PSIs use secondary diagnosis codes to detect complications and adverse events and are defined on 2 levels, provider and domain. The set of quality measures covers a variety of areas (domains) such as postoperative complications, selected technical adverse events, technical difficulty with procedures, and obstetric trauma and birth trauma.[12,13] There are a number of ways in which AHRQ QIs are used, ranging from

279

internal quality improvement to several public reporting and pay-for-reporting or pay-for-performance initiatives at the national, state, and regional levels. Provider-level PSIs are listed in Table 13.1.

In 2003, the Medicare Prescription Drug, Improvement, and Modernization Act Section 1013 authorized AHRQ to conduct and support research with a focus on outcomes, comparative clinical effectiveness, and appropriateness of pharmaceuticals, devices, and healthcare services.[13] The American Recovery and Reinvestment Act of 2009 established additional funding for this initiative, discussed in more detail later in this chapter.[14,15]

Table 13.1. Agency for Healthcare Research and Quality Patient Safety Indicators[16]

The PSIs provide a perspective on patient safety events using hospital administrative data, which are readily available and relatively inexpensive to use, and include the following 27 measures:

1. Hospital-Level Patient Safety Indicators (20 indicators)
   - Complications of anesthesia (PSI 1)
   - Death in low mortality DRGs (PSI 2)
   - Decubitus ulcer (PSI 3)
   - Failure to rescue (PSI 4)
   - Foreign body left in during procedure (PSI 5)
   - Iatrogenic pneumothorax (PSI 6)
   - Selected infections due to medical care (PSI 7)
   - Postoperative hip fracture (PSI 8)
   - Postoperative hemorrhage or hematoma (PSI 9)
   - Postoperative physiologic and metabolic derangements (PSI 10)
   - Postoperative respiratory failure (PSI 11)
   - Postoperative pulmonary embolism or deep vein thrombosis (PSI 12)
   - Postoperative sepsis (PSI 13)
   - Postoperative wound dehiscence in abdominopelvic surgical patients (PSI 14)
   - Accidental puncture and laceration (PSI 15)
   - Transfusion reaction (PSI 16)
   - Birth trauma—injury to neonate (PSI 17)
   - Obstetric trauma—vaginal delivery with instrument (PSI 18)
   - Obstetric trauma—vaginal delivery without instrument (PSI 19)
   - Obstetric trauma—cesarean delivery (PSI 20)

2. Area-Level Patient Safety Indicators (7 indicators)
   - Foreign body left in during procedure (PSI 21)
   - Iatrogenic pneumothorax (PSI 22)
   - Selected infections due to medical care (PSI 23)
   - Postoperative wound dehiscence in abdominopelvic surgical patients (PSI 24)
   - Accidental puncture and laceration (PSI 25)
   - Transfusion reaction (PSI 26)
   - Post-operative hemorrhage or hematoma (PSI 27)

(Reprinted from *Patient Safety and Quality: An Evidence-Based Handbook for Nurses.* AHRQ Publication No. 08-0043. Agency for Healthcare Research and Quality, Rockville, MD. http://www.ahrq.ga/qual/nurseshdbk/)

The National Quality Forum

The National Quality Forum (NQF) was proposed in 1998 by the President's Advisory Commission on Consumer Protection and Quality in the Health Care Industry. Created as part of an integrated national quality-improvement agenda, NQF is a private sector standard-setting organization with more than 375 members representing multiple sectors of the healthcare system including consumers, purchasers, physicians, nurses, hospitals, and accrediting and credentialing groups. There are 18 nursing organizations represented, including the AANA, which became the second nursing organization to become a member in 2001.[17] The NQF operates with a mission to improve the quality of American healthcare by (1) setting priorities and goals for performance improvement, (2) endorsing national consensus standards for measuring, (3) publicly reporting on performance, and (4) promoting education and outreach programs.[18]

NQF endorsement, which involves rigorous, evidence-based review and a formal consensus development process, has become the gold standard for healthcare performance measures. Major healthcare purchasers, including the Centers for Medicare & Medicaid Services, rely on NQF-endorsed measures to ensure that measures are scientifically sound, relevant, and help standardize and raise the bar for performance across the industry. The NQF functions through voluntary consensus process and has endorsed some 500 products, including performance measures, indicators, and practices for facilities that provide surgery and anesthesia.[11]

The Surgical Care Improvement Project

The Surgical Care Improvement Project (SCIP) is a Medicare-sponsored partnership of organizations seeking to improve patient care by reducing surgical complications. Areas of focus include surgical site infections, adverse cardiac events, deep vein thrombosis, and postoperative pneumonia. Process variables such as prophylactic antibiotics, beta-blockers, and blood glucose control have been identified by the project.

Each SCIP target area is advised by a technical expert panel. These groups provide extensive clinical and technical expertise as well as resources to ensure that SCIP measures are fully supported by evidence-based research. The SCIP quality measures are aligned with both Joint Commission and Medicare requirements and reflect guidelines, standards of care, or practice parameters. Medical information from patient records is converted into a rate or percentage that is used to benchmark hospital performance among local, regional, state, and national benchmark competitors.[7]

The AHRQ, NQF, and SCIP initiatives all highlight preventable medical errors. Medication error reporting and prevention has been an important emphasis in quality and safety initiatives. Anesthesia practitioners must take leading roles in the clinical research, practice, and cultural changes required to reduce medication errors. Anesthesia specialists are often personally responsible for drug administration and already have effective patient safety standards, guidelines, and practice protocols in place. Furthermore, the specialty has been able to effectively design monitors and ventilation systems and to greatly reduce death due to hypoxia or ventilatory failure in anesthetized patients. Unfortunately, according to data submitted to SCIP, surgery patients are 3 times more likely to experience a harmful medication error than patients anywhere else in the healthcare system.[7]

281

Recognizing the need for communication and teamwork, the Council on Surgical and Perioperative Safety was incorporated in August 2007. This body is a unique coalition of 7 professional organizations representing key members of the surgical team including the American Association of Nurse Anesthetists, the American Association of Surgical Physician Assistants, the American College of Surgeons, the American Society of Anesthesiologists, the American Society of Perianesthesia Nurses, the Association of Perioperative Registered Nurses, and the Association of Surgical Technologists. The council and its member organizations have a combined total of more than 250,000 surgical healthcare team members and represent more than 2 million healthcare practitioners. The Council on Surgical and Perioperative Safety promotes excellence in patient safety in the surgical and perioperative environment. Surgical procedures performed under anesthesia are associated with the highest intensity level of care and necessitate the combined team effort of many highly competent individuals to be successful.[19] The Council on Surgical and Perioperative Safety has endorsed safe surgery principles that include issues such as fire safety, evidence-based standards, patient transfer, standard nomenclature, workplace violence, and medication errors.[19]

Quality Improvement Methodologies

Quality improvement is defined as a systematic, data-guided activity designed to bring about immediate improvement in healthcare delivery. In the past 2 decades, quality improvement methods have evolved to emphasize the importance of identifying processes with unsatisfactory outcomes, measuring key problems, using analysis to devise a new approach, integrating a redesigned approach for the process, and measuring subsequent performance to determine if the process change was successful. A *quality improvement strategy* is any intervention aimed at reducing the quality gap for groups of patients that are representative of those encountered in common practice. Objectives for measuring healthcare quality consist of (1) determining the effects of healthcare on desired outcomes; (2) assessing the degree to which healthcare adheres to processes based on scientific evidence or agreed to by professional consensus and; (3) is reflective of patient preferences.[19,20]

Several strategies have been proposed for improving quality, safety, and clinical outcomes. W. Edwards Deming, PhD, promoted constant and systematic analysis and measurement of process steps in relation to capacity or outcomes or total quality management. His model incorporated the view that the entire organization must be committed to quality and improvement to achieve the best results. Total quality management involves organizational management, teamwork, defined processes, systems thinking, and change to create an environment for improvement.[3] In healthcare, continuous quality improvement is used interchangeably with total quality management. Continuous quality improvement has been used as a means to develop clinical practice and is based on the principle that there is an opportunity for improvement in every process and on every occasion. Quality assurance and its component, QI, originated in engineering and manufacturing where systems theory, statistical process control, and continuous quality improvement were combined with general management methods. Many hospital-based QA programs focus on issues identified by regulatory or accreditation organizations, such as checking documentation, reviewing the work of oversight committees, and studying credentialing processes. Both QA and QI have been adopted by healthcare systems and serve as the building blocks for current quality initiatives.

Measuring and Assessing Quality

Health system performance measures often reflect the 6 dimensions of quality outlined in the IOM report, *Crossing the Quality Chasm*.[22] Dimensions address to what extent a process is safe, effective, patient-centered, timely, efficient, and equitable.

Measurement is a critical part of testing and implementing change. Competent measures tell a team whether proposed changes actually led to improvement. Although quality improvement occupies an uncertain territory between clinical care and research, the difference is extremely important. Research and quality improvement may vary in purpose and process, but the key element for both is the translation of information into operational constructs. Although measurement for improvement should not be confused with measurement for research, the assessment of the results should meet principles of reliability and validity.[23]

Table 13.2. Comparing Concepts of Research and Quality Improvement[23]

Component	Quality improvement	Research
Purpose and scope	Examine processes to guide actions. Process-specific issue	Generate new knowledge. Test hypotheses. Generalizable to other situations, settings
Tests	Single, predetermined indicators	Many sequential, observable tests
Design	Focus on processes	Scientific framework Well controlled
Subject selection	Convenience subpopulation of patients specific to indicator Collect large amounts of data	Based on design, power analysis, statistical models. Gather "just enough" data to learn and complete another cycle
Duration and results	Can take long periods of time to obtain results Used by institution or organizations	"Small tests of significant changes" accelerates the rate of improvement Formally presented, available to others

(Adapted with permission from Beyea et al.)

A comparison of these concepts is outlined in Table 13.2.

Performance is influenced by structural factors both internal and external to an organization. Donabedian's structure/process/outcome model, frequently cited in research on measures of healthcare quality, defines structural measures of quality as the professional and organizational resources associated with the provision of care, such as staff credentials and facility operating capacities. Process measures of quality refer to the things done to and for the patient by practitioners in the course of treatment. Outcome measures are the desired states resulting from care processes, which may include reduction in morbidity and mortality and improvement in the quality of life.[1,3]

The first step in assessing quality requires identification of strategies by which any actual change can be identified and measured. Generally a pilot-testing period follows, during which qualitative and quantitative data are analyzed. Data are evaluated to determine the probable effects that changes will have on the system. Finally, based on the experiences, some action is taken to implement the change, complete a system redesign, and continually evaluate the change in the improvement cycle.[21] The scientific method generally involves planning a test, conducting the test, and studying the results. Quality management has adapted this

Table 13.3. Principles of Quality Management[21]

Focus on the consumer.	Services should be designed to meet the needs and expectations of targeted population. An important measure of quality is the extent to which needs and expectations are met.
Understand work as systems and processes.	Providers need to understand the service system and its key processes in order to improve them. Using tools of process engineering allows simple visual images of these processes and systems.
Teamwork	Work is accomplished through processes and systems in which different people fulfill different functions. It is essential to involve the people who fulfill these functions to understand changes that need to be made, the effective implementation of the appropriate processes, and the development of ownership of the improved processes and systems.
Focus on the data.	Data are needed to analyze processes, identify problems, and measure performance.
Develop action plan	Changes can then be tested and the resulting data analyzed to verify that the changes have actually led to improvements.

method, expanding it by adding an action plan. Table 13.3 lists the characteristics or principles of quality improvement that must be attendant to analysis.[16,21]

Outcomes can be described from several perspectives. As measurements or variables, outcomes describe the result or effect of particular interventions. When a patient is the focus, measurement may be the effect of a method of treatment. For the patient who undergoes an anesthetic, a desirable outcome might be defined as discharge from the facility within a predetermined period of time. Other examples of outcome measures include the incidence of morbidity and mortality, complication rates, patient satisfaction, length of stay, and overall cost.[3,21] Quality tools used to define and assess problems with healthcare are seen as being helpful in prioritizing quality and safety problems and focusing on systems, not individuals. Currently, several methods or tools are used to link outcomes and improvement.

The Plan-Do-Study-Act Approach

The Plan-Do-Study-Act (PDSA) approach is the first of many paradigms in common use to effect positive change or outcome. The primary feature of this model is the cyclical nature of effecting and assessing change, most effectively accomplished through small and frequent PDSAs before changes are made throughout the system.[1,3,21] The purpose of PDSA quality improvement efforts is to establish a functional or causal relationship between changes in processes, specifically behaviors and capabilities, and outcomes. The PDSA cycle starts with determining the nature and scope of the problem, what changes can and should be made, a plan for a specific change, who should be involved, what should be measured to understand the

impact of change, and where the strategy will be targeted. Change is then implemented and data and information are collected. Results from the implementation study are assessed and interpreted by reviewing several key measurements that indicate success or failure. Action is taken on the results by implementing the change or beginning the process again.[21]

Root-Cause Analysis

The Root-Cause Analysis (RCA) is a commonly used paradigm that assesses reported incidents and differentiates between active and latent errors. Such analysis would ideally result in policy change that would eliminate reoccurrence. It also serves as a basis to suggest system changes, including reducing risk and improving communication. Root-Cause Analysis is used extensively in engineering and more recently in healthcare. The technique formalizes investigation and problem-solving approaches focused on identifying and understanding the underlying cause(s) of an event. The Joint Commission requires RCA to be performed in response to all sentinel events and expects the organization to develop and implement an action plan consisting of improvements designed to reduce future risk of events and to monitor the effectiveness of those improvements.[16,24,25]

Root-Cause Analysis is a technique used to identify trends and assess risk that can be used whenever human error is suspected, with the understanding that system failure, rather than individual factors, is likely the root cause of most problems (a W. E. Deming quality principle). A similar procedure is the critical incident technique, where after an event occurs, information is collected on the causes and actions that led to the event.[24] Critical incident investigation was first used as a technique to improve

285

safety and performance among military pilots. The focus on critical incidents allowed investigators to observe the differences between behaviors that led to success and failure. More recently, a modified critical incident technique has been used to interview anesthesia practitioners to obtain descriptions of preventable incidents and to record and discuss untoward incidents.

An RCA can be described as a reactive assessment that begins after an event, retrospectively outlining the sequence of events, charting causal factors, and identifying root causes to completely examine the event. Those involved in the investigation ask a series of key questions, including what happened, why it happened, what were the most proximate factors causing it to happen, and why those factors occurred. Answers to these questions help identify ineffective safeguards and causes of problems so similar problems can be prevented. It is important also to consider events that occurred immediately before the event in question because other remote factors may have contributed. The final step of a traditional RCA is developing recommendations for system and process improvement(s), based on the findings of the investigation.

Additionally, it is critical to consider how to differentiate system from process factors, without focusing on individual blame because this bias may distract the team from investigating systems and process factors that can be modified through subsequent interventions.[25]

The Six Sigma System

The Six Sigma System, originally designed by the Toyota Corporation as a business strategy, involves improving, designing, and monitoring the production process to minimize or eliminate waste, optimize satisfaction, and increase financial stability.

Six Sigma has been used successfully in healthcare to decrease defects, variations, and operating costs as well as to improve outcomes in a variety of settings. The performance of a process is used to measure improvement by comparing the baseline process capability (before improvement) with the process capability after piloting potential solutions for quality improvement.

The primary methods used with Six Sigma inspect process outcomes and count the defects, calculate a defect rate per million, and use a statistical table to convert defect rate per million to a σ (sigma) metric. This method is applicable to analysis processes much like pretest and posttest studies. A second method uses estimates of process variation to predict process performance by calculating a σ metric from the defined tolerance limits and the variation observed for the process. This method is suitable for analytic processes in which the precision and accuracy can be determined by experimental procedures.[16,26]

Overlapping Six Sigma methodology is a secondary process, different in that it is driven by the identification of customer needs, and it aims to improve processes by removing activities that do not add value or that contribute to waste. This methodology depends on root-cause analysis to investigate errors and then to improve quality and prevent similar errors. Factors involved in the successful application of the process in healthcare include eliminating unnecessary daily activities associated with overly complicated processes, work-arounds, and repeated work efforts.

The key elements of Six Sigma are also related to the Plan-Do-Study-Act model. The plan phase of PDSA is related to defining core processes, key customers, and customer requirements of Six Sigma. The do phase of PDSA is related to measuring performance of Six Sigma, and the study phase of PDSA is related to analysis of Six Sigma. The act phase of PDSA is related to improving and integrating Six Sigma.[16,26]

Failure Modes and Effects Analysis

Failure Modes and Effects Analysis is an evaluation technique used to identify and eliminate known or potential failures, problems, and errors from a system design, process, or service before they actually occur. Failure Modes and Effects Analysis is used prospectively to identify potential areas of failure and retrospectively to characterize the safety of a process by identifying those areas of failure and incorporating the staff's point of view. Failure Modes and Effecs Analysis is dependent upon a multidisciplinary approach, integrated incident and error reporting, decision support, standardization of terminology, and education of caregivers. This method is often used by hospitals to evaluate alternative processes or procedures as well as to monitor change over time. The process supports requirements of the Joint Commission mandating that accredited healthcare providers conduct proactive risk management activities to identify and predict system weaknesses and adopt changes to minimize patient harm on 1 or 2 high-priority topics a year.[16,25,27]

For example, one of the Joint Commission's National Patient Safety goals is to improve the effectiveness of communication among caregivers.[10] The Joint Commission identifies miscommunication as the root cause of approximately 70% of all sentinel events. Because healthcare involves multiple disciplines, a means of standardized interdisciplinary communication is critical to enhance quality of care and promote patient safety. Although communication is an essential component of all healthcare curricula, each discipline has its own terminology, expectations, and idiosyncrasies relative to communication, all of which can have an impact on the effectiveness of communication across disciplines.[27,28] In situations in which the patient is at risk for adverse errors, team collaboration is essential and critical information must be accurately communicated. Collaboration among physicians, nurses, and other healthcare professionals increases awareness of the type of knowledge and skills of those working cooperatively in complementary roles, sharing responsibility for problem solving and decision making, leading to improved patient care.[29]

Situation-Background-Assessment-Recommendation Method

In an attempt to standardize and improve communication among healthcare personnel, the model of interdisciplinary communication, known as Situation-Background-Assessment-Recommendation, or the acronym, SBAR, is gaining increased attention. The model consists of 4 components: situation, background, assessment, and recommendation, as described in Table 13.4. SBAR allows for an easy and focused way to set expectations for what will be communicated between members of the team, an essential factor for developing teamwork and fostering a culture of patient safety.[28]

Patient care scenarios using the human patient simulator provide an opportunity to teach practitioners to effectively use a standardized communication method. Human patient simulation is a teaching strategy that allows practitioners to develop new or refine existing skills in a realistic clinical situation via high-fidelity technology without posing risk to a patient. The use of simulation can

---

Table 13.4. Components of the SBAR Model of Interdisciplinary Communication[7]

Situation	Statement of what is happening at the present time that has triggered the situation
Background	Information that puts the situation into context and explains the circumstances that have led to the situation
Assessment	Statement of the communicator's ideas about the problem
Recommendation	Statement of what should be done to correct the problem, by when, and by whom.

---

contribute to patient safety and optimize outcomes of care, as well as provide learners with opportunities to intervene in clinical situations that are rare or unusual.[1]

Crew Resource Management

To enhance teamwork many organizations have adopted the principles of Crew Resource Management, originated by NASA and used in the aviation industry to respond to simulated disasters. Often managed through the use of simulation, the crew resource management training model focuses on leadership, decision making, communication, and team training. It also provides a review of general competencies that can be transferred from team to team in ever-changing team structures in various healthcare settings such as operating rooms, emergency departments, or intensive care units.[28,30]

Practice Standards

The self-regulating health professions in the United States are mandated to ensure that licensed practitioners provide safe and effective care. A standard is an expectation of practice, a mandated rule of sorts, used as a basis of comparison for measuring or judging value or quality. In nurse anesthesia practice, for example, standards are used to determine whether a certain level of care is provided. From the aspect of quality improvement, standards may be viewed as expectations that drive the achievement of certain behaviors as a means of self-regulation and accountability to ensure quality performance.[31]

The AANA has established standards for CRNA practice. As noted in an earlier chapter of this text, standards evolve through consideration of existing research evidence and consensus opinion. Standards serve to (1) provide direction and a framework for the evaluation of practice, (2) describe the profession's accountability to the public, and (3) delineate performance outcomes for which a nurse anesthetist is responsible. Standards also establish an expected level of patient care and enable the measurement of a nurse anesthetist's competency. Standards have been used to evaluate and ensure quality and manage individual and institution risk.[31]

The push for transparency and accountability is driving public reporting of performance data and demands that information be incorporated in the credentialing of healthcare practitioners. In an effort to promote high-quality care, the federal government and other payers are incorporating requirements that individual practitioners document their performance outcomes against benchmark data.[1,31] Standards of practice set the foundation for many of these benchmarks.

Public Reporting of Quality Data

Public purchasers including Medicare and Medicaid are increasingly adopting new quality-oriented measures that emphasize public reporting of provider performance. The Patient Safety and Quality Improvement Act of 2005 requiring that critical information be accurately communicated was enacted in response to reports that preventable medical errors result in billions of dollars in increased healthcare costs, disability, and death. The purpose of the act was to create a legal structure in which healthcare providers could voluntarily disclose information about preventable adverse events, learn from mistakes, and avoid them in the future.[32,33] The goal of Congress in enacting the Patient Safety and Quality Improvement Act was to create opportunities for providers to share patient safety information with independent entities, called patient safety organizations, which analyze and aggregate patient safety data from multiple providers and use it to identify patterns that suggest underlying causes of patient risks and hazards.

The Tax Relief and Health Care Act of 2006 created a pay-for-reporting program, called the Physician Quality Reporting Initiative, within Medicare.[34] The Physician Quality Reporting Initiative established a financial incentive for physicians and other health practitioners to participate in a voluntary quality reporting program. Eligible participants include doctors of medicine, doctors of osteopathy, physician assistants, nurse practitioners, clinical nurse specialists, and Certified Registered Nurse Anesthetists and anesthesiologist assistants. The Physicians Quality Reporting Initiative quality measures relate to important processes of care that are linked to improved healthcare quality outcomes. They are evidence- and consensus-based measures that reflect the work of national organizations involved in quality measure development, consensus endorsement, and adoption. These include the American Medical Association (AMA) Physician Consortium for Performance Improvement, the NQF, the Ambulatory Care Quality Alliance, and other physician and nonphysician professional organizations, including the AANA. The Physicians Quality Reporting Initiative is considered a transitional step in the development of a pay-for-performance program that will use evidence-based quality measures to financially reward quality efforts.[34,35]

Performance Measurement

Measuring performance is central to quality improvement because it provides information on current and past performance that can help guide future improvement efforts. In particular, performance measures can distinguish between good and substandard performance. Accordingly, the development and application of performance improvement measurement (PI) is essential to improving the quality of care. It is one of the first steps in the improvement process and involves the selection, definition, and application of performance indicators. The indicators and guidelines for clinicians are more challenging because they must reflect what is actually feasible in a given setting.

290

Performance improvement addresses human performance within organizations at the individual, process, and organizational levels. It uses a systematic method that has 5 stages: (1) getting agreement on the project goal from the clients, stakeholders, and PI practitioner; (2) conducting a performance needs assessment (identifying performance gaps and their root causes); (3) designing the interventions to close the gap; (4) implementing the interventions; and (5) evaluating the change in the performance gap.[21,36]

Quality is an elusive term. However, it can be thought of as 3 points on a triangle. The points are: (1) defining quality, (2) measuring quality, and (3) improving quality. Defining quality means developing statements regarding the input, process, and outcome standards that the delivery system must meet. Such statements are used to define expected quality in all aspects of healthcare. Measuring quality consists of measuring the current level of compliance with standards. Improving quality involves using appropriate methodologies to close the gap between the current and expected levels of quality. Quality improvement uses quality management tools and principles to understand and address system deficiencies and may be simple or complex.[1,36]

Although both quality improvement and performance improvement take a systems view, a noticeable difference between them is that performance improvement places more emphasis on human performance and quality improvement focuses on processes. Both quality assurance/quality improvement and performance improvement emphasize standards, but the former is more systematic and comprehensive. In quality assurance/quality improvement, standards are classified into 3 domains: technical, clinical (evidence-based), and administrative. Quality assurance recognizes that standards must be in place and met for these inputs, processes, and outcomes in order to maximize the potential for desired health outcomes.[1,20] Performance improvement is most often applied to worker performance expectations, and clinical indicators are a well-recognized performance factor.

Comparative Effectiveness

The American Recovery and Reinvestment Act of 2009[15] authorized funding that directed the IOM to develop broad-based priorities for implementing comparative-effectiveness research (CER). These funds are managed by the National Institutes of Health, the Department of Health and Human Services, and the Agency for Healthcare Research and Quality. To prioritize initiatives, the IOM committee placed particular emphasis on questions regarding the clinical effectiveness of care. Funded agencies are required to obtain input from professional organizations and the public in formulating a research agenda.[37]

The basic purpose of CER is to accelerate the discovery of the best approaches to personalize care, develop management strategies for individual patients, and gain clearer understanding of the difference in effectiveness of a therapeutic approach among patient groups.[37-39] Although CER methods are not entirely new, the initiative supports research that is more comprehensive and relevant to actual clinical decisions than traditional clinical research.

There is tremendous potential in the power of CER; however, critics argue that a number of troubling issues and difficult questions remain. When assessing efficacy, randomized controlled trials (RCTs) are considered to be the gold standard. However, a sufficient number of studies of important clinical questions may not be available. A wealth of useful information does exist in observational studies and other sources. Observational studies, unlike RCTs, do not involve any intervention with study participants. They measure health outcomes as they naturally occur in real-world populations. Systematic evidence reviews are structured analyses of available evidence from a comprehensive literature search with a detailed evaluation of the quality of studies. Decision models are formal analytic frameworks that may incorporate costs, the value of outcomes, and the probabilities for particular benefits and harms to assess the overall benefits and costs of treatment alternatives.[38,39] The challenge is to balance the need for practical, clinically relevant measures with the equally important need for theoretical integrity and comprehensiveness.

Comparative research has also drawn criticism for its potential to eliminate treatment options, yet most health experts agree that it is an important tool for integrating healthcare services. However, acceptance by key stakeholders is essential, and some practitioners consider CER a threat to the personalization of care. Research further suggests that merely providing information to healthcare practitioners results in only a modest behavioral response. Therefore, efforts to alter providers' behavior need to combine CER with aggressive promulgation of standards and changes in financial and other incentives. As an emerging trend, CER is predicted to accelerate the translation of evidence into everyday care, enhance the opportunities for doctors and patients to define value, and allow providers and patients to communicate with researchers and policymakers about clinically important issues earlier in the research process. The ultimate goal focuses on improving individual health as well as limiting healthcare spending.

Implications for Anesthesia

In the next few years, AHRQ plans to spend $34.5 million on projects aimed at implementing innovative approaches to integrating CER findings into clinical practice and healthcare decision making. There is a substantial need to generate new knowledge. Engaging in CER offers several advantages for hospitals and providers including CRNAs. Once the research is disseminated, hospitals and clinical practitioners will be on the front lines of implementing and ensuring translation into practice.

Quality efforts in anesthesia provide a prime example of putting evidence-based standards into practice. In the mid-1980s, both the AANA and the American Society of Anesthesiologists (ASA) developed standards of practice. Providers had an incentive to follow the standards because deviations exposed them to malpractice liability. After standards were adopted, mortality rates were substantially reduced. Subsequently, the IOM noted that anesthesia professionals have emerged as strong leaders in creating systems built on foundations of sound safety principles.[9]

In anesthesia practice, many clinical decisions are not rooted in large comparative effectiveness trials that demonstrate efficacy, effectiveness, and efficiency. *Efficacy* refers to the potential benefit or risk of a treatment under ideal circumstances in a specific patient population. Effectiveness refers to the actual benefit of that treatment in usual care settings in a broad patient population. *Efficiency* incorporates the financial costs and savings of the alternatives.[40,41]

292

Application of CER is particularly challenging for the delivery of anesthesia care considering the already low level of adverse outcomes. CER often requires a defined high-risk patient population, detailed protocols, mandates for specific care, and studies designed to use the targeted intervention. Furthermore, many people are involved with the patient throughout the surgical process and many things are not easily or clearly attributable to one individual provider. Efforts to measure both professional and organizational performance are also difficult for anesthesia providers.

Although clinical indicators are increasingly promoted by professional organizations, the characteristics and validity of clinical anesthesia indicators are not well defined.[40-42] A recent meta-analysis to clarify the number, characteristics, and validity of indicators available for anesthesia care identified 108 anesthetic indicators, of which 53 related to surgical or postoperative ward care. Most were process measures (42%) or outcome measures (57%) assessing the safety and effectiveness of patient care. To identify possible quality issues, most clinical indicators were used as part of an internal hospital comparison or professional peer-review process. Of the clinical indicators, 60% relied on expert opinion as the primary means of validation. The authors concluded that indicators tended to be viewed as quality improvement tools rather than true measures of clinical practice and patient outcomes in anesthesia. Most clinical outcome indicators were used as indirect measures that triggered further steps to determine potential quality concerns.[43-44]

Currently, anesthesia data collection is guided by using AHRQ patient safety quality indicators. The complications of anesthesia indicator is intended to capture cases flagged by external cause-of-injury and complications codes for adverse effects from the administration of therapeutic drugs, as well as the overdose of anesthetic agents used primarily in therapeutic settings.[12,13]

Recently, anesthesia professionals have worked with other specialty societies through the AMA-sponsored Physician Consortium for Performance Improvement to develop measures that meet requirements for evidence-based medicine and other criteria for NQF endorsement. Both the AANA and the ASA provided input in the development of clinical measures such as perioperative antibiotic administration, blood-glucose stability, and maintenance of normothermia for anesthesia provider reporting. Beginning in January 2010, the hospital prospective payment system requires that all hospitals report selected measures in order to receive full Medicare annual payment updates. Reportable provider measures must be aligned with endorsed hospital measures. Table 13.5 outlines the NQF-endorsed anesthesia reporting measures for 2010.[45]

Although quality improvement efforts in anesthesia should be aligned with broad healthcare quality improvement initiatives, anesthesia departments should adopt practices that meet specific operational needs. However, anesthesia practitioners should also understand that reimbursement in the future will be linked to both outcome measures and demonstrated compliance with process variables.

Pay for reporting or performance is a popular strategy currently in use for public and private payer reimbursement for both institutional and individual physician providers. Pay-for-performance programs represent a substantial shift from traditional service-based reimbursement to a system of

---

Table 13.5. National Quality Forum-Endorsed Anesthesia Reporting Measures for 2010

Measure 30 – Administration of prophylactic antibiotics: timely preoperative care

Measure 76 – Prevention of catheter-related bloodstream infections: central line sterile technique

Measure 193 – Perioperative temperature management: patients undergoing surgical or therapeutic procedures under general or neuraxial anesthesia of 60 minutes duration or longer, except patients undergoing cardiopulmonary bypass

---

(From Health and Human Services, Centers for Medicare & Medicaid Services, Anesthesiology Center. http://www.cms.gov/center/anesth.asp.)

performance-based provider payment using financial incentives to drive improvements in quality of care. Pay-for-performance strategies currently comprise basic structure and process metrics (as opposed to outcome metrics) that set relatively low performance thresholds; however, through CER, pay-for-performance strategies that align reimbursement allocation using evidence-based data and positive reinforcement are anticipated to produce large-scale improvements in quality and cost efficiency. As a result, pay-for-performance incentives will most likely remain a mainstay of healthcare reimbursement.[40,45,46]

The recent establishment of the ASA Anesthesia Quality Institute (AQI), a national clinical database initiative, seeks to validate anesthesia process and outcomes in order to guide data-driven performance improvement.[46] Furthermore, the data registry will strive to achieve multiple goals, including clinical research, benchmarking, and public reporting. The AANA has been successful in negotiating language with CMS ensuring that "eligible professionals" (such as CRNAs) are reflected in all CMS communications regarding AQI reporting.[46-48]

Reform

With the release of The IOM's *To Err Is Human: Building a Safer Health System*[9] and *Crossing the Quality Chasm: A New Health System for the 21st Century*,[22] the healthcare landscape has changed irrevocably. The focus on specific quality concerns of patient safety provides a strong impetus for change throughout the healthcare system. Furthermore, the IOM's recommendations for changes in the healthcare delivery system launched groundbreaking initiatives for reform.

The nation recently engaged in a great debate about the future of healthcare in America. Stakeholders agree that the US healthcare system is complex, expensive, and often inefficient. Although America leads the world in technological innovations, as of 2010, more than 40 million citizens have no health insurance coverage at any one time. The United States spends almost twice as much of its gross domestic product on healthcare as the United Kingdom, yet for some sectors of the population, health status measures are worse than those in some developing countries. In addition, the satisfaction of the American

293

people with its healthcare system is lower than for most English-speaking countries. Escalating healthcare expenditures in the United States exceed $2 trillion a year. In 2008, nearly 50 million Americans did not have health insurance, and another 27 million were underinsured.[49]

Current payment mechanisms reward the provision of narrowly defined services and increased product volume, independent of appropriateness or health outcomes. There are significant data gaps on the effectiveness of medical interventions and processes of care. Furthermore, there are few integrated analyses of existing data or new research on the comparative efficacy and cost-effectiveness of healthcare diagnostics or therapeutics. Many federal and state laws are inconsistent or at cross-purposes and frequently inhibit the coordination of care among various providers or more effective use of physicians, nurses, and other practitioners.[17,20] Most of the reform discussions center on recommendations to simplify and rationalize federal and state laws and regulations to facilitate organizational innovation, support care coordination, and streamline financial and administrative functions. Further proposals include the development of a health information technology infrastructure with national standards of interoperability to promote data exchange. Additionally, the creation of a national health database with the participation of all payers, delivery systems, and others who own healthcare data.[49]

Although experts agree that effective deployment of health information technology is essential for collecting data on outcomes that guide quality improvement, successful and comprehensive electronic health information networks are few and underutilized. Only 17% of US physicians and 8% to 10% of US hospitals have a basic electronic health record system. Far fewer have or routinely use sophisticated and comprehensive technology-based systems that would allow efficient use of data to solve quality-related problems.[17]

Lagging quality of care has been a persistent problem and challenge for health policy makers. The coverage, cost, and quality problems of the US healthcare system are evident. Sustainable healthcare reform must go beyond financing expanded access to care to substantially change the organization and delivery of care.

In March of 2010, the Patient Protection and Affordable Care Act (PL 111-148) was signed into law. Although controversial, eliciting much debate among policy experts and the public alike, the bill is intended to change the US healthcare system during the next 10 years by focusing on value and quality to patients, not just lowering costs.[50] Despite considerable uncertainty about the effects of the new law, it seems an extraordinary achievement that will continue to evolve through its implementation.

Summary

Quality improvement requires 5 essential elements for success: (1) fostering and sustaining a culture of change and safety, (2) developing and clarifying an understanding of the problem, (3) involving key stakeholders, (4) testing change strategies, and (5) continuous monitoring of performance and reporting of findings to sustain the change.

The pursuit of value in healthcare will require changes in structure, delivery, measurement, and accountability. Evidence-based practice and clinical indicators are emerging strategies to achieve those goals that, in turn, facilitate clinical decision-making, intervention, and outcome measurement.

Quality incentives pervade the recent legislation with mandates to identify gaps where no quality measures exist as well as existing quality measures that need improvement, updating, or expansion. The reform legislation places a huge emphasis on public reporting and pay-for-performance programs. Quality is integral to various payment programs, including payment incentives tied to reducing avoidable readmissions and reducing healthcare-acquired conditions, and provisions for many demonstration projects on payment tightly linked to better care and better patient outcomes. Healthcare practitioners, including CRNAs, have the opportunity to participate in these projects and to contribute to CER initiatives.

To understand systems improvement, it is important to be familiar with the factors that influence it. Healthcare providers must recognize and improve patient care processes and find mechanisms that enhance performance and quality outcomes.

CRNAs must continue their contributions to the specialty through participation and leadership of future quality initiatives, remaining at the forefront of developing clinical standards and evidence-based clinical practices, testing performance measures, and implementing system improvements. Above all, CRNAs must understand that quality is not achieved by doing different things. It is achieved by doing things differently; to redefine systems, processes, and outcomes; to measure, monitor, manage, and maximize value. The provision of excellent patient care is impossible absent attention to its quality.

Cutting costs while attempting to improve quality and increase access to care will require extensive creativity and willingness to accept substantial changes in the delivery of healthcare services. CRNAs and other practitioners will be challenged by changing environments and the need to adapt practices that meet professional and personal goals as well as public accountability. Moving toward and securing a culture of safety, efficiency, quality, and accountability throughout healthcare will require a paradigm shift in which value is measured in patient outcomes. The increased focus on patient-centered care and value-based purchasing links payments to value related to the whole patient experience and also recognizes shared accountability among providers. The shift will require unprecedented collaborative effort in order to transform the current environment of care. Additionally, strategies are being developed to ensure the implementation of methods to use clinical data and information as well as research evidence to improve practice and value to patients.

There are enormous challenges to redesigning the healthcare system, including a need to balance the competing views and needs of purchasers, patients, and healthcare professionals. To influence change and improve patient safety and quality demands a willingness to alter existing complexity and inefficiencies in processes and delivery structures. It requires the integration of technology, delivery models, evidence-based education, and lifelong learning, professionalism, and collaboration. It requires commitment and advocacy for improved patient care outcomes, performance monitoring and measurement, and effective management of costs.

The challenge of creating consensus is significant but surmountable. The reward is reform and modernization of how the United States finances and delivers healthcare. The ultimate goal is to ensure real value, better quality care, and improved health of Americans.

295

References

1. Martin-Sheridan D, Mastropietro C. Improving quality in the 21st century. In: Foster SD, Faut-Callahan M, eds. *A Professional Study and Resource Guide for the CRNA*. 1st ed. Park Ridge, IL: AANA Publishing Inc; 2001:503-527.

2. Walton M. *The Deming Management Method*. New York, NY: Perigree, The Berkeley Publishing Group; 1986:28, 33-35.

3. Donabedian A. *An Introduction to Quality Assurance in Health Care*. New York, NY: Oxford University Press; 2003:46-56, 56-61, 91-93.

4. Berkowitz E. Medicare and Medicaid: the past is present. *Health Care Financ Rev*. 2005;27(2):11-23.

5. Jost TS. Medicare and the Joint Commission on Accreditation of Healthcare Organizations: a healthy relationship? *Law Contemp Problems*. 1994; 57(4): 15-45.

6. Bhatia A, Blackstone S, Nelson T, Ng TS. Evolution of quality review programs for Medicare: quality assurance to quality improvement. *Health Care Financ Rev*. 2000;11(7):68-75.

7. Bratzler D. SCIP today and SCIP tomorrow: looking ahead to 2010. Paper presented at: Oklahoma Foundation for Medical Quality Teleconference; November 11, 2009; Oklahoma City, OK. http://www.cfmc.org/hospital/hospital_scip.htm. Accessed April 26, 2010.

8. The Joint Commission. Sentinel Events Statistics. http://www.jointcommission.org/Library/annual_report. Accessed December 10, 2009.

9. Kohn LT, Corrigan JM, Donaldson MS, eds, Institute of Medicine. *To Err Is Human: Building a Safer Health System*. Washington, DC: National Academies Press; 2000:39, 48, 80.

10. The Joint Commission. Improving America's Hospitals: The Joint Commission's Report on Quality and Safety 2008. http://www.jointcommission.org/Library/annual_report. Accessed November 2008.

11. Consensus Development Process. www.qualityforum.org/Measuring_Performance/Consensus_Development_Process.aspx. Accessed November 18, 2009.

12. Farquhar M. AHRQ quality indicators. In: Hughes R, ed. *Patient Safety and Quality: An Evidence Based Handbook for Nurses. Vol 3*. 2008. Rockville MD: AHRQ Publications; 2008:50-53.

13. Agency for Healthcare Research and Quality. Guide to the Prevention Quality Indicators. http://www.qualityindicators.ahrq.gov/downloads/pqi/pqi_guide_v31.pdf. Accessed December, 2009.

14. Medicare Modernization Update Overview. Prescription Drug, Improvement, and Modernization Act. PL 108-173. 2003. www.cms.hhs.gov/MMAUpdate/. Accessed November 20, 2009.

15. The American Recovery and Reinvestment Act PL 111-5. 2009. www.cms.hhs.gov/ARRAUpdate/

16. Hughes R. Tools and strategies for quality improvement and patient safety. In: Hughes R, ed. *Patient Safety and Quality: An Evidenced Based Handbook for Nurses. Vol 3*. Rockville, MD: Agency for Healthcare Research and Quality; 2008:1-18.

17. Steinbrook R. Health care and the American Recovery and Reinvestment Act. *N Engl J Med*. 2009;360(11): 1057-1060.

18. AANA members named to National Quality Forum. *AANA Newsbulletin.* March 2008. http://www.aana.com. Accessed November 6, 2009.

19. Council on Surgery and Perioperative Safety. www.cspsteam.org/. Accessed November 18, 2009.

20. Shi L, Singh D. *Essentials of the US Health Care System.* 2nd ed. Jones & Bartlett Publishers: 2009:3-15.

21. Varkey P, Peller K, Resar RK. Basics of quality improvement in health care. *Mayo Clin Proc.* 2007;82(6):735-739.

22. Institute of Medicine. Crossing the quality chasm: a new health system for the 21st century. Washington, DC: National Academy Press; 2000.

23. Beyea SC, Nicoll LH. Is it research or quality improvement? *AORN J.* 1998;68(1):117-119

24. Anderson B, Fagerhaug T. *Root Cause Analysis: Simplified Tools and Techniques.* Milwaukee, WI: American Society for Quality, Quality Press; 2000:50-59.

25. Hendrickson K, Dayton E, Keyes M, Carayon P, Hughes R. understanding adverse events: a human factors framework. In: Hughes R, ed. *Patient Safety and Quality: An Evidenced Based Handbook for Nurses.* Vol. 1. Rockville, MD: Agency for Heathcare Research and Quality; 2004: 47-66.

26. Guinane C, Davis N. The science of Six Sigma in Hospitals. *Am Heart Hosp J.* 2004;2(1):42-48.

27. Burgmeier J. Failure mode and effect analysis: an application in reducing risk in blood transfusion. *Jt Comm J Qual Improv.* 2002;28(6):331-339.

28. Østergaard H, Østergaard D, Lippert A. Implementation of team training in medical education in Denmark. *Qual Saf Health Care.* 2004;13(Suppl 1):91-95.

29. Haig KM, Sutton S, Whittington J. SBAR: a shared mental model for improving communication between clinicians. *Jt Comm J Qual Patient Saf.* 2006;32(3):167-175.

30. Powell SM, Haskins RN, Sanders W. Improving patient safety and quality of care using aviation CRM. *Patient Saf Qual Healthc.* 2005;2(4):28-33.

31. Tunajek S. Standards of care in anesthesia practice. In: Foster SD, Faut-Callahan M, eds. *A Professional Study and Resource Guide for the CRNA.* 1st ed. Park Ridge, IL: AANA Publishing, Inc; 2001:256,265-275,281-282.

32. Conn J. It's one step toward quality. *Mod Healthc.* 2005;35(32):6-7.

33. US Department of Health and Human Services. Patient Safety and Quality Improvement Act of 2005 Statute and Rule. www.hhs.gov/ocr/privacy/psa/regulation/. Accessed November 16, 2009.

34. Centers for Medicare & Medicaid Services. Statute/Regulations/Program Instructions. PQRI Statutory Authority. Tax Relief Healthcare Act of 2006.www.cms.hhs.gov/PQRI/05_StatuteRegulationsProgramInstructions.asp. Accessed November 16, 2009.

35. Medicare "Pay for Performance (P4P)" Initiatives [press release]. Baltimore, MD. Centers for Medicare & Medicaid Services. January 31, 2005. http://www.cms.hhs.gov/apps/media/press/release.asp?Counter=1343. Accessed December 8, 2009.

36. Massoud RMF. Advances in quality improvement: principles and framework. *QA Brief.* 2001;9(1):13-18. http://www.reproline.jhu.edu/english/6read/6pi/pi_advances/piadvances1.htm Accessed March 18, 2010.

297

37. Iglehart J. Prioritizing comparative-effectiveness research: IOM recommendations. *N Engl J Med.* 2009; 361(4):325-328.

38. Alexander GC, Stafford RS. Does comparative effectiveness have a comparative edge? *JAMA.* 2009;301(23): 2488-2490.

39. Teutsch SM, Berger ML, Weinstein MC. Comparative effectiveness: asking the right questions, choosing the right method. *Health Aff.* 2005;24(1):128-132.

40. Posner K, Domino K. Anesthesia risk, quality improvement and liability. In: Barash P, Cullen B, Stoelting R, Cahalen M, Stock C. eds. *Handbook of Clinical Anesthesia.* 6th ed. Philadelphia, PA: Lippincott Williams & Wilkins; 2009:28,31-33.

41. Smith D, Fleisher L. Approaches to quality improvement in anesthesia care. In: Longnecker D, Brown D, Newman M, Zapol W, eds. *Anesthesiology.* 1st ed. New York, NY: McGraw-Hill Professional. 2008:452-464.

42. McIntosh CA, Macario A. Managing quality in an anesthesia department. *Curr Opin Anaesthesiology.* 2009;22(2): 223-231.

43. Kheterpal S. Perioperative comparative effectiveness research: an opportunity calling. *Anesthesiology.* 2009; 111(6):1180-1182[editorial].

44. Haller G, Stoelwinder J, Myles PS, McNeil J. Quality and safety indicators in anesthesia: a systematic review. *Anesthesiology.* 2009;110(5):1158-1175.

45. Health and Human Services, the Centers for Medicare & Medicaid Services. Anesthesiologist Center. http://www.cms.gov/center/anesth.asp. Accessed May 12, 2010.

46. Hannenberg AA, Warner MA. The registry imperative. *Anesthesiology.* 2009; 111(4):687-689.

47. Lagasse R, Johnstone R. Pay-for-performance in anesthesiology. In: Lake CL, Johnson JO, McLoughlin TM, eds. *Advances in Anesthesia.* New York, NY: Mosby. 2008:67-101.

48. Purcell F. 2009 Medicare issues final rule on anesthesia payments, 2010 fee schedule, other critical CRNA issues. *AANA NewsBulletin.* 2009;63(12): 16-19.

49. Arrow K, Auerbach A, Bertko J, et al. Toward a 21st-century health care system: recommendations for health care reform. *Ann Intern Med.* 2009; 150(7):493-495

50. Initial Guide on Major Health Reform for CRNAs. Federal Issues & Actions News. March 26, 2010. http://www.aana.com. Accessed June 3, 2010.

298

Study Questions

1. Define 5 components of quality assessment methods and develop a plan to implement them in your department of anesthesiology.

2. Why is it essential for a quality assessment plan to be linked to outcome assessment?

3. Discuss necessary components to developing evidence-based practice clinical indicators.

4. Discuss the role of anesthesia providers in clinical indicator development.

5. Describe how simulation can be applied as a training tool to improve patient safety and outcome.

6. Identify the roles and responsibilities of the patient safety organizations responsible for quality measurement indicators.

7. Discuss how comparative effectiveness research findings might be used to maximize the impact on clinical and health policy decisions.

8. What is the difference between quality assurance studies and clinical research activities?

The Politics of Healthcare

CHAPTER 14

Federal Healthcare Policy: How the AANA Advocates for the Profession

Nancy Bruton-Maree, CRNA, MS
Rita M. Rupp, RN, MA

Key Concepts

- Research supports the position of the American Association of Nurse Anesthetists (AANA) that changes in the Tax Equity and Fiscal Responsibility Act of 1982 rules favoring less restrictive conditions for payment would allow flexible allocation of anesthesia personnel and provide a more efficient service to consumers.

- Deferring to state law in reference to physician supervision of nurse anesthesia in the proposed rules and regulations for hospital reimbursement from Medicare would be consistent with language used by the Centers for Medicare & Medicaid Services for other healthcare practitioners.

- The AANA has actively lobbied for changes in Medicare reimbursement rules and regulations that would promote the profession of nurse anesthesia while maintaining patient safety and a quality standard of care.

- Since the inception of healthcare reform, the AANA has taken a proactive position in support of legislation that ensures consumers a choice of provider and accountability in healthcare.

Continues on next page.

Key Concepts (continued)

- The AANA has guarded the ability of Certified Registered Nurse Anesthetists to compete in the healthcare marketplace through supporting antitrust and antidiscrimination legislation.

- More than 75% of all graduates of anesthesia programs during the last decade have received federal money, either as direct student aid or indirectly through new program start-up funds or faculty-assistance plans.

- The AANA supports development of teaching rules similar to the ones afforded to medical anesthesia residency programs as a means to reimburse CRNA clinical faculty who teach in nurse anesthesia educational programs. This type of incentive would enhance the viability of nurse anesthesia education.

A number of federal initiatives in the 1980s and 1990s had a major impact on the nurse anesthesia profession. Sponsored legislation and regulatory advocacy were most often brought to the attention of policy makers by the American Association of Nurse Anesthetists (AANA) or state organizations in the form of annual legislative agendas. Issues most often related to equity in reimbursement, regulatory recognition, quality of care, insurance, antitrust, and antidiscrimination. This chapter will address the advocacy role of the AANA in a select number of these federal healthcare initiatives. Before discussing each of these areas in detail, I have provided some background on the Medicare program as it relates to the issues of supervision and medical direction of Certified Registered Nurse Anesthetists (CRNAs).

Understanding the Medicare Program

The Medicare program is divided into 3 major sections, which are commonly referred to as Medicare Part A, Medicare Part B, and Medicare Part C. Medicare Part A outlines the rules and regulations by which hospitals and ambulatory care facilities are reimbursed for services, supplies, drugs, and equipment provided to Medicare patients. Medicare Part A does not include any reimbursement that goes directly to anesthesiologists, nurse anesthetists, or anesthesiologist assistants (AAs). As of this writing, the Medicare Part A regulations require physician supervision of CRNAs as a condition for hospitals, ambulatory surgical centers (ASCs), and critical access hospitals (CAHs) to be eligible to participate and receive reimbursement from Medicare.[1-3]

Medicare Part B sets forth the payment regulations for healthcare professionals who are eligible to receive direct reimbursement through the Medicare program. The requirements that must be met to receive reimbursement from Medicare Part B are distinct and separate from Medicare Part A. Currently there are 2 types of reimbursement provisions for anesthesiologists under Medicare Part B related to their working with CRNAs. These provisions include payment for medical direction and medical supervision of anesthesia services.[4] If Medicare is billed for medically directed anesthesia services by an anesthesiologist, he or she must be directing no more than 4 concurrent procedures involving residents, CRNAs, or AAs.[4] The 7 conditions of payment enacted as a result of the Tax Equity and Fiscal Responsibility Act of 1982 (TEFRA) must be followed (Table 14.1).[5-7] In these medically directed cases, the anesthesiologist receives 50% of the payment for each case that he or she is medically directing, and a medically directed CRNA administering the anesthesia receives the other 50%.[8]

Medicare Part B also includes a provision for payment to anesthesiologists for medical supervision of nurse anesthetists who are administering anesthesia.[4] Although current Medicare statutes define the conditions for medical direction, there is no specific definition for medical supervision. Medical supervision is indirectly defined in 42 CFR §414.46 as "if the physician medically supervised more than four concurrent anesthesia services, CMS bases the fee schedule amount on an anesthesia specific CF and three base units."[4] Clearly, the current statutes recognize the level of involvement required for a physician to be medically directing a case, and situations wherein the physician is providing supervisory services.

The current payment methodology for medically supervised anesthesia cases is:

305

Table 14.1. Medicare Program Conditions for Physician Payment of Medically Directed Anesthesia Services[5-7]

Original Rules
42CFR §405.552 Conditions for payment of charges: Concurrent anesthesiology services.
(a) (1) For each patient, the physician:
(i) Performs a pre-anesthetic examination and evaluation;
(ii) Prescribes the anesthesia plan;
(iii) Personally participates in the most demanding procedures in the anesthesia plan, including induction and emergence;
(iv) Ensures that any procedures in the anesthesia plan that he or she does not perform are performed by a qualified individual as defined in program operating instructions;
(v) Monitors the course of anesthesia at frequent intervals;
(vi) Remains physically present and available for immediate diagnosis and treatment of emergencies; and
(vii) Provides indicated postanesthesia care.

Proposed Rules
42CFR §415.110 Conditions for payment: Medically directed anesthesia services.
(a) (1) For each patient, the physician:
(i) Performs a preanesthetic examination and evaluation, or reviews one performed by another qualified individual permitted by the state to administer anesthetics;
(ii) Participates in the development of the anesthesia plan and gives final approval of the proposed plan;
(iii) Personally participates in the most demanding procedures of the anesthesia plan;
(iv) Ensures that any aspect of the anesthesia plan not performed by the anesthesiologist is performed by a qualified individual as specified in operating instructions;
(v) Monitors the course of anesthesia at intervals medically indicated by the nature of the procedure and the patient's condition;
(vi) Remains physically present and available for immediate diagnosis and treatment of emergencies; and
(vii) Provides indicated postanesthesia care or ensures that it is done by a qualified individual as described in paragraph (a)(1)(iv) of this section.

Current Rules
42CFR §415.110 Conditions for payment: Medically directed anesthesia services.
(a) (1) For each patient, the physician:
(i) Performs a preanesthetic examination and evaluation;
(ii) Prescribes the anesthesia plan;
(iii) Personally participates in the most demanding aspects of the anesthesia plan including, if applicable, induction and emergence;
(iv) Ensures that any procedures in the anesthesia plan that he or she does not perform are performed by a qualified individual as defined in operating instructions;
(v) Monitors the course of anesthesia administration at frequent intervals;
(vi) Remains physically present and available for immediate diagnosis and treatment of emergencies; and

Continues on page 307.

Table 14.1. Medicare Program Conditionsa for Physician Payment of Medically Directed Anesthesia Services[5-7] (continued)

(vii) Provides indicated postanesthesia care

(b) Medical documentation. The physician alone inclusively documents in the patient's medical record that the conditions set forth in paragraph (a)(1) of this section have been satisfied, specifically documenting that he or she performed the preanesthetic exam and evaluation, provided the indicated postanesthesia care, and was present during the most demanding procedures, including induction and emergence where applicable.

---

1. Physician anesthesiologists are paid at a base of 3 units (with an additional 1 unit if they were present during induction). This represents payment for physician involvement in the presurgical anesthesia services.[4]
2. Both CRNAs and AAs are reimbursed at 50% of the total fee if a physician is involved in the medical supervision/direction of the case.[8]

The requirement for CRNAs to be reimbursed through Medicare Part B is that they must meet the state licensure requirements in the state in which they practice and they must be currently certified by the Council on Certification of Nurse Anesthetists or the Council on Recertification of Nurse Anesthetists.[9] Also, they must have graduated within the last 18 months from a nurse anesthesia program that meets the standards of the Council on Accreditation of Nurse Anesthesia Educational Programs, and they must be awaiting initial certification.[9]

Nurse Anesthesia Reimbursement

In 1983 the Prospective Payment System (PPS) legislation was passed in an effort to control hospital costs to the Medicare program.[5] The law provided that all services by providers other than those reimbursed through Medicare Part B would be bundled into a hospital diagnosis-related group payment.[5] The caveats for CRNAs in this law were several: (1) It would be impossible for the anesthesia component of payment to cover the full cost of hospital-employed CRNAs; (2) Unbundling of services and payment was prohibited; and (3) Anesthesiologists who had been billing for CRNA services under Part B by considering them a physician service could no longer bill through this mechanism.[5] Simply put, CRNA services were, for all practical purposes, nonreimbursable.

Because of the potential negative impact of the PPS legislation on nurse anesthetists, the AANA advocated the following legislative changes.[5]

1. A provision allowing a temporary pass-through of hospitals' CRNA costs for a 3-year period, which would ensure that hospitals would not lose money on CRNA services.
2. A single exception to the unbundling provisions of the law for anesthesiologist-employed CRNAs, because it was questionable if anesthesiologists could bill for CRNA services under the new provision.
3. Inclusion of direct reimbursement for CRNAs in the Omnibus Budget Reconciliation Act (OBRA) of 1986, to become effective January 1, 1989, with the 2 temporary provisions being extended

307

to the effective date of the legislation. Two payment schedules were incorporated in the law—one for CRNAs not medically directed by anesthesiologists and the other for CRNAs working under anesthesiologists' medical direction.

As a part of OBRA 1989, Congress mandated a study of reimbursement mechanisms that would not serve as disincentives for using CRNAs.[5]

Tax Equity and Fiscal Responsibility Act of 1982

In 1982 TEFRA was enacted into federal law as a means to control escalating Medicare costs for hospital-based services, which included anesthesiology, pathology, and radiology. Among the many cost concerns that TEFRA addressed was a need to ensure that an anesthesiologist demonstrated that he or she provided certain services as part of a given anesthetic to qualify for payment for medical direction of a CRNA. Before the enactment of TEFRA, anesthesiologists could bill for their services in conjunction with medical direction of hospital-employed CRNAs without demonstrating that they provided specific services to qualify for such payment. Although the 1976 Medicare manual did require that the "physician be close by and available to provide immediate and personal assistance and direction," it stated that availability by telephone did not constitute direct, personal, and continuous service.[5] Because some anesthesiologists failed to comply with Medicare rules, and because the number of anesthetics administered by CRNAs that could be supervised and billed by anesthesiologists had no limit, some private payers began refusing to reimburse for more than 2 concurrent procedures.[5] In addition, the

Medicare Inspector General's Office expanded its search for fraudulent practices for anesthesia billing.[5]

In 1983 the Health Care Financing Administration (HCFA; now the Centers for Medicare & Medicaid Services, or CMS) published the final rules implementing TEFRA relative to payment for anesthesiology physician services.[5] In instituting the rules, HCFA chose a 4:1 ratio of medical direction, limiting payment to anesthesiologists to no more than 4 concurrent procedures administered by CRNAs. The rules implemented 7 conditions that an anesthesiologist must satisfy if he or she was to obtain reimbursement for the medical direction of CRNAs. These original conditions are listed in Table 14.1.

In its comments on the proposed TEFRA rules, the AANA expressed concern that the limitation of concurrent procedures reimbursable on a charge basis should not be linked to presumptions about the quality of anesthesia services furnished by CRNAs under a physician's general supervision. The published response by HCFA was as follows:

> The distinctions we are making are between physician services to providers and individuals, not between good and bad anesthesia services. Anesthesia administered by non-physician anesthetist is a covered service, reimbursable on a reasonable cost basis. Therefore the criteria for 'medical direction' should not be interpreted as standards of practice or standards of quality, but rather as a description of those elements of common medical practice that are expected to be present when a physician has significant involvement with an individual patient.[10]

Even though the AANA was successful in obtaining this clarification from HCFA, the TEFRA conditions of payment for anesthesiologists have been inappropriately interpreted by many as quality-of-care standards for the practice of anesthesia instead of reimbursement criteria for anesthesiologists. The regulations have served to create disruptions in the overall delivery and flow of services in the operating room, causing needless and costly delays to the government and ultimately to consumers. In some cases, anesthesiologists have used the medical direction conditions of payment in negotiations with hospitals as justification to adopt the anesthesia care team model of practice. Assertions that the medical direction conditions are standards of care and ensure a better level of quality than the care provided by a solo CRNA practitioner have been successfully used by anesthesiologists to support the anesthesia care team model, but such assertions are not supported by valid scientific research.

By 1996 the AANA believed that changes in healthcare and healthcare reimbursement favoring less restrictive conditions would allow flexibility in allocation of anesthesia personnel and more expedient service to consumers. In addition, studies began to support the opposite of the anesthesiologists' promotion that medical direction of CRNAs provided a higher quality of care. For example, the 1992 Center for Health Economics Research report to the Physician Payment Review Commission (PPRC) recommended the following: "Refinements to the TEFRA provisions should be considered in view of the reductions in payments to the anesthesia care team. In particular, opportunities for increasing the flexibility of role functions should be reviewed. Considerations should also be given to the appropriateness of promulgating specific practice standards within a payment policy."[11] The Center for Health Economics

Research report went on to say, "With the implication of a capped payment, the Health Care Financing Administration should consider whether to review the TEFRA requirements to see if modifications of the TEFRA rules would permit greater efficiencies without decreasing the quality of care."[11]

In 1993 the PPRC Report to Congress on "Payments for the Anesthesia Care Team" noted: "The use of the anesthesia care team seems to be determined by individual preferences for that practice arrangement. There appear to be no demonstrated quality of care differences between the care provided by the solo anesthesiologist, solo CRNA, and the team."[11]

In a study of medical direction conducted at a Los Angeles county hospital, findings concluded, "Anesthesiologists and nurse anesthetists in this study agreed in their perceptions that more than 70% of these cases did not need medical direction."[12] The report further noted, "Even though this study was from one practice setting, it suggests that excessive medical direction may be contributing to the higher costs of anesthesia care teams. Revision of medical direction guidelines (TEFRA), focusing on patient and operative factors, is recommended to preserve the anesthesia care team as a practice option, while making it more cost effective."[12] In another study of medical direction, the findings were as follows:

> Significantly, the protocol groups appear to have no difference from the retrospective group in all outcome criteria, meaning that medical direction can be reduced without a reduction in quality. This can result in a significant cost reduction when physician time is considered. It is possible to significantly reduce the costs of anesthesia care teams through reduction of unnecessary

medical direction and revision of TEFRA guidelines. This study may have other applications in terms of provider job satisfaction and the ability to use physician resources most effectively.[13]

In 1997, based on studies such as the ones just described, the AANA initiated as part of its legislative agenda a congressional lobbying effort to revise the TEFRA conditions of payment for medical direction of CRNAs by anesthesiologists. In 1998 the AANA shifted its focus from legislative strategies for revision of TEFRA to revision through regulatory change. Healthcare reform, contrary to earlier predictions, brought an increase in surgical and anesthesia case numbers, and managed care companies put emphasis on increased operating room efficiency without a decline in quality of care. The TEFRA conditions, in many instances, hindered efficient utilization of operating rooms. Because the TEFRA conditions were not tied to quality of care, the AANA, as did other healthcare organizations, used legislative and regulatory change as the avenue to advocate positively for the public as well as for its members.

In a 1998 joint meeting that included the American Society of Anesthesiologists (ASA), the AANA, and the HCFA, proposals were advanced by both the AANA and the ASA for revisions to 7 conditions of payment for physician medical direction. The ASA and the AANA reached consensus on a revised recommended set of medical direction requirements that are listed as proposed revisions in Table 14.1.[6] However, it came to the AANA's attention in a 1998 publication called *Anesthesia Answer Book—Action Alert* that the ASA had second thoughts about the agreed-upon revisions.[14] The response by HCFA to the concerns posed by the ASA membership and several state anesthesiol-

ogist societies was to retain the current requirements established in 1983.[5] Then the HCFA decided that the medically directing physician must be present at induction and emergence for general anesthesia but only if applicable for other types of anesthesia, such as regional anesthesia.[7] The CMS (formerly HCFA) plans to study the medical direction issue further, welcomes comments, and may propose changes in the future.

Because fraud has been elevated to a level of serious concern (as it relates to the misapplication of the 7 conditions), all providers should have a complete understanding of practice parameters allowable in a medically directed situation. An anesthesiologist who is concurrently directing the administration of anesthesia to not more than 4 surgical patients cannot ordinarily be involved in furnishing additional services to other patients. However, addressing an emergency of short duration in the immediate area, administering an epidural or caudal anesthetic to ease labor pain, or periodic rather than continuous monitoring of an obstetrical patient does not substantially diminish the scope of control exercised by the physician in directing the administration of anesthesia to the surgical patients.[9] It does not constitute a separate service for the purpose of determining whether medical direction criteria are met. Furthermore, while directing concurrent anesthesia procedures, a physician may receive patients entering the operating suite for the next surgery, check or discharge patients in the recovery room, or handle scheduling matters without affecting fee schedule payment.[9]

It is important to note the last requirement of the current rules in Table 14.1: the statement requiring the anesthesiologist to document that his or her medical direction involvement is a part of the final language

Table 14.2. Medicare and Medicaid Programs: Hospital Conditions of Participation[2]

Current Language
Medicare and Medicaid Guide
Subpart D – Optional Hospital Services
42CFR §482.52 Condition of participation: Anesthesia services.
If the hospital furnishes anesthesia services, they must be provided in a well organized manner under the direction of a qualified doctor of medicine or osteopathy. The service is responsible for all anesthesia administered in the hospital.
(a) Standard: Organization and Staffing.
The organization of anesthesia services must be appropriate to the scope of the services offered. Anesthesia must be administered by only
(1) A qualified anesthesiologist;
(2) A doctor of medicine or osteopathy (other than an anesthesiologist);
(3) A dentist, oral surgeon, or podiatrist who is qualified to administer anesthesia under State law;
(4) A certified registered nurse anesthetist (CRNA) as defined in §410.69(b) of this chapter who is under the supervision of the operating practitioner or of an anesthesiologist who is immediately available if needed; or
(5) An anesthesiologist's assistant, as defined in §410.69(b) of this chapter, who is under the supervision of an anesthesiologist who is immediately available if needed.
(b) Standard: Delivery of services.
Anesthesia services must be consistent with needs and resources. Policies on anesthesia procedures must include the delineation of preanesthesia and postanesthesia responsibilities. The policies must ensure that the following are provided for each patient:
(1) A preanesthesia evaluation by an individual qualified to administer anesthesia under paragraph (a) of this section performed within 48 hours prior to surgery.
(2) An intraoperative anesthesia record.
(3) With respect to inpatients, a postanesthesia follow-up report by the individual who administers the anesthesia that is written within 48 hours after surgery.
(4) With respect to outpatients, a postanesthesia evaluation for proper anesthesia recovery performed in accordance with policies and procedures approved by the medical staff.

Proposed Language
42CFR §416, 482, 485, and 489
42CFR §482.45 Condition of participation: Surgical and anesthesia services.
If the hospital provides surgical or anesthesia services, they are provided through the use of qualified staff. The patient receives appropriate pre- and post-procedure evaluations, and all care is accurately documented.
(a) Standard: Staffing.
(1) Surgical procedures are performed only by practitioners with appropriate clinical privileges.
(2) Anesthesia is administered only by a licensed practitioner permitted by the State to administer anesthetics.

Continues on page 312.

311

Table 14.2. Medicare and Medicaid Programs: Hospital Conditions of Participation[2] (continued)

(b) Standard: Evaluations.

    (1) A comprehensive assessment of the patient's condition is performed before surgery, except in emergency cases where a modified assessment is acceptable.

    (2) A preanesthesia evaluation by an individual qualified to administer anesthesia is performed prior to the administration of anesthesia.

    (3) A postanesthesia evaluation for proper anesthesia recovery is performed by an individual qualified to administer anesthesia.

(c) Standard: Documentation of care.

    (1) The comprehensive or modified presurgical assessment described in paragraph (b)(1) of this section is entered in the patient record before surgery, except in emergency cases, where the assessment may be entered following surgery.

    (2) A properly executed informed consent form for the operation is entered in the patient's record by the hospital before surgery, except in emergency cases where the delay needed to obtain consent would place the health or safety of the patient in serious jeopardy.

    (3) The hospital maintains a complete, up-to-date operating room register.

    (4) The hospital writes or dictates an operative report describing complications, reactions, length of time, techniques, findings, and tissues removed or altered immediately following surgery and enter it in the patient's record promptly following surgery.

    (5) The hospital maintains an intraoperative anesthesia record and enters it in the patient's record promptly following surgery or any other procedures requiring anesthesia.

    (6) The hospital writes a report of the results of the postanesthesia evaluation described in paragraph (b)(3) of this section and enters it in the patient's record promptly following completion of the procedure for which anesthesia was required.

312

that became effective January 1, 1999. Of particular importance in the compliance arena is the CMS's imposition of specific documentation requirements for the medically directing anesthesiologist.[7] This documentation requirement by the CMS was at the recommendation of the AANA. The AANA asked the CMS to revise the medical documentation requirement, thus mandating that the physician alone personally documents the record. The AANA's rationale for the request was that the CRNA should not have to document the physician's participation because the CRNA may not agree concerning the extent of the physician's participation in the case.

The AANA continues to monitor the impact that the TEFRA rules for physician reimbursement for medical direction of CRNAs have on operating room efficiency, patient care, and CRNA practice. Making changes in these conditions for payment has been difficult for the AANA because these conditions do not affect CRNA reimbursement for anesthesia services. It is difficult for a healthcare provider organization to implement change regarding another provider's mechanism of payment; therefore, change in the TEFRA conditions for payment may come incrementally as more evidence supports the problematic impact they have on operating room efficiency and cost.

Since the inception of the medical direction guidelines, the AANA has influenced changes in the TEFRA conditions for physician medical direction payment and reimbursement for CRNA services in the following ways:

- The adoption of a medical direction ratio of 1:4 rather than 1:2
- A published statement by HCFA that the criteria for medical direction should not be considered quality-related standards, but rather, payment criteria
- Adoption of 1998 revisions that facilitate flexibility in practice
- A published requirement that the physician document his or her personal and inclusive involvement in satisfying the conditions for medical direction payment
- Adoption of a 50% split in payment by the anesthesiologist and CRNA for a case, as long as the ratio of medical direction does not exceed 1:4
- Adoption of a 50% split in payment between the anesthesiologist and CRNA when the medical direction ratio is 1:1

Supervision: Medicare Conditions of Participation

The original Medicare regulations require physician supervision of CRNAs as a condition for hospitals, ambulatory surgery centers (ASCs) and critical access hospitals (CAHs) to receive Medicare payment (Tables 14.2-14.4).[1-3,15,16] These regulations do not require that a CRNA be supervised by an anesthesiologist.

During the 1990s, the AANA pursued a revision of these Medicare conditions of participation that would remove the physician supervision requirement for CRNAs and instead defer to state statutory rules and regulations related to licensure. Currently, 31 states have no physician supervision or direction requirement concerning CRNAs in nurse practice acts, board of nursing rules and regulations, medical practice acts, board of medicine rules and regulations, or their generic equivalents. Clearly this is an indication that many states, as a matter of public policy, do not believe it is necessary to require physician supervision of CRNAs.

In December 1997, HCFA released for comment proposed revisions to the Medicare Conditions of Participation for Hospitals, ASCs and CAHs. These proposed revisions would eliminate the requirement for physician supervision of CRNAs, deferring instead to state law (See Tables 14.2-14.4).[1-3,15-17] The AANA supported these proposed revisions to the Medicare and Medicaid rule for facility reimbursement for the following reasons:

- The proposed rule brings HCFA into compliance with 42 USC section 1395, which prohibits "any Federal officer or employee to exercise any supervision or control over the practice of medicine or the manner in which medical services are provided, or over the selection, tenure, or compensation of any officer or employee of any institution, agency, or person providing health services; or to exercise any supervision or control over the administration or operation of any such institution, agency, or person."[18]
- Routinely, HCFA defers to state policy regarding licensure and practice acts regarding healthcare practitioners. Deferral by HCFA to state law on the issue of physician supervision comports with other portions of the proposed rule as it relates to other healthcare practitioners as well as to prior HCFA policy.[18] Executive Order No. 12612 (October 27, 1987) directs executive departments and federal

313

Table 14.3. Medicare and Medicaid Programs: Ambulatory Surgical Services (ASC) Conditions of Participation[1]

Current Language[a]

§416.42 Condition for coverage—Surgical services.

Surgical procedures must be performed in a safe manner by qualified physicians who have been granted clinical privileges by the governing body of the ASC in accordance with approved policies and procedures of the ASC.

(a) *Standard: Anesthetic risk and evaluation.*

   (1) A physician must examine the patient immediately before surgery to evaluate the risk of anesthesia and of the procedure to be performed.

   (2) Before discharge from the ASC, each patient must be evaluated by a physician or by an anesthetist as defined at §410.69(b) of this chapter, in accordance with applicable State health and safety laws, standards of practice, and ASC policy, for proper anesthesia recovery.

(b) *Standard: Administration of anesthesia.* Anesthetics must be administered by only—

   (1) A qualified anesthesiologist; or

   (2) A physician qualified to administer anesthesia, a certified registered nurse anesthetist (CRNA) or an anesthesiologist's assistant as defined in §410.69(b) of this chapter, or a supervised trainee in an approved educational program. In those cases in which a non-physician administers the anesthesia, unless exempted in accordance with paragraph (d) of this section, the anesthetist must be under the supervision of the operating physician, and in the case of an anesthesiologist's assistant, under the supervision of an anesthesiologist.

(c) *Standard: State exemption.*

   (1) An ASC may be exempted from the requirement for physician supervision of CRNAs as described in paragraph (b)(2) of this section, if the State in which the ASC is located submits a letter to CMS signed by the Governor, following consultation with the State's Boards of Medicine and Nursing, requesting exemption from physician supervision of CRNAs. The letter from the Governor must attest that he or she has consulted with State Boards of Medicine and Nursing about issues related to access to and the quality of anesthesia services in the State and has concluded that it is in the best interests of the State's citizens to opt-out of the current physician supervision requirement, and that the opt-out is consistent with State law.

   (2) The request for exemption and recognition of State laws, and the withdrawal of the request may be submitted at any time, and are effective upon submission.

[57 FR 33899, July 31, 1992, as amended at 66 FR 56768, Nov. 13, 2001; 73 FR 68812, Nov. 18, 2008]

Proposed Language[b]

Part 416

Subpart C—Specific Conditions for Coverage

42CFR §416.42 Conditions for coverage: Surgical services.

(b) *Standard: Administration of anesthesia.* Anesthesia is administered only by a licensed practitioner permitted by the State to administer anesthetics.

---

[a] As adopted, from 47 FR 34082 (August 5, 1982; effective September 7, 1982), and at 57 FR 33878 (July 31, 1992; effective August 31, 1992).

[b] From 62 FR 66730 (December 19, 1997).

agencies from limiting the policy discretion of the states to the extent possible, unless the federal statute "contains an express preemption provision or there is some other firm and palpable evidence compelling the conclusion that the Congress intended preemption of State Law, or when the exercise of State authority directly conflicts with the exercise of Federal authority under the Federal statute."[18]

"Requiring supervision can increase surgeon concerns about liability. These concerns, no matter how unwarranted, sometimes serve to increase cost. There are instances in which hospitals or ASCs with limited financial resources nevertheless feel compelled, because of surgeon liability concerns, to hire anesthesiologists to supervise CRNAs."[18]

- "The proposed rule will not mandate changes in personnel in hospitals or ASCs. There will be no dramatic change in the way anesthesiologists, other physicians, and nurse anesthetists work in hospitals or ASCs, simply by virtue of the deferral to state law on supervision. In addition, nothing in the HCFA proposed rule would prevent a state legislature from enacting a physician requirement if they chose to do so."[18]
- "Supervision is unnecessary, as evidenced by the numerous states that do not require supervision but still maintain high-quality anesthesia care."[18]
- "HCFA's proposed rule confirms earlier HCFA intentions in the 1994 draft regulation removing supervision for hospitals, the 1997 draft regulation removing supervision for ASCs, and the 1995 Medicare reform package as agreed to by the Senate Finance Committee."[18]

- "CRNAs have the education and training to practice without physician supervision."[18]
- "No significant differences in quality of care between anesthesia outcome providers have been documented or proven."[18]
- "The federal government explicitly recognizes the value of CRNAs. CRNAs are reimbursed under a number of programs and they are the predominant anesthesia personnel in the military."[18]
- "Federal law does not require that anesthesiologists supervise or 'medically direct' CRNAs. What federal law does require is that if anesthesiologists supervise CRNAs, and want to bill for that supervision, anesthesiologists must satisfy the 7 criteria listed in section 405.552. This is a critical distinction, because it is important to bear in mind that the Medicare requirements for medical direction are payment criteria only, and do not mandate any particular practice arrangement."[18]
- "Nurse anesthetists were the nation's first anesthesia personnel, giving anesthetics for more than 100 years. Nurse anesthetists are clearly qualified as anesthesia providers, even without physician supervision."[18]

The ASA opposed the HCFA proposal and called for a national study comparing anesthesia outcomes between the 2 provider groups. However, undertaking such a study, which would have cost taxpayers approximately $15 million, was considered and rejected by the Centers for Disease Control and Prevention (CDC) in 1990. At that time, the CDC concluded that poor anesthesia outcomes were so rare that it would be a waste of government money to conduct an anesthesia outcomes study.[19]

315

Table 14.4. Medicare and Medicaid Programs: Critical Access Hospital Conditions of Participation[3]

Current Language[a]

Part 485

Subpart F—Conditions of Participation: Critical Access Hospitals (CAHs)

42CFR §485.639 Conditions of participation: Surgical services.

Surgical procedures must be performed in a safe manner by qualified practitioners who have been granted clinical privileges by the governing body of the CAH in accordance with the designation requirements under paragraph (a) of this section.

(a) Designation of qualified practitioners. The CAH designates the practitioners who are allowed to perform surgery for CAH patients, in accordance with its approved policies and procedures, and with State scope of practice laws. Surgery is performed only by—

    (1) A doctor of medicine or osteopathy, including an osteopathic practitioner recognized under section 1101(a)(7) of the Act;

    (2) A doctor of dental surgery or dental medicine; or

    (3) A doctor of podiatric medicine.

(b) Anesthetic risk and evaluation. A qualified practitioner, as described in paragraph (a) of this section, must examine the patient immediately before surgery to evaluate the risk of anesthesia and of the procedure to be performed. Before discharge from the CAH, each patient must be evaluated for proper anesthesia recovery by a qualified practitioner as described in paragraph (a) of this section.

(c) Administration of anesthesia. The CAH designates the person who is allowed to administer anesthesia to CAH patients in accordance with its approved policies and procedures and with State scope of practice laws.

    (1) Anesthetics must be administered only by

        (i) A qualified anesthesiologist;

        (ii) A doctor of medicine or osteopathy other than an anesthesiologist, including an osteopathic practitioner recognized under section 1101(a)(7) of the Act;

        (iii) A doctor of dental surgery or dental medicine;

        (iv) A doctor of podiatric medicine;

        (v) A certified registered nurse anesthetist, as defined in §410.69 (b) of this chapter;

        (vi) An anesthesiologist's assistant as defined in §410.69(b) of this chapter; or

        (vii) A supervised trainee in an approved educational program, as described in §413.85 or 413.86 of this chapter.

    (2) In those cases in which a certified registered nurse anesthetist administers the anesthesia, the anesthetists must be under the supervision of the operating practitioner. An anesthesiologist's assistant who administers anesthesia must be under the supervision of an anesthesiologist.

(d) Discharge. All patients are discharged in the company of a responsible adult, except those exempted by the practitioner who performed the surgical procedure.

Continues on page 317.

[a] From 60 FR 45851 (September 1, 1995), as amended at 62 FR 46037 (August 29, 1997)

Table 14.4. Medicare and Medicaid Programs: Critical Access Hospital Conditions of Participation[3] (continued)

Proposed Language[b]

Part 485

Subpart F—Conditions of Participation: Critical Access Hospitals (CAHs)

42CFR §485.639 Conditions of participation.

(c) Administration of anesthesia. The CAH designates the person who is allowed to administer anesthesia to CAH patients in accordance with its approved policies and procedures and with State scope of practice laws.

Anesthesia is administered only by a licensed practitioner permitted by the State to administer anesthetics.

    (vii) A supervised trainee in an approved educational program, as described in §413.85 or 413.86 of this chapter.

  (2) In those cases in which a certified registered nurse anesthetist administers the anesthesia, the anesthetist must be under the supervision of the operating practitioner. An anesthesiologist's assistant who administers anesthesia must be under the supervision of an anesthesiologist.

(d) Discharge. All patients are discharged in the company of a responsible adult, except those exempted by the practitioner who performed the surgical procedure.

[b] From 60 FR 45851 (September 1, 1995), as amended at 62 FR 46037 (August 29, 1997); 62 FR 66763 (December 19, 1997, Proposed Rules).

Throughout the comment period, while HCFA deliberated on its final revisions to the Medicare and Medicaid conditions for participation, the AANA vigorously lobbied HCFA in support of the proposed supervision rule. The Association emphasized that thanks to advancements in pharmaceuticals, monitoring technology, and anesthesia provider education, anesthesia care today is safer than ever before, with approximately 1 death for every 240,000 anesthetics, compared with 2 deaths for every 10,000 anesthetics just 20 years ago.[19]

It is important to understand the efforts that the AANA put forth to advocate its position on the supervision issue. These include but are not limited to the following:

- Representatives of the AANA met with many key government personnel to advocate the position of CRNAs on the issue of supervision, including HCFA analysts, the administrator of the HCFA, members of Congress and their staffs, the secretary of the Department of Health and Human Services (HHS), members of the White House staff, staff of the Office of Management and Budget, and a host of others.

- As the ASA's opposition to the proposed rule increased, together with the delay in HCFA announcing the final rule, the AANA called on Sen Kent Conrad (D, North Dakota) and Congressman Jim Nussle (R, Iowa) to introduce legislation to require HCFA to implement the new regulations related to CRNA supervision in the hospital conditions for payment for participation in the Medicare program.

- The AANA retained outside legislative consultants to assist in the promotion of its legislative initiatives.

- The AANA retained public relations consultants, who assisted in the following endeavors to increase the public's awareness of the vital role that CRNAs play in anesthesia delivery in this country. advertising in many publications, including the Capitol Hill newspaper *Roll Call* and *USA Today;* assisting with media training for AANA officers and staff, who have appeared on radio programs and have been interviewed by a variety of publications; and developing radio advertisements for use in Washington, DC, to garner support for the AANA's position.

- The AANA retained grassroots consultants to assist in gaining letters of support for the new regulation from key members of Congress.

The effects of these advocacy efforts yielded an extensive base of support from a broad healthcare sector and the public. Support for the proposed rule came from the American Hospital Association, National Rural Health Association, Federation of American Health Systems, St. Paul Fire and Marine Insurance Company, Kaiser Permanente (Central Office, California and Oregon Kaiser System), and numerous rural hospitals across the country. The list of national and health professional associations, individual nurses and physicians, and members of the public at large that wrote letters to the HCFA and the CMS on this issue is exhaustive.

From the beginning, the ASA used as one of its major arguments that a change in this rule would be detrimental to Medicare beneficiaries. In an effort to obtain the views of a sample population of senior citizens, the AANA commissioned a survey of Medicare patients conducted in October 1999 by the independent research firm Wirthlin Worldwide, which revealed the following: (1) 88% of Medicare beneficiaries surveyed would

be comfortable if their surgeon chose a nurse anesthetist to provide their anesthesia care; (2) 81% surveyed preferred a nurse anesthetist or had no preference between a nurse anesthetist or anesthesiologist when it came to their anesthesia care; and (3) 62% of those surveyed found it acceptable for the nurse anesthetist to not be supervised by the surgeon, but to work collaboratively with the surgeon who would be present throughout the surgery.[20]

On March 9, 2000, after deliberating for more than 2 years, the CMS announced that removal of the federal requirement that nurse anesthetists must be supervised by physicians when administering anesthesia to Medicare patients would be forthcoming. The final rule was to be published in the *Federal Register* in June 2000; however, the rule was not published in June as anticipated. The rule remained on hold through the following months with periodic reports that it was in progress at the Office of Management and Budget. The AANA continued to press the administration to publish the rule. Because Congress did not complete its budget and legislative work until late in the year, implementation of the rule remained vulnerable to legislative threats from the ASA, which was pushing for a legislatively mandated study that, if enacted, would preempt implementing a final rule.

It was not until January 18, 2001, with the approval of the Clinton administration, that the rule was published in the *Federal Register* and it was scheduled to become effective March 19, 2001.[15-17] The rule eliminated the federal requirement for physician supervision of CRNAs as proposed in the December 19, 1997, rule. However, on March 19, 2001, the effective date was delayed 60 days by the new Bush administration for purposes of review.[21] On May 18, the rule was further delayed for 180 days

318

to explore alternatives for implementation.[22] On July 5, 2001, CMS published a proposed rule that would maintain the existing supervision requirement but allow a state's governor, in consultation with the state's boards of medicine and nursing, to request an opt-out or exemption from the physician supervision requirement, consistent with state law.[23]

The AANA submitted extensive comments to the CMS concerning the July 5, 2001, proposed rule. The essence of the AANA position was that the CMS should reinstate the January 18, 2001, rule, which removed the federal supervision requirement and deferred to the states on the regulation of CRNAs. The AANA noted in its comments that it agreed with the initial approach reflected in the December 19, 1997, proposed rule and the January 18, 2001, rule, which articulated the need to focus on outcomes of care and work toward eliminating unnecessary procedural requirements. The AANA further noted that it believed the CMS had been moving in the right direction toward streamlining outdated requirements and embodying an approach that more accurately reflects clinical practice while maintaining high quality of care.

> In the January 18, 2001 rule, HCFA (now CMS) agreed with the AANA regarding virtually every major issue that was raised. These arguments were stated succinctly by HCFA in the January 18, 2001 *Federal Register,* leaving the AANA, hospitals, and supporters of the rule in Congress to assume that the 180-degree turnaround was not due to policy issues but rather political considerations.[24]

The AANA also noted considerable support from external entities for HCFA's proposed rule of December 19, 1997, and the January 18, 2001, final rule:

> The AANA has worked diligently with several administrations to bring about the January 18 rule change—a change supported by the American Hospital Association, the Federation of American Hospitals, Premier, Inc., VHA, Inc., the National Rural Health Association, the Center for Patient Advocacy, the TREA Senior Citizens League, the American Nurses Association, Mutual of Omaha, United Healthcare of Arizona, dozens of individuals, hospitals, and many others. Several state governors have also written HCFA/CMS to support the approach reflected in the January 18 rule....The primary opposition to the January 18 rule change came from organized medicine, though physicians at CMS did approve the adoption of the January 18 final rule. Opponents to implementation of the January 18 rule have tried to exploit the unfounded fear that CRNAs would be providing anesthesia care without physician involvement if the rule were implemented. That is not the case, as existing Medicare Conditions of Participation require that every Medicare patient be under the care of a physician.[24]

Ultimately, however, the CMS published in the November 13, 2001, *Federal Register* its final rule concerning the federal Medicare and Medicaid physician supervision requirement for CRNAs.[25] The November 13 rule amended the requirement in the Anesthesia Services Condition of Participation for Hospitals, the Surgical Services Condition of Coverage for Ambulatory Surgical Centers, and the Surgical Services Condition of Participation for

319

Critical Access Hospitals. The November 13 rule, which is virtually identical to the July 5, 2001, proposed rule, took effect immediately upon publication.

The rule allows states to opt out of or be exempted from (the terms are used synonymously) the federal physician-supervision requirement. For a state to opt out of the federal supervision requirement, the state's governor must send a letter of attestation to the CMS. The letter must attest that: (1) The state's governor has consulted with the state's boards of medicine and nursing about issues related to access to and quality of anesthesia services in the state; (2) It is in the best interests of the state's citizens to opt out of the current federal physician-supervision requirement; and (3) The opt-out is consistent with state law.[25] A governor's opt-out request takes effect immediately upon submission to the CMS.[25]

Additionally, the rule states that a governor can request at any time that a previously granted opt-out be withdrawn.[25] Such a request would be effective upon submission to the CMS.[25] Less than 1 month after the rule took effect, Iowa became the first state to opt out of the federal supervision requirement.

Finally, in its November 13 rule comments, the CMS states that the Agency for Healthcare Research and Quality (AHRQ) will "conduct a study of anesthesia outcomes in those states that choose to opt-out of the CRNA supervision requirement compared to those states that have not."[25]

The AANA supports the AHRQ conducting a scientific study of anesthesia outcomes of CRNAs and anesthesiologists working alone but strongly believes that CRNAs must be fairly represented in defining the design parameters and methodology of such a study. A scientifically valid study should be governed by the following principles:

- It should compare important anesthesia outcomes of patients receiving anesthesia from unsupervised CRNAs with those receiving anesthesia from anesthesiologists personally providing the service. Any scientifically valid anesthesia outcomes study of CRNA practices must include anesthesiologists practicing without CRNAs (as indicated in the CMS July 5 proposed rule). Otherwise, there will be no valid basis for comparison of CRNA and anesthesiologist outcomes.

- It should be designed by a team of qualified researchers representing all stakeholders including, at a minimum, CRNAs, anesthesiologists, the HHS, and the AHRQ or other designated agency, with no single group having a majority.

Since Iowa's opt-out in 2001, Nebraska and Idaho (March 2002), Minnesota (April 2002), New Hampshire (June 2002), New Mexico (November 2002), Kansas (April 2003), Wisconsin (June 2005), North Dakota (October 2003), Washington (October 2003), Alaska (October 2003), Oregon (December 2003), Montana (January 2004), South Dakota (March 2005), Wisconsin (June 2005), California (July 2009), and Colorado (September 2010) have become opt-out states.[26] The AHRQ has conducted no studies in the states that have chosen to opt out of the CRNA supervision requirement.

Montana Gov Judy Martz was granted an opt-out for her state in January 2004, but in May 2005 new Gov Brian Schweitzer reversed the opt-out.[26] When Governor Schweitzer did this, he did not cite any evidence to justify his decision.[26] After the governor and his staff became familiar with the reasons that justified the original opt-out, Governor Schweitzer restored the opt-out in June 2005.[26] This opt-out is still in effect.

Throughout the 4 years that the federal physician-supervision issue engaged the healthcare community, many individuals and organizations worked for the removal of this requirement. The AANA clearly recognized that the efforts of many different groups and individuals outside of the Association who believed the initial proposed rule was the right thing to do for patients and the healthcare system were essential to HCFA's decision to remove the supervision requirement in the final rule published on January 18, 2001. To its colleagues in the nursing community who worked tirelessly in support of this effort, AANA said thank-you for staying the course. The Association noted that it believes that the removal of restrictive barriers to the legitimate practice of nursing serves the public's interest and is sound healthcare policy.

Other Medicare Reimbursement Issues

Code Split

In December 2002, AANA was successful in convincing CMS to split the procedure codes between CRNAs and AAs.[27] The split in codes between CRNAs and AAs is important because any benefits that CRNAs obtain would work to the benefit of AAs, and if the AHRQ conducts a study of anesthesia safety, as suggested in the final supervision rule, CRNAs would have to be split from AAs to provide clarity between anesthesia providers.[27]

Medicare Prescription Drug Improvement and Modernization Act

On December 8, 2004, the Medicare Pre-scription Drug, Improvement, and Modernization Act of 2003 became law.[28] This bill provides senior citizens with a prescription drug benefit and provides several types of healthcare provider reimbursement increases. The first of these is relief from the projected Part B reimbursement cuts projected for 2004 and 2005.[28] The projected cuts were 4.5% for the physician conversion factor and 3.6% for the anesthesia conversion factor.[28] Beginning in January 1, 2004, the Part B conversion factor for physician services increased by 1.5% and in 2005, the Part B physician services conversion factor increased another 1.5%.[28] These increases provided millions of additional dollars for CRNAs.[28] The bill broadened eligibility criteria for hospitals to be designated CAHs. This last provision is important because CAHs are eligible for reasonable cost-based reimbursement from the CMS to hire a CRNA.

Split Billing

An issue that was addressed jointly by the AANA and ASA in 2004 was split billing. Split billing describes a situation in which the anesthesiologist is medically directing a CRNA, and at some point the CRNA is released from the case and the anesthesiologist personally completes the case.[29] Medicare regulations have been unclear how to bill for this situation. The anesthesiologist is not personally performing the case nor is it a nonmedically directed case with respect to the CRNA, since the anesthesiologist has performed all 7 conditions of medical direction.[29] Even after considerable discussion between AANA and ASA, this reimbursement issue remains unresolved.

Pay for Performance

Because healthcare costs and expenditures continue to grow faster than the economy,

321

Medicare, as well as private payers, question what value patients get for their additional money.[30] Answering this question gives rise to a movement promoted by Medicare and other healthcare payers to promote a system of incentives for providers to more clearly demonstrate a more visible link between the service provided and the benefit derived through improvements in the quality of healthcare for patients.[30] This movement is called pay for performance, and this will affect reimbursement for CRNAs, as it will any practitioner reimbursed by Medicare and health insurance companies.[30]

The nonpartisan Medicare Payment Advisory Commission (MedPAC) bases pay for performance on 4 types of measures: process measures, designed to improve patient outcomes; outcome measures, providing information on how care affects patients; structural measures, such as provider certification and continuing education; and patient experience measures, which assess whether patients' needs are met.[30] Contribution by CRNAs and other anesthesia providers have made anesthesia extremely safe, which poses problems for pay for performance. Establishing further incentives that improve anesthesia quality is a difficult task because anesthesia complications are rare. The extremely rare occurrence of anesthesia complications creates little data to use to identify applicable and useful anesthesia quality measures.[30] Although the task will be difficult, the AANA is undertaking the project by utilizing AANA committees and panels. The AANA has demonstrated its commitment to Congress to work on this issue.[30] Identifying pay-for-performance measures is an ongoing task for AANA as well as other providers of medical care.

Prevention of Medicare Payment Cuts

The AANA has lobbied diligently to prevent cuts in Medicare payment for anesthesia services. Any cut in payment to physicians in Part B Medicare affects CRNAs equally. Rationale for preventing cuts in Part B payment is based on the fact that Medicare has consistently undervalued anesthesia services relative to market rates when compared with its reimbursement for other services. The Government Accountability Office (GAO) reported in 2005 that Medicare anesthesia payment was 67% lower than private payment measured across 7 types of anesthesia services common to both Medicare and private markets.[31] Additional rationale is that Medicare pay for performance will not make up the loss.[31] The 1.5% quality reporting incentive payment, which started in July 2007, does not offset the cuts projected in the future.[31] Last, cutting anesthesia payment would have effects on other aspects of the healthcare system critical to Medicare beneficiaries, such as access out-of-pocket expense.[31]

Teaching Rules

Teaching anesthesiologists can bill using what has been called for many years "anesthesia teaching rules." Until recent years, teaching rules have not applied to teaching CRNAs. Medicare established anesthesia teaching rules to pay for anesthesia services, which involve student nurse anesthetists and anesthesiology residents without paying the learners themselves.[32] The anesthesia teaching rules for anesthesiologists can be summarized as follows:

- Medicare reimburses qualified anesthesia providers for treating a Medicare beneficiary. A qualified provider may be an anesthesiologist or a qualified anesthetist, who is defined as a CRNA or an AA medically directed by an anesthesiologist.[32]

- Medicare reimburses for anesthesia services delivered by an anesthesiologist medically directing certain personnel according to medical direction payment rules. An anesthesiologist may claim a medical direction payment of 50% of an anesthesia fee in cases where he or she has preformed the 7 steps of medical direction while medically directing the work of a CRNA or an AA. An anesthesiologist may claim medical direction for up to 4 simultaneous cases.[32]

- Medicare does not reimburse students for providing care.[32]

- A teaching anesthesiologist providing services to a patient involving 1 student, either a medical anesthesia resident or student nurse anesthetist, may bill Medicare for 100% of a fee.[32]

- A teaching anesthesiologist providing services to 2 patients, each involving medical anesthesia residents, may bill base units plus a share of discontinuous time for each patient's case.[32]

- A teaching anesthesiologist providing services to 2 patients, each involving student nurse anesthetists, may bill 50% of each case. This reimbursement for cases involving student nurse anesthetists is somewhat less than the reimbursement for cases involving medical anesthesiology residents as just described.[32]

- A teaching anesthesiologist who provides services to 1 or more patients and is medically directing 1 or more teaching nurse anesthetists, each of whom is involved with student nurse anesthetists, may bill the cases as being medically directed provided that the teaching anesthesiologist has met the 7 conditions for payment for medical direction.[32]

Although CRNAs do not have teaching rules, Medicare authorizes 2 forms of payment for teaching CRNAs. Both of these payment forms were obtained because of advocacy by the AANA for such payment. These are as follows:

1. A nonmedically directed teaching nurse anesthetist providing service for 2 patients, each involving nurse anesthesia students, may bill base units plus a share of discontinuous time for each patient's case.[33]

2. A nonmedically directed teaching CRNA providing service to a patient involving 1 student nurse anesthetist may bill 100% of a fee.[33]

The policy that allows payment to a teaching nurse anesthetist who is continually present with a student nurse anesthetist is current policy that is included in the July 31, 1992, final CRNA fee schedule regulation, but not specifically included in the Medicare Carriers Manual.[32]

Even though nurse anesthesia students are registered nurses experienced in critical care nursing and closely supervised by qualified teaching anesthesiologists or CRNA faculty, Medicare pays less than 100% of the fee for services in which students are involved in 2 or more concurrent cases.[32] This is the way Medicare shifts healthcare costs to anesthesia groups and hospitals. Medicare also pays teaching anesthesiologists more money for 2 cases involving medical anesthesia residents than for 2 cases involving nurse anesthesia students. Law also allows Medicare to pay additional direct graduate medical education money for resident physicians but not for education of advanced practice registered nurses.[32]

323

Because of the disparity in reimbursement for anesthesiologist faculty and CRNA faculty, the AANA has sought fair, equitable teaching rules for nurse anesthesia program directors and clinical faculty. This has been an incentive for the AANA since 2002. Certainly, of greatest interest to the AANA is that teaching rules would be such that patient safety would be maintained, which would require the continued high clinical practice standards demanded of an accredited nurse anesthesia program.

In 2006 Rep Philip English (R, Pennsylvania) introduced the Medicare Academic Anesthesiology and CRNA Payment Improvement Act of 2006 (HR 6184), which was cosigned by Melissa Hart (R, Pennsylvania), Earl Pomeroy (D, North Dakota), Thomas Allen (D, Maine), Frederich Boucher (D, Virginia), Sheila Jackson (D, Texas), John Conyers (D, Wisconsin), and Bart Stupak (D, Michigan).[33] This bill, had it passed, would have reversed Medicare payment reductions in anesthesia education and would have promoted equitable treatment of teaching anesthesiologists vs teaching CRNAs and anesthesiology resident physicians vs student nurse anesthetists.[33] This bill did not disadvantage one anesthesia professional over another, and it would have helped the educational system meet growing demands for anesthesia professionals.

The ASA, however, did not support the revisions in teaching rules that the AANA wanted. Instead, the ASA pressed the CMS to allow teaching anesthesiologists to bill for reimbursement according to teaching rules used by surgeons.[34] A change in this manner would allow teaching anesthesiologists to bill 100% for supervision of 2 anesthesia residents for 2 concurrent cases.[34] The CMS rejected this proposal but did allow the teaching anesthesiologists to

bill base units plus discontinuous time for up to 2 concurrent cases utilizing anesthesiology residents.[34]

At the time that HR 6184 was introduced, the ASA supported HR 5246 introduced by Rep E. Clay Shaw Jr (R, Florida) and HR 5348 introduced by Rep Pete Stark (D, California)[35,36] These bills would have benefited only teaching anesthesiologists and anesthesia residents.[35,36] None of these bills were passed.

The AANA continued to lobby for reform and equity for teaching rules that would allow equitable reimbursement for both teaching anesthesiologists and teaching CRNAs. In 2007 the AANA and CRNAs advocated for Congress to include in its Medicare package the provisions of HR 6184.[37] However, no change was made in the Medicare anesthesia payment teaching rules during that year.

Although from 2002 until 2008 various bills were introduced to make payment for teaching anesthesiologists and teaching CRNAs equitable, it was not until July 9, 2008, that HR 6331 passed both houses of Congress. This bill passed the House of Representatives with a vote of 355 to 59 and the Senate with a vote of 60 to 30.[38,39] President George W. Bush vetoed this bill, but Congress overrode the president's veto on July 5, 2008, making the bill law effective January 1, 2010.[40]

The bill HR 6331 does not specify exact teaching rules that will apply to nurse anesthesia teaching programs. Specifically, the bill states: "Treatment of Certified Registered Nurse Anesthetists - With respect to items and services furnished on or after January 1, 2010, the Secretary of Health and Human Services shall make appropriate adjustment to payments under the Medicare program under title XVIII of the Social Security Act for teaching certified registered nurse anesthetists to implement a policy with respect to teaching certified registered nurse anesthetists that—(1) is consistent with the adjustments made by the special rule for teaching anesthesiologists under section 1848(a)(6) of the Social Security Act, as added by subsection (a); and (2) maintains the existing payment differences between teaching anesthesiologists and teaching certified registered nurse anesthetists."[41]

Wanda Wilson, CRNA, PhD, AANA president at the time HR 6331 was passed, stated that under Section 139, between the time of the passing of the bill and January 2010 (email communication, July 10, 2008):

> [T]he Medicare agency must conduct a regulatory proposal, public comment, and final rulemaking process so that this statutory language may be made into detailed payment rules which are critical to the patients, practice and profession of nurse anesthesia. Seventeen months sounds like a long time to do this work; in fact, it is scarcely more than a wink in Washington time. Nurse anesthesia educational program directors, educators, clinical practice administrators and others will certainly be called upon by your AANA to help the Medicare agency carry out this critical task.

Standards for Health Plans/Provider Nondiscrimination Language

From the inception of managed care reform, the AANA adopted a proactive position in support of the following: (1) legislation ensuring that consumers have healthcare choice and accountability and (2) health plans that include provider nondiscrimination language prohibiting health plans from arbitrarily excluding providers based solely on their licensure or certification. The rationale for this position was that discrimination in any form would limit access, choice, and marketplace competition for CRNAs. The key concepts that the AANA strongly supports for all health plans are: (1) Patients have the fundamental right to choose their healthcare providers, (2) Patients have a right to information, (3) Patients and their healthcare providers have a right to due process, and (4) Healthcare providers should be protected from unjustified liability.

In 1994 the AANA strengthened its position on nondiscrimination by healthcare plans through membership in a coalition of nonphysician providers. Since 1997 the Association has served as chair of the coalition working for the adoption of the Patient Access to Responsible Care Act (PARCA), which reflects the key principles of managed care reform outlined in the preceding paragraph. The PARCA alliance's major work resulted in the Patient Access to Responsible Care Act of 1997, introduced by Congressman Charlie Norwood (R, Georgia).[42] Although this bill was ultimately unsuccessful, in 1999 both the House and Senate passed a comprehensive proposal for managed care reform. However, it was not until 2001 that patients' rights legislation moved to its next important stages of evolution. In August 2001, patients' rights legislation was approved by the Republican-majority House of Representatives with President Bush's support; a more expansive bill passed the Democrat-controlled Senate (S1052), but President Bush indicated he would veto this legislation.[43]

Both the Senate and House bills include key provisions backed by the AANA and PARCA, including language insisting on provider nondiscrimination and point-of-service assurance. Both bills also ensure that during internal and external appeals

325

processes at least 1 qualified healthcare professional who delivers the service in question—whether it is a physician or a non-physician provider—will be represented on the review panel. Previous versions had only physicians doing the reviews. Although both the House and Senate measures are largely similar, Republicans and Democrats appeared willing to go to the mat to secure victory for their own perspectives on whether to make managed care plans liable for their decisions. The issue remained unresolved as 2001 came to a close.

The AANA maintains its leading role in efforts to move final passage of effective patients' rights legislation. The PARCA coalition continues today, and the AANA continues to play a leadership role in it.

Antitrust

Over the years, CRNAs and their state associations have been vigilant in monitoring both state and federal regulation for situations that would jeopardize a CRNA's ability to compete in the marketplace. Most often these situations involve CRNAs being coerced into unfavorable work or salary arrangements, or employment arrangements that could substantially affect their ability to practice.

In his 1998 book, *Not What the Doctor Ordered: How to End the Medical Monopoly in Pursuit of Managed Care*, Jeffrey C. Bauer[44] offered a compelling view of how some physicians attempt to control the healthcare market:

> The CRNA story illustrates perfectly the benefits of competition from qualified non-physician practitioners and the harmful effects of doctors' anticompetitive efforts to control the market. In particular, it shows why persistent enforcement of antitrust law, something very different from health reform,

is needed to protect consumers' welfare from doctors' monopoly when acceptable substitutes are available. Nursing's early leadership in anesthesia was perfectly logical because anesthetic services require the professional skills at which nurses excel: monitoring patients, making decisions, and taking actions (which commonly includes administering medications). Nevertheless, state medical societies began challenging nurse anesthetists' rights to practice since the time of the Flexner Report, promoting legislation that would prevent anyone other than a physician from administering anesthesia. Doctors' efforts to eliminate or control the competition included not-so-subtle efforts to discredit nurse anesthetists in the eyes of the public.

More specifically, there are situations in which antitrust ramifications are readily apparent. The first involves independent CRNAs who may function as independent contractors. As such they compete directly with physician anesthesiologists. Consequently, weakening of antitrust laws and regulations would not serve CRNAs well when competing for market share. A second example could be cited by CRNAs in anesthesia care team practice, where under the guise of facility reorganization they are not offered a stable employment situation, salary, or benefits.

The AANA's federal lobbying activities related to antitrust have focused on opposing any legislation that weakens antitrust laws or any changes to the Federal Trade Commission antitrust guidelines as they relate to physicians. The AANA's efforts have also included opposing legislation that eliminates the protection that nonphysician providers have under the antitrust laws from anticompetitive treatment by anesthesiologists and health plans. A recent example of the AANA's advocacy for maintaining strong federal antitrust enforcement and protection was exemplified in the AANA's opposition in 1999 to antitrust bill HR 1304 (Rep Tom Campbell, R, California). Basically, HR 1304 would have created a broad new antitrust exemption for physicians and healthcare providers to negotiate terms, fees, and conditions with health plans, without fear of antitrust sanction.[45]

The AANA has a long history of monitoring legislation and regulatory change in antitrust law that could negatively affect CRNA practice. For example, in 1993 the AANA testified in opposition to President Clinton's Health Security Act provisions, which would have granted an antitrust exemption to providers to negotiate collectively with regional alliances over fee schedules to be paid under certain fee-for-service plans. Although CRNAs were included in the definition of providers in the Clinton bill, CRNAs have historically had less negotiating power than physicians and therefore would have been at risk of being excluded from the fee-negotiation process.

Certified Registered Nurse Anesthetists have the ability to compete in the healthcare marketplace because of their cost-effectiveness and the quality of care they deliver. They can, however, only continue to do this if they have a level playing field on which to compete. The AANA believes the current antitrust laws are intended to preserve competition and promote consumer welfare. Expanding antitrust exemptions beyond what current law permits would only serve to undermine these objectives by eliminating competition, limiting consumer choice, and increasing costs to consumers.

Nurse Anesthesia Education Funding

A primary mission of the AANA is to support the education of students and CRNAs. The AANA has been very active over the last decade in securing from federal sources this necessary and vital support for educational programs. There are 2 primary sources from which this money is derived. The first is from the Nurse Education Act. This act was established under Title VIII of the Public Health Service Act. The program has provided funding for grant programs administered by the Division of Nursing under the Health Resources and Services Administration at HHS. Historically funding has gone to nurse anesthesia students, faculty, and new programs. This federal program has served the nurse anesthesia community well in the past, and its continuation remains a high priority for the AANA. In 2007, nearly 87% of nurse anesthesia educational programs received traineeship funds.[46]

Nurse anesthesia education was historically allocated as a line item of funding. In 1998, as part of the reauthorization of Title VIII, Congress replaced it with language allocating nurse anesthetist education a minimum percentage of total Title VIII funding. The legislated set-aside of 4.38% of Title VIII funds for nurse anesthetist education, about $3 million in fiscal year 2001, expired at the end of fiscal year 2002. Funding provided in fiscal year 2001 totaled $1.9 million in grants to 8 schools, plus $1 million in traineeship grants to 66 schools. Reauthorization of Title VIII is of crucial concern to nurse anesthesia education because of the importance of federal funding to expanding nurse anesthesia programs, especially during this time of acute shortage of anesthesia providers.

327

Debate over the Title VIII funding allocation has been characterized by sharp disagreements among nursing organizations over nursing funding, rather than on the perspective that nursing education funding generally should increase. There is a disparity in the amount of money the federal government spends on medical education as opposed to nursing education. In a written communication from AANA Associate Director of Government Affairs Ann Walker-Jenkins (July 15, 2008), this disparity in spending was defined as about $56 to medical education for every $1 to nursing education.

In 2002 the Nursing Advisory Panel proposed cuts in Title VIII money to advanced practice nurse education funding.[46] Another recommendation of this panel was for the Division of Nursing to have wider latitude in allocating resources designated for nursing education.[46] For CRNAs, this would mean a reduction in funding from about $2 million for improving CRNA schools and $1 million for nurse anesthesia traineeship money.

In a personal telephone communication with Frank Purcell (July 14, 2008) it was disclosed that since 2002, approximately $3 million to $4 million of Title VIII money that has been allocated to advanced practice nurse education has gone to nurse anesthesia educational programs. This money funds nurse anesthesia traineeships, as well as nurse anesthesia education and practice grants to establish new programs and expand existing programs. The AANA requests yearly and has been successful in persuading Congress to include report language with health funding legislation advising the Department of Health and Human Services to make this allocation. The exact sums awarded, however, depend on the actual successful competitive applications for Title VIII funds.

The other primary source of funding for nurse anesthesia comes from the Medicare program. To ensure a stable and adequate supply of qualified health professionals to care for the nation's elderly population, especially those in rural and medically underserved urban areas, Medicare has historically paid hospitals for their share of the cost that they incur in connection with approved educational activities. Hospitals that operate approved nursing and allied health programs are eligible for reimbursement under the Medicare Nursing and Allied Health Education Program.

However, with the movement of most nurse anesthesia programs to university-owned programs, reimbursement of training costs has been seriously curtailed by changes made to the inpatient and outpatient PPS and the current nursing and allied health regulations that will reimburse hospital-operated programs only for the net costs of clinical training programs. The effect of these requirements is a 55% decrease in 8 years in the number of nurse anesthesia programs receiving Medicare funding. Additional curtailments in reimbursement for CRNAs involved in clinical supervision of students occurred with the enactment into law of Medicare direct reimbursement of nurse anesthetists. Before the provisions for direct reimbursement, the full services of CRNAs, including clinical supervision of students, were reimbursed on a reasonable cost basis. Since direct reimbursement was implemented, Medicare will reimburse a teaching CRNA for the anesthesia service only if the CRNA is supervising the student in a 1:1 ratio and is present in the anesthetizing area during the entire case with the student. No reimbursement is provided for either service if the CRNA is supervising students in a 1:2 ratio unless the CRNA is nonmedically directed. Now that HR 6331 is law, reimbursement for CRNA faculty should increase; however, the amount and extent of that reimbursement will be subject to proposed and final rules adopted by Medicare (Wanda Wilson, CRNA, PhD, email communication, July 10, 2008).

The AANA has addressed these reimbursement/funding issues as part of its federal agenda. Clearly, the lack of payment provisions discourages healthcare facilities from becoming involved in nurse anesthesia educational programs if they cannot recover the costs of CRNA clinical instructors. The AANA believes that Medicare education funds should be utilized to promote a cost-effective health workforce with an appropriate balance of physicians, nurses, and related healthcare professionals. Services provided by advanced practice nurses such as nurse practitioners, clinical nurse specialists, and CRNAs have the greatest potential for increasing accessible, affordable, high-quality healthcare services to Medicare beneficiaries. Advanced practice nurses cost much less to prepare and, overall, are lower-cost providers in the marketplace than their physician colleagues. Second, the AANA believes that the nursing component of the Medicare education funds should be made available to education programs as well as to institutions currently eligible for Part A reimbursement.

Summary

There are many other legislative issues that the AANA has lobbied successfully, including military incentive pay and direct assistance to state organizations involved in particular issues of reimbursement, recognition, and practice rights. The primary mission of the AANA—to support member well-being through effective advocacy—has been quite successful. In fact, in 1999 the AANA Office of Federal Government Affairs was named by *Fortune* magazine as one of the most effective lobbying groups on Capitol Hill—a tribute to both the AANA's professional personnel and to its members who value effective advocacy efforts on their behalf. Furthermore, many other professional organizations look to the AANA's experience and expertise to formulate, organize, and deploy their own legislative plans. Clearly, the AANA must continue to be highly visible and influential in both federal and state governments on matters of public policy pertinent to its members and the patients they serve.

Most important to appreciate is the notion that a legislative agenda is only as successful as those involved in its implementation. This advocacy effort, although managed through the AANA's Washington, DC, office at the direction of the AANA Board of Directors, is possible only through the dedicated efforts of the AANA's members. It is the members themselves who provide grassroots efforts, participate in local and national campaigns of elected members of Congress, provide congressional testimony, participate in public relations campaigns, write letters, make phone calls, organize communications systems, provide funds to the CRNA Political Action Committee, and meet personally with leaders of business, industry, and governmental bureaucracies. We can never lose sight of the concept that an organization is only as strong as its members, and their grassroots involvement is absolutely essential to achieving success in the public policy arena.

329

References

1. Condition for coverage—surgical services. *Fed Regist.* 1992;57:33899. 2001;66(219):56768. Codified at 42 CFR §416.42.

2. Condition of participation—anesthesia services. *Fed Regist.* 1986;51:22042. 1992:57;33900. 2001;66(219):56769. Codified at 42 CFR §482.52.

3. Condition of participation—surgical services. *Fed Regist.* 1995;60(170): 45951. 1997;62(168):46037. 2001;66 (138):39938. Codified at 42 CFR §485.639.

4. Additional rules for payment of anesthesia services. *Code Fed Regul.* 42 CFR §414.46. October 1, 2004:678-679.

5. Gunn IP. Nurse anesthesia: a history of challenge. In: Nagelhout JJ, Zaglaniczny KL, eds. *Nurse Anesthesia.* 3rd ed. St Louis MO: Elsevier Saunders; 2005:1-29.

6. Conditions for payment: medically directed anesthesia services. *Fed Regist.* 1998;63:30884-30885. To be codified at 42 CFR §415.110.

7. Conditions for payment: medically directed anesthesia services. *Code Fed Regul.* 42 CFR §415.110. May 20, 2010.

8. Medicare Reimbursement. AANA website. http://www.aana.com. Accessed June 11, 2010.

9. Anesthesia Billing Guide. Centers for Medicare & Medicaid Services. Hingham, MA: NHIC, Corp; August 2009:6.

10. Responsible charges for anesthesiology services. *Fed Regist.* 1983;48: 8928. Codified at 42 CFR §405.553.

11. *Physician Payment Review Commission 1993. Annual Report to Congress.* Washington DC: Physician Payment Review Commission; 1993:Chap 11.

12. Fassett S, Calmes SH. Perception by an anesthesia care team on the need for medical direction. *AANA J.* 1995;63(2); 117-123.

13. Stein CS. A patient-based approach to medical direction within the anesthesia care team. *AANA J.* 1994;62:359.

14. ASA disagrees with AANA, in part, on medical direction. *Anesthesia Answer Book Action Alert.* Park Ridge, IL: American Society of Anesthesiologists;1998:1-2.

15. Condition of participation: surgical and anesthesia services. *Fed Regist.* 1997; 62(244):66758. Was to be codified as 42 CFR §482.45.

16. Ambulatory surgical services: condition for coverage—surgical services. *Fed Regist.* 1997;62(244):66755. Was to be codified as 42 CFR §416.42.

17. Conditions of participation: specialized providers: condition of participation: surgical services. *Fed Regist.* 1997;62 (244):66763. Was to be codified as 42 CFR §485.639.

18. Foster SD. Comments of the American Association of Nurse Anesthetists on the proposed rule regarding the Medicare and Medicaid program; Hospital conditions for participation, provider and supplier approval. Park Ridge, IL: American Association of Nurse Anesthetists; 1998.

19. Centers for Disease Control and Prevention. In: *Quality of Care in Anesthesia.* Park Ridge, IL: American Association of Nurse Anesthetists. 1998:sect 1.

20. Nine out of 10 Medicare patients are comfortable with nurse anesthesia care. AANA Advocacy [advertisement]. Park Ridge, IL: American Association of Nurse Anesthetists; 2000.

21. Medicare and Medicaid programs: hospital conditions of participation; anesthesia services: delay of effective date. *Fed Regist.* 2001;66(53):15352.

22. Supplementary information. *Fed Regist.* 66(97):27599.

23. Medicare and Medicaid programs; hospital conditions of participation: anesthesia services. *Fed Regist.* 2001:66(129):35395.

24. Chambers DA. Comments of the American Association of Nurse Anesthetists on the proposed rule; Medicare and Medicaid programs; hospital conditions of participation; anesthesia services; 66 FR 35395 (July 5, 2001) File code HCFA-3070-P. Park Ridge, IL: American Association of Nurse Anesthetists; 2001.

25. Medicare and Medicaid programs: hospital conditions of participation: anesthesia services. *Fed Regist.* 2001;66(219):56762-56769.

26. Federal supervision rule/opt-out information. American Association of Nurse Anesthetists website. http://www.aana.com. Accessed February 25, 2011.

27. Hebert D. Election 2002—what it means for nurse anesthetists. *AANA NewsBull.* 2002;56(11):11.

28. Purcell F. CRNAs and the new Medicare act. *AANA NewsBull.* 2004; 58(01):10-12.

29. Purcell F. AANA, ASA petition CMS for "split billing" fix. *AANA NewsBull.* 2004;59(7):16-17.

30. Purcell F. What is "pay for performance"? *AANA NewsBull.* 2005;59(5): 15-16.

31. Keep Medicare strong: stop Medicare anesthesia cuts. March 2007. American Association of Nurse Anesthetists website. http:/www.aana.com. Accessed February 25, 2001.

32. Purcell F. Medicare and CRNA education. *AANA NewsBull.* 2005;59(2): 14-15.

33. Medicare Academic Anesthesiology and CRNA Payment Improvement Act of 2006. HR 6184. 109th Cong, 2nd Sess (2006).

34. Purcell F. CMS cuts part B—For now. *AANA NewsBull.* 2003;57(12). http://www.aana.com. Accessed May 12, 2010.

35. To Amend Title XVIII of the Social Security Act to Restore Financial Stability to Medicare Anesthesiology Teaching Programs for Resident Physicians, HR 5246, 109th Cong, 2nd Sess (2006).

36. Medicare Anesthesiology Teaching Funding Restoration Act of 2006, HR 5348, 109th Cong, 2nd Sess (2006).

37. Purcell F. The new Congress and CRNA education. *AANA NewsBull.* 2007;61(3):26-27.

38. House passes Medicare legislation reversing Part B cut: Includes anesthesia teaching rules. American Association of Nurse Anesthetists website [membership required]. www.aana.com. June 23, 2008.

39. Senate passes Medicare legislation with teaching rules provision: President vetos bill, Congress' override votes soon. American Association of Nurse Anesthetists website [membership required]. www.aana.com/fga hotline.aspx. July 14, 2008.

40. Medicare payment relief, teaching rules reforms become law as Congress overrides President's veto. American Association of Nurse Anesthetists website [membership required]. www.aana.com/fgahotline.aspx. July 15, 2008.

331

41. Improvements for Medicare anesthesia teaching programs, §139 in Medicare Improvements for Patients and Providers Act of 2008. HR 6331, 110th Cong. 2nd Sess (2008).

42. Summary of HR 1415 (Norwood) Patient Access to Responsible Care Act of 1997 "PARCA." Health Administration Responsibility Project website. http://www.harp.org/h1415sum. htm. Accessed July 30, 2008.

43. S1052 – Bipartisan Patient Protection Act. White House Office of Management and Budget website. June 21, 2001. http://www.whitehouse.gov/omb/legislative/sap/107-1/S1052-s.html. Accessed January 19, 2010.

44. Bauer JC. *Not What the Doctor Ordered: How to End the Medical Monopoly in Pursuit of Managed Care*. 2nd ed. New York, NY: McGraw-Hill; 1998.

45. Quality Health-care Coalition Act of 1999. HR 1304. 106th Cong, 1st Sess (1999).

46. Hebert DE. Nursing advisory panel proposes cuts to advanced practice education funding. *AANA NewsBull*. 2002;56(7):15.

Acknowledgment

The author of this chapter has relied on selective source documents developed by the AANA staff in the Park Ridge, Illinois, and Washington, DC, offices in the course of writing this chronology of federal legislative advocacy. I gratefully acknowledge the expert contributions and commitment of these professional staff members.

332

Study Questions

1. Describe the functions of Medicare Part A and Part B. Distinguish between medically directed and nonmedically directed payment systems. Supervision is a term used in both Parts A and B, yet has different meanings in both parts. Describe and distinguish each.

2. What barriers exist that make revision of the 7 conditions for reimbursement for physician medical direction difficult?

3. How has TEFRA been inappropriately interpreted? How has that affected the practice of CRNAs?

4. Describe some of the more important reasons AANA has given CMS to support the removal of physician supervision.

5. What is the significance of provider nondiscrimination language in healthcare plans?

6. List 3 reasons related to anesthesia practice why CRNAs should support strong federal antitrust legislation.

7. What are teaching rules and how would the implementation of such rules for nurse anesthesia faculty encourage hospitals to become clinical sites for nurse anesthesia programs?

CHAPTER 15

Asserting Influence in Healthcare Policy

David E. Hebert, JD

Key Concepts

- Understanding the role that the American Association of Nurse Anesthetists (AANA) and Certified Registered Nurse Anesthetists (CRNAs) play in the political and legislative arenas is fundamental to the protection of nurse anesthesia practice.

- Becoming politically active requires a basic understanding of the political process, governmental agencies, and the role citizens play in the democratic and legislative process.

- Charting the path of state and federal agencies in the development of health policy is critical to understanding where and when CRNAs must intervene.

- Influencing change in state and federal legislative outcomes requires vigilant staff and member participation.

- A glossary of terms related to the legislative process appears at the end of this chapter after the summary.

Politics is not a spectator sport. State and federal legislators can only represent and serve you well if you educate them on health issues through legislative and political involvement. The decisions made in Washington, DC, and in state capitols affect you and your profession. The purpose of this chapter is to provide information on how the American Association of Nurse Anesthetists (AANA) is involved in political and legislative arenas, how you can become politically active, how state and federal governments determine health policy, and how state and federal legislative processes can be influenced.

State and federal legislators' interests reflect their political views, careers, and personal experiences. Individuals who have had a career in healthcare understand the role of nurse anesthetists; however, many of those outside the healthcare professions do not. It is your job to educate them.

336

American Association of Nurse Anesthetists Involvement in National Politics and Legislation

Political Activity
In 1983, the AANA registered the AANA Separate Segregated Fund, its political action arm, with the Federal Elections Commission. The AANA volunteer structure of this effort includes an 8-person political action committee (CRNA-PAC). The purpose of the CRNA-PAC is to promote and facilitate the accumulation of voluntary contributions from members of the AANA or others who may legally be solicited by the fund. Distributions from the fund are made by the committee to support candidates in elections that have national importance. The committee directs distributions from the fund to support candidates who serve in key

positions and have the responsibility to shape the nation's healthcare policies. The CRNA-PAC has become a strong and vibrant political action committee and is one of the top healthcare PACs in the nation. According to data released by the Federal Election Commission on April 25, 2011, the CRNA-PAC gave $519,450 to federal candidates in the 2010 election cycle, ranking 18th in total contributions among health professional associations. For total donation figures for other associations and a wealth of information on the influence of money in politics and how it affects policy and citizen's lives, visit www.opensecrets.com, the Center for Responsible Politics website.[1]

Legislative, Regulatory, and Policy Activity
The AANA represents the interests of its CRNA members to federal legislative and regulatory officials. The voice of the AANA is strong because it represents 90% of the CRNAs and student registered nurse anesthetists in the anesthesia profession. The legislative positions that AANA lobbyists champion come from the policies adopted by the AANA Board of Directors. Recommendations to the Board come from individual CRNAs, state associations, and resolutions passed at the AANA Annual Meeting. As effective as the Association is at representing member views, the personal communication of CRNAs with legislators is required to enhance the credibility of the Association message.

American Association of Nurse Anesthetists Office of Federal Government Affairs
The AANA Office of Federal Government Affairs, in Washington, DC, opened in July 1990. Its role is to help shape federal healthcare policies and create a favorable

legislative and regulatory environment for the nurse anesthesia profession. In addition, it develops draft position papers and statements for approval by the AANA Board of Directors. Information on federal government affairs is shared with the AANA membership via both print and electronic publications. The AANA Department of Federal Government Affairs monitors and works on a variety of issues. Table 15.1 lists activities of and contact information for the professional staff in the Department of Federal Government Affairs.

Table 15.1. American Association of Nurse Anesthetists Department of Federal Government Affairs

The professional staff in the AANA Department of Federal Government Affairs monitor and work on a variety of issues, including but not limited to:

Medicare Reimbursement Issues in Congress and the Centers for Medicare & Medicaid Services

Medical liability/tort reform

Managed care

Reauthorization of the Nurse Education Act

Reauthorization of the Higher Education Act

Reauthorization of the National Health Services Corps

Military pay and promotions

Veterans Administration (VA) pay and promotions

Indian Health Service pay and promotions

Agency for Healthcare Research and Quality (AHRQ) Practice Guidelines, including pain management, cataracts, and AIDS

AHRQ research

Accountable Care Act (ACA)

Contact: AANA Office of Federal Government Affairs
25 Massachusetts Avenue, NW Suite 550
Washington, DC 20001-1450
Telephone: (202) 484-8400
Fax: (202) 484-8408

337

Federal Political Network and Director Program (FPD)

Many CRNAs have a close legislative and political relationship with their individual members of Congress. The AANA has formalized that relationship with the development of a "key contact network." The purpose of the network is to provide CRNA legislative contacts with timely information about legislation of interest that the AANA would like members of Congress to support. Examples include introduction of legislation, cosponsorship of legislation, voting for legislation, or amending legislation to include AANA-endorsed provisions. When appropriate, CRNA legislative contacts may be asked to attend local fundraisers for their member of Congress when the CRNA-PAC has contributed to that member's campaign.

In order to supervise that key contact, the AANA instituted a Federal Political Director (FPD) program in each state. The FPD is generally appointed by the state president to be the federal political "eyes and ears" for CRNAs as well as the formal liaison to the AANA Federal Government Affairs Office (in concert with the state president). When the AANA needs help in getting CRNAs to contact Capitol Hill, it is the job of the FPD to solicit as many telephone calls, letters, or telegrams into federal offices as possible from members on issues important to the AANA. The FPD may also be asked to provide guidance to the CRNA-PAC about whom to support in congressional races. In addition, the FPD often will work with other CRNAs in the state to get CRNAs involved in campaigns. It is important to make the distinction that the FPD does not take the place of the key contact. The key contact is the individual whom the FPD recruits to be the political contact to a particular senator or representative. This key contact needs to develop a strong working relationship with the member of Congress and his or her staff. This is generally accomplished by telephone and visits to the district office and/or trips to Capitol Hill during the AANA Mid-Year Assembly. Although on some occasions the FPD may be the key contact, particularly in a small state where there may not be enough CRNAs to handle multiple tasks, whenever possible, the FPD is essentially the "grassroots" coordinator finding key contacts for the various members of that state's congressional delegation. CRNAs will be contacted throughout the year and asked to contact their members of Congress to cosponsor a bill, oppose a bill, sponsor an amendment, oppose an amendment, speak to the Association or possibly write a letter to the Centers for Medicare & Medicaid Services (CMS) or other federal agencies on behalf of the AANA.

How You Can Become Politically Active

Politics is the use of power for change. Although politics is not always nice or fair, healthcare professionals must become adept at managing the political process. Otherwise, someone else may exert power on policy decisions that will have a detrimental impact on professional practice and reimbursement.

Although political activity takes time and energy, it is the best investment you can make in a career. Politics is an integral part of our lives. On a daily basis, our personal relationships involve the art of negotiation and compromise—the essence of politics. In addition, professional relationships revolve around power, teamwork, and creating policies, which are also characteristic of politics. Skills that can be learned by participating in the political process will be useful tools in both your personal and professional lives.

To be a player in the game of politics, the first thing to do is get on the playing field. Do not make the common mistake of thinking that you have to commit to a major amount of time to political activity to make a difference. Any effort you can con- tribute will make a difference. Start by de- termining a reasonable time commitment, one that can be realistically followed and completed. Table 15.2 offers suggestions of ways to become politically involved.[2]

Table 15.2. Ways to Become Politically Involved

Join your state and/or national associations and participate in their government relations or political action committees.

Become active in the League of Women Voters, which often is involved in voter registration drives and "get out the vote" campaigns during elections.

Join your state Democratic or Republican party so that you can pay your "political dues" to the party structure. This is important if you ever want to run for political office.

Make a financial contribution to your state and/or national association's political action com- mittee.

Approach local talk show hosts about healthcare issues that you care about or call in to talk to health guests on television shows.

Volunteer to speak on healthcare issues to local elderly and consumer organizations.

Build a coalition of individuals like you, so that you have the additional power of a collective voice. Then use the coalition as a legislative network for lobbying on issues.

Participate in professional research, because the database that research provides is key to the shaping of healthcare policy.

Run for elective office.

Campaign to get appointed to a board, commission, or other decision-making body that will influence health policy.

Invite key decision makers to visit your place of work. There is no more effective way to teach decision makers about the importance of the job you do than by showing them firsthand.

Write an article on a healthcare issue for your local newspaper.

Continues on page 340.

> **Table 15.2. Ways to Become Politically Involved (continued)**
>
> If a legislator or other decision maker does something important on a healthcare issue of concern to you (such as successfully championing your bill through the legislative process), arrange a media "photo opportunity" at which the decision maker is given an award by your state or national association for his or her efforts.
>
> Participate in a formal or informal legislative/political internship or fellowship. At the local level, contact your city councilperson's office or mayor's office about volunteer positions. At the state level, call your state association or the office of your state representative and senator to find out if there are any programs. At the federal level, contact the AANA or the offices of your member of the House of Representatives and your 2 members of the Senate.
>
> Host a candidate's night at a meeting of your local or state association to discuss health policy issues.
>
> Participate in a candidate's election campaign.

340

Working on a Campaign

When most people think of political action, they usually think of working on an election campaign. Political campaigns can be exhilarating, frustrating, and sometimes exhausting. Part of the reason for the frustration is that most campaigns are chaos. You can imagine how difficult it is to orchestrate every one of the paid staff, in addition to hundreds of volunteers. The exhilaration comes from knowing that you have played a part in electing someone to office who cares about the same issues, including health issues, that you do. Helping to get someone elected who can support the nurse anesthesia profession is exhilarating and professionally satisfying. Even if the candidate loses the election, you will always remember the part that you played. If you would like to work on a political campaign, Table 15.3 lists some of the activities you can choose.

Networking

American society is too complex and diversified for easy consensus on most issues. Therefore, you may need to form coalitions with other groups that have a mutual interest in a given public policy. Although alliances may be necessary, approach them with caution because there is usually a price to be paid in terms of needing to compromise or to accommodate the needs of the other groups in the coalition. It is a political call whether or not the benefits of a coalition outweigh the inherent negatives.

There are areas you should consider before formally associating with other groups. You should make sure that there is an even division of responsibility. You also want to make sure that you can trust the judgment of your partners. There is nothing worse than finding out that you are associated with a campaign that is unethical or irresponsible. By the same token, you do not want to join every coalition. There are limits to how

Table 15.3. Campaign Activities

Before Election Day

Stuffing envelopes with the candidate's campaign literature

Putting up yard signs for your candidate

Distributing campaign literature door-to-door

Canvassing door-to-door to determine voter opinions

Staffing phone banks to urge voters to vote for your candidate

Chauffeuring the candidate to functions (This is an especially good time to talk about health-care with candidates, because you literally have a captive audience.)

Writing policy papers for the candidate to use

Participating in mass mailing efforts to registered voters or a targeted audience

Serving as the candidate's representative at functions

Building a base of your colleagues so, for example, you can have a "Tuesday CRNA Night" at the campaign headquarters during which CRNAs do all the necessary tasks, such as answering the phones, stuffing envelopes, and answering mail

Hosting a "meet and greet" function for the candidate in your home

Holding a fundraiser for the candidate in your home

Making a financial contribution to the candidate

On Election Day

Staffing phone banks to remind voters to vote on election day

Distributing your candidate's campaign literature at polling places (contingent on election laws)

Providing transportation and babysitting services to voters

Watching the polls (to ensure that the voting process is carried out according to the election laws)

Hosting a victory party for your winning candidate

much your organization can do. You should also be concerned about appearing to be active on too many fronts. Being overextended can damage your credibility in the legislative arena as much as being inactive. Specific parameters should be set when you join a coalition. At a minimum, the coalition ought to be restricted to a specific issue, event, or period. If no such limitations are established, you may find yourself in a situation you cannot easily escape later.[3] Table 15.4 lists the steps for a successful coalition.[4]

Potential Legislative Benefits of Political Activity

Political and legislative activity are the flip sides of the same coin. Always keep in mind that politics may help you achieve your healthcare policy objectives because the political arena provides access to decision makers. Your relationship with key decision makers may help influence their decisions on vital health policy issues. Your political activity on behalf of a candidate will not always result in the elected candidate voting the way you want, but it does give you the

---

Table 15.4. Steps for a Successful Coalition

Define and agree on the goal—why is this legislation necessary?

Establish guidelines and rules for the coalition. All groups are free to act for themselves, except when they use the name of the coalition.

Define tasks.

Establish a coordinating committee.

Organize resources to complete the necessary elements of the campaign.

Keep everyone together and focused on the one area of agreement. Do not let areas of difference or other issues cause infighting.

Keep jealous feelings to a minimum. Make sure everyone feels involved and assure them that their individual interests are well represented.

Watch legislators' attitudes toward your group to ensure that they are positive.

Establish effective communication methods for educating the public. It is important that the coalition speak with one voice.

Try to meet at least once a month, if possible, to keep apprised of activities.

Keep members informed with a regular update.

Investigate any legal requirements that may apply to your coalition, such as lobbying requirements.

opportunity to eloquently make your case to the candidate. Table 15.5 lists some tips regarding political activity.

Potential Personal Benefits of Lobbying

Life can be difficult enough without having to find time to lobby. Yet the professional and personal benefits are worth the effort. Aside from the satisfaction of helping your

---

Table 15.5. Tips for Political Activities

Do:

Build a professional image, and remember that you never get a second chance to make a first impression.

Work on developing your writing and speaking skills.

Learn all you can about a candidate's positions before you volunteer to work on his or her campaign.

Make realistic time commitments about what you can offer a campaign.

Follow through on your commitments responsibly.

Have business cards with you at all times for networking.

Work to expand your network by recruiting other volunteers.

Vote and encourage others to vote.

Don't:

Be afraid to volunteer for a low-level task.

Neglect traditional political organizations.

Forget to get very clear directions about what the campaign's expectations are regarding your job responsibilities and time commitments.

Be discouraged if it takes time to work up to more senior roles in a campaign.

Put off getting involved until the timing is perfect—it never will be.

Forget to take fair credit for the work that you have done.

Bring your own political issues to the table. Remember, when you are working on behalf of nurse anesthesia, those are the issues to focus on.

343

profession, it can help you personally. If you have ever had your own ambition to run for political office, this is a great way to get started. You can learn the process, find out how decisions are made, and perhaps most importantly, meet people who can help you in a future political career. Perhaps your son or daughter would like to have an internship on Capitol Hill during the summer— getting to know your legislator is the first step. Legislators receive dozens of applications for internships. Knowing the legislator in advance can help. Or maybe a member of your family would like to apply for a nomination to a military academy. Members of Congress make nominations to West Point and the Naval and Air Force Academies. So knowing your legislator can have other added benefits as well.

How State and Federal Governments Determine Health Policy

As state legislatures take greater initiative in determining health policy, many organizations are taking their first steps into state government affairs. With the exception of Nebraska, state legislatures consist of 2 houses: the senate (commonly referred to as the upper house) and, depending on the state, either the house or assembly (commonly referred to as the lower house). Bills are identified by state, house of origin, and number (ie, California Senate Bill 1, cas1; Nebraska Legislative Bill 3, ne13; New York Assembly Bill 3695, nya3695. State legislatures adopt resolutions and bills. Some resolutions are adopted only by one house, and others are adopted by both houses. The substance of resolutions varies; some are used to express legislative concern about a specific issue, and some are simply congratulatory. Most states do not require action by the governor for resolutions to

become officially adopted.

Although each legislature has its own unique set of rules and procedures, most bills follow the same general path: introduction, consideration by the first house, consideration by the second house, and consideration by the governor.

Bill Introduction
The state legislative process begins when a bill is introduced. In most states, bills may be introduced only by members or committees of the legislature. In about half the states, bills may not be introduced until the legislature convenes. The remaining states allow the introduction of bills before the official convening date for presession study. This practice is called prefiling.

Committee Referral and Action
After introduction, bills are referred to a committee for public hearing. The number, structure, and operating procedures of committees are unique to each state. Some states use a joint committee system to review bills, but most states have separate committees in each house dealing with specific subjects, such as health. Committees usually have the authority to recommend that bills be passed as introduced, passed as amended, substituted by the committee, or killed. Often, bills that would cost money or have some other financial consequence are reviewed by 2 committees; a policy committee reviews the substance of the bill and the fiscal committee reviews the financial aspects of the bill.

Floor Action
Many bills do not receive committee approval and thus proceed no further. The bills that are approved by committees (as introduced. amended, or substituted) proceed to the floor for consideration by the entire

chamber. The chamber may pass the bill in the form recommended by the committee(s), amend the bill and pass it, or kill it. When a bill is passed by the chamber of origin, it is sent to the second chamber and the procedure is repeated: committee referral, committee action, and floor action in the second chamber. As in the chamber of origin, bills may be approved, amended, substituted, or killed in committee or on the floor. Bills that are amended in the second chamber return to the chamber of origin for concurrence. If the chamber of origin concurs with the amended version of the bill passed by the second chamber, the bill is eligible to be sent to the governor for signature. If the chamber of origin does not concur, the second chamber may withdraw the amendments. If the second chamber does not withdraw the amendments, a conference committee is appointed to resolve the differences between the chambers. The report of the conference committee must be approved by both chambers for the bill to move on to the governor.

Governor's Actions

When a bill is approved and passed by the legislature, it is sent to the governor. In most states, the governor may sign a bill into law; veto all or part of the bill (line item veto); or, depending on whether the legislature is in session or adjourned, let the bill die without signature or let it become law without signature.

Vetoed bills are returned to the chamber in which they were introduced. The legislature may pass bills that have been vetoed by the governor if a specified majority of both chambers (usually two-thirds) votes to override the veto. Figure 15.1 provides a flow chart of a typical state legislative process.

Federal Legislative Process

Members of Congress lead lives with long and sometimes difficult hours. The stress of maintaining a residence in their home district as well as one in the nation's capital can be challenging. Unless it is a politically "safe" district, meaning that the member of Congress generally has no problem getting elected or re-elected because of the political make-up of the district, many in Congress spend countless hours campaigning for election or reelection. Along with their congressional responsibilities, they spend their lives going from meeting to meeting, depending on their staff for information and guidance.

Nowhere are policy and process more intertwined than in the Congress of the United States. Skillful legislators use the legislative process to advance their policy goals. Sponsors often amend the wording of a bill to keep it from being referred to a hostile committee. For instance, an anti-abortion amendment may be added to a House appropriations bill and may be germane because it restricts federal funding for abortions. Procedural techniques and policy interact at many stages of the legislative process. "Legislation is like a chess game more than anything else," Representative John D. Dingell (D-MI) has said. "It is a seemingly endless series of moves, until ultimately someone prevails through exhaustion, or brilliance, or because of overwhelming public sentiment for their side."[5] The decision of which committees receive a bill for consideration is based on the determination of the parliamentarian.

By the mid-1980s, the federal budget deficit and the complex special budget process that Congress devised for dealing with it resulted in the increased use of omnibus bills. Rather than separate bills going all the way through the normal legislative

345

Figure 15.1 Typical State Legislative Process

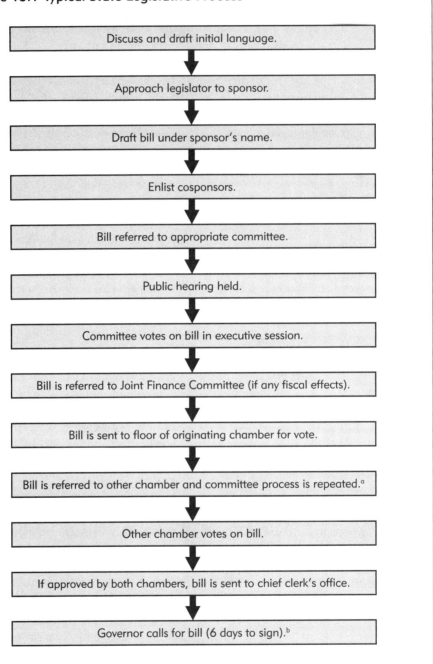

Discuss and draft initial language.

Approach legislator to sponsor.

Draft bill under sponsor's name.

Enlist cosponsors.

Bill referred to appropriate committee.

Public hearing held.

Committee votes on bill in executive session.

Bill is referred to Joint Finance Committee (if any fiscal effects).

Bill is sent to floor of originating chamber for vote.

Bill is referred to other chamber and committee process is repeated.[a]

Other chamber votes on bill.

If approved by both chambers, bill is sent to chief clerk's office.

Governor calls for bill (6 days to sign).[b]

[a] If the bill is revised by the other chamber, it returns to the originating chamber. The originating chamber may concur with, disapprove of, or modify changes. Bills can go back and forth between chambers several times.
[b] If the bill is not signed before the end of the session, it is pocket vetoed and sent back to both chambers for override.

process, many often unrelated proposals were packaged in a single, large piece of legislation. These so-called omnibus budget reconciliation bills contained literally hundreds of provisions that were supposedly necessary to develop an overall budget plan for the year. The opportunities to debate and amend these bills are often severely limited. Consequently, omnibus bills allow measures that would not normally be approved as separate bills to get adopted. Sometimes this global approach contains provisions that benefit CRNAs, and sometimes it contains provisions that harm CRNAs. A positive example is the authority for CRNAs to receive direct Medicare reimbursement, included in the Omnibus Budget Reconciliation Act of 1986.

Legislative Vehicles

There are 4 basic forms in which legislative proposals may be introduced: bills, joint resolutions, current resolutions, and simple resolutions. Bills are the most common form. They are prefaced by "H.R." in the House and "S." in the Senate, followed by a number assigned based on the order of the bill's introduction during a congressional session. Joint resolutions may originate in either the House or Senate and are labeled "H. J. Res." or "S. J. Res." followed by a sequential number. The most common use of a resolution is to continue an existing law. A resolution is subject to the same procedure as a bill, unless it is proposing an amendment to the Constitution. If this is the case, then it must be approved by two-thirds vote of each chamber and be sent directly to the administrator of general services for submission to the states for ratification. Constitutional amendments are not presented to the president for signature. Concurrent resolutions are designated by "H. Con. Res." or "S. Con. Res." They must be approved by both the House and Senate before they can become effective. A concurrent resolution does not require the president's signature and does not have the force of law. It expresses the opinion of Congress and is used for matters affecting the operations of both chambers. Simple resolutions are designated "H. Res." or "S. Res." They are used for matters concerning the operation of only one chamber and are adopted only by that chamber. They may also be used to create a special investigating committee, change chamber rules, or express the sense of the chamber on specific issues.

Drafting Legislation

Legislation can be drafted by congressional staff or legislative counsels at the request of individual members or committees. Legislation is also drafted by executive branch departments and agencies as well as by interest groups. Much of the legislation dealt with by Congress in any year is composed of bills reauthorizing expiring laws, bills appropriating money to run the federal government, and bills submitted by the president and the executive branch to implement the administration's programs. Pursuant to the Constitution, revenue legislation originates in the House. By custom, appropriations legislation also originates in the House. All other bills may originate in either chamber.

Introduction and Referral of Bills

Members of the House of Representatives are elected for 2-year terms and senators are elected for 6-year terms. The length of each Congress mirrors the length of a House term—2 years. Each Congress conducts its business in 2 regular sessions that begin in January of successive years. For example, the first session of the 112th Congress convened on January 3, 2011, and is scheduled

347

to adjourn on December 8, 2011; the second session of the 112th Congress is expected to convene in early January 2012 and will likely adjourn in late September, allowing time for members of Congress to return to their respective districts or states and prepare to run for reelection. Of the many bills introduced in the House and Senate, only a fraction are reported by committees and fewer are enacted into law. Although only a small fraction of all health bills are eventually enacted into law, they stimulate vigorous debate on the future of healthcare policy. Any bill that has not received final congressional approval when Congress adjourns automatically dies and must be reintroduced in the next Congress and begin the entire process again.

To become law, proposed legislation must be approved in identical form in both the House and the Senate. The bill is subject to delay, defeat, or substantial modification. "It is very easy to defeat a bill in Congress," President John F. Kennedy once observed. "It is much more difficult to pass one."[6]

Any bill or resolution must be introduced by a representative or senator when Congress is in session. There is no limit to the number of bills a member may introduce. The legislative leader of a proposal is the key to its survival. The fact that a bill has a high-ranking sponsor automatically escalates its importance as a piece of legislation.

A House member may introduce a bill or resolution by handing it to the clerk of the House or placing it in a box called the "hopper" at the front of the House chamber. Senators usually submit their proposals and accompanying statements to clerks in the Senate chamber or may introduce their bills from the Senate floor. If objection to the introduction of the bill is offered by any senator, introduction of the bill is postponed until the next day. It is not uncommon for a representative and a senator to sponsor "companion" (identical) bills, each introducing his or her version simultaneously in the respective chamber. This is done to encourage both chambers to consider the measure simultaneously to dramatize the importance or urgency of the bill and to show broad support for it.

The House or Senate bill is then numbered, referred to the appropriate committee(s), labeled with the sponsor's name, and sent to the Government Printing Office for copies to be made. A representative or senator who is interested in actively promoting legislation often seek cosponsors. This allows other legislators to jointly introduce the bill and indicate their support for it. Bipartisan sponsorship can be very important, as can endorsement by members of the committee to which the bill will be referred. There is no limit on the number of cosponsors that can be added to a House or Senate bill or resolution. A bill written in the executive branch and proposed as an administration measure usually is introduced by the chairman of the committee that has jurisdiction over the bill's subject matter.

Committees and Subcommittee Structure

Committees are the heart of the legislative process. They have existed in the House and the Senate since 1789, and have allowed for a division of work and orderly consideration of legislation. The size of the Senate (100 members) and the House (435 members) makes it extremely difficult for all members to consider each piece of legislation. Consequently, each chamber has established its own committees to study and consider legislation. In turn, committees have established subcommittees to allow even further division of work.

Both the House and Senate have standing (permanent) committees and special (select) committees. There are 22 standing committees in the House and 16 in the Senate. Each standing committee has jurisdiction over certain subject areas of legislation, and all legislation that would affect that particular area of law is referred to that committee of jurisdiction. The number of select committees changes. The select committees are usually investigative in nature, convene for the duration of the matter under investigation, reach a decision or make recommendations, and are then dissolved.

The real work of the legislative process takes place in committees and subcommittees, including research, investigation, and public hearings. This is the time to contact your elected legislator and let him or her know your stand on the bill. At this stage you have the most ability to influence the movement of a bill. If legislators receive numerous letters in support of a bill, they relay that to the subcommittee or committee chairman and that often expedites action on the bill. Conversely, if legislators receive numerous letters opposing the bill, they will convey that fact to the subcommittee or committee chairman and the bill may die in committee without any action being taken.

Membership ratios of majority to minority parties on committees are determined at the beginning of each Congress and are generally based on the ratio for the entire membership of each chamber plus the political judgment of the majority party. Individuals are assigned to committees by caucus of the respective parties, and these assignments are confirmed by a floor vote. A member usually seeks election to the committee that has jurisdiction over a field in which he or she is most qualified and interested.

Subcommittees and committees are responsible to their parent bodies. However,

because of the complexity of their assignments, they have substantial independence and autonomy. The chairman of a committee or subcommittee is a dominant figure in the legislative process because he or she can set the agenda for committee meetings, set up the hearings, and hire the staff. When a bill is referred to a committee, the chairman can either guide it through his or her committee or sit on the bill and effectively kill it.

In Congress, seniority is power. Members rank in seniority in accordance with their appointment to the committee. The majority member having the most years of service in Congress is usually designated chairman. The most senior member of the minority party is ordinarily designated as "ranking minority member." Better committee assignments and bigger committee staffs usually go hand-in-hand with tenure on Capitol Hill. Subcommittee seniority is generally assigned in a similar way, with the full committee determining subcommittee membership and maintaining the same majority to minority ratios. In general, senators may serve on 2 major legislative committees and 1 lower-ranking committee. In the House, a representative usually serves on 2 committees.

Committee Jurisdiction

Formally, a bill is to be referred to the appropriate committee by the speaker of the House or the presiding officer of the Senate. Informally, the parliamentarians of the 2 chambers act on behalf of the speaker and the Senate presiding officer and actually refer the bills to committees. Bill sponsors may indicate their preferences for referral, although custom, chamber rules, and committee jurisdiction generally govern. In turn, the chairman of the committee will refer the bill to one of its subcommittees un-

350

less the chairman decides to have the full committee act on the proposal. The 1970s witnessed a reform of the seniority system, resulting in restraints on committee chairmen and a diffusion of power from committee chairmen to subcommittees. Each committee has its own method of determining where the predominant policy role and power are exercised, at the full committee or the subcommittee level.

When a bill contains language that cuts across the jurisdiction of 2 or more committees, it may get a referral to multiple committees. In the Senate, multiple referrals are implemented by unanimous consent agreements. In the House, referral authority remains with the Speaker. There are 3 types of multiple referrals. First, there is "sequential referral," the most common form, which allows one committee to take action first and then refer the bill on to the second committee. Second is "joint referral," where a bill is referred, within specific time limits, successively to one committee and then to another. An example of joint referral would be bills that deal with Medicare Part B, for which both the House Commerce Committee and the House Ways and Means Committee share jurisdiction. Third, there is "split referral," where a bill is referred to several committees, each having jurisdiction over specific parts of the bill. Multiple referrals often can kill legislation because several committees are unlikely to agree on a version of the bill or even to report the bill at approximately the same time, if at all. On the other hand, when several committees report a multiply referred bill, the chances of that bill's passage can be greatly enhanced.

Failure of a committee to act on a bill is equivalent to killing it; the measure can be withdrawn from the committee's purview only by a discharge petition signed by a majority of the House membership on House

bills or by adoption of a special resolution in the Senate. Discharge attempts rarely succeed. The full House and Senate seldom question a decision of a committee not to report a bill.

Hearings and Referrals

The first committee action taken on a bill usually is a request for comment by interested agencies of the government, such as the Department of Health and Human Services (HHS) on health bills. This gives the committee a preliminary indication if it should have the relevant subcommittee hold hearings on a bill. The committee chairperson may then refer the bill to a subcommittee for study and hearings, or it may be considered by the full committee. Hearings provide the opportunity for members of Congress; executive branch staff; and representatives of industry, interest groups, and academia to formally present their views and positions on the legislative topic. Panels of witnesses are often scheduled together to hear similar perspectives at the same time or to probe the conflicting points of view of the panelists. Witnesses usually give prepared comments and then answer questions from the subcommittee members. The time that each subcommittee member has to ask questions is usually limited by the chairman. Verbatim transcripts of hearings are recorded and generally printed for committee and public use, and they are often available online.

Depending on the nature of the bill, hearings may be conducted for a few hours, for several days, or for weeks. The timing and duration of subcommittee hearings depend largely on the discretion of the subcommittee chairman. Most hearings are held in open session. Often a hearing is broadcast on C-SPAN or the Internet. More frequently, the subcommittee chairman limits the number and type of individuals and organizations that may testify. This is done either to expedite the subcommittee's deliberations or to create a particular attitude at the hearings; for example, only those in favor of a chairman's bill are asked to testify. There has also been an increase, in recent years, in the number of field hearings that are held in the subcommittee chairman's district or state.

On completion of the hearings, the subcommittee "marks up" the bill, which means amending the bill. During this step, a member may offer amendments that he or she supports. As a rule, informal votes are taken on each amendment to obtain a consensus. Because of the political trade-offs and controversies that occur during markups, they are often closed to the public. The subcommittee has several options regarding actions it may take on the bill. It can:

- Fail to take action or complete action on a bill.
- Report it favorably without amendments.
- Report it favorably with amendments.
- Reject the bill.
- Report it unfavorably or without recommendation.
- Report favorably on a "clean bill." If amendments are adopted that are substantial, the subcommittee may order a "clean bill" introduced, incorporating all amendments in new bill language. The original bill then is put aside and the "clean bill" is then reintroduced, assigned a new number, and referred to the full committee.

Full Committee Action

After a subcommittee approves a bill, the full committee can choose from the same options for action that the subcommittee had. Although the full committee can du-

plicate the subcommittee's procedures by holding hearings and markup sessions, it seldom does so. Committee discussion is more general, and although amendments may be offered, they are normally fewer than those considered in subcommittee. Committees generally rely on and accept the conclusions of the subcommittee. The full committee then votes on its recommendation to the full House or Senate. This procedure is called "ordering a bill reported." Occasionally a committee orders a bill reported unfavorably, but most of the time a report calls for favorable action because the committee can effectively kill a bill simply by failing to take any action.

When a committee sends a bill to the chamber floor, it explains its reasons in a written report, which accompanies the bill. Often, committee members opposing a bill issue dissenting minority statements that are included in the back section of the report. The points made in the dissent section typically signal where the areas of contention are that will arise on the House or Senate floor. The rules of the House and Senate specify some aspects of the contents of reports; for example, they must show changes in existing law. These reports may also include an analysis of the legislative language and a statement of the committee's reasons or intent for passing the bill. In addition, the written statements from government agencies are ordinarily included in the report.

After a bill becomes law, there may be confusion or disagreement about the meaning of the actual legislative language. The committee report is often used to try to determine the legislative intent of the bill. For example, when the executive branch writes regulations or the courts rule on legislation, they often rely on the report background if the law itself is not clear. Each

351

report is given a number; for example, House Report 112-1 designates the first House committee report of the 112th Congress. Report language is often used by lobbyists to protect their association's interests. For example, the annual health appropriations bill only lists how much money is to be spent for nurse anesthesia educational programs. The accompanying report contains directives to the federal agency that implements the law on how the money is to be spent.

Floor Action

When the full committee has approved a bill, it is reported back to the chamber where it originated. Accounts of floor debate and action taken in each chamber are published daily in the *Congressional Record*. The differences between House and Senate floor procedures are largely due to the Senate's smaller size, which allows greater opportunity for informal arrangements. The larger, more complex House emphasizes rules and precedents. In the House, the completed committee bill is sent to the House Rules Committee to establish the length of time for debate and to determine whether floor amendments will be allowed. Because debate is restricted and the amending process frequently limited, the House is able to dispose of legislation more quickly than the Senate. The Senate, although it has rules and procedures, more often operates by unanimous consent. Each Senate member, even the most junior, is offered a deference rarely seen in the House. The privileges of engaging in unlimited debate, the filibuster, and offering unrelated amendments are highly cherished traditions in the Senate that are not permitted under House rules. Given these conditions, the Senate may spend days considering a measure that the House has debated and passed in a single afternoon.

Except for the House Rules Committee review, procedures are generally similar in the House and Senate. The bill is placed on a calendar for a vote. When, and sometimes whether, a bill is brought to the floor depends on many factors, including other legislation awaiting action, how controversial the measure is, and whether the leadership judges its chances for passage to be improved by immediate action. For example, the leadership may decide to delay taking up a controversial bill until its proponents can gather sufficient support to guarantee its passage. A bill is brought to floor debate by varying procedures. If it is a routine bill, it may await the call of the calendar. If it is urgent or important, it can be taken up in the Senate either by unanimous consent or by a majority vote. The policy committee of the majority party in the Senate schedules the bills that it wants taken up for debate. In the House, debate precedence is granted if a special rule is obtained from the Rules Committee. House debate is limited by the rule under which the bill is considered. Senate debate is usually unlimited. It can be halted only by unanimous consent or by a "cloture" vote, which requires a three-fifths majority of the entire Senate. Cloture limits senators to 1 hour of debate.

Voting on bills may occur repeatedly before they are finally approved or rejected. The full House or Senate must approve, alter, or reject the committee amendments before the bill itself can be put to a vote. In addition, floor amendments may be offered to further certain objectives. First, members may offer floor amendments to dramatize their stands on issues, even if there is little chance that their amendments will be adopted. Second, some amendments are introduced at the request of the executive branch, a member's constituents, or special interests. Third, some are tactical tools for gauging sentiment for or against a bill. Fourth, others are used to stall action on a bill. Finally, some amendments may be designed to defeat the legislation. A common strategy is to try to load a bill with so many unattractive amendments that it will eventually collapse under its own weight. Another strategy is to offer a "killer" amendment that if adopted would cause members who initially supported the bill to vote against it on final passage. Conversely, amendments known as "sweeteners" may be offered to attract broader support for the underlying measure.

The Senate has 3 different methods of voting: voice vote, a standing vote (called a division), and a recorded roll call vote to which members answer "yea" or "nay" when their names are called. The House uses voice and standing votes but has replaced the time-consuming roll calls with an electronic voting device to record the "yeas" and "nays." Another method of voting, used in the House only, is the teller vote. This is when members file up the center aisle past counters; only vote totals are announced. The teller vote is rarely used now, however. The most common method of voting in both the House and Senate is voice vote.

The House votes on the rule for the bill, various amendments, and then the bill itself. The Senate votes on various amendments and then the bill. Final approval of a bill requires a majority vote of the members present.

Action in the Second Chamber

After a bill is passed in one chamber, it is sent to the other chamber for action. This body may take one of several steps. First, it may pass the bill as is. Second, it may send the bill to its committee of jurisdiction for study or alteration. Third, it may reject the entire bill and advise the other chamber of that fact. Finally, it may simply ignore the bill while it continues work on its own version of the same legislation. Frequently, one chamber may approve a version of a bill that is greatly at variance with the version already passed by the other chamber, and then substitute its amendments for the language of the original bill. This retains, in effect, only the other chamber's bill designation, without the original substance.

Often the second chamber makes only minor changes in the first chamber's bill. If the first chamber agrees to these changes, then the bill is sent to the president for signature. However, if the first chamber does not agree to the second chamber's changes, then the bill is sent to a conference committee to reconcile the differences in the chambers' versions. The chamber that physically possesses the bill requests a conference. If the other chamber does not agree to a conference, then the bill dies.

Conference Committee

Sometimes known as the "third house of Congress," the conference committee usually consists of senior members (conferees) from the committees that have reported the bills. However, designated sponsors of major amendments to the bills also may be appointed to the conference committee. Conferees are appointed by the presiding officer of the Senate and the Speaker of the House. The number of conferees may vary, usually ranging from 3 to 9 members from each chamber, depending on the complexity of the bill involved. There does not have to be an equal number of conferees representing each chamber. A majority vote controls the action of each group, so a large representation on one side does not give that chamber an advantage.

353

Theoretically, conferees are not allowed to write new legislation when reconciling the 2 versions before them, but this curb is sometimes bypassed. Many bills have been put into acceptable compromise form only after new language has been approved by the conferees. Some of the hardest bargaining in the entire legislative process takes place in the conference committee, and the ironing out of differences may go on for days, weeks, or even months. The real constraining factor for conferees is that the chambers that they represent must accept the compromises. When the conferees have reached agreement, they prepare a conference report embodying their recommendations to each chamber.

The conference report must be approved by each chamber. Consequently, approval of the report is approval of the compromise bill. If no agreement is reached by the conferees, or should either chamber not accept the conference report, the bill dies.

Presidential Action

After a bill has been passed by both the House and the Senate in identical form, it is sent to the White House for action. The president has 4 options. First, the president may sign the bill, date it, and write the word "approved" on the document. The Constitution requires only the president's signature. The president may allow the bill to become law without signature. This occurs if the president takes no action for 10 days (Sundays excepted) when Congress is in session. Third, the president may "pocket veto" the bill. This occurs if Congress passes a bill and then adjourns before the president has had the 10-day option to return the bill with a veto. In this instance, the bill will not automatically become law. Fourth, the president may veto the bill within the 10-day option and return it to

Congress with a message stating the reasons for the veto. The message is sent to the chamber that originated the bill. If no action is taken there on the veto message, the bill dies. However, Congress can attempt to override the president's veto and enact the bill. The overriding of a veto in each chamber requires a two-thirds vote of those present, who must number a quorum and vote by roll call. If the president's veto is overridden, the bill becomes law, otherwise it dies.

When bills are passed and signed, or passed over a veto, they are given public law numbers in numerical order. They are identified by the Congress that passed them and by the law number, for example, Public Law 101-802 means the 802nd public law passed by the 101st Congress.[7-9] Figure 15.2 designates the flow of legislation through the House and Senate.

Practical Politics

The previous discussion explored the textbook method by which Congress passes legislation. However, the legislative process is anything but predictable or orderly. Legislation can be modified at the last minute. Informal conference committees in which Senators and members of the House meet in private often dictate how a bill will become final. Often the staff of the committees that have authorization over a particular bill will meet to hammer out the final details.

In recent years, the House and Senate leadership offices have driven the respective agendas of their political parties. This means that the Senate majority leader and House speaker have often determined the shape and form of the political agenda and bills on major issues have often been written at the leadership level, avoiding the traditional committee process.

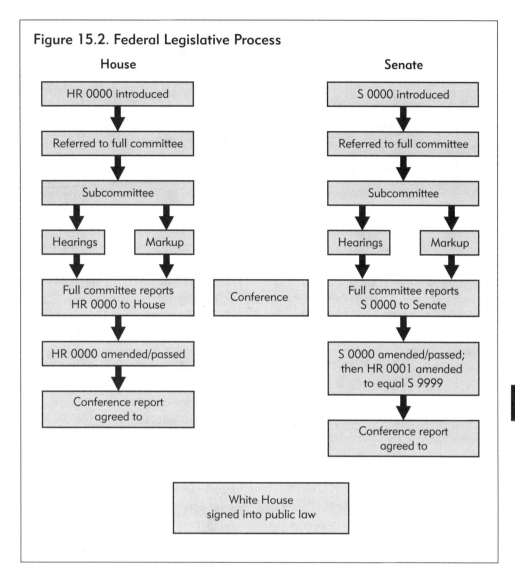

Figure 15.2. Federal Legislative Process

355

Federal Regulatory Process

All rules start with Congress passing, and the president signing, a public law creating a federal program. The law defines the goals of regulatory programs, identifies the agency responsible for achieving them, and contains substantive and procedural guidance as to how the agency is to conduct its work. Rules fill in the details of legislation, with Congress retaining an oversight function. The law usually authorizes the agency to formulate rules to carry out the purposes of the law. For example, within the Department of Health and Human Services, Medicare and Medicaid rules are handled by the Centers for Medicare & Medicaid Services. The agency of jurisdiction prepares draft rules, which are published in the *Federal Register* each federal working day. The Administrative Procedures Act (APA) establishes a 2-step procedure that an agency ordinarily uses for rule making.

First, an agency must publish in the *Federal Register* a notice of proposed rule making, which contains the text of the proposed rules or a description of the subjects and issues involved and an invitation for the public to comment on the rules. Concerned individuals and organizations may submit written comments on the proposed rule, usually within a 30- or 60-day comment period. The comments help bring to the agency's attention information that the agency may not have taken into account in drafting the proposed rule. The content of the final rule may be influenced by the views presented during this period. For example, a CMS-proposed Medicare rule on physician payment reform, which had a major impact on CRNA reimbursement as well, received 95,000 written comments. A significant number of those comments were from CRNAs.

Second, an agency carefully considers the public's comments and, if the agency still believes a rule is necessary, adopts a final rule. Before the issuance of a final rule, however, further internal review is done at all levels of the agency and by the White House's Office of Management and Budget. The final rule, with a statement of its basis and purpose, is usually published in the *Federal Register* with a comment period of 30 to 60 days before its effective date.

Increasingly, rules and rule making play a pivotal role in the policy process by transforming legislative provisions into a blueprint for regulatory program operations. More often than not, the rule-making process is transformed into a battleground of contending interests, where major political and policy issues deferred during the legislative process are resolved, at least until the rules that emerge are themselves challenged. It is not unusual for rule making by an agency to stimulate interest groups to demand new legislation.

How You Can Influence the Legislative Process

The following information references the federal level, but it is usually applicable to the state level as well.

What Is Lobbying?

"Congress shall make no law . . . abridging the freedom of speech, or of the press; or the right of the people peaceably to assemble, and to petition the Government for a redress of grievances." (1st Amendment to the United States Constitution). The right to petition government is as old as our Constitution and it is essentially the right of the citizen to "lobby" Congress.

Lobbying is trying to persuade decision makers to enact measures, such as legislation, favorable to your cause. Alternately, you may want legislation defeated or repealed that is unfavorable to your cause. You are an expert on healthcare; typically your legislator is not. Your lobbying efforts involve sharing information with a legislator that he or she would not normally have easy access to. The primary resource to obtain answers to remaining questions is from your professional organization. Normally, whoever asks you to lobby (including the AANA or state association) will provide you with these facts, along with the call for action. You should never be asked to lobby without being armed with the necessary facts.

Methods of Lobbying

The different methods of lobbying include *scheduling* a personal visit with the legislator or the health staff person in the district or the state or federal office, calling the legislator or the health staff person, corresponding with the legislator or the health staff person, or *testifying* at hearings.

How to Make an Appointment for a Personal Visit

Call the legislator's office directly, or call the US Capitol switchboard, which can connect you to the legislator's office. The number for the US Capitol switchboard and other useful federal government information is provided in Table 15.6. When you connect with the office, first ask for the legislative assistant (LA) for health. Tell the LA that you are a CRNA constituent of the legislator and that you want to meet with the legislator for 15 minutes on a specific date to discuss a particular health issue. The health LA may make the appointment for you with the legislator's scheduler or may refer you directly to the scheduler. Make sure you write down the name of the LA and the scheduler and get a specific time, meeting room number, and building; for

example, 10:00 AM in Room 205 in the Hart Senate Office Building. Leave your name and mobile phone number where you can be reached if the legislator needs to cancel the meeting. If you request it in advance, the legislator's office can usually arrange for a photographer to be present to take your picture with the legislator. An autographed picture is always a nice memento of your visit, and most offices will be happy to send it to you when developed. If a picture is being taken, request 20 minutes for your visit. Table 15.7 provides many useful tips for personal visits to legislators.

Telephoning

When time is short on an issue, a telephone call may be necessary. Call the legislator at an appropriate time in his or her office. If the legislator is not available, then ask to

Table 15.6. Useful Federal Government Telephone Numbers

US Capitol Switchboard	202-224-3121
Senate Floor Information (Democrats)	202-224-8541
Senate Floor Information (Republicans)	202-224-6191
House Floor Information (Democrats)	202-225-7400
House Floor Information (Republicans)	202-225-7430
Library of Congress	202-707-5000
Federal Register	202-741-6000
Senate and House Bill Status	202-225-1772
The White House	202-456-1414
Department of Health and Human Services	202-690-7000
Centers for Medicare & Medicaid Services	410-786-3000

Table 15.7. Tips for Personal Visits to Legislators

Do:

- Make an appointment rather than dropping by because it will greatly increase your chances of meeting with the legislator. Be brief. Expect no more than 15 minutes for the meeting.

- In scheduling your appointment, give as much notice as possible, at least 2 weeks.

- When you call for an appointment, tell the scheduler what you want to talk about so the legislator may ask the staff member who handles that topic to sit in on the meeting.

- If the legislator is unavailable when you want to meet, it is definitely worthwhile to meet with the health legislative assistant. He or she can become your best friend in the office. Rest assured that if you try to circumvent or ignore staff, you will find it difficult to get staff cooperation in the future.

- Before making your appointment, find out if other nurses have already made appointments. Team lobbying is more effective. If you are in a group, select a spokesperson to lead the discussion.

- Be punctual.

- Be professional in your appearance and approach. Carry business cards with you so that you can network at all times.

- Address legislators by "Representative" or "Senator" until they tell you to call them something different.

- Identify yourself immediately as a constituent and a CRNA when you meet with the legislator; public officials meet too many people to remember everyone.

- Assume that legislators do not understand your issue; if they do they will tell you, if they do not you have saved them from looking foolish.

- Have an outline of the points that you want to make.

- If you cannot answer a question knowledgeably, tell the legislator that you or your association will send him or her the information as soon as possible and then do so.

- Do not take up the entire 15 minutes with your presentation; allow at least 5 minutes for the legislator to ask questions.

- Listen carefully to the legislator's view on your issue.

Continues on page 359.

Table 15.7. Tips for Personal Visits to Legislators (continued)

- "Make the Ask." Always remember to request the legislator to help promote support with his or her colleagues on your issue. What is it you want them to do?

- Ask for your legislator's advice on ways to lobby your issue.

- Ask the legislator what the opposition says about your issue and rebut the arguments if you can.

- Ask your legislator to keep an open mind on your issue even if he or she states opposition to your point of view. Remember that controversial legislation and regulation usually result in compromise. Be ready with alternatives or solutions as well as with criticisms.

- Leave your legislator with a 1-page fact sheet on the issue, your position, and exactly what you want him or her to do. Provide articles or data that back up your view, if possible.

- Keep the door open for further discussion even if the legislator's attitude appears to be negative. Leave on a positive note.

- Follow up with a thank-you letter for the visit and again include a summary of the points that you made.

Don't:

- Be angry if the legislator cannot meet with you when it is convenient for you; make another appointment or meet with the health legislative assistant, who is generally the one who will make recommendations on whether to support or oppose your request. It is important to develop a good working relationship with this individual.

- Visit your legislator at home without an invitation.

- Call your legislator off the floor of the chamber unless it is truly an emergency.

- Visit the legislator more than once on an issue in a short period of time, unless you have something new to say.

- Expect an on-the-spot endorsement of your bill or issue.

- Portray your personal opinion on an issue as that of the Association; if your personal position differs from the Association's, make that clear to the legislator. It is better to avoid bringing up issues outside of the AANA agenda.

- Let a legislator sidetrack you on another issue for the entire meeting so he or she does not have to address your issue.

Continues on page 360.

359

Table 15.7. Tips for Personal Visits to Legislators (continued)

- "Cry Wolf" on every issue; overreacting diminishes credibility.

- Forget that the impression that you leave is as important as the substance of your discussion.

- Repeat off-the-record comments of one legislator to another--keep them confidential.

- Criticize your legislator for introducing a bill that you dislike, without finding out if the legislator is serious about pushing the bill.

- Bring up other issues outside of the AANA agenda. Remember, you're representing the nurse anesthesia profession in the meeting.

- Be offended if you don't always get what you request. Either by virtue of the politics of the issue or due to other demands, the legislator may not always be able to help you. But remember it is vitally important to maintain a cordial relationship so you can "live to fight another day."

---

speak to the health LA. Clearly state your name, that you are a CRNA constituent, the bill number, and what action you want the legislator to take, for example, "I am Jane Doe, a CRNA constituent of the senator's. I'm calling about S.1, the reauthorization of the Nurse Education Act, which I support. I would like him to vote in favor of the bill when it comes up for committee action tomorrow. Thank you."

Corresponding with the Legislator
Letter writing techniques are provided in Tables 15.8 and 15.9, and a sample letter is demonstrated in Table 15.10.

Correspondence to the Hill
Given enhanced security issues, handwritten letters are delivered to Congress only when they have been carefully screened at a location away from Capitol Hill. This means that handwritten letters, though effective, can be delayed. If your issue is urgent, there is no substitute for a telephone call, although email can also be effective.

Testifying at Public Hearings
An effective presentation by a CRNA at a health hearing could have a great impact on the ultimate fate of a bill. During hearings on legislation, representatives from professional associations, special interest groups, the executive branch, academia, and interested members of Congress are invited to speak. The audience can be expected to be members of Congress, members of the press, congressional staff members, and lobbyists for organizations interested in the bill. The number of people in the audience will depend on the controversial nature of the legislation. At the federal level, hearings are usually scheduled in the morning because the House and Senate normally go into session around noon. Once Congress is in session, there is always a chance that a floor vote will require committee members to leave to go vote, which has a disruptive effect on the hearing.

The twofold objective of association testimony is to inform and persuade. What you have to say is important, but how well you

---

Table 15.8. How to Address a Letter to a Legislator

House member: The Honorable _____
                U.S. House of Representatives
                Washington, DC 20515

Senate member: The Honorable _____
                U.S. Senate
                Washington, DC 20510

President: The Honorable _____
                President of the United States
                Washington, DC 20500

---

say it is just as important. Your presentation can be very effective because you will be speaking as one directly affected by the proposal being considered, because you have special knowledge of the subject, or because you represent the viewpoint of many CRNAs. Your appearance increases the likelihood that your association will be consulted on other issues. A hearing can be instrumental in establishing permanent lines of communication with legislators.

Scope of Testimony

Every piece of testimony should include the following:

1. Identification of individuals appearing
   a. Name, title, and place of work
   b. Background to establish credibility as a witness
   c. Identity of the organization and constituency you are representing
2. Identification of legislation or issue
   a. Specify bill by number, issue by title.
   b. State your position briefly and early.
   c. Paraphrase your understanding of the intent or purpose of the legislation or issue.
3. Areas under consideration
   a. Define them.
   b. If supportive, explain why.
   c. If opposed, state why and give alternatives if any exist.
4. Lengthier explanation of your position and your rationale
5. Summation including what you would like to see accomplished
6. Thanks for being allowed to present your views

Tables 15.11 and 15.12 provide more useful information for testifying. The importance of individual congressional committees to health issues varies with changing circumstances, such as committee jurisdiction, the personality and political strength of individual committee chairmen, and the current prominence of an individual health issue during a session of Congress. For the most part, however, the most influential committees are those that deal with the funding of discretionary health programs like the Nurse Education Act (appropriation and budget committees) and those that deal with the financing of entitlement programs like Medicare and Medicaid (authorization committees). Table 15.13 contains descriptions of the health-related commit-

361

Table 15.9. Tips for Letter Writing

Do:

• Contact your own representative and 2 senators. As a constituent, you have a better chance of influencing their actions than you would by writing to the entire Senate and House of Representatives.

• Consider the factor of timing. Try to write when the bill is still in committee and awaiting action.

• Address the letter properly.

• Write legibly or type your letter for easiest reading.

• Use your personal stationery unless you have been asked to write on your association's or employer's letterhead.

• Sign your full name and address to the letter so you can be contacted back. Envelopes are sometimes lost. Be sure the address that you give is in the legislator's district.

• Write to your legislator at his or her office rather than at home, so your correspondence is filed to receive a response and for future reference.

• Mention the fact that you have a personal connection with the legislator (if indeed you do) because the staff member reading the letter will be more inclined to forward it directly to the legislator.

• Stick to one subject per letter and limit the letter to one page, if possible. If you need to include copies of articles or research data, attach them to the letter.

• Identify the bill number and popular name, if possible, for example, S. 1, the reauthorization of the Nurse Education Act.

• Clearly state your position and why you have taken that position in the first paragraph.

• Personalize the effect of the bill on you, your family, your practice, your community, your state. Form letters and petitions are not considered as valuable as personal letters.

• Request the legislator to communicate his or her position on the bill to you.

• Write to say thank you for a favorable vote to let your legislator know that you appreciate a job well done. Make sure to mention helpful staff in your thank-you letter.

• Send copies of your letters to legislators and their responses to the AANA Washington, DC office.

Continues on page 363.

Table 15.9. Tips for Letter Writing (continued)

Don't:

- Become a "pen pal" and write on every issue being considered.

- Apologize for taking up the legislator's time—it is what they are elected for.

- Send a copy to a senator when you have written to a representative or vice versa.

- Be insulted if you receive a form letter in reply—legislators receive thousands of letters. After few letters have been received regarding a particular issue, a standard form letter is written by a staff member and approved by the legislator. This form letter is then sent as a reply to all those people writing about that issue.

- Send form letters or petitions, unless it is the only way a contact will be made.

- Forget to write and say thank you when legislators do something you approve of.

- Postpone writing; there is never a truly convenient time.

Table 15.10. Sample Letter to Senators

The Honorable (name of senator)
Address
Washington, DC 20510

Dear Senator_____:

    I am writing to express my strong support for S.1, the bill to reauthorize the Nurse Education Act. I would like you to cosponsor this important bill because it provides funds for nurse anesthesia educational programs, student traineeships, and faculty development.

    The education of certified registered nurse anesthetists (CRNAs) is especially important now because of the severe shortage of anesthesia providers in this country. The CRNA shortage has affected your district as evidenced by_____.

    I appreciate your consideration of this critical piece of legislation and hope you will cosponsor it. It would appreciate hearing from you regarding your position on this issue.

Sincerely,

Table 15.11. Preliminary Information Necessary Before Testifying

Before you testify on a bill, you should have been provided with the following information by your staff person:

- What are the key provisions in the legislation?

- What are the arguments on both sides of the issue?

- Who are its supporters and opponents?

- What is the bill's impact on your practice?

- Has there been any prior hearing on this topic before the panel? Can you get copies of those earlier testimonies?

- What other interest groups and associations are testifying and what are their concerns with the legislation?

- What are the concerns of the individual committee members?

- Will the legislation have a significant impact on any of the constituents of the committee members?

- Does the chair have a special interest in the bill?

- What amendments are expected to be offered during the markup process? Will the amendments alter your association's position? Do you need to propose any amendments?

- What arguments will be used to oppose your association's position? Your testimony should counter those arguments.

- What are the committee's rules of the procedure?

- What districts are represented by the committee members?

- Has your staff suggested "friendly questions" to the committee members that they may ask you to help you expand on your testimony?

Table 15.12. Do's and Don'ts of Testifying

Do:

- Arrive promptly. Witnesses will usually be allowed to enter a hearing room first, before the public. When you arrive, inform committee staff that you are there.

- At the state level, you may need to fill out a witness registration slip, where you indicate whether you are for or against the bill. Persons who wish to speak indicate so on the registration slip. At the state level, if you have traveled some distance to appear and will be returning home that day, note that fact on the registration slip. The committee chair will often call such witnesses early in the hearing to allow for their travel home.

- Be prepared to wait. There may be other bills heard before yours. It is also difficult to judge how long each speaker will take. Do not be surprised if you have to wait for some time before being called.

- If possible, bring a copy of the bill with you. This will allow you to refer to specific sections in your presentation or when answering questions.

- Providing copies of written testimony to the committee is advised even for those who present oral testimony. At the federal level the committee staff will inform you of how many copies of testimony are necessary for the committee.

- A longer written testimony will usually be submitted for the record. You will usually be presenting 5- or 10-minute remarks that are a brief summary of the lengthier text. Rehearse your presentation thoroughly and time it. Do not exceed your time limit under any circumstances. In fact, some committee rooms have green, yellow, and red lights to let you know how you are managing your time. Regardless of where you are in your prepared remarks, when the red light goes on you should finish your sentence and say thank you.

- Usually the message in a piece of testimony is so vital that a script is essential for complete accuracy; however, do not use the script as a crutch, burying your eyes in it.

- Tailor the text delivery and style of your testimony to fit your own personality. It should be simple, focused, and natural. The end result should be like a conversation between you and someone you like.

- Work with the staff person who is drafting your testimony so that you are comfortable with the way the ideas are expressed. A good use of your familiar expressions and real-life examples in the testimony will make you feel better and make the testimony seem more genuine.

- Be prepared to answer questions. The association staff should go over anticipated questions that you may receive from the committee and provide you with possible answers. Hearing tough questions in advance is much better than encountering them for the first time at a hearing.

Continues on page 366.

365

Table 15.12. Do's and Don'ts of Testifying (continued)

- If you are testifying on a controversial topic, be prepared for media at the hearing. Work with your staff person on how to handle a media interview if requested.

- Your staff will not sit at the witness table with you, but they can sit right behind you in case you need some help.

- If neither you nor your staff person knows an answer to a question, admit it and offer to supply the information later for the record.

Don't:

- Assume that all committee members are familiar with all aspects of the bill. That is the purpose of the hearing. Review the specific provisions of the bill that are of concern.

- Repeat at length the points made by a previous speaker. If you have something to add to what was said, by all means do so. If not, simply note your agreement with the earlier speaker and move on to the rest of your presentation. To be effective, your presentation must be somewhat flexible. Pay attention to what other speakers are saying.

- Attempt to answer questions for which you do not have answers or facts. If you are requested to appear by a staff member of a trade association, ask the committee chair if that staff member can respond with better facts or experience that you might have. You may also offer to provide additional information after the hearing.

- Be disappointed if only one or two legislators show up for the hearing. That does not diminish your testimony—often legislators have two or more hearings scheduled for the same time. Be comforted that everything you say is going into the hearing record and will be closely studied by the committee staff.

---

tees of the Senate and the House of Representatives that have jurisdiction over the issues that are of greatest concern to CRNAs. Their jurisdictions and important subcommittees are detailed, as well as how to contact these committees. Table 15.14 tells how to obtain congressional documents, bills, reports, and public laws.

Getting More Involved in the Political Arena

Many people have a poor view of politics. Depending upon one's political point of view, the federal government may be doing too much or too little to help. But make no mistake, if CRNAs are not involved in the process, there are others who will gladly take their place. There's an old saying that "If you're not at the table, you're likely to be on the menu." This is still true today.

Get involved at the local or state level. You can spend as much or as little time as you like. Although it is always good to see CRNAs run for political office, if you do not have the time or willingness to make that commitment, there are myriad other ways

Table 15.13. Health-Related Committees of the US Senate

Appropriations

S-128 Capitol Building, Washington, DC 20510-6025; phone (202) 224-3471. Jurisdiction: All discretionary funding for federal programs
Key Subcommittee: Labor, Health and Human Services, Education, and Related Agencies, SD-186 Dirksen Senate Office Building, Washington, DC 20510; phone (202) 224-7363. Jurisdiction: Nurse anesthesia education funding, National Center for Nursing Research

Armed Services

SR-228 Russell Senate Office Building, Washington, DC 20510-6050; phone (202) 224-3871. Jurisdiction: Military funding, including CHAMPUS
Key Subcommittee: Manpower and Personnel, same address as full committee. Jurisdiction: CRNA pay and education funding; CRNA bonus pay

Budget

SD-624 Dirksen Senate Office Building, Washington, DC 20510-6100; phone (202) 224-0642. Jurisdiction: Total health funding and financing ceiling

Homeland Security and Governmental Affairs

SD-340 Dirksen Senate Office Building, Washington, DC 20510-6250; phone (202) 224-2627. Jurisdiction: Federal worker issues

Finance

SD-219 Dirksen Senate Office Building, Washington, DC 20510-6200; phone (202) 224-4515. Jurisdiction: Taxes, Medicare, and Medicaid
Key Subcommittee: Health, full committee address
Key Subcommittee: Medicare and Long-term Care, full committee address

Health, Education, Labor and Pensions Committee

SD-428 Dirksen Senate Office Building, Washington, DC 20510-6300; phone (202) 224-5375. Jurisdiction: Health authorizations and reauthorizations, including nurse anesthesia education funding

Continues on page 368.

367

Table 15.13. Health-Related Committees of the US House of Representatives

Appropriations

H-307 Capitol Building, Washington DC 20515-6015; phone (202) 225-2771.
Jurisdiction: All discretionary funding for federal programs
Key Subcommittee: Labor, Health and Human Services Education, full committee address
Jurisdiction: Nurse anesthesia education funding, National Center for Nursing Research, AIDS funding

Armed Services

2120 Rayburn House Office Building, Washington, DC 20515-6035; phone (202) 225-4151.
Jurisdiction: Military funding, including CHAMPUS
Key Subcommittee: Military Personnel, full committee address
Jurisdiction: CRNA pay and education funding; CRNA bonus pay

Budget

207 Cannon House Office Building, Washington, DC 20515-6065; phone (202) 226-7270.
Jurisdiction: Total health funding and financing ceiling

Energy and Commerce:

2125 Rayburn House Office Building, Washington, DC 20515-6115; phone (202) 225-2927.
Jurisdiction: Public health and health facilities
Key Subcommittee: Health and the Environment, full committee address
Jurisdiction: Health authorizations and reauthorizations, including nurse anesthesia education funding, Medicaid and shared jurisdiction with Ways and Means Committee over Medicare Part B

Ways and Means

1102 Longworth House Office Building, Washington, DC 20515-6348; phone (202) 225-3625.
Jurisdiction: Taxes and Medicare
Key Subcommittee: Health, full committee address
Jurisdiction: Medicare Part A and shared jurisdiction with Energy and Commerce Committee over Medicare Part B

Table 15.14. How to Obtain Congressional Documents

Bills, Reports, and Public Laws

You can request 1 copy of 6 different items (bills, reports, public laws) in writing daily from the Senate Document Room. Phone orders are not accepted. Email requests: orders@sec.senate.gov. Most documents are available online.

> Senate Printing and Document Services
> B-04 Hart Building
> Washington, DC 20510
> (202) 224-7701

Hearing Documents

House or Senate committee prints or hearing records are generally available online through the committee's website.

> The Legislative Resource Center (LRC)
> B-106 Cannon House Office Building
> Washington, DC 20515
> (202) 226-5200

The Legislative Resource Center (LRC) provides information about legislation and records for the House for congressional offices and the public. The LRC provides access to all published documents originated and produced by the House and its committees, to the historical records of the House, and to public disclosure documents.

369

to have a voice in the process. Raising money for the candidate of your choice is always a top-tier alternative. Political contributions help support the candidacy of legislators, and there's never enough money to go around, at least in the minds of politicians. Whether or not you like the idea of money in politics, it is a fact of life. It is also what will get you noticed by your legislator, governor, or member of Congress. Hosting fundraisers gets you on their list.

But whatever you choose to do, get involved. Don't stay on the sidelines. Write letters to the editor on issues of importance to the nurse anesthesia profession. Volunteer in campaigns. Attend town hall meetings. Write a brief note to your legislators a few times a year. Stop by their offices and make friends with their staff. The goal should be to ensure that the legislator knows you on a first-name basis. Remember, you need to have those relationships established before you need their help. This is an important investment for you and your profession.

Summary

I hope the information in this chapter on how the AANA is involved in the political and legislative arenas will provide you with the impetus to assert your own influence in healthcare policy. Educating yourself on the political process will give you the power to have input on the issues that will ultimately affect you. This input will allow you to educate legislators on health issues and put the democratic process in motion.

Glossary

Act: Legislation that has passed both chambers of Congress and has been signed by the president or passed by a two-thirds majority in a presidential veto override, thus becoming law.

Amendment: A proposal of a legislator to change the language or content in a bill.

Bill: Legislative proposal originating in either chamber of Congress and designated "HR" in the House and "S" in the Senate. The bill number is usually assigned in the order in which legislation is introduced from the beginning of each 2-year congressional term.

Calendar: The agenda or list of pending business before either chamber of Congress or before a committee.

Chamber: Meeting place for the total membership of the House or Senate, as opposed to committee rooms.

Cloture: Process by which debate (or filibuster) can be limited in the Senate, other than by unanimous consent. Requires the vote of 60 senators present and voting. Under cloture, each senator is limited to 1 hour of debate.

Conference Committee: The more controversial a bill may be the more likely it will pass the Senate and House in different forms. Unless either body is willing to ac-

cept the changes of the other, the two versions must go to a conference committee. This means that a committee (the number is not fixed), chosen from the originating Senate and House committees, is appointed to work out a compromise. An agreement, if reached, is known as a "conference report." It must then be approved by both the Senate and the House.

Congressional Record: Daily printed account of the proceedings of both the House and Senate chambers, with debate and statements reported verbatim.

Executive session: Meeting of a committee at which only the committee's members, and no public or press, are allowed to attend.

Federal Register: Daily printed account of the activities of federal agencies, including rule making.

Filibuster: A device used only in the Senate to delay or prevent a vote by time-consuming talk. This tactic is often used by a minority in an effort to prevent a vote on a bill that would probably pass if brought to a vote. Can be stopped only by a 60-member vote of the senators present and voting.

Law: An act of Congress that has been signed by the president or passed over a presidential veto by the Congress.

Markup: After public hearings, a subcommittee will go into executive (either closed or open) session to start the "markup" of a bill, that is, to write amendments into it, delete sections, or revise the language. Views of both sides are stated in detail, and at the conclusion of deliberation, a vote is taken to determine subcommittee action. It may decide to report the bill favorably to the full committee with or without amendments or suggest that the bill be tabled. Each member of the sub committee has 1 vote.

Omnibus bill: A legislative proposal concerning several separate but related items.

Quorum: Number of members whose presence is needed to conduct business. This would be a majority of the members, or 51 in the Senate and 218 in the House. Any member may object to the conduct of business without a quorum and thus force a roll call to bring in absentees. Roll calls are frequently used as a delaying tactic. Much legislation is passed without a quorum because it is noncontroversial. If a point of order is made that quorum is not present, the only business that can be done is either a motion to adjourn or a motion to direct the sergeant-at-arms to request the attendance of absentees.

Roll call vote: Members vote as their names are called by the clerk of the chamber.

Rule of germaneness: Used to knock out language that does not pertain to the purpose of the bill. Also used to kill an appropriation in which the expenditure has not been previously authorized by a separate bill. The Senate may impose the rule on itself under a unanimous consent agreement to limit debate on a pending matter. A two-thirds vote is necessary to retain the language.

Standing vote: An unrecorded vote taken when all members in favor of a proposal stand and are counted, and then all members opposed stand and are counted.

Veto: Action taken by the president rejecting a bill presented by Congress for signature. When Congress is in session, the president has 10 days, excluding Sundays, to veto a bill or it automatically becomes law.

Voice vote: The presiding officer of either chamber calls for "yeas" and "nays" to determine the results.

References

1. Center for Responsive Politics. PAC Contributions to Federal Candidates Election Cycle 2010. http://www.opensecrets.org/pacs/industry.php?txt=H01&cycle=2010. Accessed June 14, 2010.

2. Mason DJ, Talbott SW. *Political Action Handbook for Nurses.* Menlo Park, CA: Addison-Wesley; 1987.

3. Lederer JC. Legislate success: learn to lobby. *ASAE Association Management.* [membership]. December 2987: 29-32. http://www.asaecenter.org/Resources/AMMagCurrentIssueToc.cfm. Accessed June 14, 2011.

4. American Society of Association Executives. When you need a coalition. *ASAE Association Management* [membership]. 1990;1(1). http://www.asaecenter.org/Resources/AMMagCurrentIssueToc.cfm. Accessed June 14, 2011.

5. Pressures in Congress. *The Washington Post.* June 26, 1983:A14.

6. Oleszek WJ. *Congressional Procedures and the Policy Process.* 3rd ed. Washington, DC: CQ Press, Inc; 1989.

7. Davies J. *Legislative Law and Process in a Nutshell.* 3rd ed. St. Paul, MN: West Publishing; 1986.

8. State Net. *From Idea to Law: the State Legislative Process.* Sacramento, CA: State Net; 1989. http://www.statenet.com. Accessed June 14, 2011.

9. National Health Council. *Congress and Health.* New York, NY: National Health Council; 1989. http://www.nationalhealthcouncil.org. Accessed June 14, 2011.

371

Key References

1. Anderson JE. *Public Policymaking.* 7th ed. Boston, MA: Wadsworth Publishing; 2010.

2. Kingdon JW. *Agendas, Alternatives and Public Policies.* White Plains, NY: Longman; 2010.

3. Mason DJ, Leavitt JK, Chaffee MW. *Policy and Politics in Nursing and Health Care.* 6th ed. Philadelphia, PA: Saunders; 2011.

4. Strand M, Johnson MS, Climer JF. Surviving Inside Congress. 2nd ed. Alexandria, VA: Congressional Institute; 2010.

Challenges in Professional Practice

CHAPTER 16

The US Legal System and Issues Affecting Clinical Practice

Gene A. Blumenreich, JD

Key Concepts

- State and federal courts differ from one another in jurisdiction, traditions, rules, and body of law. The federal system deals with issues that broadly affect interstate commerce, controversies between the states, actions involving federal property or the US government, and actions between citizens of different states. Matters affecting the health, safety, and welfare of citizens generally are included within the "police" powers of states and are reserved for state governments and their courts.

- Courts do not make law the way a legislature does. Court decisions "reveal" the law as it always was and will be, before and after their decisions. Legislation affects matters that arise only after it is enacted. In choosing between conflicting parties, the judicial system applies its goals of fairness, consistency, predictability, and the effectuation of public policy.

- A professional must render care not as a reasonable person would act but with the same degree of skill and care a reasonable member of the profession would practice in the same community in similar circumstances. The members of a profession set the standard of care by which quality of care is measured. Both the courts and the legislature can change these standards should the profession render care at a lower standard than is acceptable. In specialty areas, such as anesthesia, there is a nationwide standard of care that does not vary from community to community.

Continues on next page.

Key Concepts (continued)

- In anesthesia, there is a single standard of care against which both anesthesiologists and Certified Registered Nurse Anesthetists (CRNAs) are measured.

- The theoretical basis of negligence or malpractice is that the defendant should pay for damages caused to the plaintiff because, as between the 2 parties, the one who was at fault should bear the damage.

- Anesthesia accidents, including those involving CRNAs, have become prime examples for the application of the doctrine of *res ipsa loquitur.*

Nurse anesthesia is a specialty in the legally defined profession of nursing. Consequently, it is important for Certified Registered Nurse Anesthetists (CRNAs) to have an informed understanding of the legal system that profoundly affects the way the profession is practiced. Because many challenges to nurse anesthesia practice are based on misinformation concerning the legal status of CRNAs, an understanding of the legal system and tenets guiding its function is vitally important.

Nurse anesthesia is regulated by licensing boards and by the courts, which play a role in setting the standard of care. The hallmark of a profession is its ability to set its own standard of care. Courts learn of the standard of care through expert testimony. Because experts may disagree, the courts may have to choose between conflicting testimonies. Moreover, the legislature may require new standards of care through legislation. Consequently, even though standards are set by the profession, the standard of care is affected by the legal system, including regulatory bodies of the state, the legislature through statute, and, of course, a jury's or court's determination of what the standard is.

Deference to the Healthcare Profession

Regulation of healthcare differs significantly from regulation of other industries. In most areas, regulation clearly and specifically sets forth powers, duties, and procedures. However, in medical and nursing regulation there is a large degree of deference afforded the healthcare community by both legislatures and courts. This deference is expressed in the California Nursing Act[1]:

> ...the legislature recognizes that nursing
> is a dynamic field, the practice of which

is continually evolving to include more sophisticated patient care activities. It is the intent of the legislature in amending this section at the 1973-74 session to provide clear legal authority for functions and procedures which have common acceptance and usage.

Law school students learn very early that during a trial, "law" is determined by the judge, whereas "facts" are determined by the jury if there is one or by the judge in the absence of a jury. Evidence is offered by the parties to establish the facts. However, in some cases involving the healthcare field, judges appear to rely on expert testimony for interpretation of statutes as well as facts. For instance, *Chalmers-Francis v Nelson* in 1936[2] found that "nurse anesthesia practice is not diagnosing nor prescribing ... within the meaning of the California Medical Practice Act," and in *Bentley v Langley* in 1978,[3] an anesthesiologist was permitted to testify (incorrectly) that a doctor who supervised a nurse anesthetist was responsible for the anesthesia services administered.

This special position that the courts give to healthcare can sometimes be taken advantage of. In the 1983 case of *Sermchief v Gonzales*,[4] the Missouri legislature amended the Missouri statute on nursing to permit advanced practice nurses to give routine examinations and dispense medications within a medical protocol without being under the direct supervision of a physician. The Missouri Medical Board, known as the Board of Registration for the Healing Arts, threatened criminal prosecution of nurses who carried out these activities, claiming that the nurses were engaged in the illegal practice of medicine. A group of nurses sought protection against the Board of Registration for the Healing Arts. Both the nurses and physicians seemed to be asking the court to draw "that thin and elusive line that separates the practice of medicine and the practice of professional nursing in modern day delivery of health services." Instead, the court pointed out that what the nurses were doing was, in fact, exactly what the legislature intended them to do. Because licensing is the prerogative of the legislature, the fact that some physicians thought that the legislature had authorized nurses to do something that might have been the practice of medicine was irrelevant. If the legislature said that nurses could do it, it was the practice of nursing and the medical board had no right to interfere with their practice of it.

Sources of Law

Legislature

The powers of the legislature are limited only by constitutional restrictions and the political control of the voting public. Legislation is forward looking; it affects actions taking place after its effective date. When legislation is passed, courts interpret it by trying to determine what the legislature intended. Court decisions, on the other hand, state what the law is and, theoretically, what the law always has been. When a court determines that a judicial doctrine, such as "captain of the ship," is no longer the law, every undecided case is governed by the decision, regardless of when it arose. If a state was still following the captain of the ship doctrine, and the legislature wanted to, it could pass a law that, after a certain date, surgeons would no longer be assumed to control all actions in an operating room. Cases arising before the effective date would be decided assuming that surgeons were in control and cases after the date would be decided assuming that surgeons were not in control. Only the legis-

lature has the authority to change the law as of a particular date. The legislature can reverse decisions made by the judiciary. The legislature is limited by constitutional restrictions (eg, a legislature could not adopt a law making something that has already happened a crime, or taking property, or imposing punishment without following due process and having a fair hearing). The judiciary interprets existing law, the Constitution, statutes, and prior court decisions. Judicial interpretations of the Constitution cannot be overruled by the legislature; they can only be changed by the court's reconsideration or by changing the Constitution.

Executive Branch

The executive branch enforces laws made by the legislature and interpreted by the courts. Before the American Revolution, the executive branch was headed by the monarch or his or her representative. Now the executive branch is headed by the US president or a state governor.

A part of the executive branch of government is the attorney general, who serves as the lawyer for the government. The attorney general serves 2 functions. First, as the government's lawyer, the attorney general brings lawsuits and represents the country or the state in court. Second, the attorney general gives advice to administrative agencies or departments by interpreting the law. Interpretations of the law by the attorney general are not binding on the courts. They are important, however, because they tell how the attorney general's client, the executive branch of the government, will act.

An example of an attorney general interpretation important to nurse anesthetists is the opinion of the California attorney general on whether nurse anesthetists could administer regional anesthetics. The attorney general is often asked to give opinions when there is very little authority or precedent. In 1972, the attorney general of California was asked if it was legal for nurse anesthetists to give regional anesthetics. The attorney general searched the case law and found only an isolated statement by the California Supreme Court in the 1961 case of *Magit v State of California*.[5] In Magit, 3 foreign anesthesiologists were administering anesthesia without medical licenses. The chief anesthesiologist who employed them was prosecuted for aiding and abetting the unauthorized practice of medicine. His defense was based on the case of *Chalmers-Francis v Nelson,* one of the fundamental cases upholding nurse anesthetist practice.[2] The chief anesthesiologist claimed that since California courts permitted Dagmar Nelson, who was not a licensed physician, to administer anesthesia, California law also permitted nonlicensed anesthesiologists to provide anesthesia. In upholding the chief anesthesiologist's conviction, the California Supreme Court noted that Dagmar Nelson was a nurse and nurses have a special position in the healthcare system. The Court also pointed out that the Dagmar Nelson case had been decided at a time when California did not have a nurse practice act (a nurse practice act had since been enacted). Therefore, as precedent, the Dagmar Nelson case was limited to its facts. The court found that a nurse anesthetist administering a general anesthetic was not illegally practicing medicine.

From this simple statement in Magit, the California attorney general developed a theory that, under California law, nurse anesthetists could legally administer only general anesthesia and not regional anesthetics. Although the ruling was patently absurd, nurse anesthetists in California were uneasy that the decision would be enforced by the board of nursing. Some nurse anes-

thetists had to stop administering regional anesthesia, although most believed that the attorney general's decision was incorrect.

In 1976, the California Association of Nurse Anesthetists went back to the attorney general to ask for a reversal of his prior decision. The attorney general agreed that the Magit case was not authority for his ruling. Unfortunately, the attorney general found a new problem. The legislature had passed a bill specifically giving nurse anesthetists the ability to administer regional anesthetics, but the governor had vetoed the bill. The attorney general decided that under usual rules of interpretation, the California legislature must have believed that nurse anesthetists required additional statutory authority to give regional anesthetics (or the legislature would not have passed the bill). Since the bill had been vetoed, nurse anesthetists did not receive the additional authority and must still lack the power to administer regional anesthetics. Reportedly, the California governor vetoed the bill because he thought nurse anesthetists already had the power and the bill was unnecessary.

The attorney general's ruling stood for 8 more years until, in 1984, the office finally issued an opinion that there was no prohibition against nurse anesthetists giving regional anesthesia. As can be seen, the attorney general rendered 2 incorrect decisions that were not subject to review or correction. The decisions were troublesome because they were binding on administrative agencies. Although they were not binding on the courts, nurse anesthesia practice was harmed in California in the years the ruling stood.

Administrative Agencies

Another part of the executive branch is the administrative agency. An administrative agency combines elements of all 3

379

branches of government. An administrative agency such as the Food and Drug Administration (FDA) has a legislative function in that it adopts regulations that have the force of law. The FDA also has an executive function because it prosecutes healthcare institutions that violate the regulations. Finally, it has a judicial function in that the agency conducts hearings on charges and determines guilt or innocence. Regulations issued by an administrative agency must be consistent with enabling acts and other legislation. Although an agency may clarify unclear or ambiguous terms, it cannot adopt interpretations that are inconsistent with the clear language of legislation. Licensing agencies such as boards of nursing, medicine, and pharmacy are administrative agencies and combine functions of each of the branches of government.

380

Courts

Courts do not make law the way a legislature does. Court decisions are applicable to actions whether they occur before or after their decisions. Even though courts interpret what the law always was, the fact is that society changes, and its institutions change. Consequently, the courts constantly reexamine and reinterpret statutes and the Constitution in light of current events and situations.

For example, when the antitrust laws were passed in 1890, they were intended to prevent the excesses of the robber barons of the late 19th century who manipulated prices of oil, steel, and other products. Probably, very few people in 1890 could have imagined that antitrust laws would ever be applicable to services, especially professional services. It was not until 1942—52 years after passage of the original legislation—that the Supreme Court held that the antitrust laws applied (and had always applied) to restraint of trade by physicians. Today, the antitrust laws are routinely applied to matters involving the healthcare professions.

Common Law

In some countries, the legal system is based entirely on interpretation of statutes. Former English colonies, including the United States, inherited a tradition of judge-made law along with our common language. In feudal times in England, the courts decided disputes between persons when there were no statutes or legislation. The courts decided these matters using the goals of consistency, fairness, predictability, and effectuation (what was best for public) of policy. These decisions eventually resulted in a large body of "common law" legal principles and precedents that the courts used to make individual decisions in areas not governed by statute. The English system, including the tradition of common law dating back to feudal times, forms the basis of law in every state of the United States except Louisiana. At the time of its acquisition by the United States, Louisiana had a thriving commercial port with important commercial transactions. Fairness and consistency required that Louisiana continue its system based on the continental system of statutory interpretation, rather than common law.

In feudal times, the king rode from location to location resolving disputes between his subjects. These disputes often involved the ownership and use of land. It was important to the feudal economy that there be quick and consistent resolution of these disputes because land represented wealth and capital. If land was properly used, the kingdom would prosper, but if land was unused, the kingdom would suffer. Determination of disputes between individual citizens was an important function for the king. Over time, the process of dispute resolution became institutionalized and certain of the king's assistants became judges or specialists in dispute resolution. The tradition (largely oral) of principles that these judges followed became the basis of common law. Eventually, persons seeking justice in the king's legal system were allowed to confer with other persons with experience in the system. Thus, the profession of law developed.

Goals of Judicial Decisions

In choosing between conflicting parties, the judicial system applies its goals of fairness, consistency, predictability, and the effectuation of public policy. In a democracy, the courts draw their authority from the consent of the governed. Although the judicial system must make unpopular decisions from time to time, it must always appear to be fair in its process or it will lose support. It must be predictable as well. Those who are governed by the system must be able to understand what the system expects and how the system will operate. The system must also be consistent. It would be unfair to hold one person negligent in one case and to exonerate a person in another when both were engaged in identical conduct. A system that lacks consistency is neither predictable nor fair. The legal system also attempts to encourage actions that benefit society as a whole and to discourage actions that harm society. Consequently, the common law that was inherited from England had at its heart that all members of society must act as reasonable people would act. When a member does not, he or she is responsible for any damage caused.

Although some individual court decisions may be difficult to justify, these decisions must be judged by whether they carry out the goals of fairness, consistency, predictability, and effectuation of policy. Sometimes, to carry out its ultimate goals, the legal system may produce decisions that seem incorrect. Courts may find decisions difficult when fundamental principles are in conflict. For many years, courts held surgeons liable for any activity in an operating room because the surgeon was like the "captain of a ship" and theoretically could control any action in the room. Even when it was clear that the surgeon was not in control but dependent on a number of specialists, some courts continued to apply the captain of the ship doctrine, weighing consistency and predictability more heavily than fairness. Sometimes the system simply yields incorrect decisions, as does any human system.

State Versus Federal Courts

The US legal system is divided into 2 separate and largely independent systems. The first is the legal system of the federal government, and the second consists of the legal systems belonging to each of the 50 states and the District of Columbia. Although there is some overlap in jurisdiction, the federal and state governments have their own laws, traditions, judges, courtrooms, rules, and body of law.

Certain areas have been reserved exclusively for the federal system, including matters affecting interstate commerce. From 1930 to 1995, the level of impact these activities had to have on interstate commerce to justify federal regulation had been more and more liberally interpreted. The federal government seemed unconcerned about finding a connection with interstate commerce in creating programs affecting the health, safety, and welfare of citizens. In 1995, the Supreme Court ruled that the interstate commerce clause required a more direct impact on interstate commerce to justify federal regulation.[6] Even though courts "reveal" the law as it always was and will be, judges are human and views change, so that what seemed permanent in 1930 changed in 1995.

Federal Courts

Litigants have only limited rights to choose between federal and state courts. The jurisdiction of the federal courts is limited to (1) actions brought under federal statutes, (2) actions involving federal property, and (3) actions between citizens of different states (diversity). The perception (which may or may not be accurate) is that successful plaintiffs get larger awards in federal courts.

Lawsuits Arising Under Federal Legislation

Lawsuits based on federal statutes may be brought in federal courts, and if there are related state issues to be decided, the federal courts may also decide the related state issue. Federal laws take precedence over state and local laws. If both the federal and state governments enact conflicting legislation in a particular area, the federal act prevails. Under the doctrine of *preemption*, once the federal government has enacted legislation in an area, state laws may no longer be enforced unless the federal government specifically permits states to enact legislation in the area. The doctrine of preemption ensures that the purpose of federal legislation will be carried out and not be affected by inconsistent state laws. Sometimes Congress determines that state acts would promote and not interfere with federal policy. In such cases, Congress may permit states to adopt their own regulations. For example, in the field of antitrust law, the federal government has indicated that states may also adopt legislation prohibiting restraints of trade. Numerous states have adopted "baby antitrust statutes." Similarly, in 2003, the US Supreme Court ruled that federal legislation governing plans made available to employees did not prohibit individual states from requiring that health insurance plans permit services to be rendered by "any willing provider."[7]

Suits Against the Federal Government or Its Property

The second area of jurisdiction of the federal courts is that of disputes relating to federal property or disputes to which the federal government is a party. In feudal England, the king was always right, so a person could not have a dispute with the king. The king was immune from suit. Today, this doctrine of "sovereign immunity" protects the government from being sued without its consent. However, most citizens would be very unhappy if they were to suffer damage because of the negligence of a government worker and could not be compensated because of sovereign immunity. The federal government permits lawsuits to be brought against it under most circumstances, but these lawsuits must be brought in federal courts.

Diversity

Finally, the federal government is committed to promoting interstate commerce. Because of the founding fathers' concern that state courts would give unfair advantage to citizens of their own states, the third area of federal court jurisdiction consists of situations in which a citizen of one state sues a citizen of another. Even though a matter may involve only a state issue, if the plaintiff is a resident of one state and the defendant is a resident of another, the lawsuit may be brought in the federal court if the matter involved in the controversy exceeds $75,000.

Until 1938, the federal courts had developed their own common law, and disputes in diversity cases could have different outcomes depending on whether the suit was brought in state or federal court. Since 1938, federal courts have applied state law to diversity cases as best they can. In diversity cases, federal courts are obligated to try to reach the same result as would the state court. If the state court does not have a relevant decision to give guidance to the federal court, the federal court is obligated to predict what the state court would have done if the case had been brought there.

State Courts

Matters affecting the health, safety, and welfare of citizens generally come within the "police" powers of states and are reserved for state government. This includes not only states but also cities, towns, and other local governments. As part of their police powers, states have primary jurisdiction in licensing the healthcare industry. Disputes between people arising out of agreements or contracts are usually decided under state law, as are claims by one person that he or she may have been damaged by the negligence or actions of another. Of course, nothing is straightforward in healthcare, and many issues formerly reserved to state law are now also affected by federal reimbursement policies.

Trial and Appellate Courts

Courts are either trial courts or appellate courts. Trial courts are where cases are brought and facts presented. The trial court makes determinations of the facts of the case as well as the applicable law. In certain circumstances, the trier of facts is not a judge, but a jury. The Seventh Amendment to the Constitution preserves the right of a citizen to trial by jury. Over the years, the Seventh Amendment has been interpreted to mean that in those matters in which a trial by jury was provided when the Bill of Rights was adopted, citizens still have rights to trial by jury. In other cases, litigants can choose trial by jury, but it is not guaranteed.

Trial courts are required to make decisions quickly, and in the heat of litigation mistakes sometimes occur. In both federal and state systems, decisions of trial courts can be appealed to appellate courts. The appeals process provides time for consideration and research and is intended to lead to more uniformity in court decisions. In some states there may be only one appellate court, which would be the highest court in the state. In other states, the volume of litigation may be very large and there may be levels of appellate courts. In the federal system, decisions of the trial or district courts are appealed to a court of appeals for the region in which the state is located. Decisions of the courts of appeals may be appealed to the Supreme Court of the United States, although in some circumstances, cases may be appealed directly from the trial court to the Supreme Court. The Supreme Court has the right to set its own agenda and, as such, has the right to decide which cases it will hear of the many presented to it.

In general, decisions by the trial court as to facts made either by the judge or jury are accepted because the judge or jury has had the opportunity to see the witness and determine credibility. Testimony that is reproduced in written form does not give a reader the nonverbal clues we often rely on to determine truthfulness. Did the witness look people in the eye, squirm, seem uncertain, appear uneasy, or otherwise indicate

383

that the testimony was unreliable? Consequently, the appellate courts often defer to the fact-finding of lower courts unless it is clear from the record that the finder of fact was erroneous or prejudiced. In matters of law, appellate courts are free to review any decision made by a trial court and to come to their own conclusion. Decisions of an appellate court are binding on all courts within its jurisdiction. Consequently, many of the decisions of the appellate courts are collected and published so that people will have a chance to see the law as adopted by the court.

Each state is free not only to adopt legislation that differs from that of other states but also to have its courts make their own interpretation of law. Although states may be interested in what other state legislatures and courts may have done in addressing common problems, they are not obligated to follow their decisions. Obviously, because of common backgrounds and restraints, there is more uniformity than diversity among states, but diversity does exist.

Civil and Criminal Matters

The judicial system distinguishes between civil and criminal matters. A civil matter is a dispute between 2 or more parties. Criminal matters are proceedings in which criminal statutes are at issue. In a criminal matter, the government (federal or state) is one of the parties. Legislatures enact criminal penalties providing for jail or monetary punishments for violation of the basic fundamentals of societal living (murder, robbery, etc). Another application of criminal punishment is to facilitate the enforcement of regulatory matters. To give administrative agencies authority, the legislature provides that violation of regulatory acts or rules is criminal and can be punished by

monetary penalties or incarceration. For example, in *Chalmers-Francis v Nelson* (1936),[2] one of the fundamental cases upholding nurse anesthetist practice, Dagmar Nelson was prosecuted under a criminal statute for illegally practicing medicine.

In a civil case, the courts are more concerned with compensating people for damages they have suffered because of improper actions than with punishment. It is difficult to provide absolute distinctions between criminal and civil matters, however, because legislatures have recognized that private litigation may also play an important role in public policy. To encourage private litigation, some statutes provide that litigants are entitled to a multiple of their damages. If the behavior of the defendant is reprehensible or careless, the courts sometimes impose punitive damages to discourage the defendant from engaging in harmful acts. In the antitrust area, Congress recognized that the US attorney general did not have the budget to bring every possible antitrust suit. To encourage private parties to bring antitrust actions, Congress provided that private litigants could recover 3 times their damages and receive reimbursement of attorneys' fees as well.

Civil Litigation

The 2 basic forms of civil litigation are (1) disputes over contracts and (2) claims for negligent or intentional infliction of injury, known as torts. The law of contracts allows private parties to create their own legal framework to govern their behavior. When parties enter into a contract, both parties are expected to perform their obligations. If one of the parties fails to perform the agreed obligation, the court will award damages based on the value of the performance the injured party did not receive. Tort liability, on the other hand, recognizes that each of us has a duty to act in a reasonable manner. Where our failure to act in a reasonable manner hurts or damages someone, and the damage was reasonably foreseeable, the court will award a monetary payment intended to equal the damage caused.

An illustration of the difference between contracts and torts can be seen in the 1929 case of *Hawkins v McGee,*[8] in which a physician transplanted skin to replace damaged skin on the palm of a patient's hand. The physician promised to make the hand perfect. He transplanted skin from a hairy part of the body to the palm giving the plaintiff a hairy palm. The patient sued. In this classic case, the question was not whether the physician was negligent for using skin from a hairy part of the body but whether the physician had promised (contracted) to give the patient a perfect hand, and if so, had carried out the contract. The court held that the physician had not made good on his promise and awarded damages. Damages were not based on the damage the physician had caused (the tort standard) but on the difference between a hand with hair on the palm and one that was perfect (the damage resulting from the physician's breach of contract).

Tort Liability

Standard of Care

The law of contracts governs many things concerning nurse anesthetists, including their employment, relationships with hospitals and physicians, purchases of drugs and equipment, and numerous other matters. However, when most nurse anesthetists think about the legal system, they think of the law of torts. Tort liability affects nurse anesthetists as it affects any member of society. When engaged in activities during which a failure to act reasonably can

be foreseen to result in harm, each of us owes a duty of care to others to act the way a reasonable person would act. For example, careless operation of an automobile can kill or severely injure other people. We are expected to drive automobiles as reasonably prudent persons would.

Because the courts do not understand what nurse anesthetists do, they designate nurse anesthesia as a profession. For a professional, the standard of care is more complicated. A professional must render care not as a reasonable person would act but with the same degree of skill and care as would be practiced by a reasonable member of the profession in similar circumstances. A nurse anesthetist has expertise and education that ordinary members of society do not have. This gives members of the profession the ability to largely determine the quality of care to be rendered by the profession. When a plaintiff questions whether the nurse anesthetist has rendered appropriate care, the court hears expert testimony as to what the standard is. In some areas of healthcare, the quality of care may vary from place to place. In those cases, practitioners are only held to the standard of care within their community. In specialty areas, such as anesthesia, there is a nationwide standard of care that does not vary from community to community.

Normally, only members of the profession are competent to testify as to the standard of care for their profession. Nurses testify to the standard of care in nursing; physicians testify to the standard of care in medicine. Some people erroneously assume or question whether there is a dual standard of care in the anesthesia field, one for anesthesiologists and one for nurse anesthetists. In fact, because of the nature of anesthesia and the fact that attention and proper monitoring of patients is the overwhelming factor in the safety of anesthesia, there is a single standard of care for the administration of anesthesia that is reflected not only in the reality of practice but also in standard-of-care cases. Standard of care is closely related to the quality of care. A profession that renders care at a lower standard than another will necessarily have a different quality of care.

In the anesthesia field quality of care between nurse anesthetists and anesthesiologists is uniform, and that is further evidence that the standard of care is the same. Consequently, there are cases when courts have permitted anesthesiologists to testify as to the standard of care to be followed by nurse anesthetists and cases in which nurse anesthetists have been allowed to testify as to the standard of care for anesthesiologists (*Carolan v Hill*, 1996).[9]

The standard of care for nurses is "to apply that degree of skill and learning in treating and nursing a patient which is customarily applied in treating or caring for the sick or wounded who are suffering in the same community." The Michigan case of *Whitney v Day* in 1980 is interesting because it was claimed that nurses were not entitled to a shortened statute of limitations available for professionals sued for malpractice.[10] The charge was made that nurses had to be examined on the same negligence standard as the general population. In *Whitney v Day,* the court specifically discussed the profession of nurse anesthetists. The court said[10(p711)]:

> nurse anesthetists are licensed as nurses and then they are certified after an 18 month period of study [this has, of course, been increased since the case was decided in 1980] in their specialty. Thus, they are professionals who have expertise in an area that is akin to the practice of medicine. Because a nurse

anesthetist possesses responsibilities greater than those possessed by an ordinary nurse, and because those responsibilities lie in an area of expertise in which some physicians receive full residency training, we conclude that it was not an error for the trial court to set forth a standard which . . . [incorporates the malpractice standard].

The court pointed out that the Michigan statute had been amended so that malpractice limitations were specifically made effective to nurses.

Because nurse anesthetists have been recognized as a separate professional group that establishes its own standard of care, it is understandable that the uninformed would assume that this standard of care would be different than that of an anesthesiologist. For example, in another Michigan case, *Theophelis v Lansing General Hospital* in 1985, there had been a suit against a hospital where both the nurse anesthetists and the anesthesiologist had been released from liability before trial.[11] In what really amounted to legal maneuvering in the absence of any factual information, the hospital argued that a release of the nurse anesthetists and the anesthesiologist implied that the hospital was innocent as well. The court, attempting to justify the trial court's determination to let trial proceed against the hospital, wrote: "we note for example that it would have been possible for the jury to determine that Nurse Palmer, given her limited training, was not negligent in failing to use a precordial stethoscope but that the hospital was negligent in not requiring the use of one."[11(p252)] This is sheer speculation on the part of the court and does not in any way determine that there is a different standard of care for nurse anesthetists. It does, however, illustrate what can happen when laypersons (who unfortunately include judges) are allowed to speculate, in the absence of information, about the nature of nurse anesthetists and nurse anesthesia.

More typical is the case of *Webb v Jorns* in 1971.[12] In this case involving a cardiac arrest during the course of administering the anesthetic, the court turned its attention to whether the nurse anesthetist had been negligent, specifically whether the patient had received an overdose of halothane. The expert was a physician. The testimony did not concern what a nurse anesthetist would or would not have done under the circumstances but rather whether in the physician's judgment there had been an overdose of halothane. The physician had testified that a mixture in excess of 1.5% halothane would have been an overdose, but the facts supported the position of the nurse anesthetist that the mixture had never exceeded 1.5%. Thus, the standard by which negligence was judged was a general standard based on what happens in the anesthesia area and not one that focused on whether nurse anesthetists follow different standards than anesthesiologists. It is not conceivable that nurse anesthetists would consider a maximum dosage to be 1.5% while anesthesiologists would have another maximum dose limitation.

Another case that supports the view of a single standard of care in anesthesia is *Parks v Perry* in 1984.[13] Numbness and weakness in a patient's hand was submitted to the jury under the doctrine of *res ipsa loquitur* (see the section on this topic later in this chapter) based on expert testimony that the damage would not have occurred in the absence of negligent administration of an anesthetic. No reference was made to the standard of care by nurse anesthetists or that

of anesthesiologists. Likewise, in *Yoos v Jewish Hospital of St Louis* (1982),[14] the court did not look at separate standards of care, but at what should and should not occur in the field of anesthesia.

Why is there only one standard of care in the anesthesia field? Because there is only one quality of care. Studies have shown that anesthesia incidents tend to occur because of human error or failure, not because of lack of education. Care and attentiveness are not attributes that depend on whether the practitioner is a nurse or a physician. Therefore, the standard of care in anesthesia is to be as careful and attentive as the human mind will permit.

The issue of the standard of care is a factual matter because it depends on the testimony of expert witnesses. What the expert testifies to and what the jury believes can vary from case to case. Disquieting though it may be, as a practical matter it must be recognized that the standard of professional care is determined on an individual basis for each case. Thus, to discuss standard of care requirements is to make a prediction what experts will testify and what the judge and jury will believe.

This point is illustrated by the 1990 case of *Washington v Washington Hospital Center, et al.*[15] Expert testimony as to what constitutes the standard of care cannot be based on mere speculation or conjecture but should have a factual basis. "While absolute certainty is not required, opinion evidence that is conjectural or speculative is not permitted" (*Washington v Washington Hospital Center*[15] quoting from *Sponaugle v Preterm, Inc,* 1980[16]). The testimony must show what the standard is as practiced by the profession. What a single practitioner would do does not establish the standard of care. Similarly, the testimony should not be what the expert would have done under

387

similar circumstances, but what members of the profession would do.

In the Washington case, the plaintiff was a healthy 36-year-old woman who underwent elective surgery at the Washington Hospital Center on November 7, 1987. An endotracheal tube was inserted into the esophagus rather than the trachea. It was not noticed until it was too late, and the plaintiff suffered catastrophic brain injury. The nurse anesthetist and anesthesiologist settled, and the case proceeded only against the hospital. It was claimed that the hospital was negligent in failing to provide an end-tidal carbon dioxide (CO_2) monitor, which would have allowed early detection of insufficient oxygen, arguably in time to prevent the brain injury. After a jury verdict in favor of the plaintiff, the hospital asked the trial court to rule that the expert testimony offered was insufficient and that judgment should have been entered in the hospital's favor, notwithstanding the jury verdict. The trial court refused, and the hospital appealed the decision to the District of Columbia Court of Appeals.

The plaintiff's expert had testified that the hospital deviated from the standard of care by failing to supply a CO_2 monitoring device. Among other things, the hospital claimed that the plaintiff's expert lacked an adequate factual basis for his testimony. The court noted that the standard of care was as follows[15]:

> the course of action that a reasonably prudent [professional] with the defendant's specialty would have taken under the same or similar circumstances. . . . Thus the question for decision is whether the evidence as a whole and reasonable inferences therefrom, would allow a reasonable juror to find that a reasonably prudent tertiary care hospital . . . at the time of [plaintiff's] injury in November 1987 and according to national standards, would have supplied a carbon dioxide monitor to a patient undergoing general anesthesia for elective surgery.

The plaintiff's expert had testified that the standard of care in November 1987 required a hospital to provide an end-tidal CO_2 monitor. The hospital charged that the plaintiff's expert based his opinion on inadequate facts. Even though the expert gave no testimony on the number of hospitals having end-tidal CO_2 monitors in place in 1987 and never referred to any written standards or authority as the basis of his opinion, the court concluded that his opinion, combined with other evidence concerning the standard of care, was sufficient to create an issue for the jury.

The hospital argued that end-tidal CO_2 monitors were not the standard of care. It pointed to an American Society of Anesthesiologists (ASA) policy that recommended but did not require them and standards adopted by Harvard Medical School teaching hospitals, which referred to CO_2 monitors only as an "emerging" standard. The court indicated nonetheless that the jury's conclusion should be allowed to stand based on other testimony introduced at trial. The question was what a reasonably prudent hospital would do, and "Hence, care and foresight exceeding the minimum required by law or mandatory professional regulation may be necessary to meet that standard."[15] Thus, the fact that neither the ASA nor Harvard Medical School recognized CO_2 monitors as a standard of care was irrelevant if a reasonably prudent hospital would have provided them.

To someone not familiar with anesthesia as it was practiced in 1987, the principles underlying the Washington case seem straightforward.

To those familiar with anesthesia in this period, the proof that was offered in the Washington case that CO_2 monitors were the standard of care seems pretty thin. Most practitioners would have agreed that end-tidal CO_2 monitors were not widely used in 1987 and were not part of the standard of care. Thus, a valuable lesson about the legal standard of care must be learned. Even though the standard of care is determined by practitioners, it must be found and applied by courts and juries who are subject to their own emotional demands. Those entities have substantial discretion to believe or not believe evidence and sources that practitioners might weigh differently. Standards set by professional organizations may be evidence of the standard of care, but they are not necessarily accepted as the standard of care. In addition, the courts reserve the right to determine that the level of care practiced by an entire profession may be inadequate, although this has been rare in the healthcare field.

Failure to Comply With Law or Regulation

The court's right to determine that a level of care is inadequate is similar to the ability of the legislature to set a standard of care without regard to the practices previously followed by a majority of the profession. Once the legislature enacts legislation creating the standard, it is the standard. Failure to follow a standard of care set forth in a statute is negligence in and of itself. This is known as "negligence per se." The principle of negligence per se is helpful to a plaintiff because the plaintiff does not have to offer expert testimony on the standard of care followed by the profession. *Central Anesthesia Associates, PC, et al v Worthy et*

al (1985)[17] demonstrates the application of this legal principle.

In the Worthy case, anesthesia was administered by a registered nurse enrolled as a student nurse anesthetist in a school operating at a hospital in the State of Georgia. The student nurse anesthetist was under the supervision of a physician assistant. During a tubal ligation procedure, the patient, Ms Worthy, suffered a cardiac arrest resulting in brain damage. During the cardiac arrest, only the obstetrician-gynecologist, the physician assistant, and the student nurse anesthetist were in the operating room where the surgery was being performed. At the time, Georgia had a statute that required that a CRNA administer anesthesia "under the direction and responsibility of a duly licensed physician with training or experience in anesthesia."[17] The requirement that the supervising physician have "training or experience in anesthesia" is unusual. In states where statutes require supervision, they usually only require that the supervisor be a physician. Large numbers of nurse anesthetists work with surgeons who have no training or experience in anesthesia (in fact, Georgia has since changed its law). Moreover, there is no indication as to whether this standard is higher or lower than normal practice standards. However, whatever Georgia's statute means, it does not permit a physician assistant to supervise a student nurse anesthetist.

The Worthy court held that the Georgia statute created a standard of conduct for those who are authorized to administer anesthesia. For negligence per se to apply, the person injured must be someone the statute was trying to protect. The court also held that the standard of conduct was created by the legislature to protect patients, such as Ms Worthy, from unreasonable risks associated with the administration of anesthesia. The court held that under the statute, the role of supervising a nurse administering anesthesia could not be delegated to a physician assistant. As a result, the court concluded that the defendants had violated the statute and were, therefore, negligent per se.

Other Evidence of Standard of Care

The standard of care is set by the profession except when courts may require a higher standard, if the profession sets it at an inadequate level. The legislature may also establish a standard of care in its discretion. Nonetheless, nongovernmental bodies, such as professional and accrediting agencies, hospitals, and institutions, frequently establish rules or policies that can be considered by the judge or jury as evidence of the standard of care. In certain cases, hospital or institutional rules can become binding by contract. In *Williams v St Claire Medical Center* (1983),[18] the issue presented to the court was whether a hospital owed a duty to its patients to enforce its policies and bylaws and, if so, whether a violation of these policies and bylaws constituted negligence per se. The patient suffered permanent brain damage while being administered an anesthetic by a nurse anesthetist who was not a CRNA.

The hospital's policy required that anesthetics be administered by a CRNA or a qualified physician. In addition, CRNAs were required to be supervised by the chairperson of anesthesia services and be in communication with an anesthesiologist and surgeon or obstetrician, except in emergency procedures, when an anesthesiologist was not available. At the time of the incident, the hospital, contrary to its own policies, did not have an anesthesiologist on staff, and the nurse anesthetist was not a CRNA.

The court held that when a patient consents to and authorizes an operation, he or she thereby accepts all the rules and regulations of the particular hospital at which the operation is performed. The court further held that while a patient must accept the hospital's particular rules and regulations, the patient should be able to rely on the hospital to follow its rules and regulations, ostensibly established for the patient's care. The plaintiff in this case argued that the hospital's violation of its own policies constituted negligence per se. The court refused to extend negligence per se to a hospital's policies but allowed the policies to be admitted as evidence of negligence. Similarly, in *Castillo v United States* (1975),[19] violation of institutional policy was not negligence per se but could be considered as a relevant factor in determining the extent of the duty owed to the patient.

Proving that an anesthetist failed to meet the standard of care can be difficult and expensive. The plaintiff's lawyers must obtain testimony as to the standard of care, must obtain and present evidence that the standard of care was breached, and must be able to present this to a jury in a way that will be understandable. This makes the trial of malpractice cases difficult and demanding for plaintiffs' lawyers. The economics of litigation push plaintiffs' lawyers to look for "magic bullets," which allow plaintiffs to recover, without expending the effort and costs of proving negligence. After the decision in the Worthy case was published, a number of cases followed, claiming that various routine aspects of nurse anesthesia practice violated state statutes and gave rise to negligence per se. For example, in *Mitchell v Amarillo Hospital District* (1993),[20] the Texas Court of Appeals dismissed a negligence per se case that had argued that nurse anesthesia constituted a denial of constitutionally guaranteed civil rights. Also, in *Drennan v Community Health Investment Corporation* (1995),[21] the Texas appellate courts dismissed yet another negligence per se claim that it was negligence per se for a pharmacy to dispense drugs to a CRNA.

Vicarious Liability

As hospitals evolved in the later part of the 19th century, the courts were confronted with this new entity. How they dealt with this entity demonstrates the application of fairness, consistency, predictability, and the effectuation of public policy. Part of the public policy in assessing damage for tort liability is to discourage dangerous conduct. Persons held liable should be able to adjust their conduct to avoid situations that cause damage. Moreover, persons liable either should be able to afford the damage or should be in a position to pass the cost of reimbursing injured parties on to other users of the products or services.

How did the courts award damage caused by nurses employed by hospitals but who were assisting independent contracting physicians? Nurses were often paid too little to be capable of paying for the damage their negligence might have caused. At the same time, the nurses were employed by hospitals that frequently were charitable institutions. Hospitals seldom made sufficient profit to absorb the cost of negligence of their employees. Holding hospitals liable for the negligence of the nurses they employed really meant asking contributors to the hospitals to pay patients for damages incurred. Consequently, the courts adapted to this entity by finding a new doctrine, "charitable immunity" in the existing "sovereign immunity" doctrine, an ancient

English legal doctrine that the king could not be liable because the king could do no wrong. Hospitals would not be liable for the negligence of their employees because they were performing government-like functions.

The doctrine of charitable immunity can be traced back to 1876 and the case of *McDonald v Massachusetts General Hospital*.[22] In this case, a patient claimed that he had been damaged by the actions of a doctor on the staff of Massachusetts General Hospital. The patient was receiving free care at the hospital, and the physicians and surgeons were also providing free services. Moreover, funds for Massachusetts General Hospital were derived primarily from grants and donations. Patients paid only according to their ability and not according to services they received. The Massachusetts court reasoned that the hospital was acting as if it were a government agency. Just as a government has sovereign immunity, the court held that a charity engaged in similar activities had "charitable immunity." If the grants and donations the charity solicited from the public were used to pay malpractice claims, the court worried that the public would not support the hospital, and a worthwhile activity would be denied the public. The result of charitable immunity was that patients themselves would bear the risk of negligence they encountered. However, it turned out that the courts were not willing to agree that patients who were injured at charitable hospitals could have no recourse.

One of the early principles of tort law was the doctrine of *respondeat superior*: "let the master answer." When damage is caused by a servant (later referred to as an employee), the master (later referred to as an employer) should be held responsible for it. It was the employer who controlled the way things were done and was in the best position to

391

see that the action giving rise to negligence was avoided. It was also the employer who sold the product, set the price, and earned the profit.

When *respondeat superior* was applied to nurses, the idea of holding their employer, the hospital protected by charitable immunity, responsible was not appealing. Who served in the role of "master" with regard to a nurse's negligence that occurred in a hospital? Ultimately, the courts agreed that the answer was the surgeon. It was the surgeon who attracted patients to a hospital, the surgeon who profited from the services of the hospital and its nursing employees, and the surgeon who had the apparent authority to be responsible to see that negligent actions were controlled and did not cause damage. Although the surgeon was not the employer in a strict sense, negligence of the nurse and other hospital employees was attributed to the surgeon.

In a number of cases, including *Schloendorf v Society of New York Hospital* (1914),[23] the courts held that physicians who were on the hospital's staff were not employees of the hospital and the physicians' negligence could not be blamed on the hospital. Similarly, nurses engaged in treating patients, even though paid by the hospital, were acting to benefit the surgeon and should be treated as servants of the surgeon. This developed into doctrines known as "captain of the ship" (which held that once the surgeon assumed control of the operating room, the surgeon was responsible for everything, including negligence that occurred) and "borrowed servant" (which held that a doctor may be held liable for the negligence of a hospital employee who is subject to the doctor's control).

But what about the hospital's administrative employees who are not engaged in

patient care? What control did a surgeon exercise over a billing clerk, security guard, or cook? They could not be said to be "borrowed" by surgeons. In fact, nurses did not spend all of their time on patient care; time was spent on administrative matters as well. Despite the doctrines of captain of the ship and borrowed servant, there were some activities of hospital employees for which only the hospital could be liable. In some states, persons damaged by administrative acts of hospital employees were unable to recover. In other states, the courts attempted to deal with this problem by developing exceptions to charitable immunity. When a nurse negligently injured a patient while engaged in administrative activities, only the hospital was liable, but when a nurse injured a patient while engaged in medical duties, the surgeon was liable. Even in the earliest days of the 20th century, the healthcare field was quite complicated, and because lawyers and courts do not understand healthcare, these fine distinctions led to a number of seemingly inconsistent holdings about the liability of nurses and hospital employees.

Because there were activities of their employees for which the hospitals were liable and a sense that charitable immunity would not last forever, hospitals began to purchase liability insurance. In 1957, New York began to roll back its support of the doctrines of charitable immunity and captain of the ship (*Bing v Thunig*).[24] In doing so, the court emphasized the inconsistent results of charitable immunity.

As charitable immunity died, one would have expected its companions, captain of the ship and borrowed servant, to die with it. However, they continued as the courts made difficult decisions between consistency and predictability on the one hand and fairness on the other. As the captain of the ship doctrine unfolded and was further developed by the courts, the courts realized that what was important about the relationship of the surgeon to the hospital staff was not the legal status of employer/employee (which everyone knew was a fiction) but the nature of control established by the surgeon. Where the surgeon actually controlled the negligent act, the nurse or other assistant was acting as the surgeon's agent, and the negligence of the nurse or other assistant should properly be charged to the surgeon. Moreover, to hold the surgeon liable, the surgeon had to be able to control the means, not just the outcome. Because anesthesia is a specialized area requiring additional education, surgeons do not normally control the means followed by nurse anesthetists. The type of control normally exercised by a surgeon ("Keep the patient still; keep him quiet!") is not the type of control leading to liability. Captain of the ship and its fellow travelers, such as borrowed servant, have fallen out of favor in recent years as courts have more clearly seen that an operating room is a complex byplay of professionals with areas of specialty, and that the surgeon's role is one of coordination rather than control. Increasingly, surgeons are held liable only when they actually control the means of an action that gives rise to the negligence and not when they are deemed to have assumed the helm of the operating room or to satisfy other nautical or military analogies.

Misrepresentations Concerning Vicarious Liability of Nurse Anesthetists

In the early part of the 1980s, the number of anesthesiologists in the United States increased dramatically. Certain anesthesiologists had believed that when there was a sufficient number of anesthesiologists, the healthcare community would turn to physician anesthesia and the practice of nurse anesthesia would die out. When that did not happen, some anesthesiologists began to compete with nurse anesthetists by warning surgeons of the so-called significant risks that surgeons took when operating with a nurse anesthetist rather than an anesthesiologist. This risk was based in large part on the captain of the ship theory of legal liability, even though fewer and fewer states recognized it.

In holding physicians liable for the negligence of anesthetists, the courts, except in states still following captain of the ship, do not look at whether the anesthesia administrator is a nurse or a physician but at the degree of control the physician exercises over the anesthesia administrator. Thus, a court may render different conclusions for cases that involve a physician working with a CRNA or, for that matter, a physician working with an anesthesiologist, if the physician controlled the ways and means of anesthesia in one case but not in the other. A physician or authorized provider is neither automatically liable when working with a CRNA, nor is the physician immune from liability when working with an anesthesiologist.

In *Schneider v Einstein Medical Center* (1978)[25] and *Kitto v Gilbert* (1977),[26] the court found surgeons liable for the negligence of anesthesiologists because the surgeons controlled the anesthesiologists' actions. The question, as in cases of a physician working with CRNAs, is whether the physician was in control of the acts of the anesthesiologists. This is a factual inquiry and not a conclusion of law. There are many cases in which courts have found that the surgeon was not in control of the CRNA and, therefore, not liable for the negligence of the CRNA. These include *Cavero v*

Franklin Benevolence Society (1950),[27] *Fortson v McNamara* (1987),[28] *Franklin v Gupta* (1990),[29] *Goodman v Phythyon* (1990),[30] *Hughes v St Paul Fire and Marine Insurance Company* (1981),[31] *Kemalyan v Henderson* (1954),[32] *Pierre v Lavallie Kamp Charity Hospital* (1987),[33] *Sesselman v Mulenberg Hospital* (1954),[34] *Starcher v Byrne* (1997),[35] and *Thomas v Raleigh General Hospital* (1987).[36]

Even in cases in which the surgeon was held liable, there is often evidence of individual wrongdoing on the part of the surgeon. Moreover, numerous cases hold that mere supervision or direction of a CRNA is insufficient evidence to hold a physician liable for the CRNA's negligence. See, for example, *Whitfield v Whittaker Memorial Hospital* (1969),[37] *Foster v Englewood Hospital* (1974),[38] *Elizondo v Tavarez* (1980),[39] *Baird v Sickler* (1982),[40] *McCullough v Bethany Medical Center* (1984),[41] and *Parker v Vanderbilt* (1988).[42] It is clear from the case law that in order for a physician to be liable for the acts of the anesthesia administrator, the physician must be in control of the ways and means of the administrator's actions and not merely be supervising or directing the administrator.

Consequently, court decisions concerning liability of surgeons for the negligence of nurse anesthetists have varied depending on the facts of the particular case. Where surgeons have been held to be in control of the ways and means of anesthesia, they have been held liable, and where they have not, they have not been held liable. The same principles govern liability of surgeons for negligence of anesthesiologists.

It does not make sense for either nurse anesthetists or anesthesiologists to attempt to capitalize on the errors of the other. Not only can anesthesiologists make mistakes, but surgeons can be sued when they work with anesthesiologists just as easily as they can when they work with nurse anesthetists. Case examples are *Adams v Children's Mercy Hospital* (1993),[43] *Bert v Meyer* (1997),[44] *Brown v Bozorgi* (1992),[45] *Carolan v Hill* (1996),[9] *Dunn v Maras* (1995),[46] *Kerber v Sarles* (1989),[47] *Kitto v Gilbert* (1977),[26] *Medvecz v Choi* (1977),[48] *Menzie v Windham Community Memorial Hospital* (1991),[49] *Quintal v Laurel Grove Hospital* (1965),[50] *Robertson v Hospital Corporation of America* (1995),[51] *Ruby Jones v Neuroscience Associates, Inc* (1992),[52] *Schneider v Einstein Medical Center* (1978),[25] *Seneris v Haas* (1955),[53] *Szabo v Bryn Mawr Hospital* (1994),[54] *Thompson v Presbyterian Hospital* (1982),[55] *Tiburzio-Kelly v Montgomery* (1996),[56] and *Vogler v Dominguez* (1994).[57]

The Lawyer

Although anesthesia is very safe, nurse anesthetists face occasional litigation or may require assistance to deal with regulatory boards. Courts and administrative agencies have their own rules to make their tasks flow more efficiently. Thus, nurse anesthetists may meet another element of the legal system, the lawyer. One of the biggest benefits of professional liability insurance is that it will cover the cost of a lawyer to represent the nurse anesthetist who faces suit. The lawyer provided by professional liability insurance will face a number of important, if conflicting, concerns as he or she addresses a case. Litigation can be and often is extremely expensive. Litigation is also uncertain. We all like to think that we govern our activities solely on the basis of logic; however, human beings, including those who serve on juries, are complicated. Sometimes they are affected by things that are not logical, including emotions such as sympathy for a severely damaged patient.

Finally, the parties in any given litigation matter are engaged in a complex drama in which interests and relationships often are not what they appear to be. For example, the nurse anesthetist involved in a malpractice lawsuit is provided a lawyer by the insurance carrier. The nurse anesthetist's attorney has a duty of loyalty to the nurse anesthetist. However, the lawyer is hired by the insurance company and the attorney's bills will be paid by the insurance company. Usually, this will not be the only matter referred to the attorney by the insurance company. On the other hand, nurse anesthetists are rarely involved in more than one malpractice claim. A nurse anesthetist whose practice creates enough malpractice claims to have a regular relationship with a malpractice attorney will probably lose the ability to practice either because of the inability to obtain malpractice insurance or as a result of a licensing decision. Human nature makes it likely that the attorney will have more loyalty to the insurance company than to the insured.

Sometimes there can be a conflict between the insurance company and the insured. To an insurance company, litigation is often a simple financial decision. If it is going to cost a lot in legal fees to defend a case and if a jury is likely to award a large recovery regardless of fault, then business concerns suggest that the case be settled and the risk of greater loss avoided. To a healthcare practitioner, who views himself or herself as innocent, deciding whether to settle may not be that easy. Agreeing to a settlement carries with it a number of unpleasant ramifications. The practitioner's name will be referred to the National Practitioner Data Bank. People may assume that if a practitioner settled, he or she must have done something wrong. A settlement can cause problems later on and may

have to be explained to future employers. How willing will the insurance company be to continue to provide insurance coverage for a practitioner who has cost the company a lot of money? From the insurance company's standpoint, it is easy for insureds to want the insurance company to defend their honor, no matter the cost. Insureds do not have to pay for it.

Because of these conflicts inherent in the insurance relationship, the question sometimes arises: Who does the lawyer represent? The 1991 case of *Trementozzi v Safety Insurance Co*[58] stated that the duty of a lawyer provided by an insurance company is to represent the insured and not the insurance company, even though the insurance company may pay the bills. Both the lawyer and the insurance company are obligated to act in the best interests of the insured. Lawyers are not supposed to represent clients with different interests at the same time.[59]

Nurse anesthetists must be aware of and involved in their legal defense. Even knowledgeable healthcare defense attorneys may not be familiar with the capabilities of nurse anesthetists. The insurance company may also be providing coverage for multiple defendants. Nurse anesthetists must be vigilant that their interests are being protected. They are entitled to a defense that protects their best interests, not the interests of the insurance company paying the bills.

The attorney-client privilege protects one of the oldest confidential relationships in society. Communication between attorney and client is protected because of the need of attorneys and their clients to have open, full, and frank discussions. What happens to this privilege when the attorney is representing conflicting clients? The attorney-client privilege only protects documents and disclosures that are not disclosed to third parties. If someone discloses information to persons with whom there is no privilege, then the information is not confidential and it is no longer privileged even if his or her attorney were part of the group to whom the information was disclosed.

Damages

The amount of damages awarded to a successful plaintiff depends on the type of case. In a suit based on a breach of contract, damages are based on the difference between what was promised or agreed to and what was delivered. In a tort case, damages are measured by the value of the damage inflicted by the defendant. In the healthcare field, trying to value the damage caused is a major area of dispute. As with many other areas for which there cannot be precise answers, damages are an area for the jury to answer as best it can. In the case of bodily injury, monetary damages are awarded to compensate people for damage that has no monetary value. What is the value of a chipped tooth? How do you monetarily compensate for the loss of eyesight or death? Some lawyers have been quite successful in refining techniques to increase jury awards for damage to the body. Awarding damages when harm results from a failure to meet the standard of care compensates the individual who was damaged and encourages practitioners to be careful. Damages based on the value of the injury caused, even if it is difficult to value, are called compensatory damages.

If the wrongdoing has been intentional or gives a sense of outrage, courts may award punitive, or exemplary, damages. Something more than mere negligence is required for punitive damages. There must be circumstances of aggravation, spite, or malice; a fraudulent or evil motive; or a conscious disregard of the interests of others.[60] Punitive damages are private fines imposed to punish reprehensible conduct and to deter its future occurrence.

An important aspect of punitive damages is the lack of insurance coverage. Many professional liability insurance policies do not insure against intentional acts. Punitive damages are imposed for intentional actions and therefore are not covered by insurance. Critics of the legal system contend that, in the healthcare field, when juries award punitive damages, they merely multiply their award. Because awarding compensatory damage for bodily damage has little basis in reality anyway, compensatory damage already punishes the defendant. Awarding punitive damages is just another opportunity to invite a jury to grant large awards.

Cases imposing punitive damages against nurse anesthetists are rare. The Georgia Court of Appeals, in a close 5:4 split, reversed the award of punitive damages in a 1991 case where, apparently, the anesthesia machine ran out of agent and had to be refilled during the operation.[61] Running out of an anesthetic agent in the middle of surgery is, obviously, a violation of the standard of care. Four of the 9 judges would have upheld the award of punitive damages. They reasoned that the jury had determined that the anesthesia machine would not have run out of agent if it had been checked. The failure to check the level of anesthetic was similar to failing to check the level of gas before flying an airplane. It shows such a conscious indifference to the patient's well-being that the jury was entitled to award punitive damages. On the other hand, the majority of the Court of Appeals held that there was no evidence of an intentional disregard of the rights of the patient, nor was there any evidence that the anesthesia providers knowingly or willfully disregarded the rights of the patient so as to authorize a finding of conscious indifference to consequences.

Another case involving punitive damages arose in Arkansas, where a jury assessed $3 million in punitive damages against the manufacturer of a ventilator. There was evidence that the manufacturer was aware that anesthetists using a selector valve could easily place hoses on the wrong unmarked valve, with disastrous results. In the Arkansas case, someone had incorrectly put a hose where a bag should have been connected. When the nurse anesthetist decided to change bags, she attached a hose to the wrong port. The effect of the improper connection was to permit the anesthesia machine to continue to pump air into the patient's lungs, with no way for the air to escape. The ensuing buildup of pressure and lack of oxygen resulted in damage to the patient's lungs and brain. The rule for imposing punitive damages in Arkansas is that the defendant must have known, or ought to have known, in light of the surrounding circumstances, that its conduct would naturally or probably result in injury and that the defendant continued such conduct in reckless disregard. The manufacturer claimed it was not at fault because separate acts of negligence had to occur for the accident to result. Many witnesses testified that the accident was foreseeable. The unmarked valve had been criticized in premarket tests, and other similar incidents involving the machine had been reported. The appeals court upheld the jury award of punitive damages because the manufacturer knew that the patient's life always depended on the artificial breathing supplied by the ventilator (*Airco, Inc, Appellant, v Simmons First National Bank, Guardian*, 1982).[62]

Because of the great risks involved in anesthesia, even the smallest moment of carelessness can have disastrous consequences. Nurse anesthetists can avoid the imposition of punitive damages by being able to prove that they followed procedures, such as the use of checklists designed to minimize the possibility of lapses, and by being able to document that they acted in the best interest of their patient, even after an incident occurred.

Res Ipsa Loquitur

A key element of the law of negligence is fault. Awards are made against a defendant because the defendant caused the damage. The theoretical basis of negligence or malpractice is that the defendant should pay for damages caused to the plaintiff because, between the 2 parties, the one who was at fault should bear the damage. In terms of prevention, the knowledge that one can be held liable for malpractice or negligence is supposed to make people more careful and avoid negligent actions in the future. In cases involving anesthesia, how does the patient show that the anesthetist was at fault? The field is too complicated for the average patient to understand. Sometimes the patient does not even know what happened because he or she was unconscious. As a result, many cases involving malpractice of anesthetists are decided under the legal doctrine of *res ipsa loquitur*.

Res ipsa loquitur, literally translated as "the thing speaks for itself," had its basis in a case decided in 1863 in which a barrel of flour rolled out of a warehouse window and fell on a passing pedestrian (*Byrne v Boadle*).[63] Although the injured pedestrian had not personally observed whatever went wrong on the upper floor of the warehouse, it was clear that this type of accident would not have happened without someone's negligence. Whoever caused it must have been under the control of the warehouse owner.[63]

397

The doctrine of *res ipsa loquitur* depends on 3 things: (1) the injury must occur under circumstances such that in the ordinary course of events the injury would not have occurred if someone had not been negligent, (2) the injury must be caused by something within the exclusive control of the defendant, and (3) the injury must not have been due to any voluntary action or contribution on the part of the plaintiff. Classic examples are exploding boilers, defective food in sealed containers, and various types of falling objects, including not only barrels of flour but also elevators and, in one case, a 600-lb cow.

Anesthesia accidents have become prime examples for the application of the doctrine of *res ipsa loquitur*. In an anesthesia accident, the third requisite that the plaintiff did not contribute to the accident, is almost always true, especially where the patient is unconscious. Similarly, if an anesthesia injury has occurred, the instrumentality that caused the damage will often have been within the exclusive control of the anesthetist. It is the application of the first requisite, that the event must be of a kind that ordinarily does not occur in the absence of someone's negligence, that has caused whatever theoretical disputes there may be over the application of the doctrine to anesthesia.

Although the basis of the law of negligence is fault, many accidents can occur without anyone being at fault. Someone slipping and falling, a blowout of a tire, skidding cars, and fires of unknown origin have all been held to be situations where the doctrine of *res ipsa loquitur* would not apply because it could not be said that the injury could not have occurred without negligence.[60]

Theoretically, laypeople are supposed to understand that anesthesia is an area where accidents can happen without anyone being at fault. Realistically, however, it is a tribute to anesthetists that anesthesia accidents occur so infrequently that there is a common tendency, albeit incorrect, to believe that the accident would not have occurred without someone being negligent. There is also a financial incentive for the patient to base the case on *res ipsa loquitur*. Lawsuits can be very expensive, and part of the expense is hiring expert witnesses to testify as to the standard of care. The major benefit to a patient of the doctrine of *res ipsa loquitur* is that it moves the burden of proof to the defendant.

How can a defendant-anesthetist defend a case of *res ipsa loquitur*? The defendant must introduce proof that (1) whatever instrumentalities were in the defendant's exclusive control during the operation were not those that caused the injuries and/or (2) there were ways in which the incident could have occurred other than as a result of the anesthetist's negligence. Thus, in anesthesia cases, the role of the jury becomes one of choosing to believe the defendant's expert witnesses or the plaintiff's expert witnesses as to whether the injury would have occurred without negligence.

Summary

The legal system is imperfect, as are all human systems, in its attempts to resolve disputes in a fair, consistent, and predictable manner. Nurse anesthetists should be aware of their status as professionals and the principle that the system expects them to act as other nurse anesthetists would act.

398

References

1. California Nursing Act (Cal Business and Professions Code, Chapter 6, Code 2725, 1974).

2. *Chalmers-Francis v Nelson*, 6 Cal 2d 402 (1936).

3. *Bentley v Langley*, 249 SE2d 481 (NC 1978).

4. *Sermchief v Gonzales*, 660 SW2d 683 (Mo 1983).

5. *Magit v State of California*, 57 Cal 2d 74 (1961).

6. *US v Lopez*, 514 US 549 (1995).

7. *Kentucky Association of Health Plans v Miller*, 538 US 329 (2003).

8. *Hawkins v McGee*, 84 NH 114, 146 A 641 (NH 1929).

9. *Carolan v Hill*, 553 NW2d 882 (Iowa 1996).

10. *Whitney v Day*, 100 Mich App 707 (1980).

11. *Theophelis v Lansing General Hospital*, 355 NW2d 249 (1985).

12. *Webb v Jorns*, 473 SW2d (Tex 1971).

13. *Parks v Perry*, 68 NC App 202 (NC 1984).

14. *Yoos v Jewish Hospital of St Louis*, 645 SW2d 177 (Mo 1982).

15. *Washington v Washington Hospital Center, et al*, 579 A2d 177 (DC Ct App 1990).

16. *Sponaugle v Pre-term, Inc*, 411 A2d 366 (DC 1980) (DC Ct App 1990).

17. *Central Anesthesia Associates, PC, et al v Worthy, et al*, 254 Ga 728, 333 SE2d 829 (1985).

18. *Williams v St Claire Medical Center*, 657 SW2d 590 (Ky Ct App 1983).

19. *Castillo v US*, 406 F Supp 585 (NM 1975).

20. *Mitchell v Amarillo Hospital District*, 885 SW2d 857, Texas, 1993).

21. *Drennan v Community Health Investment Corporation* (905 S.W. 2d 811, Texas, 1995).

22. *McDonald v Massachusetts General Hospital* (120 Mass 432, 1876).

23. *Schloendorf v Society of New York Hospital*, 211 NY 125, 105 NE 92 (1914).

24. *Bing v Thunig*, 2 NY 2d 656, 143 NE2d 3 (1957).

25. *Schneider v Einstein Medical Center*, 390 A2d 1271 (Pa 1978).

26. *Kitto v Gilbert*, 570 P2d 544 (Colo 1977).

27. *Cavero v Franklin Benevolence Society*, 223 P2d 471 (Cal 1950).

28. *Fortson v McNamara*, 508 So2d 35 (Fla 1987).

29. *Franklin v Gupta*, 567 A2d 524 (Md 1990).

30. *Goodman v Phythyon*, 803 SW2d 697 (Tenn 1990).

31. *Hughes v St Paul Fire and Marine Insurance Company*, 401 So2d 35 (Fla 1987).

32. *Kemalyan v Henderson*, 277 P2d 372 (Wash 1954).

33. *Pierre v Lavallie Kamp Charity Hospital*, 515 So2d 614 (La 1987).

34. *Sesselman v Mulenberg Hospital*, 306 A2d 474 (NJ 1954).

35. *Starcher v Byrne*, 687 So2d 737 (Miss 1997).

36. *Thomas v Raleigh General Hospital*, 358 SE2d 222 (WVa 1987).

37. *Whitfield v Whittaker Memorial Hospital*, 210 Va 176 (1969).

38. *Foster v Englewood Hospital*, 19 Ill App 3d 1055 (1974).

39. *Elizondo v Tavarez*, 596 SW2d 667 (Tex 1980).

40. *Baird v Sickler*, 69 Ohio St2d 652 (1982).

399

41. *McCullough v Bethany Medical Center,* 235 Kan 732 (1984).

42. *Parker v Vanderbilt,* 767 SW2d 412 (Tenn 1988).

43. *Adams v Children's Mercy Hospital,* 848 SW2d 535 (Mo Ct App 1993).

44. *Bert v Meyer,* 663 NYS2d 99 (NY 1997).

45. *Brown v Bozorgi,* 234 Ill App 3d 972, 602 NE2d 48 (1992).

46. *Dunn v Maras,* 182 Ariz 412, 897 P2d 714 (1995).

47. *Kerber v Sarles,* 542 NYS2d 94, 151 A2d 1031 (NY 1989).

48. *Medvecz v Choi,* 569 F 2d 1221, US Ct App, 3d Cir (1977).

49. *Menzie v Windham Community Memorial Hospital,* 774 F Supp 91 (Conn 1991).

50. *Quintal v Laurel Grove Hospital,* 62 Cal2d 154; 397 P2d 161 (1965).

51. *Robertson v Hospital Corporation of America,* 653 S2d 1265 (Ct App La 1995).

52. *Ruby Jones v Neuroscience Associates, Inc,* 250 Kan 477, 827 P2d 51 (1992).

53. *Seneris v Haas,* 45 Cal2d 811, 291 P2d 915 (Cal 1955).

54. *Szabo v Bryn Mawr Hospital,* 432 Pa Super 409, 638 A2d 1004 (1994).

55. *Thompson v Presbyterian Hospital,* 652 P2d 260 (Okla 1982).

56. *Tiburzio-Kelly v Montgomery,* 452 Pa Super 158, 681 A2d 757 (1996).

57. *Vogler v Dominguez,* 624 NE2d 56 (Ind 1994).

58. *Trementozzi v Safety Insurance Co,* Mass Suffolk Sup Ct Civil Action No. 90-1017B (June 26, 1991).

59. American Bar Association. *ABA Model Code of Professional Responsibility,* Rule 1,7. Chicago, IL: American Bar Association; 1983).

60. Prosser WL, Keeton WP, Dobbs WB, eds. *Law of Torts.* 5th ed. St Paul, MN: West Group; 1995:9217.

61. *Newton Hospital,* 200 Ga. App. 788; 409 SE2d 572, 1991.

62. *Airco Inc, Appellant, v Simmons First National Bank, Guardian,* 2765 Ark 486, 638 SW2d 660 (1982).

63. *Byrne v Boadle,* 159 Eng Rep 299 (1863).

400

Key References

1. A broad variety of legal issues involving CRNA practice, employment, and other professional issues can be found in the "Legal Briefs" section of the *AANA Journal.* Articles by Gene Blumenreich and other legal experts can be reviewed through the annual index of the *Journal.* All publications are available in the library or archives of the AANA in Park Ridge, Illinois.

Study Questions

1. Why is it that courts generally grant substantial deference to the healthcare community? What relationship does this behavior have to traditional definitions of professionalism?

2. Identify which court cases involving CRNAs have had major implications for the profession since the turn of the century. What is their enduring legacy to contemporary practice?

3. Using the AANA standards of care as a reference, discuss how standards developed, what external agencies have influenced them, and how technology and scientific advances have influenced their refinement.

4. Propose reasons why there is a single standard of care in anesthesia for all providers. What benefits does this fact accrue to CRNAs?

5. List the state bureaucratic agencies/bodies and other professional organizations or institutions that have a direct and compelling influence on the standard of care of CRNAs.

6. What argument would you provide a surgeon who is refusing to work with you because of the issue of vicarious liability? What is your rationale and what are the facts?

7. Define and discuss the relevance in practice of the legal doctrines of *respondeat superior*, captain of the ship, borrowed servant, charitable immunity, and *res ipsa loquitur*.

CHAPTER 17
Understanding Malpractice Litigation

Janet M. Simpson, JD

Key Concepts

- Standard of care can be defined as the level of care generally practiced by members of the profession in the same or similar circumstances (community), a deviation from which represents a risk of injury to the patient or plaintiff. Medical negligence occurs when a Certified Registered Nurse Anesthetist (CRNA) does not exercise the required degree of skill and reasonable care espoused by this standard, and "duty, breach, and causation" exist.

- The most commonly considered evidence for standard of care comes from the expert witness, who must testify regarding medical probabilities, events, or deviations.

- All CRNAs bear the responsibility to report notice or receipt of a claim or lawsuit to their insurance carrier, be available to meet with an assigned attorney, and actively assist the legal team in preparing the facts, evidence, and plan for defense.

- There are several types of depositions in which CRNAs may be involved, all of which require detailed preparation. Depositions are guided by strict protocol and can best be prepared for with careful study and planning.

- Occurrence insurance is the preferable type of liability product covering all acts occurring within the policy period regardless of when the lawsuit is filed, but it is generally much more expensive than claims-made insurance.

In the course of an active clinical career, most Certified Registered Nurse Anesthetists (CRNAs) will come in contact with the civil justice system—hopefully not, however, as a defendant. If such an occasion does arise, the CRNA must understand in detail the course of malpractice litigation and how best to prepare a defense. This chapter introduces the most common sources of claims and lawsuits filed against anesthetists and presents details regarding the frequency of suits, assertions of negligence, causes of injuries, types of injuries, and amounts of money paid in damages to the plaintiff. By studying these data, one can draw general conclusions regarding the prevention and defense of medical negligence actions. The chapter also acquaints the CRNA with the process of a medical negligence lawsuit and details what to expect during the proceedings, including guidance from the insurance carrier and attorney, depositions and trial testimony, acting as an expert witness, confidential and privileged communications, and settlement and trial considerations. Issues involving professional liability insurance and coverage benefits also are discussed.

Most importantly, this chapter will help CRNAs to appreciate the importance of communication with patients and families as a primary defense against malpractice litigation. Although the national trend demonstrates a decrease in the number of anesthesia mishaps and complications, the severity of injury from complications may be devastating. It is paramount that CRNAs appreciate the fact that effective, attentive communication with families and patients attenuates litigation risk, but only when accompanied by comprehensive and legible documentation of perioperative events.

Considerations in Negligence

The ever-present threat of a medical negligence lawsuit substantially influences the day-to-day delivery of healthcare. Reasons for the threat of suit are numerous but relate generally to consumer dissatisfaction and frustration with the healthcare system at large. The system appears insensitive and often fails to consider the effects of its actions or nonactions on the patient and the patient's family. In addition, adequate healthcare is priced beyond the means of many in society. In the United States, there are more than 50.7 million people who cannot afford health insurance (in 2009).[1] The United States spent nearly $2.3 trillion a year in 2008 on healthcare yet provides no universal coverage.[2] With these statistics, it is no wonder that many citizens hold great contempt for the system in general, as well as for the providers who seemingly represent this flawed and unresponsive system. It should also be noted that patients and their families frequently have unrealistic expectations of both the healthcare system and providers. Complicated medical and surgical procedures that do not produce desired outcomes reinforce the public's perception that failure to obtain ideal medical results constitutes negligence. In addition, litigants have unrealistic expectations both of the monetary awards that can be secured in negligence cases and the total cost of litigation itself.

These notions often overshadow the fact that, beginning in the 1980s, anesthesia mishaps have been in steady decline for both nurse and physician providers of anesthesia. The overall mortality rate has dropped from approximately 1 death for every 1,000 anesthetics given 50 years ago to approximately 323 deaths per year from all anesthetics given in the United States. As is consistently shown, there is no statistically significant difference between CRNA and anesthesiologist rates of injury and death attributable to anesthesia-related causes. These data can be accessed on the American Association of Nurse Anesthetists (AANA) website (www.aana.com) or through AANA library archives in Park Ridge, Illinois.

Components of Medical Negligence

Often one hears the term *medical malpractice* used more frequently in popular jargon than the term *medical negligence*. The former is technically incorrect, as there is no legal theory of malpractice, be it medical, legal, architectural, or related to any other discipline. There is, however, a legal theory of negligence about which the CRNA must become familiar.

Legal theories are composed of specific elements, and the plaintiff has the burden of proof for all elements of negligence. The first element in negligence is duty. The plaintiff must prove that a duty to exercise reasonable care existed between the plaintiff and the defendant, in this case the anesthetist. Anytime an anesthetist undertakes patient care, he or she must exercise reasonable care. If debate arises on this element, it generally involves whether the anesthetist entered into a professional relationship with the patient.

As an example, if 2 anesthetists with the same last name are working in the same hospital and a plaintiff sues the one who did not provide anesthetic care, the claim fails because there is no duty to exercise reasonable care flowing from the anesthetist sued by the plaintiff. That is, no patient-anesthetist relationship was ever established between these 2 individuals. Taking a less obvious example, if an anesthetic is planned for 1 PM, and the anesthetist preoperatively visited the

patient at 9 AM, can the patient prevail in a suit if her appendix ruptures between 9 AM and 1 PM? Does a duty exist between the patient and CRNA? The simple answer is probably. However, circumstances involving other required elements will likely arise to make this case defensible as well.

The second element involves breach of the anesthetist's duty to exercise reasonable care with the patient. This is the negligent act, error, or omission part of the formula. The anesthetist must act within the appropriate standard of care in providing anesthesia services to the patient. The patient's petition or complaint filed to initiate the lawsuit generally sets out the allegations of negligence. A plaintiff asserts that several actions were carried out improperly or were omitted, thus making a claim that these actions, errors, and/or omissions constituted negligence on the part of the anesthetist. For example, the plaintiff may claim the defendant should have employed a regional rather than general anesthetic technique. This allegation involves negligent professional judgment. Alternatively, a plaintiff may allege that the anesthetist improperly placed an endotracheal tube in the esophagus and failed to recognize its misplacement. This involves an allegation of technical error and a judgment or diagnostic error.

In all instances, the breach must have caused physical injury to the plaintiff, or the plaintiff's decedent, as the case may be. This represents the third element of negligence, causation. The anesthetist may have negligently administered the anesthetic, but the patient had no injury. For example, if the CRNA anesthetized the patient with a general anesthetic agent, turned on the ventilator, and left the room, this would constitute improper care. Yet, if the patient awoke at the end of the case without sequelae, a

405

lawsuit based on these circumstances would fail for lack of a causation element because there was no physical injury.

Assume the same conduct by the anesthetist, but this time the patient is injured. The surgeon nicked a ureter. Still, the case of medical negligence against the anesthetist fails because the nicked ureter and the anesthetist leaving the operating room (OR) are not linked. Again, there is no causation element. The plaintiff must prove he or she was injured as a result of the negligent conduct. An unfortunate result, in and of itself, does not raise the question of negligence. In fact, the law is to the contrary. In most jurisdictions, the healthcare provider is entitled to exercise his or her best judgment, because the public and courts understand that medicine is not an exact science. In some jurisdictions, if the healthcare provider exercises the required degree of skill, he or she is not liable for any honest error in judgment.[1] This assumes that the action carried out was an action that a reasonable healthcare provider might elect as a treatment option.

Assessing Standards of Care

For a plaintiff to proceed to a point at which a jury can consider the case, he or she must establish what the appropriate standard of care is related to the alleged negligent acts or omissions. The standard of care can be defined as that level of care generally practiced by members of the profession in the same or similar circumstances, a deviation from which represents a risk of injury to the patient/plaintiff. The "same or similar community" is also referenced by many when describing the appropriate standard of care. Be aware that the definition of community has expanded dramatically because of continuing education requirements and

because national professional groups have promulgated standards and goals for safe practice.[3] Professional groups publishing and endorsing standards hope that by reducing patient injury, the number of medical negligence claims and lawsuits will decrease through improved practice techniques. This will focus the issues and merits for attorney consideration before suits are filed and shorten the time and expense associated with litigation.[2]

There are a variety of means available to establish, for a jury's consideration, the appropriate standard of care. These include but are not limited to textbooks, authoritative treatises, professional journal articles, facility policy and procedures, standards or policy statements of professional organizations, expert witnesses, state or federal statutes, and prior case law. Textbooks, treatises, and journal articles, however, may not be sufficient by themselves to override the professionals' general practice patterns. This evidence often must be supported with expert testimony.[3]

An individual facility's policies and procedures are actually self-imposed standards. They state the standard of care expected of its healthcare providers. The rationale for these standards is generally patient safety. Therefore, if an anesthetist fails to follow anesthesia departmental policies and procedures and an adverse result occurs, there is little justification for the deviation. Such cases are difficult to defend successfully.

State or federal statutes and prior case law come into play somewhat less frequently. Legal cases that have been appealed sometimes make blanket statements of what the court considers to be the appropriate standard of care. This statement can be translated into law in future cases.

Damages

To collect money for negligent conduct, the plaintiff must establish damages. Damages may be in several forms: economic (sometimes called compensatory), noneconomic, or punitive. The petition or complaint also sets out in general terms the damages claimed in the lawsuit. Economic or compensable damages include all things lost to the plaintiff as a result of the alleged negligence and resultant injury that can be measured through economic calculations. Economic damages may include medical expenses attributable to the injury, both past and future; lost wages due to time off work to recover from the injury; and future lost wages. If the patient has died, heirs may be entitled to recover the patient's projected lifetime wages through a claim filed by the deceased's estate. Loss of household services is routinely compensated as economic damages. Some courts allow economists to testify for the plaintiff as to the economic value of more esoteric functions such as the loss of guidance a parent provides to a child. If the parent has died as a result of medical negligence, that person's minor child may be able to recover the economic loss associated with the parent's guidance and counseling. The precise calculation of economic damages varies considerably among jurisdictions. Calculations change dramatically depending on the circumstances of the parties as well. Look to your attorney for specific information on the calculation of economic damages and compare this calculation with the amount of professional negligence insurance coverage you have available.

Noneconomic damages are the intangible elements of life. They include pain, suffering, loss of enjoyment of life, and disfigurement. As between a husband and wife, noneconomic damages also include loss of consortium, or loss of sexual or other marital relations. Some jurisdictions rule that loss of affection, guidance, and counseling to an injured party's minor child fall within noneconomic damages. It is the noneconomic damage portion of awards that the plaintiff has historically tried to inflate. By injecting a medical negligence case with extreme sympathy for the injured party, the plaintiff's attorney seeks to inflate the verdict far in excess of the actual economic damages. Some states have placed caps or maximum recovery limits on the amount of noneconomic damages a plaintiff may recover. The jury is generally allowed to render any verdict it selects. The court then applies the cap, if appropriate, to reduce the noneconomic portion of the verdict.

Occasionally a defendant's conduct will be such that the plaintiff will seek punitive damages. The key words generally found in a petition or complaint that indicate punitive damages are requested include *gross, willful,* and/or *wanton.* A specific request or prayer for punitive damages may or may not be articulated in the petition or complaint. Seldom does a claim of medical negligence rise to a punitive level. Generally a court must decide whether the evidence is sufficient to allow a jury to consider awarding punitive damages. A court might allow punitive damages when a patient who is under general anesthesia and on a mechanical ventilator is abandoned by the anesthetist during the course of anesthesia. Habitual negligent conduct may also rise to punitive levels. As the word indicates, punitive damages are meant to punish the offending defendant. These damages typically are not covered by professional liability insurance and cannot be discharged through bankruptcy proceedings. The defendant is obligated to pay them personally.

407

Issues of Tort Justice

The original purpose for the tort justice system was to provide compensation and deterrence. In recent years the system has come under more frequent attack for several reasons. Critics claim the system affords variable and unpredictable compensation for injuries. Because a jury determines the dollar award, if any is to be awarded, plaintiffs with similar injuries may receive vastly different awards. Another criticism proposes that too much of the professional liability insurance premium does not reach the injured party. Rather, the premiums are used for defense costs, for operating the insurance company, or as profit for the company's shareholders. Finally, critics of the current system assert that too much of the jury award goes to the plaintiff's attorney in fees, generally 33% to 50%. Deterrence can more readily be handled, it is claimed, through effective risk management and quality improvement efforts.

There are justifications for leaving the basic tort system in place, however. If inequities exist, adjustments in the law can compensate. Allowing a jury to consider evidence on an individual's injuries provides compensation, if deserved, in an amount appropriate for the plaintiff's circumstances. A no-fault compensation system would likely decrease the costs of defending medical negligence claims, but the number of claims would likely rise dramatically, perhaps not saving any money because of the increased overall payout. There are certainly inequities and abuses in the current tort system, but without it, healthcare providers would have no opportunity to defend their reputations, and providers in high-risk healthcare areas might decide to leave practice. Also, checks in the current system make portions of the award paid to a plaintiff's attorney subject to court approval in some jurisdictions. This at least prevents the plaintiff's attorney from blatant overcharging.

The Expert Witness

The most commonly considered evidence of whether an appropriate standard of care was upheld comes from the expert witness. The court makes the determination whether a proposed expert witness qualifies as such and may testify. Some states have statutory limitations on who may testify. For instance, Kansas requires that the expert testifying on liability issues practices in the same profession at least 50% of the time within 2 years of the incident in question. This is meant to prevent physicians from retiring and spending their golden years in the courtroom supporting or criticizing the actions of others. This does not prevent a retired professional from giving an opinion on causation. All testimony must be offered on the standard of care in place at the time of the incident. This is difficult at times, because several years may pass between the incident and the filing of the lawsuit. Additional years may pass before the case comes to trial. This is especially true in cases involving minors. In some states, the statute of limitations allows filing lawsuits up to 19 years after the alleged negligent conduct.

An expert witness must testify in terms of medical probabilities or events that are more likely than not. An expert may not speculate to establish the alleged deviation. An expert must also indicate a familiarity with the standard of care. To simply advise a jury, "I administer anesthesia this way," is not sufficient. One individual's practice does not comport with the definition of an appropriate standard of care. Expert witness testimony is generally required to show both liability and causation. Causation testimony deals with what medical injuries have been incurred to date as a result of the negligent act and what will likely be suffered in the future.

An expert witness serves the purpose of informing jurors on specialized areas not within the knowledge of laypersons. Occasionally medical negligence cases are filed that can be analyzed without the assistance of medical expert testimony. As an example, if a patient falls from the OR table and is injured, a jury could well assess whether this could occur absent negligence on the part of the professionals attending the patient in the OR. Another common example involves the retained sponge or instrument. A jury can assess without expert testimony whether items should be left in a body cavity following surgery. Jurors are encouraged to rely on their own common sense and life experiences when making such judgments.

Because medical negligence actions often involve more than 1 defendant, and patient care generally involves more than 1 provider, comparative fault becomes a critical issue. Strict comparative fault means the plaintiff collects the percentage of the award assessed against each defendant. Variations apply. For example, some states do not allow the plaintiff to collect at all if that plaintiff is judged to be 50% or 51% negligent. Instances in which the plaintiff's fault may be compared include failure to return for follow-up treatment, smoking with knowledge that it causes lung cancer, or failure to follow rehabilitation instructions. The rules also vary on whether nondefendant healthcare providers' fault can be compared. Some states allow this and some do not. However, if a party settles with the plaintiff before trial, his or her negligence can be compared unless the remaining defendants have agreed to the contrary.

What to Do if Named in a Suit

Service of Process

The first involvement with a new lawsuit is service of process, meaning the delivery of the lawsuit petition or complaint to the provider. This is the document filed by the plaintiff, with the court setting out the allegations of negligence or other wrongdoing. This document may be served personally. A court representative actually locates you, generally at home or work, and personally delivers the petition or complaint along with information indicating when you must respond to the allegations to avoid a default judgment. A default judgment results when the defendant fails to respond in a timely fashion to the petition or complaint. The plaintiff's allegations are therefore deemed admitted, and judgment in the amount requested by the plaintiff is entered. As one can see, the appropriate response or answer when served process is very important.

There are other means of receiving notice of the lawsuit, including delivery via certified mail, which is an appropriate way to effect service on a defendant in most jurisdictions. Occasionally service of process is improper. The precise rules dictating proper and improper service and remedies for improper service vary among jurisdictions. Generally, if the plaintiff is trying to carry out personal service and someone leaves the documents with an office or hospital employee who is not designated with authority to receive such documents, the service is invalid. However, if the court representative leaves the documents with someone of suitable age at your home, service is valid.

There are 2 important points to keep in mind when you are served with process. First, make a note of the date, time, and

409

manner in which the documents were delivered and the date and time you received the documents if it is different from the former. An attorney will need this information. Second, notify your professional liability insurance carrier immediately that you have been named in a lawsuit and served with process. Notify your carrier initially by telephone and follow this notice with a letter advising the company of the lawsuit and enclose a copy of the suit papers received. Next, open a personal records file to keep copies of documents, letters, and other papers that will be generated during the course of litigation.

You should not ignore the service of process, as a default judgment can be entered following the time allowed for your answer to be filed with the court. In addition to the risk of default judgment, ignoring service of process places your professional liability insurance coverage at risk. Most policies contain a clause requiring you to notify the company of a claim or lawsuit so that a defense can be undertaken. Failure to comply with this requirement may void your coverage. Above all, the CRNA should speak to no one about the allegations or the case. The plaintiff's attorney may ask in deposition or trial to whom you have spoken about this case. By talking about the lawsuit with others, you may be involving them unnecessarily in the litigation process.

Some professionals want to undertake an immediate and independent investigation of the facts. Avoid this urge until you have consulted with the attorney that your insurance company appoints to the case. Certain privileged status attaches to an investigation undertaken at the direction of your counsel. Embarking on an independent investigation before conferring with counsel regarding your intended efforts may result in your work ending up in the hands of the plaintiff and plaintiff's counsel. In summary, when served with process, advise your insurance carrier of this fact. Do not speak with others regarding the lawsuit, and do not undertake an investigation of the matter without first speaking with and clearing your proposed action with your appointed attorney.

Selection of Counsel

Once advised of the lawsuit, a claims adjustor with your professional liability carrier will appoint an attorney to defend you. Selection of counsel is obviously an important aspect of defense. Some professionals, in seeking a level of comfort with the whole process, will request that a friend, neighbor, or relative be appointed to handle the case. Most adjustors resist this suggestion with good reason. Attorneys, similar to healthcare providers, specialize in their practice areas. It takes years to acquire the knowledge of medicine necessary to defend medical negligence actions. Likewise, it takes years to develop networks with potential experts around the country. It is not in your best interest for the insurance company to accede to your request and appoint an attorney friend or acquaintance.

You should feel comfortable with inquiring about the proposed attorney's background and qualifications. Professional liability carriers generally have a limited list of attorneys whom they have previously investigated relative to qualifications and past work performance. These attorneys generally limit their practice to medical negligence defense. You may want to inquire in some general areas such as an attorney's prior experience with medical negligence cases and anesthesia cases in particular.

Often more than one defendant is named in a medical negligence action and one attorney represents more than one defendant.

If you find yourself represented by an attorney who also represents a codefendant in your lawsuit, you can question this arrangement with your adjustor and the attorney if the arrangement seems inappropriate to you. The analysis made in this situation is twofold. First, do you and the codefendant have the same interests; that is, are you both employed by the same hospital or professional group, and did you both provide care to the allegedly injured party? Second, do you have conflicting interests that could result in compromising the defense of one to bolster the defense of the other? For example, did either of you disagree regarding the method of anesthesia used with the allegedly injured party?

Nurse Anesthetist's Responsibilities in Tort Action

Professional liability insurance finances your defense and provides coverage in case of monetary settlement or verdict. However, in addition to paying premiums, you have other duties under the terms of the insurance contract. As mentioned earlier in this section, you have a duty to report receipt of a claim or lawsuit so that an investigation and defense can be set in motion. You also have a duty to assist and cooperate in preparing your defense. This includes being available to meet with your attorney to discuss the facts of the case, plan a defense, and prepare for your deposition and trial. Failure to make yourself reasonably available may result in a warning that your company will no longer finance your defense and will not be responsible for a settlement or judgment. Continued failure to cooperate and make yourself reasonably available will result in the warning being carried out.

Generally, nurse anesthetists are interested in being involved in the process of discovery and in assisting with the defense. Early in the relationship, you should enter into an understanding with your attorney regarding your level of involvement. Always feel free to contact your attorney with questions or comments. You may wish to limit your involvement to periodic reports from the attorney of discovery schedules, important court dates, and settlement discussions. You may wish to assist in selecting expert witnesses by attending key depositions or by suggesting demonstrative ways to explain the technical aspects of the case to the jury. Your attorney will welcome your interest and participation. Keep in mind that anesthesia liability cases are not common and that many important issues are based on what occurs in actual anesthesia practice. Your attorney may not be familiar with anesthesia practice. Consequently, you should actively monitor your case and be aware of positions being taken.

Certain privileges attach once your attorney becomes involved in the litigation. As with the privilege of confidentiality between a healthcare provider and patient, often called the physician-patient privilege, there is a privilege of confidentiality between an attorney and client. To qualify under the attorney-client privilege, there must be true confidentiality of communications. Therefore, when you meet with your counsel, do not take your spouse or best friend along for moral support. As your attorney does not represent this person, the confidential nature of the attorney-client communications would be destroyed. A plaintiff's attorney would be entitled to ask what was said during the meeting. Also, do not describe the content of the communications between yourself and your attorney to third persons later. This too destroys the confidential nature of the communication and opens the possibility of disclosure to the opposing side.

411

A second privilege that attaches after your attorney is appointed to represent you deals with attorney work product. This means that all efforts undertaken by the attorney or someone under his or her direction and acting on the attorney's behalf are privileged and cannot be discovered by the opposing side. Therefore, any investigation that you assist with should be specifically requested by your attorney in order to remain protected and thus confidential. Investigation you may assist with includes literature searches on relevant standards of care or causation issues, review of the patient's lifetime medical records, or review of literature authored by plaintiff and defense experts.

Peer review, quality assurance, and risk management activities may or may not be protected from discovery, depending on the state and jurisdiction. However, if these activities are to be protected under the laws of any jurisdiction, they must be handled in a confidential manner. If you participated in a peer review activity or know that one was conducted on your case, advise your attorney of this fact to allow him or her an opportunity to deal with the issue before it becomes a problem.

Planning for Litigation

Within the time allowed, your attorney will prepare an answer denying the plaintiff's allegations of negligence and file this with the court. This document is general in nature and requires little, if any, input from the defendant to complete. As soon as practical, your attorney will want to meet with you to discuss the case. Be prepared to review the anesthetic record with your attorney in detail. Even experienced medical negligence attorneys have difficulty deciphering the symbols and abbreviations used on an anesthetic record. Also be prepared to discuss

other parts of the patient record that contain your notations or to which you refer when preparing for or administering an anesthetic. If you have the opportunity, review the patient record before the initial meeting. You may be able to isolate events or conditions that explain the patient's condition that may or may not have to do with anesthetic management.

In addition to the thorough record review, your attorney will want your best recollection of the events at issue. Do not prepare a written chronology unless your attorney asks you to do so. Include as much detail as possible in your oral description. Your attorney may also want a description of formal and informal relationships among all OR personnel. Laws vary from state to state regarding lines of responsibility and comparative fault principles. The better defense is one with all defendants agreeing there is no liability among themselves. If the defendants point fingers at one another and claim the other is at fault, the plaintiff wins automatically. The plaintiff does not care where the money comes from, only that money is recovered. Therefore, the best defense is a joint defense, whenever possible. Confide in your attorney any suspicions that other healthcare providers may have been at fault. Discuss this matter thoroughly with your attorney before offering testimony at deposition or trial to this effect.

During the initial interview with your attorney, a preliminary list of the plaintiff's specific allegations of negligence will be discussed. Your input into weaknesses in the case is important. Also, your attorney will ask your opinion of standard of care matters at issue. Sources of standards that support your care can be identified, namely standards of the AANA and the American Society of Anesthesiologists, facility policies and procedures, textbooks, and noted journal articles. Be certain to point out portions of the patient record that support your defense and refute the plaintiff's theories. This is the time for a frank, open discussion of the case. It is best to make a sound preliminary judgment as soon as practical regarding the likelihood of prevailing, should the case proceed to trial.

Your initial interview will also include a discussion of potential expert witnesses. Because of your expertise, you can suggest local anesthetists who are familiar with the standard of care, are articulate, and are not intimidated by direct questioning. Nationally recognized experts may also be considered, depending on the issues to be addressed. Because the standard of care for administering anesthesia is the same for both physician and nurse anesthetists, either CRNAs or physicians may be used as expert witnesses. Friends are generally not preferred as potential expert witnesses, because the jury may discount their testimony as biased. Areas of expertise beyond anesthesia may be required to fully support your patient care in a case. The causation element may be addressed by others such as a forensic pathologist, neurologist, and so on. Finally, in an initial interview, you will probably discuss the course of the litigation. This is a time for you to learn what to expect and over what time frame. Expect delays and cancellations through the discovery process. It is not clear whether these are due to the nature of litigation or the nature of attorneys. Whatever the reason, flexibility is a must. During the pendency of the litigation there will be many occasions to rediscuss and refine the items mentioned thus far. A discussion of the discovery process and deposition testimony is found later in this chapter.

Settlement and Arbitration

Sometime during the course of the action, the plaintiff may make a demand for settlement, meaning payment of a specific dollar payment that will resolve the matter without trial. Settlement discussions come in many formats, both formal and informal. Formal settlement discussions may be held outside the courtroom through mediation or arbitration. Mediation often takes on a form of shuttle diplomacy. Each side presents the strengths of his or her case and points out the weaknesses in the other side's case. This is generally done through statements of counsel. Clients are generally in attendance, along with representatives of the professional liability carriers. After listening to both sides make a presentation, the plaintiff and defense sides often separate. The mediator then meets with each side to discuss privately and candidly their chances of prevailing at trial. Demands and offers to settle are made and conveyed by the mediator.

Arbitration is different from mediation, in that the independent arbitrator may be an individual or a group. The sides present their arguments, and the arbitrator arrives at an opinion regarding the value of the case and proportionate shares of contribution, if any. Arbitration may be binding or nonbinding, depending on the agreement made before the process is undertaken. If the arbitration is binding, the parties are agreeing in advance to accept the arbitrator's judgment and forgo a trial. If negligence is found by the arbitrator, money in the amount and proportions suggested by the arbitrator is paid. Nonbinding arbitration is advisory only. It allows the parties to consider how a jury might react to the facts of the case. Both mediation and arbitration are generally undertaken when both parties are genuinely interested in settlement.

413

Court-managed settlement conferences are mandated in some states. A judge serves in a role similar to the mediator. The judge's status often influences the parties to accommodate and makes the parties feel they have aired their relative positions in open court. Both are obvious advantages when dealing with the emotions that often charge a party's judgment.

Informal settlement negotiations are generally conducted between the attorneys. You have the right to inquire about and be kept advised of this process. You may not have the right to prevent settlement under the terms of your insurance contract. When considering whether to support settlement efforts or proceed to trial and a jury verdict, there are considerations beyond the merits of the case. Is there a large sympathy factor for the plaintiff? Will trial pose a substantial personal expense in terms of time away from employment? Is there a large chance there could be a verdict in excess of policy limits?

This last item, excess verdict, brings the subject of personal counsel into discussion. Even though your attorney, paid by the insurance company, represents your interests, there may be times when it is prudent to undertake the personal expense of consulting with additional counsel. If punitive damages are claimed or if there is a great chance that a jury could reach a verdict against you in excess of your policy limits, your personal assets are exposed to judgment. Punitive damages are generally not covered by insurance, and the company may be reluctant to offer the money necessary to settle the case. A personal attorney can make an independent evaluation of these factors and advise you accordingly. You may request that the personal attorney press the insurance company to settle the case so that you avoid exposure of personal assets.

Before and During a Trial

Assuming the lawsuit is moving to trial, anticipate extensive preparation beforehand. You will need to review the medical records and know their contents thoroughly. Allow time to read depositions of all witnesses before the trial begins. Feel free to take notes regarding aspects of testimony that can be improved or attacked. Note the style of questions posed by plaintiff's counsel. Conduct any final research and review your attorney's research as it applies to standard of care and causation issues.

Assist in gathering anesthesia equipment, anatomical models, or other items that will help educate the jury about your role as an anesthetist. Juries appreciate a witness who takes time and effort to teach them about the subject matter. Your testimony has a much greater impact on the jury when you use demonstrative aids. The jury remembers what you show them longer than what you tell them. This way you demonstrate to the jury that you are knowledgeable about the equipment and procedures. Be absolutely positive that all demonstrative aids brought to the courtroom function properly.

Make yourself available for extensive conferences with your attorney before trial, as your attorney will want to prepare you for testimony before the jury. Generally this includes actual practice situations where you are asked to respond to questioning. All of the exhibits and means to use each will be reviewed. Preparation is a key element to success at trial. Spend the time necessary to prepare adequately. Know the medical record and listen to your attorney.

Personal attendance is required every day of the trial, and it is important for you to assist your attorney with the defense. Attendance also shows the jury that you care about the outcome of the litigation. Depending on the complexity of the issues and

414

the number of parties, an average medical negligence case may last 1 to 4 weeks. If you do not live in the city where the trial will be conducted, discuss your personal expenses associated with room, meals, and so on ahead of time. Your insurance policy probably does not cover these items. They will likely be your personal responsibility.

Dress professionally for the trial. This means a jacket and tie for the men and suits or dresses for the women. Avoid wearing flashy clothing or jewelry and driving an expensive car to the courthouse. Jurors can become offended by an obviously expensive lifestyle. Always conduct yourself professionally in the courtroom. Appear interested in the proceedings and remember that the jurors are constantly evaluating you, whether you are testifying or not.

After a verdict is rendered, the losing side may take an appeal to a higher court. The specific circumstances and implications of an appeal are so individual that I cannot speak to them here. Should an appeal be taken in your case, look to your attorney to explain all possible results and ramifications.

Deposition and Trial Testimony

Types and Purposes of Depositions

Attorneys use depositions in the discovery process of any major piece of litigation. Specific rules governing the procedure are set out in every state and vary somewhat among the jurisdictions. Generally, depositions are conducted outside the courthouse, by agreement of the parties. The witness swears to tell the truth, and a certified court reporter takes down every word spoken during the deposition. Attorneys ask questions, and the witness, or deponent, answers. The stress of these proceedings is most often relieved by adequate study and preparation before the event.

The deponent may provide valuable information to a medical negligence case for several reasons. First, the deponent may have been present when the events in question occurred. The deponent may have treated the individual at another time, making him or her knowledgeable about the plaintiff's condition. In these types of situations, the deponent is a fact witness. There is no anticipation on anyone's part that the deponent will become a defendant in the lawsuit. A fact deposition is limited to questions involving who, what, when, and where.

A second form of deposition involves the defendant who has knowledge about not only the facts but also a rationale for decisions, treatment, and judgments carried out with the patient. As a defendant, your answers to questions are the crux of the case. You will spend a substantial amount of time preparing for the deposition before it occurs. Tips for depositions, included in this section, are particularly applicable to the defendant deponent.

In a third type of deposition, the deponent may be an expert witness, someone with no personal knowledge of the facts. The expert witness generally has been selected by a party to testify because of his or her background and education. This makes the person uniquely qualified to offer opinions about the facts of the lawsuit. The expert witness reviews medical records, other deposition testimony, procedural documents, and any other relevant information. He or she then offers opinions on the appropriate standard of care, causation, damages, or other related topics that are beyond the knowledge of laypersons.

Depositions are not always exclusively categorized within 1 of the 3 areas mentioned

415

here. For instance, a fact witness may later become a defendant. The fact witness may also have opinions about the appropriate standard of care or causation based on his or her knowledge of the events or experience. A defendant certainly testifies about facts but may also have opinions about the appropriate standard of care or causation. The expert witness must interpret facts in order to supply the opinion testimony. The boundaries of your testimony should be considered before the deposition begins.

There are multiple reasons for taking depositions and multiple uses for them once they have been completed. Understanding an attorney's intent helps prepare you to offer testimony in the most favorable light. Beginning with the fact witness deposition, the testimony establishes a sequence of events that can later be evaluated. Did the healthcare providers make appropriate judgments in treating the patient? Did any single act or series of actions lead to the injury? The deposition makes the testimony immortal. If a witness is unavailable for live trial testimony, the deposition can be read to the jury. A witness may be unavailable because of distance from the trial location, death, or injury. If the deponent does appear at trial and changes his or her testimony from the sworn statements given in the deposition, an attorney can point out the changes to the jury. The attorney may suggest a variety of reasons for changing the testimony, such as the deponent has a poor memory, is trying to protect someone, or is simply lying at one time or the other. An attorney may suggest to the jury that the witness is not credible.

Preparation for Deposition

Before agreeing to give deposition testimony, a nondefendant anesthetist should fully investigate the possible ramifications of the

deposition. Could you become a defendant after the testimony? If the answer is yes, or you are not sure of the answer to this question, you should advise your professional liability insurance carrier that your deposition has been requested. Tell the insurance representative that you are concerned you may become a party to the lawsuit. Request that an attorney be appointed to prepare you for the deposition and represent you at that proceeding. If there is no chance or likelihood that you will be added to the lawsuit, you may be working with a defense attorney who represents another healthcare provider to prepare for the deposition. Note that rules allowing contact between a healthcare provider and attorney vary from state to state and must be considered before discussions of a patient's treatment are undertaken. The Health Insurance Portability and Accountability Act (HIPAA) has also imposed limitations on disclosure of protected healthcare information. Before discussing the case with an attorney not representing you in a lawsuit, you must be sure an appropriate release or court order exists allowing you to share the confidential patient information.

Documents reviewed in direct preparation for your deposition and relied on for testimony can be reviewed by opposing counsel. Therefore, only review those documents before your deposition that your attorney agrees are appropriate. As an example, if your attorney has asked you to provide a narrative of the events at issue and you review this document to refresh your recollection for the deposition, that document may be discoverable by opposing counsel. The same is true for research materials you may locate and review to support your actions and opinions.

If you have an opportunity to attend one or more depositions before yours, it will help you to be comfortable with the process. You will be able to appreciate the attorney's manner of questioning and direction for theories of liability.

Giving a Deposition

In general, a deposition is not a time to explain everything that you believe is relevant. Save that detail for trial. Rather, in a deposition, answer only the question that is asked. Answer truthfully, but answer yes or no when possible. Avoid nods of the head and gestures, because the court reporter can only take down actual words. Explain your answer with detail only when necessary. Make sure your responses are clear. Remember that the plaintiff's expert opposing your position and the expert retained to support you will read the deposition. It should be medically correct in all respects. You are not giving a deposition to help the opposing side. Do not suggest areas of questioning or help the attorney ask the question.

If you do not understand a question, say so or ask the attorney to rephrase it. Do not answer a question that you do not understand. Sometimes the correct answer is that you do not know or do not remember the specific information sought. Do not guess or speculate about an answer. If, at the conclusion of the process, you believe the plaintiff's attorney has failed to ask you questions on an important aspect of the case, do not worry. That does not preclude you from commenting on the subject at trial. This is the plaintiff's attorney's opportunity to learn all information that he or she believes is relevant and important to the plaintiff's case. Deposition is generally not the time for you to win the case. Save your arguments for the jury.

There are 3 means to testify regarding involvement with a patient. First, you can testify to things you remember. If an event was

catastrophic, you may well remember details clearly. If the patient's care was not appreciably different from that of any other patient and a substantial amount of time has passed, you may not remember the case at all. Second, you may testify to what is found in the patient care record. Although you may not specifically remember that the patient's blood pressure was 120/80 mm Hg on arrival in the postanesthesia recovery area, the chart indicates that is the fact. Therefore, you can say without hesitation what the blood pressure reading was at that time. Similarly, with other aspects of your documentation, you can refer to the record when answering questions. Third, you can testify from habitual conduct. Many things that you do every day are not documented. One cannot document every single aspect of care. However, if you routinely perform a function, you can say you are sure to have performed that act in this case simply because it is your habit. Do not hesitate to testify to facts that fall within your habit, routine, or custom of practice. On the other hand, if you claim something is your habit when it is not, you open the door to otherwise irrelevant but potentially harmful testimony of what you may or may not have done on certain other occasions.

Because brain injury or brain death and other respiratory complications are often the issues when an anesthetist is a defendant in a medical negligence action, a plaintiff's attorney will try to establish events on a minute-by-minute basis. Discuss with your attorney before the deposition how to approach this subject. Hypoxia and brain injury occur and become permanent within a very few minutes. Therefore, the plaintiff's attorney will attempt to show inappropriate judgments, inattention, or negligent conduct during the critical minutes. Anesthetic records generally provide an accounting of vital signs every 5 minutes. Establishing exactly what occurred between the recorded vital signs is often difficult. Healthcare personnel use terms that may seem harsh to laypersons. Consider your phraseology and discuss key terms with your counsel before a deposition. As an example, brain-damaged infants are often called "bad babies" in informal conversation. A plaintiff's attorney can make you seem cruel and insensitive for associating a negative term with a helpless infant who has been irreparably damaged owing to negligence.

Only parties to the lawsuit, including the plaintiff and defendant, their attorneys, the court reporter, and the witness, may attend depositions, absent agreement among the parties to the contrary. It is common to take a short break every hour or so. As a witness, you do not want to become overly tired when answering questions. Breaks help refresh you and help keep your mind focused. You can confer with your counsel out of earshot of all others anytime you desire. You have the opportunity to review your deposition after the reporter has transcribed it. Take that opportunity to make a careful and detailed review and to correct any errors that have been made.

Trial Testimony

Your second opportunity to testify is at trial. Needless to say, you will spend considerable time with your attorney in preparation. The same cautions apply at trial as in your deposition. In addition to your words, the jury will evaluate your demeanor. You may be called to testify by the plaintiff to establish the events at issue. Seldom can the plaintiff describe to the jury what transpired in the OR. Healthcare providers must set the stage for the plaintiff to attempt to prove his or her theories of negligence and show the injury and

damage that resulted. Trial testimony is extremely individualized depending on the facts, attorney preference, strengths of the witness, and trial strategy, among other things. This is the main event. Do not spare time in preparation, and be sure to listen to your attorney's advice.

Tips for Avoiding Litigation

Goals set by every CRNA include helping patients to the best of one's ability, avoiding injury, and avoiding involvement as a defendant in a medical negligence action. Avoiding litigation begins with anesthesia education. Attitudes of respect for the patient and caution in treatment decisions set the stage for your career and directly affect your involvement in situations where medical negligence might occur. One cannot prevent a patient from suing. One can, however, be in the best possible position to defend oneself should a suit be filed. This attitude and manner of conducting oneself may deter some attorneys from actually filing the lawsuit.

Communication With Patients and Families

Patients and families should all be treated with respect. Surgery and anesthesia are major events in a person's lifetime; consequently, the patient and family deserve time and attention to properly prepare and decrease their anxiety. It cannot be stressed enough that should major patient complications arise perioperatively, especially those associated with a negative patient outcome, families should be informed immediately. Events can be described in general terms and the CRNA should provide a clear description of what treatments, therapies, interventions, and follow-up care has been planned for the patient. The CRNA should be available periodically throughout follow-up care and should be actively involved in discussions with the family regarding the patient's progress. Often patients and families sue based not on patient outcome alone but also on the provider's perceived lack of sensitivity or understanding of the gravity of the situation.

Obtaining Informed Consent

A patient's memory for details and discussions of informed consent is poor.[5,6] However, the discussion should go forward with family members in attendance if the patient desires. The entire process should be documented. List the family members present, for example, husband, aunt, adult daughter, and so on. List the risks of the anesthetic that are discussed. Death, although a rare event, should also be mentioned as a risk. List the options of anesthetics discussed. If one option is discarded in favor of another based on patient preference, document this fact. If the option of anesthetic technique selected by the patient is not as advisable as the discarded option, detail this discussion in the patient record. Anesthetic options assume that more than one technique can safely be accomplished taking into account the patient's condition and requirements of the surgeon.

Many institutions employ a consent form for the anesthetic similar to the one the patient signs authorizing the surgical procedure.[3] The consent form validates that the anesthetist explained the risks and options associated with the procedure and that the patient knew and accepted this information before agreeing to proceed. These forms are helpful in defending patient claims of no knowledge of possible death or injury associated with the anesthetic. If an institution provides separate surgical and anesthesia consent forms, both should be signed by the patient. In those cases, the surgical consent alone may not provide sufficiently broad consent for anesthesia.

Documenting Review of Patient Records

The patient's medical history should be taken carefully and comprehensively and compared with the documented physician history (by the surgeon or referral physician). If an anesthesiologist or other CRNA has completed the patient's history and physical examination, be sure to document on the chart or OR record that you have been apprised of that information before you administer the anesthetic. By assuming duty for the case, you assume responsibility for all perioperative activities, including a competent anesthesia workup.

More and more institutions are using electronic records. If you are not using that technology, the findings of the respiratory, cardiovascular, and airway examinations are most relevant for anesthetists, because failed intubations account for a large number of anesthetic mishaps. Anticipating potential airway difficulties via a competent and documented airway examination will generally result in avoiding patient injury and exposing oneself to litigation. A special anesthesia checklist with blanks for elaborating on information received is an excellent method for documenting the procedure. As always, equipment and machine checks should be documented on the anesthetic record, as this information attests to proper function and acquisition of baseline physiologic data.

Do not limit your ability to prove that you provided standard of care services to a patient by failing to document actions in the OR or any other anesthetic setting. Fill out the record completely regardless of whether the case involves sedation and monitoring

419

or a complicated general anesthetic procedure. Sophisticated monitoring of cardiorespiratory status is now commonplace. The information from these monitors must be recorded on the patient record frequently to show that you were aware of the readings and that they fell within normal parameters. If the readings are outside normal parameters, an adjustment in the anesthetic should be reflected on the record as well. Similarly, if the electronic record is not an accurate reflection of what is happening, record your explanation.

In an emergency situation the patient becomes the priority, providing less time for detailed record keeping. During these periods, make short (even cryptic if necessary) notes of vital signs, monitor readings, and medications. Once the emergency has passed, complete the anesthetic record as soon as possible. If the patient can safely be left in the care of others, find a quiet place to sit and complete your anesthetic record without distraction. If the timing of events is only approximate, indicate that fact. Review the record carefully to see if all information available has been included. Avoid leaving large gaps in vital signs or monitoring readings. If the original record is illegible, rewrite the entire anesthetic record in clear handwriting immediately after the crisis has passed and place it with the patient record. The legible record should contain the same information but with more detail than the illegible original. Discard the illegible copy. Do not confuse completing a record with altering an already completed record.

Do not feel restricted to document only on the anesthetic record after a crisis has occurred. To fully document the situation, you may need to complete a dictated or longhand progress note. This note should also reflect any conferences with family members after the emergency. Again, list the individuals present for the conference and the general nature of the information you relayed. Note the family response if it seems threatening or out of the ordinary for the circumstances.

Routine Postoperative Patient Follow-up

Even when there is no crisis, you will want to follow up with your patient after he or she has recovered from the anesthetic. If the patient has a complaint, you may be able to explain why the discomfort was necessary. Your obvious concern for the patient goes far toward avoiding a formal lawsuit. As before, document the substance of the postoperative visit, including all patient complaints and your response. Always make a note of the existence or nonexistence of patient complaints about pain or awareness during the anesthetic. Also be sure you have documented that you have transferred care to appropriately licensed individuals in the postanesthesia care unit or intensive care unit before beginning another case. Remember to maintain continuity in care.

Maintaining and Documenting Standards of Care

At all times, maintain familiarity with standards of care promulgated by anesthesia specialty organizations. These are the academic and clinical constructs against which your performance will be measured. Always pattern your practice in accordance with these standards and fashion your anesthesia record to reflect their implementation. If a patient wishes to file a medical negligence action, an attorney will review the case before proceeding, to determine its merits. In addition, before the filing of a lawsuit, an expert review is obtained by most reputable plaintiff's attorneys, again to assess merit. If the attorney and expert consultant can find no deviation from the appropriate standard of care on your part, based on the patient's record, there is an excellent chance the lawsuit will never be filed.

As a final point in discussing documentation, the question arises as to whether the anesthetist should prepare a set of personal notes describing some crisis event. The better response is no. The patient record should reflect the patient's condition, treatment provided, and patient's response. A set of personal notes should not elaborate on these items. Generally, an anesthetist considers writing personal notes when disagreement or conflict has occurred. Again, the better suggestion is not to undertake the effort of detailing a conflict. Personal notes prepared without advice and direction of counsel are generally subject to discovery if a lawsuit results. Calmer heads will prevail later. Memorialized conflicts will little serve anyone's purpose at that time.

Professional and community participation play a role in your likelihood of involvement in a medical negligence lawsuit. This is especially true if you live and work in a smaller community. If you live a lifestyle of helping and caring for others and maintain high personal and professional standards, prospective plaintiffs are less likely to sue, prospective plaintiff's attorneys are less likely to pursue the case, and prospective expert witnesses for the plaintiff are less likely to agree to testify. Hesitation at any one of the 3 links in the chain may result in no medical negligence action or in a failed or abandoned action.

Professional Liability Insurance

Types of Policies

In general, there are 2 types of policies written by professional liability insurance companies: occurrence and claims-made. Occurrence is by far the preferable type but is not usually available. An occurrence policy covers the insured for all acts occurring within the policy period, regardless of when the lawsuit is filed. If you purchased an occurrence policy for the calendar year 2005 and a minor child files a negligence claim in 2010, you would be covered under your 2005 policy assuming that is when the alleged negligence occurred. This is obviously favorable to the CRNA. It does, however, make long-range risk and liability planning difficult for the company that provided coverage. In this circumstance you may have had insurance coverage with this company only 1 year (2005) and only paid 1 premium, yet the company is responsible for defending the lawsuit filed against you in 2010. Moreover, in periods of inflation, the premium is based on experience in 2005, but a recovery will be paid many years later in inflated dollars.

A claims-made policy is usually much less expensive than an occurrence policy but is less favorable for the insured CRNA. Under a claims-made policy, you must have coverage at the time of the incident and continuously through the date the claim is made or the lawsuit is filed. To have coverage in the preceding example, you would have to purchase the insurance in 2005 and maintain coverage continuously with that company through 2010, the time the lawsuit is filed. Obviously the insurance company has several advantages. The early years with an insurance company are relatively low risk. It is not often that an act leading to a lawsuit and the lawsuit occur in the same policy year. Therefore, the company can collect several years' premiums before having to defend a lawsuit. Also, the company's risk begins, as above, in 2005. If you had any anesthetic mishap before 2005, it is not the

421

responsibility of this company, as you have no negative history to begin the policy period. This type of policy also encourages the CRNA to remain with one company over a long time period, stabilizing the market from the company's point of view. Terminating coverage with the company terminates the company's risk with respect to future claims or lawsuits.

There are ways for a CRNA to change professional liability insurance carriers and maintain continuous coverage. This brings into play 2 additional insurance terms: retroactive date, often called retro date, and tail coverage. The retroactive date is the date on which coverage for incidents begins. One can purchase liability coverage for a time period preceding the actual date coverage is purchased. For example, if you purchase claims-made insurance on January 1, 2002, but have practiced anesthesia since 2000, you may want to purchase coverage for events that may materialize into claims or lawsuits from 2000. In your policy, the retro date would read January 1, 2000. Any number of years of retroactive coverage is available for a quoted price. The length of time you purchase will depend on a number of individual factors, including your state's statutes of limitation and the length of time you have practiced.

At the other end of the picture is tail coverage. When one is canceling insurance for any reason, it is possible to purchase tail coverage. Tail coverage provides insurance benefits in the future for events that may have occurred during the time the insurance you are now canceling was in effect. Using the same years as before, if you maintained claims-made insurance with the same company from 2005 through 2010 and canceled, you may be able to purchase tail coverage from that company at the time of cancellation. The tail coverage would provide benefits for a specified number of years into the future, for claims and suits arising from care rendered during the policy years 2005 through 2010. The number of years for which you should have tail coverage varies, as with retro dates. Many people purchase tail coverage upon retirement or when moving to a different state where their prior company does not sell insurance. Obviously, you would want to price shop to see if tail coverage or retroactive coverage is the most economical, assuming you are continuing to practice.

Limits of Coverage

Limits of professional liability coverage have 2 components. The limits are indicated with a slash mark between 2 numbers, for example, $1 million/$3 million. This means $1 million in liability coverage is available for any 1 event in a policy year. Remember, 1 event may have more than 1 plaintiff; for example, a husband is injured and sues for physical injuries, and his wife sues for loss of consortium. Three million dollars in coverage is available for any number of events in the policy year. These coverage limits concern the payment of verdicts and settlements only. They are not typically depleted by the expenses incurred in litigation, for example, attorney's fees, deposition and expert charges, and so on. In a few states, insurance policies are available wherein expenses of litigation deplete the coverage limit. This means if it costs $100,000 to defend a lawsuit, only $900,000 would remain for a verdict or settlement. Injuries sustained as a result of anesthesia negligence can have catastrophic results. Therefore, large limits in liability coverage are recommended. An active practicing CRNA should generally not carry insurance limits below $1 million/$3 million. Some individuals recommend that the limits of liability be tailored to your geographic area and work setting. If lower limits are selected, the CRNA should understand that there may be some exposure of personal assets to attachment and liquidation in order to pay a large judgment.

Your policy details what is and is not covered in your defense. In general, however, all judgments and settlements within the limits are covered. Expenses of litigation are covered and include fees paid to your attorney, fees paid to expert witnesses, costs of depositions, costs of creating demonstrative exhibits, costs associated with collecting medical records, and numerous other expenses, which amount to a substantial expenditure when added together. Your insurance covers events occurring within the course and scope of your duties as an anesthetist. Specific exclusions may exist in your policy, and you should be aware of these to avoid practicing in a setting where you have no coverage. A policy may cover you while you practice in one state only. This would limit crossing state lines or moving about the nation in a locum tenens arrangement. A policy may cover you while working for your employer only. This would limit freelance arrangements in your spare time. Policies are limited to acts falling within the scope and practice of anesthesia services. Although not seen frequently in the anesthesia profession, a claim of improper touching or fondling of a patient may not be covered under your policy.

Insurance Carriers

Professional liability insurance coverage is available from several types of companies and sources. An obvious first choice for the CRNA to consider for medical liability insurance is AANA Insurance Services, an agency wholly owned by the AANA. This service agency was established specifically for CRNAs to obtain high-quality insurance products and as a source of expert guidance on insurance matters.

Alternatively, many groups of physicians or hospitals have collaborated to form privately owned and operated mutual insurance companies. Some groups with substantial financial backing have self-insured their prospective liability expenses and exposure. These are often health maintenance organizations, hospital chains, or state university facilities.

If coverage is not available to a CRNA through one of these means, there may be a patient compensation fund in your state. Some states operate such funds to assure the public that healthcare providers in the state will have liability coverage should a judgment be entered against them.

Finally, a joint underwriting association (JUA) may be available. This may also be referred to as a high-risk pool. The purpose of a JUA is to provide professional liability insurance for providers who in good faith are entitled to coverage but who are unable to procure even basic insurance from traditional markets.

Summary

It should be obvious to every CRNA and student registered nurse anesthetist that an in-depth knowledge of the legal system of this country, especially as it relates to medical negligence litigation, is mandatory. Both time and care should be taken by the CRNA to meticulously document his or her standard of care, become familiar with the processes of deposition and trial testimony, and know how to effectively support the attorney's effort to procure a positive outcome for the provider.

423

References

1. *Brown v United States,* 419 F2d 337, 341 (Mo cite-66085 [2] ED Mo, 1969).

2. Posner KL. Data reveal trends in anesthesia malpractice payments. *ASA Newslett.* 2004;68(6):7-8,14.

3. Garnick DW, Hendricks AM, Brennan TA. Can practice guidelines reduce the number and costs of malpractice claims? *JAMA.* 1991;266(20):2856-2860.

4. *Davenport v Ephraim McDowell Memorial Hospital, Inc.,* 769 SW2d 56 61 Ky App. (1988).

5. Lloyd A, Hayes P, Bell P, Naylor AR. The role of risk and benefit perception in informed consent for surgery. *Med Decis Making.* 2001;21:141-149.

6. Cassileth BR, Zupis RV, Sutton-Smith K, March V. Informed consent—why are its goals imperfectly realized? *N Engl J Med.* 1980;302(16):896-900.

Study Questions

1. Define the common elements that constitute claims of negligence and give practical examples of how each is operative in the anesthesia setting.

2. Discuss the different forms of damages and in what cases punitive judgments against an anesthesia provider may be upheld.

3. List and discuss some of the major roles and responsibilities that a CRNA may have in helping prepare for trial with his or her attorney.

4. What advice would you give a colleague as tips for avoiding litigation?

5. What are the differences between occurrence and claims-made liability insurance? Which is most advantageous and why?

CHAPTER 18
Administrative Management

Christine S. Zambricki, CRNA, MS, FAAN

Key Concepts

- Management and leadership are key competencies for the Certified Registered Nurse Anesthetist (CRNA) administrator.

- CRNAs' clinical expertise, advanced education, and knowledge of the standards of care in the perioperative environment provide a strong foundation for their administrative role in healthcare.

- The operations component of contemporary surgical leadership involves continual quality improvement in all domains of the operating room.

- The ability to create a talent-based organization with emotionally engaged employees is a key competency of the CRNA administrator.

Surgical services epitomize a complex clinical and administrative environment. There are few departments in the hospital that have the same impact on the institution and that span so many different service areas. The operating room (OR) has a profound impact on a hospital's net operating income and is critical to physician and patient relationships and customer satisfaction. Because of the special characteristics of surgical services, leaders in this area are some of the most visible and vital administrators in healthcare organizations. This chapter is designed to help Certified Registered Nurse Anesthetists (CRNA) who are actively engaged in leadership positions in the OR. The content will provide salient insight into the responsibilities of these roles and guidance as healthcare moves aggressively into accountable, integrated, and managed care systems. To address the different perspectives and specialized knowledge required for success, this chapter is divided into major areas of importance for the CRNA leader: Management and Leadership, Operations, Talent, Quality and Safety, and Education and Research.

Management and Leadership

Effective leaders make a difference. CRNAs wishing to assume administrative positions as leaders in the anesthesia and wider hospital community must possess and enhance their leadership knowledge, skills, and abilities. These are essential components of the administrative "toolkit," requisite to accepting additional responsibilities in healthcare.

Leadership skills are often initially used to operate and improve the perioperative domain, a vital and consequential component of the hospital enterprise as a whole. The surgical service line comprises an estimated 50% to 70% of most hospitals' net income. Ongoing healthcare reform will possibly reduce the contribution margin of surgery; however, this area unquestionably remains an important profit center. Whether for the net income generated or the substantial expense incurred, the perioperative area and its leadership remain permanently fixed under the "C-suite" microscope. However, financial considerations are only one aspect of the centrality of OR services.

Operating room services define physician and patient relationships with the hospital. They are key drivers for customer satisfaction and patient safety goals. CRNA administrators are in the position to leave a lasting legacy, good or bad, on their team members, their peers, the department, and on the greater organization. Ultimately, the manner in which the CRNA leader transforms the perioperative environment and creates the culture will affect patients and their families, the community, and in some cases, the healthcare industry.

CRNAs in leadership roles hold titles such as clinical coordinator, supervisor, manager, director, and administrator. For the purposes of this chapter, these titles are used interchangeably to mean CRNAs in positions of authority and influence. The term *perioperative* refers to the range of care that the patient experiences from preanesthetic screening and assessment through preoperative, intraoperative, anesthetic, and postoperative phases.

CRNAs are not new to administrative management responsibilities. It has been common practice for CRNAs to direct departments of anesthesia or other related service areas. As hospitals move toward clinical integration according to service lines, CRNAs are assuming broader administrative responsibilities including those in intensive care and surgical nursing units, and pharmacy and emergency room departments. Because the role of the CRNA director is no longer limited to anesthesia departments, it is more important than ever that CRNAs obtain knowledge and expertise in fields common to any hospital administrator, which most likely were not part of their original education or subsequent clinical experience.

From an internal perspective, there are 2 driving forces in hospital organizations supporting the development of an integrated governance structure for ORs and anesthesia. First, the need for quality improvement has led to a service line approach. The service line movement coordinates activities across department lines for the good of a single population of patients. For the surgical services service line, this often leads to consolidation of leadership for the anesthesia and perioperative areas. Second, as public payer reimbursement decreases, hospitals are seeking to maintain an effective management structure that focuses on broad spans of authority, reducing redundant administrative positions.

By virtue of their educational and experiential background, CRNAs bring certain skills to a leadership role and have learned to work closely with physicians—both anesthesiologists and surgeons—while delivering anesthesia care to patients in the OR. This experience is extremely useful in developing physician–staff relationships, an essential skill for effectiveness as a surgical services leader.

CRNAs are often chosen for leadership positions because they are OR-based nurse specialists with postgraduate education. Graduate level degrees bring a certain fund of knowledge to those in director positions. With a strong background in critical care nursing, CRNAs have the clinical expertise to evaluate practice in the areas of anesthesia, pain management, and surgery. This background, coupled with the individual capacity for interpersonal relations and leadership, creates many opportunities for CRNAs who wish to focus their professional careers on hospital administration.

Much is made of the distinction between management skills and leadership competencies. Both are key behaviors in perioperative governance. For the 21st century CRNA administrative manager the decision is not whether to be a manager or a leader, because the job requires competence in both realms.

Management skill is necessary for the execution phase of the commitments and change initiatives that make leadership vision and strategic direction a reality. Execution is not simple; and the devil is in the details. Management espouses transactional behaviors such as planning, organizing, coordinating, directing, controlling, and evaluating the team. In practical terms, management is what gets the department staffed, the history and physicals completed before surgery, the first cases of the day started on time, and provides the oversight for quality improvement. Management executes the plan and makes sure that the work gets done. To manage effectively, one must provide clarity on the "what" and the "why" and deliver frequent and transparent feedback on how things are going. The day-to-day oversight, direction, and control of such important tasks challenge CRNA administrators every day.

In addition to capably fulfilling their management responsibilities, the best CRNA leaders have the vision, time, ability, and focus to engage in key relationships. They take the forward-thinking risks involved in moving the enterprise to new strategic positions and accomplishments

429

through innovation. Such leadership is transformational. Competent CRNA administrative directors can, by inspiring others, achieve extraordinary outcomes for their patients, their departments, their healthcare facilities, and their profession.

The paths to professional leadership for CRNAs are diverse. A CRNA leader who demonstrates excellence in clinical practice and relationship skills may be selected for a management role when the need arises. A CRNA supervisor may be promoted to consolidate management of linked departments such as surgery, anesthesia, and preoperative and postoperative services. A nurse anesthetist may choose a leadership career path, pursuing education, training, and increases in responsibility resulting in a leadership role. In some circumstances, a CRNA leader is seemingly plucked from the masses when a leadership position is unexpectedly vacated. In the context of industry pressure to increase efficiency and effectiveness, despite the path a CRNA takes to a leadership role, the competencies required for success are identical.

CRNA directors have increasing responsibility for aligning clinical, financial, and service strategies in the institution. This may include coordination of care with out-of-hospital enterprises such as freestanding surgical centers, doctor's offices, and pain clinics. They may negotiate contracts for medical practices, perfusion services, or instrument cleaning. The CRNA director allocates capital and labor expenses and manages targeted staff shortages. In today's cost-sensitive environment, with substantial increases in responsibility there may be concomitantly reduced resources of time, money, and staff assistance. Meanwhile, the CRNA must be physically present in the OR and provide visible leadership there. Managerial and peripheral responsibilities sub-

stantially reduce the time available for this important aspect of the role; however, time in the OR yields practical information about the concerns of its inhabitants as well as the reality of operations.

The transition from clinical expert to administrator presents many challenges. CRNA leaders must adopt the corporate culture in which they work. It is more important than ever to demonstrate consistent execution with business results, rather than focusing only on clinical improvements. At times the CRNA administrator can be caught in organizational upheaval as environmental changes drive healthcare change and the entire industry evolves with 21st century realities.

Operations

Management Decision Making

The highly functioning OR is one of the best examples of interdisciplinary team cooperation in healthcare. Individuals with advanced and unique professional training come together to provide care to patients in a fixed timeframe in the closed box called an OR. This group of people working together requires a high degree of coordination and communication. Similarly, the leaders supporting the OR teams require exceptional teamwork to remove barriers and empower their teams to do what they do best. In the administrative realm leaders must often come together and develop new working relationships to solve problems.

Quality and depth of administrative leadership are reflected in relationships with key constituencies, including other units, CRNAs, nurses, surgeons, anesthesiologists, and hospital administrators. This is a major transition for the CRNA practitioner, whose anesthesia practice has been characterized by independence and one-on-one patient relationships. Reinvention is a lifelong and continuing learning process, and in this case, the CRNA may benefit from additional education focused on management, choosing a mentor, and establishing a solid support system.

Beyond the more formal aspects of preparing for the role of administrator such as graduate education and experience are the skills required to bring people together for a common cause or purpose. The administrator's job is to visualize, manage, and promote the institutional mission. That goal can only be achieved by a skillful administrator who understands concepts of interdisciplinary collaboration and the importance of personal and social interactions, and who demonstrates effective communication skills.

Building relationships with key individuals before the inevitable problems arise is not just desirable: it is essential. Table 18.1

provides a list of important contacts for the new CRNA administrator. This is a starting point, and the CRNA administrator should make every effort to meet with these individuals on a "get to know you" basis within the first few weeks of assuming a new position. Additional individuals will be added to the list based on the unique organizational structure in the hospital.

Working in the Hospital's Administrative Structure

In orienting to a new administrative position, the CRNA director must understand clearly the governance of the organization, the major players involved, and the locus and method by which decisions are made. This can be done through observation, talking to peers, and reviewing files for approval documents and memos. New relationships with critical stakeholders, both internal and external, must be forged or renewed.

431

Table 18.1. Important Contacts for the CRNA Administrator

C-suite

Chief executive officer	Chief financial officer
Chief information technology officer	Chief human resources officer
Chief nursing officer	Chief operating officer

Physician chairmen and chiefs
Anesthesiology, Critical Care Medicine, Emergency Medicine, Pathology and Laboratory Medicine, Radiology, Surgery, Surgical Specialties such as neurosurgery, orthopedics, ophthalmology and others not included in the Department of Surgery

Department directors
Facilities, Materials Management, Operating Rooms, Intensive Care Units, Planning, Purchasing, Radiology, Laboratories, Admissions and Transfer Office, Biomedical Engineering, Housekeeping, Patient Transportation

Nurse managers
Ambulatory Surgery Unit, Emergency Department, Operating Rooms, Preoperative Units, Postanesthesia Care Unit, Preoperative Testing, Surgical Intensive Care Unit, Inpatient Surgical Units

There are some obvious things that the director can do to work productively in the hospital's administrative structure. It is important that the CRNA director engage in activities that support the hospital in its entirety. In these activities, the director functions in a complementary role to the hospital mission and makes a contribution beyond his or her own parochial interests, thus increasing the director's inherent value to the organization.

One example of broadening work activity is in the arena of hospital committees. Many types of committees can be found in healthcare organizations. At the least, there will be department committees, hospital administrative committees (interdepartmental), and medical staff committees (interdepartmental). One way to get a better understanding of the needs of departments outside the OR is to be a member of a committee in another department. For example, the intensive care unit (ICU) may have a quality improvement committee. This would be an interesting and appropriate committee for a member of the anesthesia department, given the interdepartmental synergies and the clinical knowledge base required to evaluate care in this setting, particularly as it relates to the airway. Other committees suitable for CRNA administrator involvement include the pharmacy and therapeutics committee, OR committee, medical quality committee, and library committee. Through involvement on medical and administrative committees, the director will develop relationships with many key leaders and physicians throughout the organization. These relationships will lay the groundwork for a positive working environment in the future.

Another important contribution that the CRNA director can make to the hospital organization is to exhibit a willingness to take on additional responsibility. As administrative positions are vacated because of attrition, more and more chief executive officers are choosing to reassign duties rather than fill the positions. The director may receive additional areas of responsibility not related to nurse anesthesia or even the OR, such as heading up a service line initiative, Joint Commission preparation, or a new educational program. The director may not be asked whether he or she wishes to have additional responsibility; rather, it is assumed that the director will gracefully respond with the best effort to accomplish the objectives of the organization.

A CRNA executive must observe the corporate culture and develop an understanding of and respect for the conventions of administrative behavior at the institution. This must not be taken lightly. Corporate culture encompasses many different elements of hospital life. Clothing is a part of corporate culture, so is the style and format of presentations made to upper-level administrators. Respecting corporate culture does not exclude the ability to display some individualism, but to be part of the culture means embracing the major tenets and functioning within them. Some will be obvious on the first day or at the first meeting, and others may be more subtle and appreciated only over time.

As part of the greater leadership team, the CRNA administrator desiring increased responsibility must develop the ability to think beyond the context of the OR. Because of the high degree of specialization and the physical detachment inherent in their location, those in the OR and anesthesia departments risk becoming isolated and self-centered in their thinking. The director will have a responsibility to advocate for the area; moreover, this will be expected of the director at meetings and other venues for decision making. However, beyond advocacy, the director must also keep a balanced view and an open mind regarding the needs of all patients and the overall obligations of the hospital.

Competing priorities will arise over resources such as capital dollars, space, and patient beds. A CRNA director who is always focused solely on his or her area of responsibility will be viewed as narrow-minded and lacking global perspective. Worse yet, this myopia may result in poor decisions for the hospital as a whole. With the challenges of today's healthcare, the chief executive officer needs every member of the leadership team to be working for organizational benefit, not for self-interest.

Every hospital develops an organizational mission and values, goals and objectives by which the organization defines itself and its strategic direction. Despite the diversity of healthcare organizations in the United States, these organizational goals are surprisingly consistent throughout the industry. The CRNA director, functioning in a leadership position, is responsible for the alignment of departmental goals with those of the organization. This is important for 2 reasons. First, the relevance of departmental or service entities in a hospital is measured primarily by the extent to which their productivity contributes to the global goals of the hospital. Second, budget allocations in the system are often determined according to the extent to which departmental activities contribute in meaningful ways to the institutional mission.

In addition to developing broad vision in the organization, the director must become knowledgeable about the healthcare industry in general. This can be accomplished by reading industry publications such as *Hospitals and Health Networks, Health Affairs,* and *Modern HealthCare.* Another important source of information is the lay press. With increasing frequency, major newspapers and news magazines feature in-depth stories on the healthcare industry and US healthcare reform, as well as stories on medical advances and futuristic projections. The Internet is an ever-changing source of information. Knowledge about national healthcare issues will provide insight into the pressures the institution is facing from the outside. The CRNA director can anticipate changes that will affect reimbursement or services offered. Knowledge of trends in healthcare provides a common language and understanding that is expected of individuals at the director level regardless of their administrative assignment.

Traditionally, hospitals have been organized according to functional areas or disciplines (eg, nursing, medicine), and a hierarchical decision model moves issues up the ladder for resolution. This approach will not work in the OR, where professionals from multiple disciplines work in close, sometimes overlapping roles to achieve a goal. Because a smoothly functioning OR requires efficient patient flow, problem resolution must cut across disciplines and be supported by collaborative efforts that satisfy the legitimate concerns of all participants and clarify the work processes.

Tackling administrative problems can be fraught with landmines such as egos, turf, history, and money and power. One of the most important things CRNA administrators can do is to ensure that all interested parties are appropriately represented at problem-solving meetings and that the discussion environment is safe for all participants. All viewpoints must be heard so that the root cause of the problem can be identified and the final solution embraced.

433

Meetings are necessary to get things done in the hospital setting. Meetings also provide an opportunity to achieve "buy-in" from various stakeholders if the meeting is conducted in a manner that builds consensus. Table 18.2 provides suggestions for effective leadership behavior at a business meeting.[1]

Conflict may occur when people fail to understand others' rationale and motive. In many respects, professionals working in the OR have similar values. All profess to be motivated by a dedication to patient care and a commitment to values of hard work and education. These joint values can form a foundation for the development of effective interpersonal relationships.

However, perspectives among professionals may differ in some areas. In many hospitals, physicians work in a private practice model, and other staff members are employed on an hourly wage or salary. The economic necessity in private practice is to do more cases, whereas the motivation for employees may be to finish the day and go home. This difference can lead to conflict when physicians press to add additional

---

Table 18.2. Preparation and Participation in Meetings

Begin and end on time.

Create a realistic agenda.

Be prepared, participate.

Get to the point, no speeches or long stories.

Be open minded—have a sense of appreciative inquiry.

Focus on the problem, not the person.

Limit or prohibit side conversations, texting, and emails.

Pick your battles.

Support the decision and move on when the group moves on.

Encourage different points of view and explore the minority opinion.

Say it in the room, not in the hall.

Don't rush decision making.

Lob up ideas and suggestions ("How about this?" vs "I think . . .")

Slay sacred cows, challenge assumptions, honor questions.

Encourage and involve quieter members.

434

cases to the schedule. Understanding the motivation for a specific behavior often makes collaboration easier, even if one does not personally benefit from the behavior.

Another common point of conflict exists in many ORs. Because physicians are not salaried staff members, meeting time for committee work represents potential loss of income. Physicians may not want to attend meetings during the day, and the director may not want to attend meetings at night. As a result, physicians may favor quick deliberations and rapid adoption of their solution to a problem rather than spending time on in-depth analysis. This approach may frustrate salaried employees who feel the need for further discussions or more time for problem solving. For important issues, meetings must be scheduled at a time that will not interfere with office practice or OR time. Flexibility in scheduling will help the CRNA director build trusting relationships by sending the message that the input of all members of the team is worthwhile and necessary.

The nursing model of assessment, planning, implementation, and evaluation is familiar to nurse anesthetists as the foundation of nursing practice and also has application for management decision making. First, departmental problems must be identified, defined, and clarified (assessment). Collecting appropriate data and hearing all sides of the problem are important before proceeding. There are always at least 2 perspectives to every problem and usually more than 2. Data are key to depersonalizing problems and developing win-win solutions. Fixing the symptoms without fixing the underlying system problems is a short-term solution without long-term results. Once the problem is clearly understood, a solution can be devised (plan). The next step is development of a work plan with responsible parties, timelines, and tasks, and the execution of the plan (implementation). Most importantly, and a frequently missed step, is the need to follow up and ensure that the solutions in place have the desired effect (evaluation). Again, data are key to the process. Corrections may be necessary with frequent monitoring to ensure that the solution remains in place. This is a critical piece of the management decision-making process.

The following sections of this chapter highlight 2 important operational areas that may be new to the CRNA administrative manager: the OR schedule and materials management. Although these may not be in the core competency of anesthesia training or even the experiential base of a practicing CRNA, schedule and materials management are vital operational components to the successful functioning of the OR. As a leader in the OR, the CRNA administrator adds value by engaging in these broader issues of OR management.

Operations: The Operating Room Schedule

Important aspects of the CRNA leader's operational responsibilities are management activities and decisions related to the OR schedule. An efficient OR requires substantial leadership and teamwork to work through daily operational problems. This includes ensuring performance consistency of team members, instruments, supplies, and equipment. These resources must be correct to do the job, in working order, and on time.

The team charged to administer the OR schedule, or to "run the board," on a day-to-day basis commonly includes representation from OR nursing and from anesthesia with surgeon backup as needed. Every day a constant barrage of critical decisions

435

must be made, with many compromises along the way. Uncertainty, change, and sometimes chaos are part of life in the OR suite. To be successful, the CRNA administrator works with team members to bring consistency to crucial daily decisions involving the flow of people, patients, materials, and information. The OR schedule sets the framework for this daily flow. The OR Committee or a similarly named entity, is a multidisciplinary decision-making group consisting of (at a minimum) representatives from surgery, nursing, and anesthesia. This group is charged with establishing rules for conduct of the business of the OR.

As a member of the OR leadership team, the CRNA administrator is a member of the OR Committee. The OR Committee is responsible for oversight of the OR schedule, which leads to important and frequently contentious work as surgeons compete for valuable OR time.

The OR Committee sets rules for fundamental trade-offs between convenience and efficiency for OR stakeholders. To a great extent, the profitability of the institution as a whole is determined by the rules developed by the committee that governs the OR schedule.

Despite the best plans and the most complete rules, once the day starts, deviations from the schedule are normal. Emergencies must be fit into the schedule, surgical procedures are cancelled, cases go longer than scheduled, and employees have to leave work suddenly. When these things happen the CRNA administrator, as a member of the OR leadership team, must ensure that decisions are responsive, transparent, and perceived as fair and equitable. The CRNA administrator owes it to the team to support decisions and not to blame other user groups (ie, nursing staff, surgeons) for problems.

Benchmarks for general purpose ORs predict approximately 1,000 cases per OR per year, with 85% of these cases electively scheduled. Ambulatory surgery ORs may see 1,200 cases per OR per year or more. Certificate of Need (CON) states may require different volumes. By definition, elective cases are scheduled 2 or more days before the day of surgery, but an urgent case is one that should be done within 24 hours or less. A case may be designated urgent because of the medical needs of the patient or to avoid incurring an additional hospital day for the patient. The definition of emergency is that the patient is in danger of loss of life or limb if the surgery is not performed within a short period of time as defined by the OR Committee. There are rarely disagreements about what constitutes an emergency case.

The goal of OR scheduling is to complete elective surgical cases efficiently. Balance must be achieved between the requirement for convenience on the part of the surgeon and the need for the institution to conserve staff resources. Surgeons believe that when there is both a surgeon and a patient all resources should be available to begin the case. Surgeons want their procedures to be scheduled consecutively and prefer a first case of the day start, so they do not get behind in their schedule because of a preceding surgeon. Scheduling an individual surgeon's procedures sequentially reduces delays and minimizes case turnover time. The competing goals of the institution are to fit as many cases as possible into available ORs and to match the labor expense to billable hours when cases are few. This can mean OR time that is less convenient for surgeons, and they may "vote with their feet" (ie, elect to take their patients elsewhere).

One tool that OR committees use to promote efficient use of OR time is "give away time." OR committees specify "give-away time" when blocks are unscheduled and these blocks are made available to other surgeons. Block release is commonly 5 days before the day of surgery to increase the likelihood of filling the rooms, but some late-scheduling specialties such as cardiac surgery may retain the block until the day of surgery.

Most OR committees find that a system of assigning 4-hour or 8-hour blocks of time to surgeons, surgical groups, or services is most efficient. The block allocation system should leave some time unblocked so that new surgeons will be able to schedule cases, busy surgeons may add more operating time, and OR management will be able to close rooms for maintenance or upgrades. The committee reviews block assignments at least annually and sets criteria for increasing or decreasing block time. A reasonable threshold for granting more time is 85% use, and less than 70% use for taking time away. Timely release of block time for other professional activities, vacations, and other situations should not penalize the surgeon. The key to success is transparency of rules and decisions for all stakeholders.

The conduct of the OR schedule has major implications for the CRNA administrator. From actively participating in rule making and decisions at the OR Committee level to implementing these rules day to day, this is a key area of engagement for all perioperative leaders. The OR schedule closes at a predetermined time the day before. At this point cases are put on the "add-on" list, and the final schedule is reviewed for accuracy and opportunities to improve it. The schedule is checked for conflicts of surgeons or equipment and to make sure that the room assignment will accommodate the special needs of the case. ORs

might be consolidated if there are large gaps in the schedule. Case times may be adjusted to ensure "truth in scheduling" when surgeons schedule unrealistic case times. Once the schedule is finalized the CRNA administrator is responsible to ensure that sufficient staff and appropriate equipment are available to meet the needs of patients and surgeons, and that anesthesia staff members assigned to the case possess the skills and knowledge necessary to provide safe care.

Despite the best guidelines, once the day begins circumstances change, and leadership team members must step up and make decisions. Some frequently occurring challenges include finding an immediate room for an emergency patient, the hierarchy of bumping cases, urgent vs emergent designation, staffing shortages, late surgeons and patients, and surgeons who repeatedly overbook their block time. Each of these special situations has an impact on the nurses, CRNAs, anesthesiologists, and technologists working in the OR. Limiting the number of people who have authority to approve additions and changes to the schedule is wise. There must be a comprehensive and timely communication method to ensure that everyone is on the same page every minute of every day, or chaos will reign. Anesthesia departments may choose to organize CRNA services as general, specialty specific, or geographically specific. Most small ORs adopt the generalist approach because of ease of assignments and the need for all staff to share call coverage. Medium-size ORs frequently use a hybrid model in which CRNAs are organized in clusters, concentrating on a group of similar services such as cardiac, vascular, and thoracic services, with crosstraining in a second service cluster. Larger hospitals are most likely to divide CRNAs into subspecialty groups

437

concentrating in such areas as cardiovascular surgery, pediatric surgery, and neurosurgery. Regardless of how the anesthesia service is organized, every CRNA must be capable of providing a safe anesthetic for common cases such as general surgery and others likely to occur on weekends and off-shift.

Operations: Materials Management

Management of materials, both supplies and instruments, is a key driver of financial performance in the OR. The OR is the most complex area of the hospital in terms of the number and variety of items on the item list. For example, instrument trays for an orthopedic case routinely have more than 500 different items. In addition to instruments and supplies, an OR case requires fixed and mobile equipment such as ceiling-mounted microscopes and transesophageal echocardiography carts. Although anesthesia supplies and equipment are more limited, the CRNA administrator must have working knowledge of the OR supply chain and the challenges of managing the enterprise. In some cases CRNAs assume leadership roles with responsibility for the ORs in addition to the anesthesia department. In other situations inventory management for anesthesia and ORs may be integrated with a materials management function as part of the facilities department. In either case, as a member of the perioperative leadership team, the CRNA administrator is responsible to be a supportive and knowledgeable partner in reducing cost and standardizing supplies.

To provide all of the necessary supplies, instruments, equipment, and personnel for a case, the OR maintains a record of each type of surgery that lists the preferences of surgeons (preference card) or the requirements for a specific type of case (procedure

card). Preference and procedure cards also list items of interest to anesthesia including special positioning requirements, laser needs, and medications to have on hand. The card also identifies additional items such as implantable items that must be separately tracked and unique items that can be billed individually for insurance purposes.

Maintenance of preference and procedure cards is essential for continued accuracy and relevance. When a case is scheduled, the preference or procedure card generates a "pick list" that is used by personnel responsible for gathering the supplies for a given case. The system quickly breaks down if the preference or procedure card is not updated, leading to delays, frustration, and even patient harm. Many hospitals migrate from a surgeon-specific preference card system to procedure cards to achieve the advantages of surgeon standardization. This is easier said than done, because surgeons may still want special items during the case and additional items may have to be added at the last minute, leading to delays and workarounds such as notes and reminders about individual surgeon preferences. If the system is to be procedure card–based, there must be buy-in from surgeons and the willingness to enforce the cards by OR administration.

Small to medium-size ORs may use a simple system for delivering supplies to the ORs. In this case, supplies are located in a proximal area where the OR nurse gathers the items and moves them into the OR. Large surgery departments frequently use a case cart system in which a rolling cart is stocked in advance and moved to the surgical suites before surgery. Regardless of which system is used, there must be a process in place to rapidly secure additional instruments and supplies as needed by the surgeon. One of the challenges in managing the ORs' multimillion dollar inventory is the need to keep minimal inventory on hand while having additional instruments and supplies ready at a minute's notice. Because of the expense of OR inventory, the material management function requires that OR leaders apply laser beam focus to the entire supply chain process.

Continual Improvement

CRNA leaders must consistently seek to make care better through continual improvement efforts. Many hospitals embrace specific tools for improvement work and expect that leaders in the organization use this approach to solve problems in their areas of responsibility. Healthcare organizations frequently choose to employ a "toolbox" of approaches rather than adopting a single approach, expecting leaders to apply appropriate improvement techniques based on the challenges at hand. One example frequently found in the healthcare continual improvement toolbox is Six Sigma,[2] a quality-control system designed to eliminate defects in a process, such as delays in first case of the day starts. The Six Sigma philosophy focuses on continual improvement by understanding customers' needs, analyzing business methods, and instituting proper measurement approaches. Six Sigma gets its name from a statistical concept that describes the amount of variation present in a process relative to the specifications. If a process is at the Six Sigma level statistically, the variation is so small that the resulting service would be 99.9997% defect free. Another common component of the continual improvement toolbox is Lean Production,[3] which aims to remove waste and eliminate processes that don't add value to the final product, such as redundant preoperative questions by mul-

tiple caregivers. According to Lean methodology, waste is any component of a process that is non–value-added. Another definition is that waste is any part of the process that the customer would not be willing to pay for. For example, few patients would be willing to pay for the time spent in the waiting room before surgery; however, most patients would expect to pay for anesthesia and surgery time. Waste is endemic in healthcare and is likely to be the target of healthcare reform efforts in decades to come. Table 18.3 provides examples of waste in the OR that may be amenable to Lean Production tools.

Continual improvement projects have the potential to be transformational, but they are hard work. Although continual improvement efforts typically start off well, all too often they fail to have a lasting effect because team members fall back into old habits. The anatomy of improvement failure can be encapsulated in the following example.

As an example of "what not to do," the project to achieve on-time first case of the day starts begins with the formation of a team of 10 to 20 members and an improvement expert assigned to the team to guide and train them. Multidisciplinary team members, including surgeons, anesthesiologists, CRNAs, OR nurses, preoperative nurses, anesthesia technicians, OR aides, and myriad managers and supervisors are excited and collect data on their current working environment, identifying the changes most needed to achieve the stated goal (ie, achieving 100% on-time first case of the day starts). The expert develops a to-do list including action items, responsibilities, and deadlines. The staff changes processes. The expert tracks data. Leaders make this a priority, and the team makes substantial progress toward the goal (eg, achieving 80% on-time first case of the day

439

Table 18.3. Waste in the Operating Room

Categories of waste	Examples of waste
Defects: producing and correcting	Preoperative blood tests lost and redrawn
Overproduction and production of unwanted products	Routine lab tests that are not necessary, do not affect clinical decision making
Waiting	Waiting for the anesthesiologist to arrive in the room when the other members of the operating room team and the patient are ready
Not using the creativity of all employees	Operating room environment where new ideas are not considered and feedback is not solicited
Transport: moving of materials	Patient moved from phase I to phase II to phase III recovery
Inventory	Excess supplies in storage, drawers, piles
Motion: movement by workers	Searching for patients, surgeons, nurses, equipment
Extra processing	Repeat questions to patient, multiple forms requiring the same demographic information

starts). The project is declared a success, and the team's achievement is rewarded and reported throughout the organization.

Following the team's success, the expert is generally reassigned to another project, and leadership turns their attention to focus on another group. Loss of the expert can mean loss of an objective voice and the absence of expertise in sophisticated statistical analysis that allowed them to prioritize the tasks. For example, detailed data on causative factors in delaying first case of the day starts may stop being collected or analyzed. At this point the production pressure of day-to-day duties might cause individuals to revert to old habits, and the team's progress begins to regress. Other priorities, such as cost-saving initiatives reducing staff coverage, may take precedence.

The team may try to make the group look better by reporting highlights of what they hope to accomplish rather than what they actually do accomplish as performance begins to wane.

Over time, with the improvement expert gone, team members become increasingly discouraged and eventually stop caring about the project, because incentives to revert to previous behavior are more rewarding, and the process improvement is not tied to performance reviews. With the project failing and with the team reporting potential achievements, leaders may continue to communicate only about projects that are showing excellent results. Recognizing this cycle of failure, the CRNA leader is poised to prevent its occurrence through active management of the process.

The CRNA administrative manager can use several key strategies to ensure that process improvement projects have a lasting effect. First, improvement teams should have no more than 10 members, and timelines for implementing changes should be no longer than 8 weeks. Bigger teams increase the chance that competing priorities will make it hard to accomplish goals, and the longer it takes to implement the improvement, the more likely it is that other priorities will distract team members and dilute their efforts.

For optimum success the CRNA leader ensures involvement of the expert for sufficient time to motivate, educate, and sustain the team, or the CRNA administrator may be trained to take over the improvement expert role.

Regardless, the administrative manager must directly participate in the performance project rather than just providing support. He or she must observe successes and failures firsthand and make accurate assessments as to which projects are worth continuing. Performance appraisals of all staff, including the administrative manager, need to be tied to ongoing successful performance on specific improvement projects.

Health Information Technology

Health information technology (HIT) is another important realm of anesthesia operations. Comparatively speaking, anesthesia departments have been slow to adopt electronic solutions for day-to-day functions such as preanesthetic evaluation, intraoperative charting, ordering supplies, and postanesthesia care unit (PACU) order entry. Yet, HIT is a key building block of the hospital's safety, quality, and strategic framework. Both federal and state agencies require electronic health records for continued licensure or incorporate powerful financial incentives for meaningful use. Thus, hospitals and their departments are struggling to accelerate adoption of enterprise-wide HIT systems.

From a financial perspective, government regulations and payment systems provide strong incentives to adopt HIT systems and upgrade them as payment methodologies evolve. One example is the planned 2013 transition from ICD-9 (with 17,000 codes for Medicare and other reimbursement systems) to ICD-10 (with 140,000 codes). These codes appear in hospital clinical systems, research databases, and credentialing files. The additional codes will require more documentation by caregivers and aim to result in more accurate reporting for reimbursement. Training and a well-thought-out work plan for the transition are key, because hospitals risk reduced reimbursement if requirements are not met.

As a result, it is likely that CRNA administrators will be called on to implement or upgrade HIT in their departments. Options include an electronic record (a "best of breed" product specifically for anesthesia), an anesthesia electronic solution that is a component of the perioperative system, or one that is a component of a larger strategic move toward an enterprise-wide electronic medical record. If the anesthesia electronic record is a stand-alone product, it must be electronically linked to the medical information system of the hospital with bidirectional exchange of information. For example, the perioperative areas may be incorporated into an overall computerized physician order entry (CPOE) effort to improve patient safety and reduce medical errors. In addition to the ability to enter medication orders electronically in the PACU, advantages of CPOE include the ability to match orders (patient, orders, medication, and nurse),

441

to automate medication reconciliation, and to broadcast safety alerts instantaneously.

Innovation of routine HIT functions such as scheduling, record keeping, billing, and quality monitoring may have implications for the CRNA administrative manager beyond the traditional surgical information system. For example, with the movement toward patient-centered decision making, informed consent is under scrutiny. The informed consent conversation takes place in the physician's office days or weeks in advance of the procedure. At the last minute before surgery, patients sign a form attesting that informed consent has occurred. This takes place while the patient is on the preoperative stretcher, minutes away from sedation, and potentially distracted by the environment and preoperative anxiety. In the future, customized HIT systems could integrate individualized consent forms, medical information, outcomes data, and national benchmarks on performance. HIT systems also could support a computer-driven informed consent process, allowing for simultaneous interaction between the patient and the care provider.

Telehealth Services, long thought to be the bastion of outpatient clinic care, is moving to acute patient care settings and may soon have implications for the CRNA administrator. Innovations such as E-ICU monitoring systems could expand to anesthesia and perioperative areas in the future as large health systems with people and infrastructure to spare sell their capacity to smaller, rural health facilities. Hospitals that offer E-ICU add staff and sell ICU monitoring equipment to smaller hospitals to address rising healthcare costs and staffing shortages while expanding access to critical care services. Electronic ICUs monitor patients 24/7 and alert intensivists to subtle changes in patient condition. These systems have demonstrated reduced length of stay, increased protocol compliance, and a reduction in morbidity and mortality. Some experts believe that there is a role for such systems in the PACU of the future.

As HIT assumes an essential role in perioperative operations, the CRNA administrator must develop a strategy for expertise in this area. System selection, ongoing education and training, maintenance, and troubleshooting require specialized knowledge. The HIT strategy for the anesthesia department has to be developed in the context of the organizational support as a whole. Options for HIT support include ensuring that there is an HIT expert in the perioperative area, using corporate HIT staff based on need, and outsourcing HIT expertise on a contracted basis. Regardless of the approach, HIT support for the perioperative environment must be expert, timely, and responsive to input from the end users.

Operating Room Information Systems (ORIS)

Information is a powerful tool for perioperative managers. The operating room information systems (ORIS) contain financial, management, and clinical information. The ideal ORIS is designed to meet the needs of the OR leaders as well as the comprehensive reporting required by the organization as a whole.

The ORIS produces both routine reports and special reports on demand. Information contained in the ORIS should be transparent throughout the organization even if on a "read only" basis. When a particular group in the OR believes that they "own" the data, problems ensue.

It is important that the ORIS have credibility with its users and that data be quantitative and capable of being graphically represented as business analytics. Business analytics are reports that make extensive use of data and statistical methods to explain and predict performance to drive decision making. Frequently, business analytics employ graphs and other models to consolidate and interpret information in a new way.

Business intelligence refers to the use of a consistent set of metrics to measure past performance and to guide management decision making. Two useful categories of reports are utilization reports and cost reports.

Operating room utilization is on everybody's radar screen. Such reports can be developed for specific ORs, groupings of ORs, specialty groups, and individual surgeons, time of the day, days, months, and years. Units of productivity include OR occupancy, number of cases, OR minutes, turnaround time, and first case of the day starts. Utilization reports will be accepted more readily if there is consensus on key definitions by an interdisciplinary group such as the OR Committee. Accurate interpretation of report findings relies on a mutual understanding of such terms as *prime time, turnover time,* and *first case of the day start.*

Cost analysis is another important use of the ORIS. OR costs are staggering when calculated based on the OR minute. Reports can be developed for the average variable cost per case broken down into categories of labor and supplies. This can be segmented by categories of procedures, individual surgeons, by surgical specialties, or for larger ORs, by distinct areas of service. Data can be compared between months and years, inpatients and outpatients. The ORIS can also pull financial information such as the cost of implants or the use of out-of-contract supplies by surgeon by case for comparative purposes.

Staff productivity monitoring is an important element of business intelligence in the perioperative area. The most sophisticated reports link payroll data such as worked hours with financial information such as billed OR hours. For example the average worked hours for CRNAs may be 8 hours per day during prime time and the average billable OR hours may be 6 hours per day during prime time, yielding a 75% productivity rate. The CRNA leader can actively manage the match of resources with revenue-producing activity by working to consolidate ORs later in the day or by having a mix of full-time and part-time staff for flexibility.

An alternative way to measure productivity is through benchmarking CRNA and anesthesiologist performance to national norms. Organizations such as the Medical Group Management Association[4] create practice dashboards, survey tools, and other national databases that can be used to analyze anesthesia practice performance. Data include information such as the cost per anesthetizing location, units or cases per provider, the revenue per anesthetizing location, and base units plus minutes per case.

Early in their tenure, CRNA administrators should familiarize themselves with the ORIS and its capabilities. The ORIS system should be user-friendly, with the ability to generate business analytics and business intelligence information based on individual query. Data are a most powerful tool in providing credible rationale to support management changes. Transparency and data integrity are critical in creating and communicating reports in the OR. As availability of data becomes known, the problem often becomes controlling the number of reports created, prioritizing the work, and ensuring that the information is useful for decision making.

443

Talent

An anesthesia department is only as good as its people. Talent management is a critical competency of the CRNA administrative manager. For any job, the best performer is vastly better than even the average performer. For roles that require daily interactions in complex relationship situations such as those of a CRNA, the distinction between the best and others is magnified. The adage "hire tougher, manage easier" is powerful advice because success and achievement are always based on talent.

Talent is the portion of a person's performance that can't be explained by training or experience. Qualities such as positivity, relationship skills, values, exactness, and work ethic are examples of talent. Talent does not refer to clinical skills and scientific knowledge: these are the result of training and experience. CRNAs train in nationally accredited programs of nurse anesthesia and earn national certification and recertification through standardized processes. Although there is variability in clinical performance, it is far easier to select team members who are clinically competent than to recruit and select team members with extraordinary talent.

Some organizations use standardized tests to evaluate an applicant for traits that suggest talent and may not be evident on interview. The interview process can then focus on educating the applicant about the culture of the organization and asking behavior-based questions to learn how the applicant will respond to various situations. Team interviews are a way of empowering existing employees by allowing them to participate in the selection of their future peers.

Another important strategy in building a high-performance department is determining the right "fit" of a talented team member in the department. Once the CRNA administrator identifies strong talent, he or she must ensure that the candidate's talents are a "fit" for the job. It is rare for a person to have talent in every area. For example, an individual may be highly talented in relationships, positivity, and ethics, but may have low talent in exactness. This person would be a better fit as greeter in the waiting room than as an anesthesia technician in the OR.

Developing Talent

Selecting talented people who are a fit for their job duties is only the first step in developing a talent-based department. For talented employees to remain emotionally engaged in the department and in their work, they must receive recognition, have the opportunity to grow and learn, and be empowered to do what they do best. Strategies to accomplish these goals include real-time, frequent, transparent communication. In the OR, employees may need support through educational programs on topics such as conflict resolution, teamwork, and resilience techniques for coping with stress and tension at work.

Mentoring is a key role of the CRNA administrator and is a valuable tool not only to the mentee and mentor, but also to the entire hospital. Whether the leader assumes the role of mentor or creates a work environment conducive to mentoring, he or she must ensure that the mentoring is a positive benefit to all involved.

Clinical training does not necessarily prepare a CRNA to be a mentor. The leader may take advantage of support and training through the hospital Human Resources Department to structure the mentoring experience. Mentor volunteers are more likely to put in the time and effort necessary, and matching mentors and mentees who have something in common can contribute to success. Mentees often select their mentors informally once they know who can offer the best fit for their professional goals. Mentees may choose more than one mentor at a time to offer options.

Mentoring should begin with communication about how often to meet, what the mentee is looking for, and what the mentor has to offer. The best success occurs when both parties commit to trust and communication, and education on conflict-management skills is helpful. The mentee should be receptive to feedback, eager to learn, and have a positive outlook toward the experience. Both parties should understand that mentoring eventually ends to avoid misunderstandings.

The Critical Role of the CRNA Administrative Manager as Leader

There is a strong correlation between leadership effectiveness and employee engagement and productivity. Despite the multitude of leadership competencies that have been described in the literature, there is evidence to suggest that development of a "vital few" attributes differentiates great leaders from good leaders. These vital few behaviors include developing others, results-driven performance, and communication.[5] These 3 behaviors have been found to be the most important in establishing an environment in which employees are emotionally engaged. Vision, drive, experience, the ability to articulate a clear path, and a dose of charisma are additional characteristics found in the best leaders.

Quality and Safety

Establishing a culture of quality and safety is a critical responsibility of the CRNA leader. Adverse healthcare events continue to be a leading cause of death and injury in hospitals despite evidence-based preventive methods. Anesthesia department leaders commonly address anesthesia-related adverse outcomes such as chipped teeth, peripheral nerve injury, and corneal abrasion. Less obvious are the complications beyond the OR to which anesthesia may have contributed.

The anesthesia department can be instrumental in contributing to the patient's health beyond the OR and throughout the hospital stay. For example, methicillin-resistant *Staphylococcus aureus* (MRSA) was first identified 50 years ago and continues to have a major impact in terms of lives lost and healthcare costs. According to a landmark study by Eber et al,[6] hospital-acquired infections caused by organisms like MRSA killed 48,000 Americans in 2006 and cost the nation more than $8 billion to treat. The OR is a high-risk environment because MRSA commonly attacks patients via central-line–related bloodstream infections, urinary catheter–induced infections, ventilator-related pneumonia, and surgical-site infections. The study found that people who developed ventilator-acquired pneumonia after surgery stayed an average of 14 extra days in the hospital at an additional cost of $46,000 per person. In 11% of the cases, the patient died as a result. The anesthesia department plays a substantial role in preventing these infections. The CRNA administrator provides leadership to ensure adherence to practices such as hand washing and ventilator, antibiotic, central line, and urinary catheter protocols.

Many national organizations have come forward to set improvement priorities and develop evidence-based consensus guidelines to improve patient safety in healthcare institutions and in surgical services specifically. These include the Institute for

445

Healthcare Improvement,[7] The Joint Commission,[8] the American College of Surgeon's National Surgery Quality Improvement Program,[9] and the National Quality Forum.[10] Their recommendations may be specific to the OR or directed throughout the healthcare facility.

The Surgical Care Improvement Project (SCIP)[11] is a unique partnership of organizations focused on improving quality in surgical care by reducing surgical complications. SCIP is sponsored by the Centers for Medicare & Medicaid Services in collaboration with other national partners including the American Hospital Association, Centers for Disease Control and Prevention, Institute for Healthcare Improvement, The Joint Commission, and others.

The CRNA administrator attends to safety measures with implications for the OR and beyond that support a culture of safety. One example is the Institute for Healthcare Improvement's 5 Million Lives Campaign with a "central line bundle" of 5 steps to help prevent catheter-related bloodstream infections and a "ventilator bundle" that describes a series of 4 care steps to prevent ventilator-acquired pneumonia.[11] The Joint Commission's National Patient Safety Goals (NPSGs)[12] include goals to improve patient identification and the effectiveness of caregivers. The National Quality Forum–Endorsed Set of Safe Practices[13] includes recommendations for surgical-site infection prevention, wrong-site, wrong-procedure, wrong-person prevention, teamwork training, skill building, culture measurement, feedback, and intervention. Organization-wide awareness of performance gaps in any of the measures and manager accountability for safety are keys to preventing healthcare death and injury.

Culture of Safety

The Institute of Medicine (IOM) used a quote from the 18th century poet Alexander Pope "to err is human" as the title of its sentinel report on the magnitude and genesis of medical errors in hospitals.[14] This book, along with the subsequent 10 quality reports comprising the "Quality Chasm Series," is essential reading for the CRNA administrator.

Increasingly, hospital leaders are devoting efforts toward creating a culture of safety in which every team member feels comfortable raising concerns about the patient care plan. David Marx's work on creating a Just Culture[15] provides guidelines for promoting individual accountability in a nonpunitive environment. The importance of teamwork[16] and the need to create high-reliability organizations[17] in establishing a culture of safety is clear. The best organizations ensure that every team member is treated with dignity and respect; empowered to use their knowledge, skills, and abilities to make decisions; and encouraged to carry out their professional responsibilities with accountability. These safety practices are at odds with the disruptive clinician behavior sometimes seen in the OR.

Disruptive behavior is defined as anything that a clinician does that interferes with the orderly conduct of hospital business, from patient care situations to committee meetings.[18] Although there is evidence that physicians are more frequently disruptive than other healthcare team members, disruptive behavior by CRNAs has the same negative effect on patient safety. Examples of CRNA disruptive behavior include failure to address safety concerns expressed by another caregiver; resistance to standardized procedures; and demeaning behavior such as disrespectful or profane language, outbursts of anger, and comments that undermine a patient's trust in other caregivers or the hospital. The impact of disruptive clinician behavior goes beyond workforce turnover and low morale. Disruptive behavior has a direct impact on patient safety and cost.

The CRNA administrator should collaborate with other perioperative leaders to craft a "Universal Code of Conduct in the Operating Room." The code should clearly describe unacceptable behavior, include language forbidding retaliation, and should be identical for all OR staff including surgeons, anesthesiologists, CRNAs, and residents. The plan should be formally adopted by medical staff bylaw and department policy, and all staff and physicians should be trained about the behavioral expectations of the code, including what to do when disruptive behavior occurs.

At the same time, the CRNA leader must attend to, monitor, and manage conduct that elicits an inappropriate disruptive response. These include foot dragging, passive-aggression, marginal competence, or lack of preparation. The administrator is also accountable for the absence of anesthesia and OR staff when a surgeon and patient are waiting. Voluntary reporting of inappropriate behavior is not an adequate measure of compliance with agreed-upon standards, because of fear of reprisal and sociocultural factors that may prevent people from coming forward. The CRNA, in collaboration with an interdisciplinary team of surgical services leaders, must have a well-designed plan to monitor compliance with the code, including regular cultural surveys of staff and physicians, focus groups, and rounding. Code enforcement must be unfailing, timely, and consistent. Preventative strategies such as training in conflict resolution, communication, and stress management can have a substantial impact, improving the environment of safety.

Programs have been developed to support the culture of safety and improve patient outcomes, including safety checklists and processes requiring caregivers to communicate safety concerns and make measurable improvements. One such process is the Comprehensive Unit–Based Safety Program (CUSP).[19]

Originally created for the ICU environment, CUSP is designed to improve safety culture and encourage learning from mistakes to protect future patients. The first step is to educate staff on the science of safety and safety culture. Next, 2 key questions are asked: How is the next patient going to be harmed on this unit? How can we prevent this harm from occurring? Most of the time, the answer to the second question relates to communication and teamwork. A senior executive such as the CRNA administrator assists the team to learn from defects by answering 4 questions:

1. What happened?
2. Why did it happen?
3. How can we fix the problem?
4. How do you know the risks were actually reduced?

Patient and environmental safety is an essential responsibility of the CRNA administrator. Fortunately, there are national tools available to assist the leader to establish a culture of safety, enforce safe practices, and monitor safety behavior and outcomes.

Education and Research
One of the pillars of a strong perioperative environment is the commitment to training in the department. There are 2 foci in the CRNA administrator's leadership realm relative to training. The first is the responsibility of leaders to create an environment

447

in which the team members learn and grow. This dimension includes such areas as new hire orientation and staff development. The second focus is the responsibility of leaders to welcome learners and trainees and to provide them with role models and dedicated teachers who act as coaches and gatekeepers for the profession.

Both CRNA educational programs and anesthesiology residencies require clinical sites for quality instruction. Clinical experience is critical to the development of fully trained professionals, and all instructors must embrace the opportunity to optimize the students' learning. The safety of future patients lies in the hands and hearts of today's clinicians as clinical experts and teachers.

The Community

The hospital is an essential part of the community. The CRNA leader may be called upon to be the face of the hospital and meet with members of the community to communicate information about the institution. The quality and scope of services and the impact of operations will affect the lives of families nearby. As the hospital expands services and departments, members of the leadership team will serve as ambassadors to educate the community about the new offerings. Even the slightest change in the physical plant must be vetted with community members in focus groups and neighborhood meetings.

Philanthropy is another area of community responsibility for the CRNA administrator. The philanthropy component of leadership has 2 spokes. First and fundamentally, as an engaged leader and a role model for others, the CRNA must show his or her commitment to the hospital through generous giving to philanthropic initiatives and attending philanthropic events. This is not an option. The CRNA leader must sup-

---

Table 18.4. Behaviors of the CRNA Administrator as an Ambassador for the Organization

Do not speak for the organization unless authorized to do so.

Remember that you are an ambassador for the organization 24 hours a day.

Consume little or no alcohol when at organization functions.

Anticipate issues, questions, and materials you might need for community meetings.

Accept all feedback with respect, diplomacy, and graciousness and report it to your boss.

Follow up in a timely manner if you have promised to do so.

Be alert for talented people who may be interested in joining the team.

Be on time and stay late; these are valuable opportunities to make a positive impression.

Support the organization's positions and be prepared for complaints.

Others will notice how you treat staff and those in entry level positions.

---

port the leadership team and advance projects that will make the hospital successful. Second, the CRNA has an important role as a philanthropy ambassador, developing donor relationships, giving tours, and providing educational presentations to achieve philanthropic goals. Raising money is not the responsibility of the Philanthropy Department alone; it is a shared duty among all hospital leaders.

Healthcare organizations aim to be community centers for people, whether they are healthy or sick. Retail, dining services, health-related education, medical screening events, and even classes for healthy cooking are examples of ways in which the hospital draws community members to the facility. These offerings are essential marketing tools so that patients will choose the facility when they are ill.

It is important that hospitals establish relationships with elected officials at the local, state, and federal levels. In the role of ambassador, the CRNA leader must set aside partisan views and reach out to elected officials on behalf of his or her organization to further community support for the goals and objectives of the institution. The CRNA leader may also be called upon to establish relationships with public servants such as the local police department, fire department, and emergency medical services. An opportunity to support this sphere of the community is in offering training for airway management to first responders.

Regardless of the context of community relations, when a CRNA moves to a position of responsibility in an organization, he or she represents the organization in a different way than as a staff CRNA. As a leader and an ambassador for the hospital or healthcare institution, the CRNA administrator must adopt certain behaviors that convey a professional understanding of his or her representative duties in the community at large. Positivity and optimism are essential attitudes, as are the behavioral guidelines suggested in Table 18.4.[20] Being an ambassador for the organization is a source of pride and fulfillment. It is a role that prepares the CRNA administrator to be successful at higher levels in the organization. The CRNA leader should approach this responsibility conscientiously, with an understanding of the bigger organizational aims and a commitment to represent the hospital in warm and professional manner.

Summary

The OR, and therefore the management of the OR, is subject to scrutiny unknown in other parts of the hospital. Explosive change has descended on the healthcare industry, and its impact is already felt in hospitals and ORs. The CRNA director must respond to a wide range of internal and external influences that characterize the healthcare industry. Key managerial aspects of the role include working in the administrative structure of the organization, conducting financial planning and analysis, and securing appropriate staffing. The CRNA director must be well-prepared, remain flexible, support inquiry, and most of all, view responsibility as a challenge and opportunity for productive change.

449

References

1. Wallace L. *21st Century Governance.* Modified from "Sample Rules of Engagement: Meetings." Signature Resources Inc; 2010:68.

2. Brassard M, Finn L, Ginn D, Ritter D, Kingery C. *Six Sigma Memory Jogger II: A Pocket Guide of Tools for Six Sigma Improvement Teams.* Salem, NH: GOAL/QPC Products; 2002.

3. Hadfield D, Holmes S. *The Lean Healthcare Pocket Guide: Tools for the Elimination of Waste in Hospitals, Clinics and Other Healthcare Facilities.* MCS Media, Inc; 2006.

4. Medical Group Management Association website. http://www.mgma.com. Accessed January 4, 2011.

5. Trinka J. What's a manager to do? *Industrial and Commercial Training.* 2005;37(3):154-159.

6. Eber MR, Laxminarayan R, Perencevich EN, Malani, A. Clinical and economic outcomes attributable to health care–associated sepsis and pneumonia. *Arch Intern Med.* 2010;170(4):347-353.

7. Institute for Healthcare Improvement website. http://www.ihi.org. Accessed August 1, 2010.

8. The Joint Commission 2010 National Patient Safety Goals (NPSGs). Joint Commission website. http://www.jointcommission.org/standards_information/npsgs.aspx. Accessed August 1, 2010.

9. The American College of Surgeons National Surgical Quality Improvement Program. http://www.acsnsqip.org/. Accessed May 24, 2011.

10. *National Quality Forum Safe Practices for Better Healthcare 2009 Update: A Consensus Report.* Washington DC: National Quality Forum; 2009. http://www.qualityforum.org/Topics/Safety_pages/Patient_Safety.aspx.

11. Institute for Healthcare Improvement. http://www.ihi.org/IHI/Topics/PatientSafety/SurgicalSiteInfections/Resources/SurgicalCareImprovement Project.htm. Accessed January 4, 2011.

12. The Joint Commission. Standards. http://www.jointcommission.org/standards_information/npsgs.aspx. Accessed April 3, 2011.

13. Agency for Healthcare Research and Quality. National Quality Forum. Safe practices for better healthcare: a summary. http://www.ahrq.gov/qual/nqfpract.htm. Accessed April 5, 2011.

14. Committee on Quality of Health Care in America, Institute of Medicine, Kohn LT, Corrigan JM, Donaldson MS. *To Err is Human: Building a Safer Health System.* 1st ed. Washington DC: The National Academies Press; 2000.

15. Marx D. The Just Culture Community Moderated by Outcome Engineering. http://www.justculture.org. Accessed July 31, 2010.

16. Wilson KA, Burke CS, Priest HA, Salas E. Promoting healthcare safety through training high reliability teams. *Qual Saf Health Care.* 2005;14:303-309.

17. Weick KE, Sutcliffre KM. *Managing the Unexpected.* San Francisco, CA: Jossey-Bass; 2001.

18. Porto G, Lauve R. Disruptive clinician behavior: a persistant threat to patient safety. *Patient Saf Qual Healthcare.* 2006;July/August:24. http://www.psqh.com/julaug06/disruptive.html.

19. Pronovost P. Safer Care website. www.safercare.net. Accessed July 31, 2010.

20. Wallace L. *21st Century Governance.* Modified from Ambassador Duties of Board Members. Signature Resources Inc; 2010:69.

CHAPTER 19

Financial Management

Christine S. Zambricki, CRNA, MS, FAAN

Key Concepts

- The history of healthcare reimbursement is instructive to understanding contemporary challenges of healthcare financing.

- Tracking financial performance and achieving financial objectives through positive performance to budget is required of healthcare leaders today.

- Certified Registered Nurse Anesthetist administrators are accountable for financial performance in their domain of responsibility.

Every organization has financial solvency as an objective. This is essential in healthcare but often not expressed in the mission or vision statement of a nonprofit organization. Indeed, it is the ultimate and fundamental goal of any institution. Without achieving financial goals, other objectives related to patient care, quality and safety, employee engagement, and community service cannot be met. To contribute to these objectives, the Certified Registered Nurse Anesthetist (CRNA) director must achieve financial targets.

Healthcare organizations are under pressure to provide high-quality surgical care at the lowest possible cost. Operating rooms have always been considered a substantial source of revenue, and hospitals have historically increased the number of operating rooms to improve profitability. With the American system of healthcare undergoing dramatic change from paying for episodes of care to managing the healthcare of entire populations, the operating room (OR) suite is being seen more and more as an expensive hospital resource that must be expertly managed.

The CRNA administrator is a driving force behind efforts to improve the financial and operational performance of the anesthesia department and thus, the OR as a whole. To do this, the CRNA leader must use financial and operational information to make sound decisions that improve outcomes. Relevant data to accomplish this responsibility include financial reports for the anesthesia department, the surgical enterprise, and the entire organization. To understand the importance of information in financial reports and to interpret it correctly, it is helpful to briefly review the background of hospital reimbursement during the past 50 years.

Context

Spending for healthcare in the United States has been growing faster than the economy for many years, presenting a challenge for the federal government's 2 major health insurance programs, Medicare and Medicaid. The federal government generally leads the way in payment methodology for all payers including those in the private sector. Advocacy with federal government insurance programs is a priority for the nurse anesthesia profession because private insurance plans have often adopted anesthesia payment methodologies based on Medicare/Medicaid policy. Thus, a brief review of the evolution of government healthcare programs during recent decades will precede the detailed discussion of the CRNA director's core elements of fiduciary responsibility.

Historically hospitals were nonprofit businesses, charging patients and insurers for the cost of services plus a small margin or "cost-plus." In fact, facilities designated as *critical access hospitals* continue to charge this way today. When Medicare and Medicaid laws were passed in the 1960s, this charge-based system continued with all hospitals establishing charges for every reimbursable service. Successful hospitals increased the volume of billable services and captured these services with an increase in charges.

Problems appeared almost immediately after the passage of this sweeping healthcare legislation because there was more demand for healthcare than anticipated, and patients as consumers had no incentive to control use or cost.

Medicare replaced the cost-plus system with a diagnosis-related group (DRG) reimbursement methodology in 1983. Known as the prospective payment system (PPS) the patient's discharge diagnosis determined the assignment of a DRG resulting in a fixed

452

payment regardless of the amount of resources used. Incentives shifted, and successful hospitals reduced expenses for a given DRG classification and worked to ensure accuracy in DRG coding.

In the 21st century, government programs account for more than half of all US healthcare spending and are a growing burden on the federal budget, which is running annual deficits of more than $1.4 trillion. Medicare cost about $509 billion in 2009, an increase of almost 9% from the previous year.[1] By 2020, projections estimate that about $1 of every $5 spent in the United States will go to healthcare, a proportion far greater than in any other industrialized nation. In 2010, with healthcare expenditures approaching 17% of the gross domestic product, major healthcare reform legislation was passed adding substantially to the number of insured people including Medicaid beneficiaries. Spurred by incentives to reduce healthcare spending, healthcare reform drove a number of strategies, including the promotion of accountable care organizations (ACOs).

ACOS are healthcare providers or groups of providers organized to coordinate and improve care in a population of patients. To rein in the growth of medical spending, the system rewards ACOs if costs are reduced in a group of patients over time. ACOs give financial incentives to hospitals, physicians, and clinics to work together and demonstrate extensive coordination of care. With this system, hospitals achieve success by working in a network of providers to reduce the amount of healthcare resources, including inpatient hospitalization and surgery for a given patient. With a fixed payment to an entity in the ACO per a given population of patients, cost reduction remains a powerful incentive for a hospital's financial success.

Because the payment for healthcare services for the population is made to the ACO, it is important for the CRNA administrative manager to remain involved and knowledgeable regarding the portion of payment allocated for anesthesia services, the value of CRNA services, and the eligibility of CRNAs to participate as providers in the ACO. In the context of ACOs, hospital leaders expect the anesthesia department to improve financial performance by reducing cost and optimizing operational efficiency.

The growth of healthcare spending in the long term will be determined primarily by growth in the cost of medical care per person. Although the aging of the population will also contribute to future spending growth, the programs' costs per beneficiary are growing faster than both the increase in beneficiaries and the increase in the US economy. As cost-effective providers of high-quality anesthesia services, CRNAs are key to support the goals of healthcare reform. Sentinel studies in *Health Affairs*[2] and in *Nursing Economic$*[3] clearly demonstrate that CRNAs provide anesthesia care that is as safe as any alternative model and that CRNAs are the most cost-effective anesthesia care providers. According to the Institute of Medicine Report "The Future of Nursing,"[4] all barriers should be eliminated that prevent advanced practice nurses, including CRNAs, from practicing to the full scope of their training. This recommendation supports the goals of healthcare reform by allowing the healthcare industry to take full advantage of the benefits of using CRNAs. Hospitals and ACOs will then be free to choose the best anesthesia care delivery system to meet local requirements, taking into account case mix, surgeon preference, and community needs.

453

To be successful in new healthcare financing paradigms, the CRNA administrative manager uses hospital accounting systems that track the cost of resources and services provided during the perioperative period. This is known as managerial or cost accounting because the information assists in making managerial decisions.

Cost Behavior

Familiarity with common financial constructs is necessary to participate fully as a member of the hospital administrative team. The distinctions between fixed and variable costs, direct and indirect costs, and controllable vs uncontrollable costs are relevant when discussing financial performance.

In cost accounting, there is a distinction between fixed and variable costs. Fixed costs do not change when the volume of service changes. The position of the CRNA administrative manager is a fixed cost in the department because it does not change with either 100 or 200 surgical patients on a given day. Variable costs change in proportion to the volume of services. For example, the cost of anesthetic drugs is variable, because this cost will increase if there are 200 surgical patients on one day compared with 100 patients the next. Semifixed costs vary with the volume of output, but they change only when a trigger point is reached. For example, one CRNA may be sufficient to cover in-house call on the midnight shift until the number of cases being done on midnight shift reaches 800 per year, at which time a second CRNA is necessary. Semivariable costs are costs that may be proportional in some ranges and fixed in others. For example, a CRNA coordinator runs the board during the day shift (fixed) and works extra hours at the end of the shift to complete cases (variable).

Surgeons may request that financial statements be reworked to eliminate fixed costs and to only consider the contribution margin, or the difference between gross revenue and variable costs. Although the contribution margin is helpful to determine the break-even threshold or per-case impact on profit, it does not tell the full story of the cost of doing business. Contribution margin can be a helpful tool for managers in making "keep or drop" decisions. For example, if the demand for a new resource such as an OR exceeds the available time, then the OR Committee may look at contribution margin to determine the best strategic option. The department may choose to keep a service with a positive contribution margin even if it realizes a negative total profit, when indirect costs are factored in, if the contribution margin offsets part of the fixed cost. For example, if the institution has invested in a lithotripter, and each individual lithotripsy case has a positive contribution margin with a negative net income, keeping the service will offset the costs of the lithotripter investment.

Direct Versus Indirect Costs (or Expenses)

To control expense it is useful to recognize the difference between direct and indirect costs. Direct costs can be linked to specific departments, such as the cost required to provide anesthesia care to obstetrical patients. This cost includes all staff and supplies required to run the department. Because direct costs are traceable to a particular department, they are not allocated to other departments.

Indirect costs are also part of the statement of operations. They are added to direct costs to arrive at the department's total expenses. Indirect costs, or overhead, cannot be traced easily to a single department. Examples of indirect costs include ground maintenance, heating and cooling of the healthcare facility, and the costs of the cafeteria and hospital administration. Because indirect costs are not directly traceable to a unique department in the hospital, these costs are allocated to individual departments, usually in a somewhat arbitrary manner. The indirect expense line is an important one for the CRNA administrator to track every month, because the indirect allocation may begin to creep up toward the end of the budget year when the organization attempts to achieve budget projections. Hospitals should employ a systematic, equitable, and transparent approach to allocation of indirect costs based on published factors.

The true cost of business for the organization can be predicted only if both direct and indirect costs are considered. Clinical leaders may balk at accepting indirect costs in financial analysis and request that operating margin be reported. Operating margin is derived from subtracting total direct expenses from gross revenue. Operating margin is useful in evaluating department performance and in pointing out the importance of controlling direct expenses in relationship to gross revenue. If the operating margin is declining year after year, the CRNA administrative manager may "drill down" in financial records and find out why. The problem may relate to execution of the business plan, increased competition, or increased costs. The manager may also track improvement using operating margin. However, without allocation of indirect costs to all departments using some formula (which is often disputed), the enterprise as a whole will substantially under-report the cost of doing business. Indirect costs are often greater than direct costs, and even with every individual department showing

a positive operating margin, the institution theoretically could still be bankrupt.

Controllable Costs

Controllable costs are costs that can be influenced by the CRNA administrative manager's decision making. For example, if the hospital is a Level 1 trauma center and hospital policy requires that a CRNA be in house at all times, the cost of the CRNA is an uncontrollable fixed cost for the manager. In contrast, the CRNA administrative manager controls daily staffing costs through strategies such as scheduling rules for vacation and offering unpaid time off when case volume is low. Similarly, the CRNA administrative manager has some control over the variable cost of supplies.

From a 20,000 foot view, there are several drivers of controllable costs for the institution as a whole. Many of these are not under the direct influence of the CRNA administrative manager; therefore, they are considered to be uncontrollable costs from his or her perspective. Case mix and case volume at the facility are major determinants of controllable costs for the institution. Surgeon preference, and to some extent, patient preference decide the type and amount of cases. Such decisions are highly influenced by the strategic and marketing plan of the hospital and the leadership of the surgical specialty. Although the CRNA administrative manager participates in planning for new types of cases, these decisions are not truly under the control of the anesthesia department. Decisions to develop special anesthesia competencies, such as a pain service, are made by the anesthesia leaders and are considered part of their controllable costs.

The quantity and type of resources used to treat patients also are controllable costs. These choices are primarily under the

455

control of the treating physician, although they may be influenced by cost-control measures initiated by the CRNA administrative manager. For example, the physician may request that transesophageal echocardiogram (TEE) be available for major vascular procedures. This request represents an uncontrollable cost from the perspective of the CRNA administrative manager. The CRNA may have some control over the cost by developing processes to reduce TEE probe breakage, although the cost of TEE service in total is not a controllable cost to the CRNA leader.

Another factor determining controllable costs is the fixed medical facility costs of capital equipment and construction. For example, if the hospital approves a hybrid OR for endovascular procedures, the depreciation for this room is an uncontrollable cost for the CRNA administrative manager, although it is a controllable cost for the hospital. Fixed medical facility costs are subject to budget constraints set by hospital administration and department management. It is highly unusual that all requests for fixed capital equipment or construction can be approved in a given year. The best leaders develop a fair methodology for evaluating and comparing capital equipment requests by using criteria such as impact on patient safety, growth, and return on investment.

The cost of the resources needed to treat the patient is, to a certain extent, a controllable cost. Even though physicians determine the quantity and type of resources used in many cases, they are less likely to choose the brand or the vendors. The role of the CRNA administrative manager is to educate physicians about the cost of various choices and to work with the medical staff to negotiate the lowest possible price with vendors of equipment and supplies. Many hospitals have an interdisciplinary value

analysis team that collectively determines the best value for purchasing on behalf of the hospital.

The significant factor in managing controllable costs is the efficiency with which the CRNA administrative manager stewards patient care resources such as materials and staff. Important components of daily management are making efficient use of these resources and reducing all forms of waste. As previously mentioned, Lean[5] tools target the elimination of waste and may be very useful in improving clinical and administrative efficiency.

Knowledge of the different types and components of cost is necessary for realistic preparation of budgets. Identifying direct costs, understanding cost behavior, and reducing controllable costs are a large part of the CRNA administrative manager's responsibility in the financial arena.

Other Cost Terms

Other cost terms such as future costs, avoidable costs, incremental costs, sunk costs, and opportunity costs are commonly part of the financial nomenclature. Definitions and examples of these terms are included below.

Future costs are those costs calculated based on newly approved products and services. Future costs are easy to overlook but must be anticipated as a part of management decision making because historical data do not take into consideration the impact of new clinical offerings. These modifications in the type and volume of services will change the financial picture in the future, sometimes substantially.

Avoidable costs are the variable costs that may be avoided if a particular course of action is not taken. For example, if a decision is made to eliminate the obstetrics department, then the cost of CRNA salaries and anesthesia supplies for epidural service is an avoidable cost. Fixed costs are usually unavoidable in the short term but the variable costs associated with the change may go down immediately.

Incremental costs are the opposite of avoidable costs. Incremental costs are the variable costs of personnel and supplies associated with the additional volume of new business such as the additional staff necessary if a pain service is approved.

Sunk costs are retrospective costs that have already been incurred and cannot be recovered. Past decisions drive sunk costs, such as the previous purchase of equipment that must be paid for whether or not it continues to be used. Sunk costs can be either fixed or variable and should not influence decision making to the same extent as future costs.

Opportunity costs represent the difference between 2 options when leaders choose from several mutually exclusive choices. For example, the opportunity cost is $1 million when the administration decides to use an 800–square-foot space as a staff lounge rather than a new OR that will generate $1 million in net revenue. Because opportunity costs are not restricted to monetary costs, the real opportunity cost of this decision may also include lost time for patients and surgeons as they wait for an available OR and surgeon satisfaction.

Revenue

Although cost reporting is well-developed as a financial tool, revenue reporting in individual departments in the hospital is rarely an exact measure of the income generated by anesthesia services. It is essential for the CRNA administrative manager to understand the value and worth of CRNAs' services and to establish a process to accurately track revenue streams.

Revenue to the department comes from 2 sources. First, the hospital facility reimbursement for a patient theoretically includes a component for the surgery including nonprofessional anesthesia expenses. Second, the professional reimbursement for anesthesia provider services reflects the intensity (base units) and time (time units) of the care delivered. In the Medicare system "Part A" refers to hospital payments and "Part B" is reimbursement to qualified professionals such as physicians and CRNAs. Historically, CRNAs were the first nurses to be recognized for Medicare "Part B" payment.

Hospital facility reimbursement is allocated throughout the hospital by the finance department. Although the overall profitability of the hospital enterprise is known, the allocation of payments to individual departments is less of an exact science.

In contrast, the professional reimbursement theoretically should accurately reflect the services provided. However, this cannot be taken for granted. The CRNA leader must monitor the entire process for revenue capture of professional services to ensure that the department is being paid properly for services rendered. Without this oversight, it is possible that problems exist such as poor documentation, coding errors, insurance rejections, and an unacceptable accounts receivable balance. The anesthesia department has the most interest in this issue and the most to lose if it is not done properly.

Accurate revenue information is important to the fidelity of budgeting and business forecasting. Revenue tracking may include routine visits to the medical director of major insurance companies to resolve problems and clarify areas of coverage. It is essential that CRNA administrative managers understand financial reports and actively

457

manage revenue capture efforts to maximize appropriate income for the department.

Budget

The budget is a management tool used to plan and control the department's operations. CRNAs often fear that budgeting is one aspect of hospital administration for which they are ill prepared. Some dread the budgeting process and believe the result to be restrictive and even arbitrary. The reality is that a well-constructed budget can be a useful tool. The budget represents a pact between the leader and the hospital to run their areas of responsibility for a specified time (usually 1 year) for a specified amount of money.

The administrative manager makes a commitment to both revenue and expenses when the budget is completed, and this plan serves as a template for performance throughout the budget cycle, usually for a period of 1 year. Because performance will be measured relative to budget, rather than to the previous year's performance, it is essential that the budget be realistic and achievable. Errors in projections of revenue from perioperative areas can have substantial financial implications for the institution as a whole.

The budget process usually begins with a timetable for completion. This cycle may begin 3 to 6 months before the beginning of the hospital's fiscal year. An early timeline is necessary because the budget must be approved by the hospital governing board before the beginning of that budget year. There are many components and related deadlines for the completed budget package. The CRNA administrative manager must be mindful of completing each budget deadline on time, because the process proceeds in a lockstep manner, and each departmental budget influences the whole.

There are 2 types of budgets that are part of the financial planning process—the capital budget and the expense or operational budget. The processes for developing each of these budgets may proceed simultaneously because they are 2 separate processes with separate regulations for funding in hospitals. There is a relationship between the two, as will be discussed later in this chapter.

Capital Budget

The capital budget determines how the organization should make expenditures in long-term investments such as new and replacement equipment, new buildings, and major renovations. Thus, the capital budget addresses both equipment and construction dollars. Most hospitals have guidelines classifying items that fall into the capital budget by either dollar amount or depreciation life. For example, an institution may determine that capital budget items are purchases that exceed $500. A hospital may categorize as capital any equipment that has a depreciation life of 5 years or more. The American Hospital Association provides guidelines regarding depreciation of medical equipment. It is important in the OR environment to be clear how the hospital classifies instrument trays. Although in aggregate the tray may exceed the capital threshold for cost, individual instruments contained on the tray may be less than that amount. Instruments may be part of the capital budget or the operational budget depending on this determination.

As competition for capital dollars becomes more intense, it is prudent to prepare a strategy for capital purchases for a period of 2 to 5 years. In this way, hospital administration can be informed of potential expenditures and gain a thorough understanding of anticipated needs. Throughout the year, it is advantageous to obtain quotations and review equipment on an ongoing basis. This is necessary to avoid the last-minute rush of contacting sales representatives and securing accurate pricing. It is not unheard of for capital dollars to be reallocated at the end of the year to fund other projects; therefore, the earlier in the year a purchase can be made, the more likely the funding will be available. Another factor in timing capital purchases relates to the accounting method used by the hospital. If capital purchases are made at the end of the fiscal year but paid for in the next fiscal year, it must be clear to which fiscal year the expense will be allocated.

Many creative methods are used to fund equipment purchases. Equipment can be purchased outright through capital funds, either with cash or using a payment system over time. Some manufacturers offer a "lease-to-buy" option. The actual cost of total payments over time should be calculated and compared with the cost of cash purchase. It may not be financially advantageous to opt for the lease-to-buy. Yet, this may be a viable option if there are minimal capital dollars. Equipment can also be rented if the device is expensive and its use is sporadic, or if the organization wishes to determine whether purchase of the equipment is justified by volume. This is common with items such as lasers, lithotripters, and MRIs.

Another option to purchasing equipment is an agreement to purchase a volume of disposable items made by the same company in exchange for a reduced price or free equipment. The charge for the equipment is folded into the disposable product charge. In some cases the equipment may have to be returned when the agreement expires, or the equipment cost may be prorated based on disposable usage.

Before making a decision on the method of purchase, the director should collaborate with the purchasing department to analyze all options and determine the best approach. Special reductions in price may be available based on economies of scale when equipment and supplies are standardized throughout the organization.

When a decision is made to purchase equipment, there are many factors to consider. Services such as MD-Buyline offer national benchmarking for best price paid and other options of interest to subscribers. Many hospitals belong to large group purchasing organizations (GPOs) that secure special pricing agreements for member hospitals. Regardless of whether the price is individually negotiated or reduced through hospital group purchasing, it is unusual to pay the list price for capital equipment.

When equipment is needed, value analysis takes place to evaluate price, equipment specifications, and items such as training and maintenance contracts. Required features may be articulated in a request for proposal (RFP), which is sent to potential bidders, giving vendors information about item requirements and giving a deadline for a written response. In addition to price and features, the bid package specifies what training will be done and whether the training will take place on site. Bid packages also discuss the warranty, with a 1-year warranty commonly included in the purchase price. Some manufacturers offer an extended warranty at a reduced price at the time of purchase. Another factor to consider in the value analysis is how the manufacturer treats upgrades. Any upgrades should be available within a year of purchase at a discounted rate and installed free of charge. Upgrade features have become more im-

459

portant as computer software becomes an integral part of all equipment.

Construction Capital

Construction capital is used to renovate existing space or construct new facilities. Construction capital projections include all components of the construction or renovation process.

Architecture and engineering (A&E) work is the first step in planning a construction capital project. The cost of architecture and engineering is based on a percentage of the entire project with variability based on the contractor and the scope of the work. The process provides a realistic appraisal of anticipated construction costs before administrators seek the dollars to proceed with the project as a whole. The unique specifications for hospital and healthcare facilities are considered at this time (American Institute of Architects, Academy of Architecture for Health,[6] National Fire Protection Association, Life Safety Code[7]). Ideally, construction budgets for architecture and engineering costs should be approved first so the findings can be used to obtain an accurate estimate of project costs.

In a pinch, a general estimate of construction costs can be based on calculation of square footage. In the event that an unanticipated need arises during the fiscal year, it is critical not to wait until the capital budget cycle to seek construction estimates. During budget season, estimators are inundated with requests, and the estimate may be put together too quickly and may underestimate the actual costs. Worse yet, the estimate may not be done at all because of multiple requests.

In addition to the primary costs of A&E and construction, the capital construction project also includes the cost of the contents of the building. This includes furniture, fixtures, and equipment (FFE) as well as information technology costs. A contingency of approximately 10% will be added to the project for the purpose of funding cost overruns and unexpected expenses. When the project estimate is complete, construction capital includes the costs of architecture and engineering; actual construction costs; permits and other legal requirements; furniture, fixtures, and equipment; information technology; and a contingency pool.

An economic justification for capital expenditures incorporates projected volumes and reimbursement related to the capital outlay and associated expenses. The first step in developing an economic justification involves establishing certain assumptions about the project. For example, what volume of procedures will be added if space is created for an additional OR? What type of procedures will be done in this room? Will the patients be inpatients or outpatients and what is the reimbursement for the projected procedures? In the case of inpatients, overall hospital costs for the projected inpatient admission must be considered in addition to the OR and/or anesthesia expenses. What is the insurance mix for this patient population? Some procedures, such as open heart surgery, peripheral vascular surgery, and cataract surgery are generally performed on patients with Medicare as the primary insurance. Other procedures such as outpatient orthopedic surgery and tonsillectomy are commonly performed on patients with private insurance plans such as Blue Cross/Blue Shield. Because payer rates can vary widely, it is essential to estimate the payer mix for a given type of case. These factors are analyzed, and a recommendation is made to support the project or not based on whether the project is economically justified.

Although capital and expense budgets may be done separately, there is a relationship between the two. Ideally, the capital budget should be done first or at least at the same time as the expense budget. The capital project may have an impact on the expense budget. For example, the construction of an addition to the OR suite may necessitate closure of several rooms. Closure for a period of time will have an impact on both staffing and revenue if surgical cases cannot be done in usual numbers. It is important to consider horizontal and vertical adjacencies when a capital construction project is planned. For example, renovations in a surgical suite located below the neonatal intensive care unit (ICU) may result in serious vibration and noise. In the worst case, the neonatal ICU may have to be moved or the construction schedule delayed, resulting in additional expense to the organization.

The CRNA administrative manager must communicate plans well in advance in order to anticipate the impact of new programs and changes on other departments. For example, if the anesthesia department plans to institute an acute pain management program in the next fiscal year and will purchase syringe pumps for use postoperatively, there could be a substantial impact on other departments. In this case, some logical questions include: (1) Do nursing units have existing syringe pumps in place? If so, are they the same manufacturer and model? (2) Will more staffing be required to assess and manage patient pain with this technology? (3) Will more resources be required to gather the pumps and return them to the anesthesia department when patients are discharged? Communicating plans that could affect other departments contributes to an accurate and realistic budget plan throughout the institution.

Expense Budget

The second type of budget, in addition to the capital budget, is the expense or operational budget. Hospitals use 2 basic approaches to generate an expense budget: discretionary and flex methods. A discretionary budget allocates a static amount of money to the department at the beginning of the budget period, and this amount does not change regardless of changes in volume throughout the budget year. Across-the-board cuts are common with a discretionary budget. In the event that volume goes up with a concomitant increase in direct costs, the administrative manager will perform poorly to budget. If volume decreases, the manager will lack vital information on the proportional impact on cost and may inadvertently fail to reduce expenditures because the budget dollars remain fixed. This results in a negative net revenue because revenue will decrease while expenses stay the same.

In contrast, flexible budgeting is a tool that matches fixed and variable costs to fluctuations in volume. Thus, even though the CRNA administrative manager may begin the budget year with a certain amount of dollars available, on a monthly basis the budget will expand and contract as changes occur in case volume, vendor pricing, and other variables that affect expense.

The expense budget has several component parts, with a deadline for each following in logical sequence. The first component to be completed is the revenue projections for the year. The number and type of surgical cases to be done and their associated charges will determine the revenue side of the budget. It is imperative that the CRNA administrative manager seek input from physicians, staff, hospital planners, and administrators to arrive at realistic expectations for the coming year. The

461

anesthesia department must coordinate its planning numbers with OR projections, obstetrical case projections, and any off-site coverage projections for areas as diverse as endoscopy, in vitro fertilization, and radiation oncology.

During the process of budget development, many components are considered, such as year-to-date performance in the present fiscal year, new programs, new surgeons, and new procedures or extended hours. It is helpful to look outside the hospital to determine whether there are community factors that may play a role in determining volumes or mix of procedures. Is a local hospital planning to close? Are new surgeons joining an existing practice? Is the OR schedule so full that surgeons are taking their high-volume, low-acuity cases to a competing surgical center and electing to bring sicker patients to the hospital? Will the ratio of inpatients and outpatients remain relatively stable? Volume projections form the backbone of revenue projections, because reimbursement case mix, contractual allowances with third-party payers, and inpatient to outpatient ratios are applied to the volume projections. During the revenue planning process, there is an opportunity for input regarding current charges or the generation of new charges for new services.

The charge structure for anesthesia services has 2 basic components. The first is a "time-activity" charge based on the relative value guide (RVG) for anesthesia services. This charge calculates the professional payment of the CRNA and/or anesthesiologist, with most payers following the methodology used by the Centers for Medicare & Medicaid Services for Medicare payments. This system provides a charge schedule for time units (any portion of 15-min increments) and base units (a given number of units are assigned to every surgical procedure based on acuity). Anesthesia professionals may also professionally bill for related procedures outside of the operating room environment using medical/surgical codes. Examples of related procedures include pain management services, emergency intubations, and difficult IV starts.

The anesthesia department charges may also include a facility charge. The anesthesia facility charge includes the use of anesthesia capital equipment and consumption of supplies and pharmaceuticals. Some institutions opt to charge for supplies and pharmaceuticals using a checklist approach, and others employ bar-coding technology to automate the process. Operating rooms and postanesthesia care units generally levy a basic charge for a unit of time, such as a 15-minute or 30-minute interval, with charges added for each additional unit of time. Equipment and supplies are itemized and billed separately.

The resultant revenue projections drive the remainder of the budget process with allocation of resources sufficient to achieve these volume projections. In the OR, labor remains a high-cost budget item; however, the plethora of equipment, instruments, and supplies comprise one of the highest supply budgets in the hospital. The operating budget can now be constructed using the previously mentioned discretionary or flexible budget methods.

Budgeting Labor Costs

Labor constitutes the largest component of expense in the operational budget. Although CRNAs may practice in a number of different employment settings, many hospitals employ CRNAs to control the delivery of anesthesia services according to the standards and expectations of the hospital. The CRNA director needs an accurate mechanism for determining required staffing levels and monitoring labor productivity on an ongoing basis. To accomplish these goals, a staffing analysis is completed. It may be necessary to develop a productivity monitoring system to evaluate departmental performance on an ongoing basis.

An accurate staffing analysis is the precursor to an appropriate staffing budget. The CRNA director considers many factors when developing a staffing budget. The principles of projecting staffing dollars are the same regardless of type of staff. For some professional staff, standards exist that direct staffing requirements for a given service. For example, the AANA states that a minimum of 1 CRNA is required to provide anesthesia care for each anesthetized patient. Similarly, the Association of peri-Operative Registered Nurses recommends a minimum of 1 staff member for each surgical case. The American Society of PeriAnesthesia Nurses has developed staffing standards for perioperative areas. In this case study, the example of developing a CRNA staffing plan will be used.

The first step in creating a staffing model for CRNAs is to determine the anticipated requirements for coverage. Hospital A has 10 ORs running from 7 AM to 3 PM. There are 3 nonoperative locations that require anesthesia coverage each day. Off-site locations include radiation oncology, CT scan, MRI, endoscopy units, and the cardiac catheterization laboratory. The off-site schedule is done through a centralized appointment office, with a limit of 3 locations scheduled on a daily basis. If emergency cases need to be added for off-site services, the appointment office must call the CRNA coordinator to determine if staffing is available. CRNAs respond to all code calls in the institution as well as other requests for intubation or starting invasive lines. Two

CRNA staff are assigned to the obstetrics department on a daily basis. Between 1 and 2 cesarean delivery rooms may be running at a time. The epidural service is busy with 80% of the 3,500 deliveries per year requiring epidural catheter placement.

One CRNA is assigned to complete postoperative rounds and make postoperative phone calls per day. He or she also is responsible for quality assurance monitoring for the department. This function is rotated among staff members. One CRNA is scheduled daily to coordinate the schedule throughout the day. Off-shift coverage is provided by 1 CRNA in house on afternoon and evening shifts. There is no elective schedule beyond 3 PM. One CRNA is on call from home on afternoon and evening shifts. Historically, an on-call CRNA is called in about 10 hours per week and paid straight salary when called in. Weekends are covered with 1 CRNA in house on all shifts. A second CRNA is on call from home for all shifts. On weekends a CRNA is called in about 8 hours per weekend. CRNAs are paid $10 per hour to be on call. The department has no scheduled overtime; however, incremental overtime is sometimes required when cases exceed scheduled times or staff is called in. Historically, the department pays for 500 hours of overtime per year at time and a half. On the 4 approved holidays, 2 ORs and the obstetrics department are covered. Based on this example, how should the staffing budget be calculated?

The full-time equivalent (FTE) metric is the common denominator when calculating staffing. One FTE represents an individual who works 40 hours per week for 1 year or 52 weeks. An FTE equals 2,080 hours per year without benefit time. A part-time employee will be designated as a portion of an FTE based on the ratio of approved time to a 40-hour week. For example,

463

a part-time employee who is designated as a 0.6 FTE is budgeted to work 24 hours (of a total of 40 hours for an FTE) per week.

Staffing Calculation

1. Determine FTEs necessary for service coverage requirements: 20.2 FTEs

Table 19.1 shows the calculation of the FTEs and coverage requirements for the staffing example.

2. Calculate coverage for breaks and lunches: 2.0 FTEs

In this example, each employee receives a half hour for lunch and two 15-minute breaks. On the day shift, additional staff must cover these. On off-shift and weekends, the pace of the OR allows for self-coverage; therefore, only weekdays will be counted. Management personnel schedule their own lunches and breaks. The 15 employees on day shift require 15 hours per day (75/40 hours/week) to cover this time or approximately 2 FTEs. Another consideration is the hours that the cafeteria is open. In this case, it is open from 11 AM until 2 PM. Therefore, 2 people will have to do a total of 15 lunches plus their own which is a total of 17 lunches. This is not possible considering the time for report when intraoperative care is transferred as well as the hours of operation for the cafeteria. Only 5 to 6 lunches can be completed by each person, leaving 5 uncovered. The CRNA leader determines that using breaks between cases and management staff, this gap can be covered, and code calls and emergency intubations on the floor can also be covered.

3. Factor in CRNAs to cover benefit time for existing FTEs: 3.0 FTEs

A total of 22.2 FTEs are required for coverage as calculated above. In this example, every CRNA gets 4 weeks vacation, 1 week personal time, 4 holidays, 1 paid week for professional development. Historically, CRNAs average 4 sick days per year. This equals 38 total days of benefit time per CRNA ($38 \times 22.2 = 843.6$ d/y or 6,749 h/y). Recall that 1 FTE equals 2,080 hours; therefore, $6,749/2,080 = 3.24$, so an additional 3 FTEs are required for replacement of staff members due to benefit time. This brings the total staff CRNAs to be hired to 25.2 FTEs.

4. Add on-call pay and call-in pay and adjust for holiday coverage.

In addition to the 25.2 FTEs, the coverage for on-call and call-ins must be added,

---

Table 19.1. Staffing Calculation: Determining FTEs Necessary for Service Coverage Requirements

Description	FTEs
Coverage of 10 ORs, 2 OB and 3 off-site	15.0
Off-shift: 80/40, h/wk	2.0
Weekend: 48/40, h/wk	1.2
Management (QA and Coordinator role)	2.0
Total FTEs for coverage	20.2

FTE indicates full-time equivalent; OR, operating room; OB, obstetric; QA, quality assurance.

which is 0.45 for a total of 25.65 FTEs. Given a salary of $80 per hour, the total for regular salaries is:

25.65 FTEs x 2,080 hours/year x $80 per hour = $4,268,160.

Dollars for on-call coverage must be added. On-call is paid at $10 per hour. A total of 16 shifts are covered per week multiplied by 8 hours per shift for a total of 128 hours per week:

128 hours per week x 52 weeks per year = 6,656 hours per year x $10 per hour = $66,560.

Overtime dollars must also be added, which equal 500 hours times $120 per hour for $60,000. The difference in coverage for the 4 holidays should be subtracted from overall salary dollars. Normally 22.2 CRNAs are covering the clinical service on the day shift. Because only 4 CRNAs are needed for OR and obstetrics coverage on the holidays, 18.2 CRNAs x 8 hours x 4 holidays x $80/hour or $46,592 must be subtracted from the total salary dollars.

5. Calculate the final expense to budget.

There are many options to consider when calculating final budget dollars. In general, it is more economical to hire a proportion of part-time and contingent staff to have more flexibility in scheduling staff to match volume patterns. Instead of overtime,

the manager may determine that adjusting shifts can result in straight time coverage of late cases and add-ons. The management positions may be scheduled to cover all breaks and lunches, or anesthesia students and residents may contribute to the coverage equation.

This example calculates the final expense to budget using the methodology described above and is a starting point from which to make adjustments based on other options available for coverage. Table 19.2 shows the calculations for CRNA salary expense.

This process projects salary costs based on current practice. Strategic planning involves forecasting changes in the environment, many of which will have an impact on staffing. For example, if an additional procedure room is slated to open 6 months into the year, the calculation must be revised to include the future costs of orientation time and the addition of a new CRNA for 6 months. This may add to the benefit coverage and lunch and break coverage by only a small percentage; however, when calculating staffing, it is important to continue to add those small percentages. Otherwise the coverage will be inadequate when multiple changes occur over time. Although the CRNA director may not hire an additional 0.1 FTE, eventually these small increments add up to a part-time or full-time CRNA.

465

Table 19.2. CRNA Salary Expense

Regular salaries	$4,268,160
On-call pay	$66,560
Overtime	$60,000
Subtotal	$4,394,720
Less holidays	($46,592)
Total	$4,348,128

The basis for calculating CRNA staffing requirements is the workload volume. A productivity monitoring system can then be put into place to monitor monthly productivity of staff in relation to fluctuating workload.

As a first step to the productivity monitoring system, tasks performed by CRNA staff are identified and categorized as either variable or constant, based on the following definitions. *Variable tasks* are those performed in direct relation with changing workload. In the example, CRNAs covering ORs could be considered variable FTEs. With fewer scheduled cases, fewer CRNAs should be paid. The best performing departments aim to align worked hours as closely as possible to billable hours. Recognizing that the 2 values will never match exactly because of case cancellations, delays, and other gap events, it is important to employ strategies such as the use of contingent staff, voluntary work without pay, and other approaches to work toward matching worked hours to billable hours.

It can be an advantage to classify CRNA salaries as variable costs. During times of great expansion and increasing volume, variable costs will be adjusted upward in relationship to volume using standard cost accounting methods. On the other hand, salary dollars for variable positions may also be adjusted downward if volumes decrease.

Constant or fixed costs relative to salaries are those incurred at the same frequency regardless of changing workload. In the case study described, the afternoon and midnight coverage are constant or fixed costs. Regardless of whether there are cases or not, a CRNA must be in house and available for coverage. Again, there is a stair-step element to this coverage. If the number of emergency cases increases substantially, a management decision may be made to cover 2 ORs

in house rather than 1. Ultimately, all fixed positions, even the administrative ones, can undergo extremes in volume of work and be classified as semivariable. The advantage of classifying salary dollars as fixed is that the budget is more predictable and will not be affected by increases or decreases that aren't substantial enough to justify an addition or deletion of an FTE. The disadvantage is found in institutions experiencing rapid growth. If all of the employees are classified as fixed, no additional dollars will be justified in the budget to accommodate coverage as volume increases.

A management engineer or business manager may be helpful in developing a productivity monitoring system for the department. The development of such a system is beyond the scope of this chapter; however, there are several conventions used in setting up such a system. For each task, a time standard is set through the use of time studies. Each time standard is adjusted upward to reflect the amount of personal time, fatigue, or delay that was not captured. The fatigue factors represent the impact of physical fatigue on the time it takes to perform a task. If a task is studied throughout an entire shift, this factor does not need to be applied because the impact is included within the standard. If data collection takes place only during the early part of the day, the standard should be adjusted upward. Delay factors represent the common delays that occur in every work environment, adding to the time required to perform a given task. Tasks and time standards vary among institutions, depending on the types of activities. For example, CRNAs may cover obstetric cases, code calls, IV starts, or off-site cases, which need to be included to accurately predict the staffing complement.

Variance to Budget

Budget variances occur when behavior is not as predicted. Many hospitals require leaders to report a reason for budget variances. For example, a larger than predicted cost of overtime is a variance that may be explained by the sudden medical leave of 2 employees at the same time, requiring overtime coverage until a less expensive option can be explored. Tracking and reporting on budget variances is a disciplined approach to managing resources and planning for the future.

Financial Performance Statements

Every healthcare organization has its own method of displaying and evaluating financial performance. One of the key responsibilities of an administrator is to read, understand, and take action based on financial statements. There are commonalties in all financial reports regardless of the format used. CRNA administrative managers should familiarize themselves with several common reports that constitute the total picture of financial performance.

The hospital's balance sheet lists the organization's assets and liabilities at one point in time. This is a measure of the financial health of the organization as a whole.

The hospital's income statement or statement of operations shows how much money the hospital has made or lost during a time span such as a month or a year. The income statement lists revenues generated from clinical and nonclinical activities as well as expenses incurred for categories such as salaries, supplies, and services. The income statement also shows the net income, or profit/loss, which is the difference between the organization's revenues and expenses.

At the department level the income statement covers categories specific to the department function and accountability. This statement is a general report in tabular form that displays the relationship between departmental revenue and expense for a given period, generally a month. Prior year comparisons are often shown, as are budgeted amounts. This report aids the department director in monitoring financial activity. Hospitals use a conventional format, which is applied to hospital-wide statements as well as individual department statements. At year end, the same statement is used for a summary of annual financial performance.

Patient service revenue is an important dimension of financial performance. It may be divided according to class, such as inpatient, outpatient, and emergency patients. At the bottom of this group is a line for gross revenue.

Patient service revenue actually represents charges for department billable services rather than the payment received for those services. For example, inpatient revenue is the total amount of charges billed for supplies and services rendered to inpatients. This would be equal to the amount of money received if all inpatients and their insurers paid charges in full. However, this is almost never the case. The statement of operations will reconcile the difference between what is charged and what is paid in a line item that may be called contractual allowances or revenue deductions. Contractual allowances reflect agreements with third-party payers whereby the payment received is less than the amount charged. Reimbursement percentages are different for various insurers; therefore, the contractual allowance is calculated using department-specific payer mixes and payer reimbursement discounts. The contractual allowances are subtracted from gross patient service revenue to arrive at net patient service revenue.

467

Net patient service revenue is an important line to watch when changes in reimbursement take place. If a third-party insurer decides to change the method of billing for CRNAs, the net patient service revenue should reflect the impact of such a change. Miscellaneous revenue from items such as grants or consulting fees is then added into the net patient service revenue. The bottom line is the total operating revenue for the department.

The next portion of the statement of operations describes expenses incurred. These expenses are divided into categories. For example, salary expenses refer to the total of regular, overtime, contingent, and temporary salary expenses. It also includes professional fees and the Federal Insurance Contributions Act (FICA) payments. Detailed reports that provide a breakdown of individual components such as overtime are available. Beyond salaries, other direct expenses are batched together in the general statement. Direct expenses include supplies, pharmaceuticals, educational seminars, and other operational items. Depreciation of capital equipment, service maintenance, and other less obvious costs are also included in the financial statement.

Salary expense and other direct expenses are added together, giving total direct expenses. This is a critical line for the department director, because he or she may be considered accountable, with direct control and responsibility for this line. Cost-containment initiatives will be measured by their impact on total direct expenses.

Indirect expenses (indirects) also appear on the financial statement. As previously mentioned, indirects pay for the overhead of doing business in a large institution. They include a prorated portion of the expenses for support departments that do not generate revenue on their own. For example, the costs of departments such as accounting, financial analysis, public relations, and information services will be allocated to all departments as indirect expenses. Overall depreciation for hospital buildings and equipment may be allocated to departments using factors such as square footage. Individual departments have limited or no control over their allocation of indirect expenses. The method of allocation is often ill-defined, with seemingly higher allocations to revenue-generating departments.

Summary information is located at the bottom of the statement of operations in the form of net income. Net income is the bottom line. It is the measure of the profitability of the department. Net income is derived by subtracting direct expenses, indirect expenses, and contractual allowances from the gross revenue.

Some portions of the statement are expressed as a percentage reflecting the relationship between more than one variable. Net income percentage is net income related to revenue received. It is calculated by dividing net income by net revenue. As reimbursement drops, net income percentage will be reduced unless costs are reduced. Operating margin percentage is the relationship between operating margin and gross revenue. Operating margin divided by gross revenue results in the operating margin percentage.

The statement of operations may include cost accounting information regarding the number of billable procedures done by the department during a given time interval. The revenue per procedure can be calculated by dividing the gross revenue by the number of procedures. Similarly, direct expense per procedure is determined by dividing total direct expense by the number of procedures. This metric evaluates department performance relative to cost-containment objectives. In any healthcare environment with decreasing reimbursement, operations of the department must be actively managed to reduce the direct cost per procedure without affecting quality.

The statement of operations is an essential document for the CRNA director to review monthly. It is a report card of financial performance and will be seen throughout the organization. It contains valuable department-specific information such as direct costs, net patient revenue, and net income percentage, which will assist the CRNA director in planning and managing financial resources.

Financial Performance Review

As a companion piece to the statement of operations, some form of financial performance review will provide detail on monthly financial activity. This tool summarizes actual activity by category or account. For example, categories of items such as postage, disposable supplies, travel, IV solutions, and books will be listed. Expenditures and revenue compared with budget for month and year to date are available in this report. Year-to-date information is a cumulative total of the current month's and prior months' activity. Year-to-date information is helpful to compare current year and prior year performance. In this way, the CRNA director can obtain a sense of performance compared with the previous year and attempt to reconcile this with known changes in operations such as adding additional surgical hours, hiring additional staff to reduce overtime, or deciding to use less-expensive generic drugs.

The difference between actual expenditures and budget is reported as a variance. The financial performance review may provide a calculation of variance per-

centage, which is the percentage change in costs from actual to budget. It is obtained by dividing the variance by the budget. Many institutions require an explanation of budget variances, either positive or negative, when they exceed a predetermined threshold of 5%.

This level of detail permits the CRNA director to target the most significant positive and negative budget variances for review. It also assists in planning for next year's budget. For example, there may be a significant increase in travel and seminar expenses every August in conjunction with the Annual Meeting of the American Association of Nurse Anesthetists (AANA). This information can be used to spread expenses in the budget appropriately to minimize variance.

Financial Transaction Detail

The next level of detail in financial reporting is the financial transaction detail (FTD) report that provides specific information for activities that occur during the time period reported. The FTD does not have to be read line-by-line every month. Rather, it is a useful tool for the CRNA manager to take a "deep dive" when the financial performance report raises red flags. The FTD informs the manager of the content and derivation of its monthly expenses. Items such as the number of boxes of narcotic drugs ordered or the volume of intravenous fluid bags used appear on such a statement. This statement should be reviewed by an individual involved in materials handling for the department to ascertain whether any gross discrepancies exist between what has been charged to the department and what has been delivered. This report is also helpful in targeting areas for cost reduction and assessing the results of those efforts. For example, if an anesthesia department decides to implement a program of low-flow anesthesia delivery, one way of monitoring the program's success is to review the financial transaction detail for reductions in the purchase of inhalation agents.

In addition to financial measures, the CRNA administrative manager analyzes operational performance indicators that are both hospital-wide and department-specific. Occupancy, length of stay (case-mix adjusted), and revenue per discharge are examples of health system operational measures. Worked hours per billed OR hour, turnover time, first case of the day start, and variable cost per case are examples of operational metrics that are useful in measuring operational performance in the surgical suite.

Summary

Managing revenue and expenses is a key leadership competency. CRNA administrative managers require the knowledge, skill, and aptitude in this area to lead effectively. Beyond basic knowledge of financial management, the responsibilities of leadership effectiveness in the 21st century require the ability to interpret financial statements, understand performance ratios, and participate in the formulation of operational and capital budgets. Collaboration with other clinical departments, the finance department, and key medical staff leaders is essential to understanding and effectiveness in the financial arena.

CRNA leaders play an important role in the financial health of their institutions. Understanding the correct approach to fulfill this purpose is critical to the CRNA ad-

ministrative manager's success. Government agencies and private insurers are interested in reducing costs while preserving or increasing quality and access to care. It will remain for the CRNA administrator to balance responsibility for high-quality care with the pressures of financial performance.

References

1. Mathews AW. Embracing incentives for efficient health care. *The Wall Street Journal.* November 29, 2010: B1, B11.

2. Dulisse, B, Crowmwell J. No harm found when nurse anesthetists work without supervision by physicians. *Health Aff.* 2010;29(8):1469-1475.

3. Hogan PF, Seifert RF, Moore CS, Simonson BE. Cost effectiveness analysis of anesthesia providers. *Nurs Econ.* 2010;28(3):159-169.

4. Institute of Medicine. The Future of Nursing: Leading Change, Advancing Health. http://iom.edu/Reports/2010/The-Future-of-Nursing-Leading-Change-Advancing-Health.aspx. Accessed July 15, 2011.

5. *Going Lean in Health Care.* IHI Innovation Series white paper. Cambridge, MA: Institute for Healthcare Improvement; 2005.

6. The American Institute of Architects, Academy of Architecture for Health. http://network.aia.org/AIA/AcademyofArchitectureforHealth/Home/Default.aspx. Accessed July 15, 2011.

7. National Fire Protection Association. NFPA 101: Life Safety Code. http://www.nfpa.org/aboutthecodes/aboutthecodes.asp?docnum=101. Accessed July 15, 2011.

CHAPTER 20
Promoting Professional Wellness

Sandra K. Tunajek, CRNA, DNP
Diana S. Quinlan, CRNA, MS

Key Concepts

- Balancing personal, family, and career goals with physical and mental health is important to professional competence.

- The relationship between fitness for duty and patient safety is a key element in quality care.

- Systems and resource availability to maintain personal and patient safety in academic and clinical environments is a desirable institutional goal.

- Healthy coping mechanisms to manage stress related to the workplace are critical to professional stability.

- Research to extend knowledge of the meaning, scope, and implications of wellness as an integral component of personal competency and accountability is a professional goal.

- Strategies for preventing and treating forms of provider impairment need to be developed and integrated into professional environments.

The concept of healthy behavior that emphasizes equilibrium in life became a cultural movement in the past 2 decades. Today, the importance of a balanced lifestyle is receiving tremendous resurgence in both the medical and consumer literature and is heavily promoted in the media.[1] Furthermore, the escalating costs of healthcare, $2.3 trillion or 16% of the gross national product (GNP) in 2007,[2] have shifted the focus to wellness promotion, preventive modalities, and the importance of maintaining healthy lifestyles.

Stress is a growing concern in contemporary society. The frenzy of multitasking, the proliferation of technology and rapid communication, economic and global instability, and pressures for workplace productivity combine to create stress in life. Although advances are being made in improving quality of care, evidence is mounting to show that stress, fatigue, and productivity pressure are having an impact on the delivery of safe, high-quality healthcare.[3,4]

Research shows that stress has important human costs in terms of mental and physical illness. Stress also has major financial consequences. Stress has been shown to cost employers billions on an annual basis and commonly contributes to absenteeism, turnover, lost productivity, and health and disability claims. It has been estimated that stress is a contributing factor to 60% to 90% of all medical visits.[5]

Like many other healthcare professionals, Certified Registered Nurse Anesthetists (CRNAs) work long hours in a highly stressful environment and much like other professionals, often neglect their own health.[6] Studies show that the unique job demands of anesthesia professionals, including their responsibilities in critical situations and emergencies, enhance high levels of workplace stress.[7] Stress may be further exacerbated by an atmosphere of hostility, emotional problems, physical disability, addiction, fatigue, and lack of control over their environment. These factors can lead to impaired health, reduced job performance, and depression. Suicide among anesthetists, for example, has been noted by researchers as an indicator of the high stress level in the specialty.[8]

Nurse anesthetists are subject to many occupational stressors, both mental and physical, including workload, patient-care–related issues, environmental relationships, and technology overload.[7] Many providers internalize the stress as a coping strategy, which is effective for short-term but may not meet long-term needs.

The anesthesia profession is at considerable risk for the disease of chemical dependency or addiction, evidenced by studies that indicate that 10% of nurse anesthetists, anesthesiologists, residents, and students suffer from this illness.[9-13] These statistics were never more evident than in the untimely death of an American Association of Nurse Anesthetists (AANA) past president (1999-2000), Jan Stewart, CRNA, ARNP, in October 2002. Ms. Stewart was a highly respected and popular president during an intensely difficult period of the AANA history, the supervision legislative battle. Her tenure on the AANA Board of Directors while maintaining clinical obligations, adhering to travel schedules, and devotion to family, and her subsequent neglect of her personal health characterize the challenges and the need for nurse anesthetists to balance professional dedication and volunteerism with personal well-being.

In February 2004, the AANA Board of Directors responded to a call from the membership to consider the expansion of the existing peer assistance program into a broader initiative. As a result, the Board established financial support and a conceptual framework for what is now the AANA Wellness Program.

The 2004 initiative had 2 main objectives: (1) to establish the Jan Stewart Memorial Wellness Lecture Series to be presented at each AANA Annual Meeting and (2) to establish a broad-based wellness program that would provide services for members who experience a wide range of issues that affect their emotional and professional well-being.

Evolution of the AANA Wellness Program

Successful assessment and management of physical and mental health risks and behaviors is much like the anesthesia process, which identifies when a patient is at risk and the potential complications, discomforts, and untoward outcomes. It is about monitoring, balancing, maintaining, and responding to the shifts in the patient response. Routinely, CRNAs make these incremental adjustments in anesthesia plans and techniques to achieve the proper approach to a successful anesthetic and operative experience. Unfortunately, they are less likely to use similar skill and management of their own health and well-being.

Understanding of professional well-being and fitness for duty encompasses multiple elements. These include personal risk factors; workplace stressors; the disease of addiction; models of well-being theory and practice; individual assessment and coping strategies; and effective behaviors for a high-quality, balanced lifestyle.

As previously stated, the AANA Board of Directors acknowledged the need for more specialized resources in the area of overall wellness for nurse anesthetists and students. In part, this was to address concerns raised

by the death of Jan Stewart but also to heighten awareness of environmental stressors inherent to nurse anesthesia practice. Patient safety concerns related to the workforce shortages and workload pressures further emphasized the critical need for healthy, fit anesthesia professionals.

The AANA Wellness Program is a collaborative effort that involved discussions and work with the Board of Directors and includes the Council on Recertification of Nurse Anesthetists, the AANA Professional Practice Division, the AANA Ad Hoc Peer Assistance Advisory Committee, the Wellness Advocate, the Council on Accreditation of Nurse Anesthesia Educational Programs (COA), the Blue Ribbon Panel on Wellness, and subsequently the Council on Public Interest in Anesthesia (CPIA). These groups of experts confirmed the importance of the problems and the potential impact on patient safety and underlined the professional responsibility for protecting the public while serving the membership. Furthermore, the experts on the Blue Ribbon Panel on Wellness determined that fitness for duty is a complex interaction of biological, psychological, and social factors that may be enhanced by wellness education and the promotion of healthy behaviors.

The final recommendations included a conceptual model of wellness that integrated the following: (1) the Jan Stewart Wellness Lecture series, the first being held at the 2004 AANA Annual Meeting; (2) the development of a structural framework external to the work of the Board of Directors; (3) the incorporation of existing peer assistance activities; (4) the need for an individual assessment process; (5) a "brand" or identification logo for the program; (6) enhanced communication resources through the AANA website; and (7) educational programs to raise awareness concerning

473

substance misuse, stress management, chronic pain management, and disabilities.

On September 1, 2005, the CPIA accepted the responsibility for the development of the structural framework and the implementation of the AANA Wellness Program. The CPIA is an autonomous, independent, and multidisciplinary affiliate of the AANA with public representation that seeks to protect the public interest in matters of nurse anesthesia practice. A function of the CPIA is to monitor social and healthcare trends, quality and safety issues, and matters of interest and value to the membership. The CPIA is also the appellate review structure for the professional credentialing bodies: the Council on Certification, the Council on Recertification, and the COA.

Ad Hoc Peer Advisors

The Wellness Program expands the focus and builds on the previous work of the peer assistance advisors. In the first edition of *A Professional Study and Resource Guide for the CRNA,* Quinlan[14] lays the foundation and rationale for the development of wellness and peer assistance programs for nurse anesthetists.

More than 40 years ago an article appeared in the *AANA Journal* that suggested addiction was an occupational hazard within the anesthesia community.[15] Subsequent studies suggest that the problem, and its incidence, continues to affect the profession.[10,16]

In 1983, AANA members passed a resolution to form a task force "for the purpose of studying the impact of chemical dependency on our profession and to be a source of positive public relations concerning chemical dependency information as it affects our members."[17] The primary goals of the appointed task force were to review the feasibility of a support group for the members and to investigate the establishment of an "800" number for AANA members who needed assistance. The AANA hotline was established in 1986 and has functioned with peer assistance volunteers since that time.

The Peer Assistance Advisors continue to provide peer support, educational sessions, and current resources; coordinate the state peer advisors network; and update content for the peer assistance website. In September 2007, the committee functions were integrated into the AANA Wellness Program

The AANA has developed a position statement (Table 20.1) that recognizes addiction as a disease characterized by a chronic, progressive process that may destroy the individual, the family, and the community.[18] Although treatment of substance misuse is inherent to the wellness efforts, the program has the broader goals of fitness for duty, safe patient care, proper self-care, and the individual ability of practitioners to influence their own well-being.

The AANA Wellness Program defines wellness as mental, physical, and spiritual well-being, and the program is designed around the theme of "caring for self and others." Wellness is a framework that can be used in many ways to help us organize, understand, and balance individual growth and development. The foundation of the AANA program centers on researched components of a balanced lifestyle: social, intellectual, spiritual, emotional, physical, and occupational wellness.

Wellness as a Conceptual Framework

Wellness is most commonly described as an active process of becoming aware of and making choices toward successfully coping with life's difficulties.[19] Popular use of the term usually relates to individual responsibility for good health and an optimal state of well-being.

Table 20.1. American Assocation of Nurse Anesthetists Position Statement 1.7

Substance Misuse and Chemical Dependency

The AANA recognizes that substance misuse may lead to chemical dependency and addiction, a disease characterized by a chronic, progressive process that may destroy the professional, the family, and the anesthesia community. Chemical dependency is defined as a substance use disorder characterized by an inability or unwillingness to terminate utilization in spite of serious negative consequences. Although chemical dependency is a primary disease with genetic, psychological, and environmental influences and manifestations, a single use exposure of potent anesthesia opioids has been know to cause addiction.

The AANA is aware of the occupational risks for substance abuse development in anesthesia providers and the professional implications substance abuse may have for the practitioner. To address these issues, the AANA established the Ad Hoc Peer Assistance Advisors Committee (PAAC) to serve as a resource and support for nurse anesthesia practitioners and students.

As a component of the Wellness Program, the peer assistance advisors continue to provide encouragement and support for CRNA well-being through a) assessing the nature and impact of substance misuse and dependency on nurse anesthesia practice; b) educating nurse anesthetists, students, employers and the public about addiction; c) investigating the availability and effectiveness of treatment modalities; d) advocating research into the education, prevention, intervention, treatment and recovery of addiction; and, e) assisting individuals or organizations regarding intervention, treatment, aftercare and reentry into the workplace.

In the interest of patient safety and practitioner well-being, the Wellness Program promotes education and awareness regarding the disease of chemical dependency and strongly endorses peer assistance advocacy efforts for prevention, providing safeguards to patients, and ensuring the individual rights of nurse anesthetists among the communities of interest. As such, the AANA supports the concept of the development of comprehensive drug screening policies consistent with state and federal law and national guidelines. Through the auspices of the Wellness Program, there is a commitment to providing primary prevention education strategies, informational resources and peer assistance advocacy efforts that foster CRNA and student well-being and professional self-care.

Adopted by the AANA Board of Directors November, 1984.
Revised 1998 and 2007.

475

(Reprinted with permission from the American Association of Nurse Anesthetists.)

The term *well-being* brings to mind concepts such as happiness, self-actualization, optimism, vitality, self-acceptance, a purpose-driven life, optimal functioning, and life satisfaction. Obviously, these ideas are universally appealing and, as a result, have been studied by a number of researchers.

Models of wellness have evolved from the physical sciences of nursing and medicine as well as from anthropology, psychology, sociology, and theology; they encompass goals for optimal day-to-day living in which a balance of mind, body, and spirit is integrated into individual choices and behaviors.

476

Wellness is not a new concept. It dates back thousands of years to the earliest records in history. Aristotle is credited with the earliest philosophy of "nothing in excess," and Descartes, the father of modern philosophy, first linked body and mind to explain human function. Unfortunately, his beliefs perpetuated the development of separate paths of scientific study, with a focus on treatment after illness and less on the holistic approach.

A healthy lifestyle was first defined by the World Health Organization (WHO) in the 1970s as "a state of complete physical, mental and social well-being, not merely the absence of disease."[20] This concept led to a preponderance of theories related to healthy lifestyles, illness, human behavior, and the mind-body connection to wellness.

Many of the current studies of well-being are found in the psychological frameworks related to building strengths and resources throughout life. These include psychosocial development, the Social Learning Theory, and the Health Belief Model. The work of Erickson[21] focused on human development as a series of life challenges, primarily in the formative years. His research has been modified by Vaillant[22] and others by using self-reported studies to research positive well-being, adult behavioral change, and the direct influence on health and basic life satisfaction.

The Social Learning Theory of Bandura[23] emphasizes the importance of observing and modeling the behaviors, attitudes, and emotional reactions of others. Human behavior is explained in terms of a reciprocal theory, in which personal factors, environmental influences, and behavior continually interact. The ability of people to learn through their own experiences, and those of others, has application for health education through reinforcement of positive or negative consequences, expectations, and self-efficacy (one's belief in individual ability to change).

Social learning theory has been applied extensively to the understanding of aggression and psychological disorders, particularly in the context of behavior modification. It is also the theoretical foundation for the technique of behavior modeling, which is widely used in self-efficacy training programs.

Health Belief Model

The Health Belief Model (HBM),[24] developed in 1966, was one of the first models that adapted theories from behavioral science studies and incorporated them into managing health problems. Updated frequently, the HBM remains one of the most widely recognized conceptual frameworks of health behavior in societies around the world. The model assumes that people are afraid of diseases, or the consequences of behavior that lead to disease, and are thus motivated to avoid or change their actions. Changes in behavior depend on the perception of severity of the problem, perceived susceptibility, the benefit of change, barriers to change, and perceived self-efficacy. Largely in response to the emergence of the human immunodeficiency virus (HIV) and AIDS, a major example of HBM is reflected in healthcare settings in the routine use of gloves to prevent exposure to bloodborne pathogens.

Components of Wellness

Hettler[19] first described 6 components of wellness often presented as a hexagon: physical, emotional, occupational, social, intellectual, and spiritual. Building on his work, Witmer and Sweeny[25] studied the characteristics of healthy people throughout a life span. Their work incorporates dimensions of health promotion with behaviors that can be assessed through observation. This model became the foundation for wellness and prevention that serves as the basis for assessment, counseling interventions, and health promotion programs.

In this model, life tasks, which are interrelated and interconnected, are developed into measures of spirituality, work and leisure, friendship, love, and self-direction. Furthermore, research suggests that individual ability to articulate the value of these elements can strengthen self-reliance and well-being.

Self-Direction

Self-direction is the manner in which an individual regulates, pursues, and directs the major tasks in life. The patterns of behaviors and methods of adjusting or coping are processes that reflect personality and resilience in meeting challenges. The process of self-direction can be further subdivided into tasks (Table 20.2) that interact dynamically with a variety of life forces, including but not limited to family, community, religion, education, government, media, business, and global influence.

Deci and Ryan[26] summarized the discussion of well-being by describing the 2 main

Table 20.2. Dimensions of Self-Direction

Dimension	Description
Sense of worth	Satisfaction with self: acceptance of physical appearance, valuing unique characteristics and abilities
Sense of control	Belief of competence, confidence, self-efficacy, knowledge, skill, choice, influence, expectations, and control
Emotional awareness and coping	Able to express/disclose feelings, response to life experiences, sense of energy, appropriate response to challenges, negative emotions, and enjoyment of positive emotions
Sense of humor	Ability to laugh appropriately at oneself and others, capacity to objectively view and manage difficulties and to use humor to recognize inconsistencies and idiosyncrasies of situations
Self-care	Preventive mechanisms arranged through exercise, nutrition, stress reduction, rest, meditation, nonabuse of substances, and healthy relationships
Stress management	Self-regulation, seeing change as opportunity, monitoring of coping abilities, management of time, setting limits, support mechanisms, and realistic expectations
Gender and culture identity	Satisfaction with identity, valuing relationships, competence to cope with stress related to gender or cultural identity

approaches researchers take in understanding well-being. First, the hedonic approach includes the typical characteristics associated with well-being: subjective happiness, pleasure, and pain avoidance. The concept of well-being is equated with the experience of positive emotions vs negative emotions and with satisfaction in various domains of life. The second approach, the eudaemonic approach, describes well-being as fulfilling one's potential in a process of self-realization and includes concepts such as being a fully functioning person, meaningfulness, self-actualization, and vitality.

Positive Psychology

More recently, "positive psychology"[27] has emerged as a major theory founded on the belief that people want to lead meaningful and fulfilling lives. Everyone wants to be happy. Moreover, they have a desire to achieve things that make life worth living: a good education, financial security, a job that they like and enjoy, and strong relationships with family and friends. Their desires incorporate the attributes of hope, wisdom, creativity, future-mindedness, courage, spirituality, responsibility, and perseverance. The study of these positive emotions has shifted some psychologists' focus from deficits and pathology and now guides researchers to better understand and gain knowledge of what makes life worth living. Many of the research findings have been incorporated into workplace health promotion and prevention programs, academic journal articles, best-selling books, and medical treatment center environments with wellness programs for both providers and patients.

The science of positive psychology operates on 3 levels: the subjective level, the individual level, and the group level. The subjective level includes the study of positive experiences such as joy, satisfaction, contentment, and happiness. It is about feeling good. A positive affective experience has been shown to have a long-lasting effect on personal growth and development by undoing negative thoughts and enhancing resilience and durable personal resources.[28]

The individual level of positive psychology seeks to identify the personal qualities that are necessary to live a full and abundant life. Through studying human strengths, the capacity for love, courage, perseverance, and gratitude, one learns about achievement and the best way for self-improvement.

A Life Well-Lived

A life well-lived has been described as a combination of 3 factors: experiencing positive emotions regularly along with skills of amplifying those emotions (the pleasant life), experiencing a high level of engagement in satisfying activities (the engaged life), and using one's strengths in service of a greater whole (the meaningful life). The final level emphasizes social responsibilities, altruism, tolerance, work ethic, civility, and "giving back."[27,29]

Vaillant[22] has expanded the concepts of resilience and subjective well-being to include individuals' cognitive and affective evaluations of their lives. This author further suggests that strengthening an individual's mental health and promoting resilience to handling life's stressors not only reduces the risk of mental illness and substance use but also contributes to improved general health, well-being, and productivity, as well as a healthier society.

Scientists have recognized protective factors that may reduce risks to mental and general health. In recent years much has been learned about the importance of factors as simple as exercise, good nutrition, adequate rest, healthy human interactions, and support from peers as key to enhancing health.

Living today is very complex, making it difficult to achieve an overall feeling of well-being. Wellness is a combination of things that provide depth, meaning, and resilience in your life. It is a broad term that has a vast array of meanings, different for each and every nurse anesthetist or student. There are many challenges to maintaining a sense of wellness, and the definition will shift and change throughout the different stages of one's personal and professional life.

Self-Care in Professional Practice

A key component of the wellness program is professional self-care. Scientific theory views individuals as self-care agents with unique needs and suggests that individual self-management can be understood and facilitated.[30] Furthermore, the fundamental principles of professional behavior, accountability, and individual awareness serve to influence actions and lifestyle choices.

Self-care requires a commitment to self-awareness. It is very easy for healthcare providers to neglect caring for themselves. The seeds of burnout seem to take root early in careers with feelings of guilt if one does not adhere to an expected dedication to long work hours. Furthermore, certain personality traits may enhance the risk of burnout. Nurse anesthetists tend to be a compulsive group, filled with an exaggerated sense of responsibility, involvement, and availability.

As with most things in life, self-care means different things to different people. Generally, it involves taking personal responsibility for ensuring the maintenance of health and well-being. Studies have shown that people who neglect their own needs and forget to nurture themselves are at danger of deeper levels of unhappiness, feelings of resentment, burnout, and depression.[8]

Self-care is a choice, a conscious decision to shape a healthy lifestyle and a commitment to wellness, including self-responsibility, exercise and fitness, nutrition, stress management, critical thinking, meaning and purpose (spirituality), emotional intelligence, humor, fun and play, and effective relationships. Self-care contributes to high levels of well-being and satisfaction; more importantly, it is a positive component in caring for patients.

Multiple challenges exist for nurse anesthetists seeking to improve their health and well-being. Among the more common occupational stressors and risk factors that may cause harm are professional burnout, compassion fatigue, physical exhaustion, disruptive behaviors of coworkers, the threat of malpractice litigation, and chemical dependency. Students must also manage stressors associated with the anesthesia educational process.

Stress and Burnout

In the past 10 years researchers have been studying stress in anesthesia. A review of the literature indicates that stress is used in at least 4 different ways: as a stimulus, response, perception, and transaction.

A brief review of stress stimulation and response shows that when the body is exposed to a stressful condition, the hypothalamus sends cortico-releasing hormone (CRH) to the pituitary gland, which in turn secretes corticotropin and stimulates an increased release of corticosteroid hormone (cortisol) from the adrenal glands. This activation of the hypothalamic-pituitary-adrenal (or stress) axis characterizes the response to stress and is responsible for the physiological effects of stress through the fight-or-flight response.[31] The system is

479

self-regulating, and the response is short-term, returning to normal once the crisis has passed; however, persistent, sustained stress occurring over long periods of time results in chronic depletion of the hormonal and energy reserves of the body.

Stress has also been perceived as physiological and psychological behavioral responses to external or internal demands. Many studies in anesthesia suggest stress is caused by workplace demand.[8] Conditions such as time constraints, lack of control, responsibility, and complexity of tasks have an impact on the psychological response. Physiological and psychological responses may lead to a syndrome known as burnout. Work-related burnout is described by Maslach and colleagues[32] as emotional exhaustion, depersonalization, and reduced personal accomplishment. Individuals exhibit a combination of characteristics, such as physical, cognitive, and emotional deterioration of heath; a negative attitude; and reduced professional efficiency.[6]

Studies using self-report questionnaires found that anesthesia professionals experienced certain common symptoms: irritation, sleep disturbances, nausea, attention deficit, anxiety, drug and alcohol use, anger, and depression. Suicidal thoughts were associated with sleep disturbances.[8]

Burnout may present with frank changes in personality or as subtle changes that only the most intimate friends and partners may notice. The fundamental problem with burnout is that the people experiencing the feelings are too disconnected to recognize symptoms. The Maslach Burnout Inventory (MBI)is a well-established measure of burnout and is used as a screening and educational tool.[33]

The stress process is dynamic and underlies both environmental and individual change. Coping strategies refer to specific efforts to master, tolerate, reduce, or minimize stressful events and are discussed later in this chapter.

Fatigue

Compassion Fatigue

Empathy is a core characteristic of nurses and other healthcare professionals. Yet, caring too much for others and too little for oneself has emerged as a major consequence to the overall health and well-being of caregivers. The phenomenon has been described as compassion fatigue, secondary victimization, secondary traumatic stress, vicarious trauma, and secondary survivor stress.[34] Figley[34] defines compassion fatigue as a "feeling of deep sympathy and sorrow for another who is stricken by suffering or misfortune, accompanied by a strong desire to alleviate pain or remove its cause." Vicarious trauma is more closely associated with the "pervasive changes that occur within clinicians over time as a result of working with victims of trauma." Secondary stress is an empathic response associated with professionals and volunteers helping participants in catastrophic or major crisis events. Posttraumatic stress disorder (PTSD) is a recognized phenomenon often demonstrated by military personnel. Compassion fatigue and vicarious trauma tend to emerge as problems for professional providers such as nurses, physicians, and counselors. Secondary stress and PTSD symptoms may appear among all types of individuals.

The concept of compassion fatigue was first used in nursing publications in 1992. Subsequent studies confirmed compassion fatigue as a recognized stress response for individuals emotionally overcome by providing care to others.[34-36] Compassion fatigue is a state of tension and preoccupation with the cumulative impact of caring, an evolving syndrome encompassing multiple behaviors and symptoms that extends from frazzled tiredness and anxiety to psychological and physical illness. It is crucial that professionals who experience these associated behaviors—whether identified as burnout, vicarious trauma, or secondary traumatic stress syndrome—pay attention to the symptoms and seek ways to deal with the risks associated with sustained distress.

As CRNAs, we are exposed to multiple types of occupational hazards and stressors.[7,37] All are potential sources of personal harm or damage. Hazards produce risk and adverse consequences only if an exposure pathway exists or, once identified, the hazard is ignored. Healthcare professionals, including CRNAs, who experience tremendous physical, emotional, and work-related demands, are naturally predisposed to compassion fatigue. Like all caregivers, they spend most of their time at work with patients who are experiencing pain, traumatic incidents, surgical consequences, and fear. The exposure enhances the risk and conflict with an inability to balance objectivity and empathy.

The role of the empathetic, active listener associated with caring professionals and the self-preservation concepts of emotional detachment and objectivity, impressed on nurses during their training, create additional emotional burdens. Societal expectations, personal self-esteem, and identification with the professional role further exacerbate the conflict. Although there is a shortage of empirical literature, compassion fatigue is an acknowledged evolving consequence of caring. Observational reports from cohort studies related to traumatic events and professional burnout provide ongoing support for the increasing concern among the caring professions.[6,8]

A study on the stress of caring found that behavioral changes among healthcare providers who were exhibiting symptoms of compassion fatigue compared similarly to patients with major depression and risks for severe mood disorders.[36] Furthermore, Huggard[35] suggests that compassion fatigue can result if the caregiver lacks appropriate personal survival skills. Nurse anesthetists and other providers should acknowledge the risks and examine their willingness to seek advice and assistance for compassion fatigue. Table 20.3 provides a summary of conflicting emotions and symptoms that serve as warning for the problem and its impact on the work environment.

It is important for CRNAs to recognize the risks of emotional fatigue and to consciously practice coping skills. Positive self-care is a growing attitude among professional caregivers. Taking an intelligent approach by developing a plan of self-care and self-understanding improves harmony, unity, and a congruence of mind, body, and spirit.

Physiological Fatigue

Hospitals function around the clock, necessitating shift work for many personnel. Nurse anesthetists are not exempt from the effects of physiological fatigue and, by the very nature of their work (vigilance-based), may, in fact, be more susceptible.

Fatigue is a reduction in the capacity of the neuromuscular system to carry out its functions. Causes of fatigue include sleep deprivation, boredom, work overload, physical exhaustion, excessive work hours, and changes to circadian rhythms. Sleep deprivation and disturbances of circadian rhythm lead to fatigue, decreased alertness, and poor performance.

481

Table 20.3. Compassion Fatigue: Impact on Personal and Professional Function

Area of function	Impact
Cognitive	Reduced concentration, apathy, disorientation, perfectionism, lowered self-esteem, preoccupation, thoughts of harm to self and others
Behavioral	Impatience, feeling withdrawn, moodiness, sleeplessness, nightmares, hypervigilance, regression
Emotional	Guilt, anger, powerlessness, numbness, sadness, mood swings, fear, depression
Spiritual	Loss of purpose, skepticism, questioning life, disbelief, loss of faith
Personal relationships	Withdrawal, lack of interest, lack of trust, intolerance, isolation, over-protectiveness, loneliness
Physical	Exhaustion, muscle pain, impaired immune system, somatic complaints, weight loss
Work performance	Low morale, low motivation, task avoidance, negativity, detachment, absenteeism, poor work quality

Multiple studies have documented the impact of fatigue on medical personnel performance. Using standardized testing, investigators have found that, after a night of call, sleep-deprived physicians may have worse language and numeric skills, retention of information, short-term memory, and concentration. Performance on standardized tests may not reflect performance in medical situations. Taffinder et al[38] studied the impact of sleep deprivation on surgical residents previously trained on a laparoscopy simulator and found that after a night without sleep, surgeons were slower and more prone to errors on the simulator than those who had a normal night of sleep. Similarly, Denisco et al[39] studied anesthesia residents after a night of sleep deprivation and found that those who had been on call and were sleep-deprived scored less well on simulated critical events. Although psychomotor performance seems to be affected by sleep deprivation, data are inconsistent as to the impact of fatigue on cognitive function and are inadequate to assess its impact on clinical performance.

It is difficult to find scientific studies demonstrating that fatigue is responsible for anesthesia accidents and the mistakes in anesthesia and obstetrical settings. However, with the labor shortage and increasing demand for work productivity, anesthesia providers have reported errors in clinical management as a result of fatigue. Gaba and Howard[40] reported that, although subjective self-assessment of fatigue is generally underreported, there is reason to believe that fatigue is frequently a factor in medical incidents. Furthermore, sleep deprivation on a task that involves tracking has been shown to be equivalent to the effect of alcohol intoxication; in one study, performance of such a task after 24 hours of sustained wakefulness was equivalent to the performance with a blood alcohol concentration of 0.10%. Similar results were found in simulated driving studies, and other studies[41,42] demonstrated a significant reduction for interns' visual memory capacity during the night shift.

The Institute of Medicine (IOM) report *To Err Is Human: Building a Safer Health System*[4] focused on the numbers of patients who suffer the consequences of medical errors and recommended specific strategies to reduce or prevent such outcomes. The IOM report recommends that, to ensure patient safety, healthcare workers should work no more that 60 hours per week. The Accreditation Council on Graduate Medical Education (ACGME) has established limits on resident physicians' work hours to no more than 80 per week.

Additional research has shown that 3-shift work schedule concepts are of concern in fatigue-related error: (1) erratic shift scheduling, (2) continuous operations, and (3) sustained performance. Controlled experiments by Rosekind et al,[43] as well as simulated exercises, have demonstrated deficiencies in decision making, vigilance, reaction time, memory, psychomotor coordination, and information processing among flight crews and long-haul operations.

The AANA acknowledges the patient safety concerns associated with fatigue and sleep deprivation and has adopted Advisory Opinion 5.1[44] to assist organizations in developing strategies to minimize and manage worker fatigue.

Incivility and Disruptive Behavior

Increasingly recognized as an occupational stressor and productivity concern in all types of workplace environments, incivility supposedly is at an epidemic level in medicine and nursing. Disruptive clinician behavior is increasingly capturing the attention of healthcare policy makers, the media, and consumer advocacy groups. Studies show that disruptive healthcare environments heavily affect morale, job satisfaction, and productivity and, more urgently, are harmful to patient outcomes.[45] Recently, The Joint Commission issued a Sentinel Event Alert[46] that cited a history of tolerance and indifference to intimidating and disruptive behaviors in healthcare. Furthermore, effective January 1, 2009, The Joint Commission requires compliance with a new standard that addresses disruptive and inappropriate behaviors.

Researchers are expanding the definition of disruptive behavior to include any inappropriate or hostile behaviors, confrontations, or conflicts among healthcare providers. Disruptive behavior may be verbal or nonverbal and often involves the use of rude or angry language and facial expressions, threats, or even physical abuse. Disruptive behavior among doctors and nurses contributes to nurses leaving the profession.[47]

Statistics indicate that 1 of 5 Americans has an anger management problem, and some 2 million workers are victims of workplace violence each year. According to the US Department of Justice, almost 500,000 nurses become victims of violence in their workplace each year, and nurses are 3 times more likely to be the victims of violence than any other professional group.[48] The expression of anger in the workplace by practitioners is manifested in

483

a variety of disruptive and maladaptive behaviors that tend to persist or reassert themselves over time. Unfortunately, it is common for professionals to maintain a "culture of silence" that allows the behavior to persist or escalate into physical abuse. Individuals working in surgery and anesthesia, a highly stressful and potentially volatile environment, are often the targets of hostile, angry, and aggressive behaviors.

Disruptive behavior on the part of any provider undermines the institution's reputation, disrupts its operations, and affects the ability of other medical professionals to perform their jobs. Fortunately, recognition and awareness of the personnel consequences and impact on patient care have led administrators and managers to implement mechanisms to deal with workplace aggression and anger.

A work or learning environment is "hostile" when unwelcome and prohibited verbal, nonverbal, or physical behavior is severe and pervasive enough to interfere with an employee's work or a student's learning, or creates an intimidating, hostile, or offensive environment to a reasonable person.

Although it is the responsibility of managers to maintain a safe, nonhostile workplace, individual accountability is critical to changing the culture. Nurse anesthetists and other health professionals should engage in practices to ensure self-caring behaviors: good nutrition, adequate sleep, time off work, meditation, exercise, patience, forgiveness, and civility.

Research indicates that there is a link between feelings of agitation and negative emotions at work and job burnout among nurses. These experiences are an integral but often invisible part of the nursing work environment and are central to efforts aimed at increasing nurse retention and reducing the incidence of burnout—crucial factors in a profession facing nursing shortages, declining enrollments, increasing patient acuity, and an aging nurse population.[45,47]

Litigation Stress Syndrome

All practicing physicians and nurses are aware that they are vulnerable to malpractice claims, particularly for high-risk specialties such as obstetrics-gynecology, neurosurgery, and anesthesiology. Reports by the American Medical Association (AMA) reveal the biggest cost of litigation is the emotional injury experienced when one is sued. Highly qualified practitioners are accustomed to being in control, and the vulnerability and emotional response to a lawsuit is threatening to personal and professional self-image. Accordingly, more than 95% of individuals who are sued acknowledge some physical and/or emotional reaction.[49]

In a more recent survey, Waterman and coauthors[50] reaffirmed that being named in a medical malpractice lawsuit can produce devastating emotional disruption to physicians' professional and personal lives. Accusations of professional negligence or incompetence are very personal, threatening, and fear inducing. Furthermore, the stigma associated with a malpractice suit inflicts intense feelings of shame, guilt, and the sense of being a victim, all major threats to the practitioner's well-being. These feelings are further exaggerated by the legal process and persistent demands of establishing a no-fault resolution to the allegations.

The individual is likely to experience isolation, negative self-image, anger, increased negative moods, fatigue, and depression. Depression is fostered by the prolonged nature of the litigation, a sense of not being in control, and the associated feeling of helplessness that may lead to the use of drugs and alcohol as a coping measure.[51]

Hostility, anger, and depression are commonly associated with PTSD, and the American Psychiatric Association (APA) includes litigation stress syndrome in its treatment guidelines for PTSD.[52] European anesthesiologists have published guidelines for dealing with the aftermath of anesthetic catastrophes and advise against underestimating the psychological impact on staff after the death or serious injury of an operative patient.[53]

Interestingly, some practitioners report no adverse symptoms after a malpractice lawsuit. Although this may be a form of denial, research supports that this group of resilient practitioners report factors such as available peer support, shared communication with peers, patient disclosure, previous claims experience, and successful defense, which may offer protection against litigation stress syndrome.[51]

Support groups for those professionals involved in malpractice suits are not widespread but may be found in local or state medical societies, individual residency programs, hospital wellness initiatives, or employee assistance programs. Insurance carriers may provide access to counseling services as a component of malpractice coverage. Experts suggest that individual counseling may be needed to deal with the severe reactions and distress of malpractice litigation.

Student Stress

The anesthesia educational experience is highly stressful. The few studies available related to stress among student nurse anesthetists document the most common sources of student stress.[54-56] Findings show second-year students have less stress than do first-year students, and practicing nurse anesthetists have more coping resources than do students. The reports further emphasize the importance need for a proactive, supportive, struc... process designed to assist student nu... anesthetists in dealing with the multiple stressors inherent to their education. Failure to do so can lead to feelings of failure, low self-esteem, and helplessness, further leading to physical and mental effects that may predispose the student for chemical abuse or other inappropriate behaviors. Other studies have shown that low social support and little decision-making authority also contribute to student distress and may correlate to scholastic performance.[37]

A career in anesthesia means working in a stressful environment with unpredictable workloads, advanced technology, harsh lighting, ambient noise, frequent shifts in priorities, and difficult coworkers. The requirements for critical decision making, long working hours, altered sleep and eating patterns, and the need to juggle family commitments further increase stress levels. Students are expected to master large amounts of complex information; assess unusual patient health problems; develop independent, critical reading, listening, and thinking abilities; and to clearly articulate problem-solving solutions in a professional, confident manner.

Student nurse anesthetists are highly motivated, achievement-oriented individuals with high expectations, which further exacerbates these stressful circumstances. Furthermore, resources to assist students in coping with these new, stressful experiences may not be readily available or students may not be fully aware of the substantial impact these pressures can exert on physical and mental health. More importantly, students may be reluctant to access resources or seek assistance out of fear of appearing weak or inadequate.

Student perceptions of stress determine the impact on performance and learning. A little pressure can help students perform and achieve goals. With too much pressure, stress escalates and performance falls. The effects of stress on learning and memory, both facilitating and impairing influences, are well described in the literature.[57]

Research indicates that students and practicing nurse anesthetists develop multiple mechanisms to deal with daily stress.[37,55,56] Coping strategies can be separated into 2 categories. Positive coping skills or functional coping strategies that are commonly used consist of peer support, family support, social support, religion, exercise, clubs, spiritual beliefs, mentoring, and talking to friends.[58] Negative coping skills or dysfunctional coping strategies, such as illegal drug use, alcohol abuse, and promiscuous sexual behavior, have profound lifelong implications. The type of strategies that students use to cope with their problems will affect their well-being as well as influence their academic performance.

Students and CRNAs alike must be aware of the potential damages of stress and learn to recognize symptoms. Symptoms may include mental, social, and physical manifestations such as exhaustion, loss of or increased appetite, headaches, crying, sleeplessness, and oversleeping. Feelings of alarm, frustration, or apathy may also accompany stress. Escape through alcohol and drugs or other compulsive behaviors are often indications of severe stress. Unmanageable and ineffective coping may contribute to addiction, clinical depression, and suicidal thoughts—tragic consequences that possibly could be avoided by greater self-awareness.

Chemical Impairment

In the first edition of this *Guide* (Chapters 21 and 22), Quinlan[14] lays the foundation and rationale for the development of wellness and peer assistance programs by reviewing the history and incidence of chemical dependence in nurse anesthesia professionals. Her work summarizes theories, symptoms, and risk factors for addiction among healthcare professions as well as relationships within the workplace, including departmental responsibilities, intervention policies, and guidelines for managers. The discussion further encompasses prevention strategies, treatment options, and disciplinary processes and their alternatives, as well as mechanisms for recovery, reentry, relapse, and peer assistance efforts.

This section provides a brief overview and reemphasizes the major concern to the profession. For more in-depth information, review the first edition of *A Professional Study and Resource Guide for the CRNA* or access the AANA website for additional resources.

Chemical dependency is defined as the use or abuse of a substance by persons unable or unwilling to terminate its use. Twerski[59] has stated "regardless of who one is, what one is, how much one knows or how much one owns, there is always a vulnerability to addiction. No one is immune. High achievers—doctors, lawyers, business executives, clerics, nurses, professors—are particularly vulnerable."

There is little doubt that substance misuse among anesthesia professionals is a serious problem. A recent study notes that anesthesiology, emergency room, and psychiatric specialties have the highest rates of substance misuse of all healthcare professionals.[9] A retrospective study notes a higher incidence among anesthesiologists than other physicians.[12] There are few

486

studies specific to nurse anesthesia. However, a 1999 self-reported study by Bell et al[10] found that 9.8% of anesthetists admitted to misusing anesthesia substances. A conceptual model presented in this study showed the potential link between substance misuse and impaired practice to concerns of patient safety (Figure 20.1).

The study was replicated in 2006, with essentially the same results. Bell[16] reported

finding that 10% of the population surveyed admitted to use of anesthesia drugs found in the operating room, but also of using substances available outside the operating room environment. The study also found that initial misuse of substances for CRNAs tended to occur midcareer.

Baldisseri[9] estimates that 10% to 14% of all healthcare professionals misuse drugs or alcohol at some time in their careers.

487

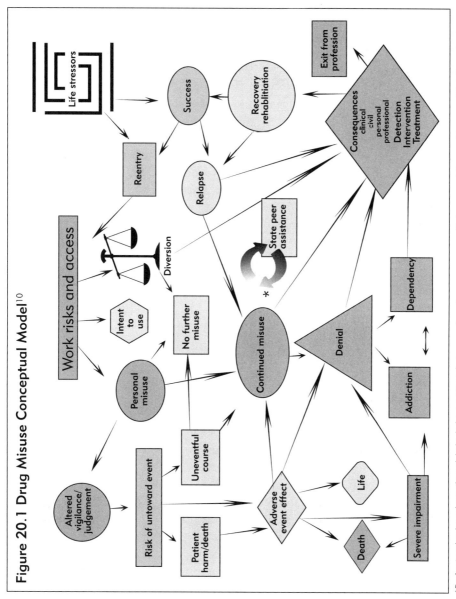

Figure 20.1 Drug Misuse Conceptual Model[10]

*Professionals who voluntarily seek help do have options that may reduce the consequences. State peer assistance advisors provide information in understanding prevention, treatment, state regulations, alternative disciplinary programs, nurses assisting nurses programs, and reentry to practice. (Adapted with permission from Bell.[10])

Substance misuse among residents is well recognized, with identified risk factors as family history of dependency, prior use, occupational stress, and ready availability of potent narcotics.[11]

The AMA and the APA recognize dependency and addiction as a diagnosable, treatable disease. The disease model is based on the concept that in order for addiction to develop, there must be a drug that is readily available and an urge to use that drug. This urge or craving is part of the neurochemical makeup of the individual and has its foundation in the central nervous system neuroreceptors. Stress has been found to be a contributing factor and, when linked with certain genetic predispositions or familial dysfunctions, the risk of becoming addicted escalates dramatically. Anesthesia professionals are at particular risk because of the accessibility of highly potent drugs.

A cascade of behavioral changes occurs when an individual begins to use drugs or alcoholic substances, and these conditions progressively deteriorate over time. The signs and symptoms vary depending on the stage of dependence and the drug of choice. For the healthcare professional, evidence of the disease on the job usually indicates a late stage of addiction. Often the problem is not discovered until the anesthetist is found unconscious or dead.

Denial is the most difficult obstacle to overcome for both chemically addicted healthcare workers and their colleagues. Denial is a normal psychological defense mechanism that operates to protect oneself from awareness of difficult or painful feelings, facts, and ideas. Denial can keep us in balance. But, when related to addiction, the denial is taken to an extreme and becomes unhealthy and an obstacle to recovery.

Enabling refers to anything that family, friends, employers, or others do that allows the addict to avoid experiencing the consequences of drinking or drug use. Because a career is a precious commodity, colleagues are often reluctant to suggest a coworker suffers from dependency. A "conspiracy of silence" develops in order to protect a job or reputation or to avoid embarrassment for the individual and oneself.

The most common mechanism for persuading an individual to seek assistance for an addiction is known as an intervention. Interventions are appropriate when concerned family members or colleagues can no longer helplessly observe the impaired anesthetist's decline or when they feel there is a justifiable concern about the abuser's welfare. For healthcare professionals, intervention and treatment may be a condition of maintaining licensure. According to the Johnson Model of Intervention, the intervention must be tailored to the specific circumstances of the individual.[60] This requires the training and experience of professionals.

The predominant format for facilities in the treatment of chemical dependence is abstinence-oriented and introduces a "Twelve Step" program. Inpatient or residential treatment programs offer the best options for the healthcare provider.

For CRNAs who have successfully completed treatment and are in active recovery from drug addiction, reentry into the workplace may be contemplated. The time away from the job will depend on multiple factors, including the drug of choice, the disciplinary process, the quality and efficacy of treatment, and adequacy of aftercare, among others. After treatment, but before reentry, the health professional should adapt to the new life with the aid of an aftercare contract. These contracts are generally developed while the addict is in initial treatment and are continued as a follow-up therapeutic plan. They act as a bridge of continued care when the recovering anesthetist returns to the workplace.[61]

Specific considerations for reentry to practice must include elapsed time, legal constraints, licensure, credentials, clinical and cognitive skills, emotional readiness, job availability, insurability, and willingness to return to the practice environment.

More information, resources, and assistance regarding chemical dependency, treatment, and recovery are available through the AANA Wellness Program.

Peer Support

Stress is an inevitable part of most working environments and can greatly affect the physical, psychological, and intellectual health of the workforce. Clearly, physical and mental illness, alcoholism, and drug dependency can be debilitating to the individual and may pose a threat to safe patient care. The decision to seek treatment can be even more difficult for professionals. Many times the professional will seek treatment only because of an intervention prompted by a licensing body or other regulatory agency.

Boards of nursing are mandated to protect the public from incompetent providers. Traditionally, regulatory boards dealt with chemically impaired physicians and nurses through disciplinary sanctions against their license to practice. Since the 1970s, boards have increasingly implemented alternatives to disciplinary sanctions, particularly in circumstances with no evidence that the behavior placed patients at risk.[14]

The National Council of State Boards of Nursing developed model guidelines for nondisciplinary alternative programs to help state boards of nursing develop a process for impaired nurses and most state boards of nursing have adopted the recommendations into state-based programs. Nurse anesthetists are eligible to participate in such programs.[61] State physicians' professional assistance programs offer similar programs. These alternative programs look beyond the licensure violations to the cause of the behavior. Furthermore, they benefit the public by intervening to prevent harm to patients; assisting the boards in holding nurses and physicians accountable through monitoring programs; and, with early identification and treatment, retaining experienced practitioners in the profession.

Most regulatory agencies use a treatment model built around professional peer support and confrontation. Professional recovery meetings, which include Caduceus-like groups (self-help recovery groups specifically for healthcare professionals), are a part of the treatment discharge plans of many professionals and function as the contracted monitoring entity for the state professional licensing boards.

Peer support is a system of giving and receiving assistance based on respect, shared responsibility, and mutual understanding. It is about relating to another's situation through shared experiences and about fostering relationships that promote growth, recovery, and wellness. Peer support is an inclusive model of positive decision making that allows people to fulfill their own needs. More importantly, participants learn how to change and control their behavior and how to define and react to problems and opportunities.

Alcoholics Anonymous (AA) is one of the original models of peer support. It operates under the principle that those who have experienced and overcome alcoholism are more effective in helping other recovering alcoholics. Today, peer-to-peer assistance

489

support has expanded to numerous settings, disciplines, and issues and has proved to be tremendously important to helping people move through difficult situations.

Peer support, whether in a structured group or a one-on-one setting, is based on the rationale that peers help themselves by helping others, and people who have overcome adversity develop special sensitivities and skills. In peer assistance, a peer or colleague acts as a friend, mentor, or trusted counselor, often providing emotional support, aid, or courage. The concept evolves from the "wounded helper" tradition that has deep historical roots and is the foundation of modern mutual-aid movements.[62]

A growing consensus in the field defines a peer as someone with knowledge of recovery from having experienced it. Peers may also share gender, ethnicity, religious orientation, disease diagnosis, or profession. Accordingly, peer credibility tends to be based on firsthand knowledge and expertise transformed into service to others. The strength of peer support groups lies in enhancing the effectiveness of existing treatment or counseling systems and providing a supporting link for successful self-care and improved health and wellness.

Peer mentoring networks can be found in a broad range of support systems, including programs for blind people, drug and alcohol addiction, cancer, smoking cessation, patients who had a stroke, disease prevention, and eating disorders, and in many other health-related areas. Peer mentoring programs also exist in many educational settings for both students and faculty, and there are a multitude of emerging programs for dealing with such life stressors as malpractice suits, gambling debt, divorce, and bankruptcy.

Confidential referral and monitoring programs are available in most states for physicians, nurses, pharmacists, dentists, and podiatrists with alcohol and/or other drug abuse or dependence or a dual diagnosis of addiction and mental illness. These programs ensure that impaired professionals receive the help they need as quickly as possible. Peer support groups as a component of these programs have been shown to help reduce the incidence of relapse. Alternative programs and peer support give affected practitioners a chance to interact with others, feel accepted, and strive to reenter the workplace as valued members of the community. Furthermore, there is growing evidence that professional association-sponsored peer assistance programs, in collaboration with disciplinary boards, appear to offer the best balance between protecting the public and the rights of the practitioners. By allowing immunity for the impaired provider who cooperates fully with the program, these programs also provide education and consultation services and professional advocacy support groups to facilitate the recovery and reentry to practice.

The consequences of compassion fatigue, burnout, sleep deprivation, toxic work environments, and substance misuse among professionals require that professionals care and support each other. Peer support is crucial to overcoming emotional, cultural, and regulatory barriers, but more importantly, it offers huge opportunities to prevent unfortunate outcomes, provide education, and promote the possibilities of change and transformation through advocacy and service.

Coping Options

Our culture teaches that we should be independent, self-reliant, rugged individualists—traits that promote resilience and strength of character. We live in a society that identifies with the strong and successful and with those who can take control and function rationally, seemingly without demonstrating feelings. Certainly, nurses are required to develop detachment skills and expected to remain objective and to appear in control. Yet they also are expected to maintain a nurturing ability to engage with the patient, to assess and interpret both verbal and nonverbal expressions of stress and pain, and to deal with the stress of trauma and death.

These persistent stressors, combined with increasing workloads and other external stressors imposed by economic, social, and biological factors, eventually exhaust our capacities to cope. Persistent stress can compromise our immune systems, affecting our physical and mental health. Anesthetists and other healthcare practitioners function in a high-risk, stressful environment that requires vigilance, exact performance, and productivity pressure, further emphasizing the great need for the development of good coping skills.[63-65]

There are individuals who seem to have remarkable resilience, remaining healthy despite high stress levels. Conceptually, hardiness is a personality dimension that "develops early in life and is reasonably stable over time, though amenable to change and probably trainable under certain conditions."[66] These individuals have a well-developed sense of life and work commitment, possess a greater feeling of control, and are more open to change and challenges. Research shows they tend to interpret stressful and painful experiences as a normal aspect of existence, part of life that is overall interesting and worthwhile. According to Fredrickson,[28] positive emotions broaden one's thought-action sequence and "prompt individuals to pursue novel, creative, and often unscripted paths of thought and action." In addition to broadening one's perspective, Fredrickson believes that the emotions of joy, love, contentment, and interest also build one's personal coping resources.

Psychological factors that affect individual coping ability include personality and behavior patterns. Furthermore, personality features such as self-efficacy expectancies, psychological hardiness, optimism, and a sense of humor are believed to have positive effects on our coping ability and our health.[67]

Resilience refers to an individual's capacity to withstand stressors, persistent negative moods, or long-term behavioral dysfunction. The primary underlying mechanism in the hardiness-resiliency process involves how stressful experiences are interpreted, usually based on the context of one's entire life experience. The central process in building resilience is the training in and development of adaptive coping skills and involves maintaining flexibility and balance in one's life.

Recommendations for building resilience and protecting the emotional well-being of helping professionals include setting realistic goals, developing problem-solving skills, creating a positive view of strengths and abilities, talking to others and seeking social support, and enhancing coping skills such as task-focused behaviors, and positive self-care.[28,67,68]

Positive Self-Care

Positive self-care is about having a personal commitment to ensure that one is functioning at one's best. Appropriate sleep, adequate amounts of water, nutritious food, exercise, and emotional and spiritual support are essential components for coping. If one goes without these essentials for any length of time, the body's operating system is undermined and adverse consequences may result.

491

Active coping (dealing with the actual stressful situations or events) can be strengthened by seeking information, seeking social support, seeking professional help, changing environments, planning activities, and reframing the meanings of problems.

Reactive coping (dealing with one's own thoughts and feelings) can be facilitated by offering accessible professional and peer counseling as well as workplace support groups such as employment assistance programs.[68] Stress-reduction strategies such as educational seminars, laughing, playing, exercising, and meditation are seen as positive coping mechanisms.[6,69]

The emerging concept of mindful meditation is an increasingly popular focus and is receiving both medical and academic attention. Mindfulness is an interesting and unique way of living and dealing with stress. It originated as a Buddhist concept, but it is now incorporated into many stress management programs as well as the complementary health prevention options now available in established medical centers. Mindfulness-Based Stress Reduction, developed by Jon Kabat-Zinn,[70] a recognized researcher at the University of Massachusetts, uses meditation practices that teach participants to respond to stressful situations in a focused manner, while simultaneously observing their own reactions and emotions in a nonjudgmental way. By using simple stress-reducing techniques such as deep breathing, muscle relaxation, or focused imagery, one can purposefully "unhook" from stressful situations and create a more relaxed state of mind. By being aware of thoughts and living consciously in the moment and effectively sensing the world around you, it is possible to make life more satisfying.

Mindful meditation is a way to quiet and calm the mind and helps restore and maintain a sense of personal balance and develop the skills to avoid emotional and physical depletion. This is important not only for persons who are facing stress-related conditions but also for persons who want to avoid physical or professional burnout.

Critical incidents are highly stressful threatening situations or events—either perceived or real—that have sufficient power to overwhelm an individual's ability to cope. After having been exposed to traumatic stress, healthcare workers may experience a range of reactions, including deterioration of job performance, personality change, anxiety states, relationship discord, grief reactions, depression, substance misuse, and suicidal thoughts. These effects can be immediate, can appear later, or both.

Critical Incident Stress Management (CISM) is a comprehensive, integrative, multicomponent crisis intervention system commonly used by large industries or organizations. It consists of multiple crisis interventions, tailored to the incident, from the precrisis phase through the acute crisis phase and into the postcrisis phase. Interventions in CISM may be applied to the individual, small functional groups, large groups, families, organizations, and even communities.[71]

Critical Incident Stress Debriefing (CISD) is a process that prevents or limits the development of posttraumatic stress in people exposed to critical incidents. Critical incidents related to healthcare most often involve injury to or death of a patient or coworker. Professionally conducted debriefings help people cope with and recover from an incident's aftereffects. Besides enabling participants to understand that they are not alone in their reactions to a distressing event, CISD provides them with an opportunity to discuss their thoughts and feelings in a controlled, safe environment.

Optimally, CISD should occur within 24 to 72 hours of an incident.[71,72]

Studies have shown that early intervention by both professionals and peers who are specially trained, and who follow an established standard of stress intervention techniques, positively affects recovery from traumatic stress. Experts believe that debriefing can help individuals improve their coping abilities and dramatically decrease the occurrence of PSTD.

Healthcare organizations have become increasingly aware of the toll that unique occupational stressors take on the quality of patient care and the safety of healthcare workers. Today, CISM systems and processes are being included in requirements for policy development, education and training, and resource programs to assist healthcare professionals in managing critical incident situations.

Balancing Personal and Professional Responsibility

Much like planning and adjusting appropriate anesthesia techniques, CRNAs can choose to do things that may create balance in their own lives. Achieving and maintaining balance can be incredibly difficult when one considers the daily onslaught of demands and the unique set of challenges facing an anesthetist. This is especially true when a CRNA also juggles multiple family demands or other external activities.

Balance is stability, from managing time correctly to eating healthily to being mindful in one's thinking, choices, and actions. Balance helps facilitate busy everyday lives. There are many ways to help achieve a degree of balance and optimal healthy lifestyle. For example, time management, eating right, working out regularly, getting enough sleep, and practicing ways to deal with stress all enable one to achieve balance more easily.

Effective assessment begins with choices and enacts a vision of what we most value for ourselves, our families, and our patients. Assessment is a goal-oriented process that involves not only knowledge and abilities of the practitioner but also the personal values, attitudes, and habits that may affect the success of choices and experiences.

Many wellness experts advocate for the principles of self-care that are taken from a mix of personal experience, wellness literature, and expert advice (Table 20.4). But it is the individual professional who must take responsibility for interpreting the environment that influences personal well-being.

It is important to not allow external factors to dominate choices or to manipulate the body's emotional and physical status. Nurse anesthetists should be accountable for developing strategies to decrease stress levels, to avoid negative moods and loss of control, and to build resilience and balance in order to live a healthy life.

Nurse anesthetists are critical members of the healthcare team. There is a severe lack of evidence-based research on wellness in this cohort of sought-after high-risk practitioners. Further studies are needed that measure and predict CRNAs' ability to cope with the conflicting emotions of their chosen careers.

Summary

It has been said that one-half of all causes of death in the United States are due to lifestyle and behavioral factors.[73] Most risk factors for the top 10 causes of death in the United States can be controlled through a basic series of lifestyle changes. Behavioral patterns can influence risk for premature mortality and morbidity, allowing primary prevention and behavior change as the preferred approach to decreasing disease states

493

Table 20.4. Principles of Wellness

Principle	Description and benefits
Create a long-term vision of your life.	Avoids being overwhelmed by tumult and confusion. Helps construct a roadmap on which a sense of accomplishment is achieved.
Connect to your colleagues.	Getting to know your coworkers provides positive support and enhances relationships.
Enjoy what you do.	Ability to laugh and see the moment as humorous is paramount in dispelling intermittent feelings of anxiety and self-doubt.
Physical well-being	Physical activity improves ability to cope with the sleep disturbances that are common among shift workers.
Keep in touch with friends and family.	Creates and maintains a healthy bond with immediate family, friends, or mentors, which is essential for support and renewal.
Manage your time efficiently.	The demands of our careers are unique and present challenges to mental and physical health.
Make plans.	Create things to look forward to: time with your children, traveling abroad, reunions, reading a good book—anything you enjoy.
Take time for yourself.	Downtime—as little as 5 minutes or as long as the weekend—refuels your sense of self.
Be realistic.	Avoid overburdening your schedule, maintain adequate sleep, maintain health, and value and commit to the things and the people you enjoy.

and improving quality of life. There has been a documented interest in preventing morbidity and mortality through specific behavior change approaches. Health behavior research has grown over the last 2 decades, with theoretical approaches to change being applied in practical ways.

Wellness encompasses elements from the physical, mental, emotional, social, and spiritual dimensions of health. Wellness is often viewed holistically and is associated with happiness, security, comfort, good health, and a purposeful quality of life. Contemporary views of individual well-being are focused on developing strategies related to personal responsibility for self-care and a balanced, healthy lifestyle.

The public and the anesthesia community have the expectation that providers will report for work fit for duty and be able to perform their duties in a safe, appropriate, and effective manner that is free from the adverse effects of physical, mental, emotional, and personal problems.

A growing body of science shows the critical effects of a sustained stressful work environment and suggests that healthcare workers need to develop essential knowledge, skills, and attitudes for making decisions concerning personal fitness and wellness behaviors. Additionally, heightened concerns for competence among healthcare providers, the increasing reports of provider impairment, and the growing public demand for accountability from the healthcare professions has refocused the anesthesia community on the need for optimal levels of physical, emotional, and mental fitness for duty.

Among policy makers there is a building consensus toward transforming professional attitudes and changing institutional policies to encourage healthcare providers to seek help for unhealthy behaviors. Research is growing to address wellness characteristics in both patient and provider populations. Much has been achieved, but there is further need for studies and the use of consistent measures to track wellness among anesthesia professionals over time.

Creating a career in the nurse anesthesia profession is a challenge and requires a workable balance between professional and personal responsibilities. Anesthesia is a field that brings great professional satisfaction but has specific issues that can cause increased stress. Identifying potential pitfalls and actively working to avoid them will help ensure a healthy and long-standing career.

All individuals and families are at risk of stress and situational distress. To build and maintain well-being, CRNAs need to develop self-understanding, coping skills, resilience, and effective use of social support.

Perhaps it is best summarized in the words of Sarah Stewart Gomes,[74] daughter of Jan Stewart, who stated in a video presented to the 2004 Annual Meeting membership, "In sharing experiences we can create possibilities from even the darkest of tragedies. My vision for my mother's legacy is that we grant each other permission to take care of each other."

Caring for ourselves and others is a critical component of personal and professional well-being. Commitment to wellness is the foundation, the first steps along the path of a journey that is an obligation—to ourselves, our work, our profession, and the public.

References

1. Jamner MS, Stokols D, eds. *Promoting Human Wellness: New Frontiers for Research, Practice, and Policy.* Berkeley, CA: University of California Press; 2001.

2. Rosdahl CB. Kowalski MT. *Textbook Basic Nursing.* 9th ed. Philadelphia, PA: Lippincott William & Wilkins; 2007:51.

3. Clancy CM. Sleepless in the hospital: evidence mounts that tired caregivers may compromise quality. *J Patient Safety.* 2007;3(3):125-127.

4. Kohn KT, Corrigan J, Donaldson MS. *To Err is Human: Building a Safer Health System.* Washington DC: Institute of Medicine report. National Academies Press; 2000.

5. Golden R. Counting the costs of stress. *New York Times.* September 23, 2004.

6. Vahey DC, Aiken LH, Sloane DM, Clarke SP, Vargus D. Nurse burnout and patient satisfaction. *Med Care.* 2004;42(2 suppl):57-66.

7. Perry TR. The Certified Registered Nurse Anesthetist: occupational responsibilities, perceived stressors, coping strategies, and work relationships. *AANA J.* 2005;73(5):351-356.

8. Nyssen AS, Hansez I. Stress and burnout in anaesthesia. *Curr Opin Anaesthesiol.* 2008;21(3):406-411.

495

496

9. Baldisseri MR. Impaired healthcare professional. *Crit Care Med.* 2007;35(2; suppl):S106-S116.

10. Bell DM, McDonough JP, Ellison JS, Fitzhugh EC. Controlled drug misuse by Certified Registered Nurse Anesthetists. *AANA J.* 1999;67(2):133-140.

11. Collins GB, McAllister MS, Jensen M, Gooden TA. Chemical dependency treatment outcomes of residents in anesthesiology: results of a survey. *Anesth Analg.* 2005;101(5):1457-1462.

12. Paris RT, Canavan DI. Physician substance abuse impairment: anesthesiologists vs other specialties. *J Addict Dis.* 1999;18(1):1-7.

13. Trinkoff AM, Storr CL. Substance use among nurses: differences between specialties. *Am J Public Health.* 1998;88(4):581-585.

14. Quinlan D. Peer assistance—parts I and II. In: Foster S, Faut-Callahan M, eds. *A Professional Study and Resource Guide for the CRNA.* Park Ridge, IL: American Association of Nurse Anesthetists; 2002:425-484.

15. Lundy JS, McQuillen FA. Narcotics and the anesthetist: professional hazards. *AANA J.* 1962;57:75-77.

16. Bell D. Current state of drug misuse by CRNAs: prevalence, attitudes, and controversies. Presented at: AANA Peer Assistance Advisors workshop; May 19, 2007; Park Ridge, IL.

17. Annual business meeting minutes. AANA Annual Meeting; August 21, 1983; New Orleans, LA [archives]. Park Ridge, IL: American Association of Nurse Anesthetists; 1983.

18. AANA Position Statement Number 1.7: Substance Misuse and Chemical Dependency. Park Ridge, IL: American Association of Nurse Anesthetists; 2007. http://www.aana.com. Accessed December 15, 2009.

19. Hettler B. Wellness: encouraging a lifetime pursuit of excellence. *Health Values* [now *Am J Health Promotion*]. 1984;8(4):13-17.

20. World Health Organization. Glossary of Humanitarian Terms. http://www.who.int/hac/about/definitions/en/. Accessed April 20, 2010.

21. Erickson EH. *The Life Cycle Completed.* New York, NY: WW Norton & Co; 1997.

22. Vaillant G. Positive emotions, spirituality and the practice of psychiatry. *Mens Sana Monogr.* 2008;6:48-62.

23. Bandura A. *Social Foundations of Thought and Action: A Social Cognitive Theory.* Englewood Cliffs, NJ: Prentice-Hall; 1986.

24. Becker MH. *The Health Belief Model and Personal Health Behavior.* Thorofare, NJ: Slack; 1974.

25. Witmer J, Sweeney T. A holistic model for wellness and prevention over the lifespan. *J Counseling Dev.* 1992;71:140-148.

26. Deci EL, Ryan RM. *Intrinsic Motivation and Self-Determination in Human Behavior.* New York, NY: Plenum Press; 1985.

27. Seligman ME, Csikszentmihalyi M. Positive psychology: an introduction. *Am Psychol.* 2000;55(1):5-14.

28. Fredrickson BL. The value of positive emotions. *Am Scientist.* 2003;91:330-335.

29. Gable SL, Haidt J. What (and why) is positive psychology? *Rev Gen Psychol.* 2005;9(2):103-110.

30. Radziewicz RM. Self-care for the caregiver. *Nurs Clin North Am.* 2001;36(4):855-869.

31. Spickard A Jr, Gabbe SG, Christensen JF. Mid-career burnout in generalist and specialist physicians. *JAMA.* 2002;288(12):1447-1450.

32. Maslach C, Schaufeli WB, Leiter MP. Job burnout. *Annu Rev Psychol.* 2001;52:397-422.

33. Maslach C, Jackson SE, Keiter MP. *Maslach Burnout Inventory Manual.* 3rd ed. Palo Alto, CA: Consulting Psychologist Press; 1996.

34. Figley CR, ed. *Compassion Fatigue: Coping With Secondary Traumatic Stress Disorders in Those Who Treat the Traumatized.* New York, NY: Brunner/Mazel; 1995.

35. Huggard P. Compassion fatigue: how much can I give? *Med Educ.* 2003;37 (2):163-164.

36. Joinson C. Coping with compassion fatigue. *Nursing.* 1992;22(4):116-120.

37. Kendrick P. Comparing the effects of stress and relationship style on student and practicing nurse anesthetists. *AANA J.* 2000;68(2):115-122.

38. Taffinder NJ, McManus IC, Russell RC, Darzi A. Effect of sleep deprivation on surgeons' dexterity on laparoscopy simulator. *Lancet.* 1998;352(9135):1191.

39. Denisco RA, Drummond JN, Gravenstein JS. The effect of fatigue on performance of a simulated anesthetic monitoring task. *J Clin Monit.* 1987;3 (1):22-24.

40. Gaba DM, Howard SK. Patient safety: fatigue among clinicians and the safety of patients. *N Engl J Med.* 2002;347 (16):1249-1255.

41. Dawson D, Reid K. Fatigue, alcohol and performance impairment. *Nature.* 1997;388(6639):235-237.

42. Rollinson DC, Rathlev NK, Moss M, et al. The effects of consecutive night shifts on neuropsychological performance of interns: a pilot study. *Ann Emerg Med.* 2003;41(3):400-406.

43. Rosekind M, Graeber R, Dinges D, et al. *Crew Factors in Flight Operations: IX. Effects of Planned Cockpit Rest on Crew Performance and Alertness in Long-Haul Operations.* Houston, TX: NASA; 1994.

44. Advisory Opinion Number 5.1. Patient Safety: Fatigue, Stress, and Work Schedule Effects. *Professional Practice Manual for the Certified Registered Nurse Anesthetist.* Park Ridge, IL: American Association of Nurse Anesthetists; 2005.

45. Tunajek S. Workplace incivility part I: anger, harassment, and horizontal violence. *AANA Newsbull.* 2007;3:30-31.

46. Joint Commission. Sentinel Event Alert: Behaviors that undermine a culture of safety. 2008; http://www.jointcommission.org/SentinelEvents/SentinelEventAlert/sea_40.htm. Accessed June 12, 2008.

47. Aiken LH, Clarke SP, Sloane DM, Sochalski J, Silber JH. Hospital nurse staffing and patient mortality, nurse burnout, and job dissatisfaction. *JAMA.* 2002;288(16):1987-1993.

48. American Psychiatric Nurses Association. Workplace Violence: APNA 2008 Position Statement. http://www.apna.org/files/public/APNA_Workplace_Violence_Position_Paper.pdf. Accessed April 20, 2010.

49. Charles SC. Malpractice litigation and its impact on physicians. *Curr Psychiatr Ther.* 1986;23:173-180.

50. Waterman AD, Garbutt J, Hazel E, et al. The emotional impact of medical errors on practicing physicians in the United States and Canada. *J Comm J Qual Patient Saf.* 2007;33(8):467-476.

51. Olson K. Recognizing the symptoms of malpractice stress syndrome. *Psychiatr Times.* 2000;17(4):17-20.

52. *Practice Guidelines for the Treatment of Patients With Acute Stress Disorder and Posttraumatic Stress Disorder.* Washington, DC: American Psychiatric Association; 2004.

53. Gazoni FM. Life after death: a resident's perspective. *Anesth Patient Safety Found Newslett.* 2006;21(1):7-8.

54. McDonough JP. Personality, addiction, and anesthesia. *AANA J.* 1990;58(3):193-200.

55. Perez EC, Carroll-Perez I. A national study: stress perception by nurse anesthesia students. *AANA J.* 1999;67(1):79-86.

56. Wildgust BM. Stress in the anesthesia student. *AANA J.* 1996;54(3):272-278.

57. Sandi C, Pinelo-Nava MT. Stress and memory: behavioral effects and neurobiological mechanisms. *Neural Plast.* 2007;16(6):1-20.

58. Tunajek S. Student stress: a question of balance. *AANA Newsbull.* 2006;60(5):20-21.

59. Twerski AJ. *Addictive Thinking: Understanding Self-Deception.* 2nd ed. Center City, MN: Hazelden Press; 1997.

60. Johnson VE. *Intervention: How to Help Someone Who Doesn't Want Help.* Center City, MN: Hazelden Press; 1986.

61. Wilson H. Compton M. Reentry of the addicted Certified Registered Nurse Anesthetist: a review of the literature. *J Addict Nurs.* 2009;20(4):177-184.

62. Tunajek S. Peer support: validity and benefit. *AANA Newsbull.* 2007;61(5):29-31.

63. Judkins SK. Stress among nurse managers: can anything help? *Nurse Res.* 2004;12(2):58-69.

64. Rowe MM. Teaching health-care providers coping: results of a two-year study. *J Behav Med.* 1999;22(5):511-527.

65. Tunajek S. Compassion fatigue: dealing with an occupational hazard. *AANA Newsbull.* 2006;5:25-26.

66. Maddi SR. The story of hardiness: twenty years of theorizing, research and practice. *Consult Psychol J.* 2002;54:173-185.

67. Lyubominsky S, Sousa L, Dickerhoof R. The costs and benefits of writing, talking, and thinking about life's triumphs and defeats. *J Pers Soc Psychol.* 2006;90(4):692-708.

68. Sapolsky RM. *Why Zebras Don't Get Ulcers: An Updated Guide to Stress, Stress-Related Diseases, and Coping.* 3rd ed. New York, NY: WH Freeman; 2004.

69. Finkelstein C, Brownstein A, Scott C, Lan YL. Anxiety and stress reduction in medical education: an intervention. *Med Educ.* 2007;41(3):258-264.

70. Kabat-Zinn J. Mindfulness-based interventions in context: past, present, and future. *Clin Psychol Sci Pract.* 2003;10(2):144-156.

71. Everly GS Jr, Mitchell JT. *Critical Incident Stress Management (CISM): A New Era and Standard of Care in Crisis Intervention.* Ellicott City, MD: Chevron Publishing; 1997.

72. Dyregrov A. The process in psychological debriefings. *J Traum Stress.* 1997;10(4):589-604.

73. Centers for Disease Control and Prevention. Behavioral Risk Factor Surveillance System Survey Data. Atlanta, GA: Centers for Disease Control and Prevention, 2008. http://cdc.gov/BRFSS/smart/2008.htm Accessed April 20, 2010.

74. Gomes SS. *About Wellness* [videotape]. Park Ridge, IL: American Association of Nurse Anesthetists; 2004.

498

Study Questions

1. What wellness and peer assistance activities, research, and efforts have been made over the past few years by the AANA on behalf of its members? How does this compare with other nursing organizations, and how do you apply this progress in your own practice setting?

2. Develop an explanation of stress and wellness that you can use for implementing stress management techniques for yourself and colleagues.

3. What are innovative methods of conducting research on the topic of wellness for CRNAs and students?

4. How would you explain the higher incidence of substance abuse in the anesthesia community than in the general population? Are anesthesia providers more prone to abuse of certain substances? If so, what do current trends indicate they may be?

5. Discuss the link between professional accountability, negative behaviors, and factors for patient risk or harm.

6. Peer support is based on the rationale that people who have experienced an adverse event can assist others in understanding and coping with similar circumstances. Discuss the value and types of peer support networks.

499

CHAPTER 21
Ethical Decision Making in Anesthesia

Marcia Sue DeWolf Bosek, RN, DNSc

Key Concepts

- Ethical situations require Certified Registered Nurse Anesthetists (CRNAs) to consider professional and personal values, think about what is the right thing to do, identify options, and act upon the selected "right" option.

- Nonmaleficence, or to "do no harm," is a fundamental goal guiding a CRNA's actions.

- Beneficence requires that an action be implemented that will bring about good for the patient.

- Justice is concerned with equity or fairness in the distribution of scarce healthcare resources.

- Advocating for the welfare of patients is a responsibility CRNAs must uphold.

- CRNAs will need to consider each ethical situation as a unique event involving specific values, customs, policies, and nuances.

Nurse anesthetists face many problems and make many choices during their daily clinical practice. Although all problems are not ethical problems and all choices are not moral choices, ethical problems do occur that require nurse anesthetists to consider their professional and personal values, identify options, and act upon the selected "right" option. This chapter is concerned with issues of healthcare ethics and the role of Certified Registered Nurse Anesthetists (CRNAs) in promoting humane, caring resolutions to these difficult ethical quandaries.

The case study exemplars presented in this chapter are real ethical situations that CRNAs described during a research study funded by the American Association of Nurse Anesthetists (AANA) Foundation investigating how CRNAs resolve clinical ethical situations. Because every clinical situation is unique, and no single, definitive, universal treatment protocol exists, the reader is cautioned not to get sidetracked by critiquing the specific clinical details, such as which drug was used. Rather, the reader should use the cases to promote thinking specifically as well as broadly about the ethical issues, values, and duties.

The terms ethics and morals are derived from Latin and Greek words meaning custom. Within each society, customs are developed. Although a custom may be sanctioned by one society, the custom may not be evaluated as being acceptable by other cultures or societies, for example, slavery, cannibalism, or polygamy. Every CRNA possesses a set of moral customs influenced by family, neighborhood, religious community, and educational background. Similarly, every clinical practice setting also has a unique set of moral customs. Thus, the potential exists for ethical situations to occur when various customs and their associated beliefs conflict.

The Advanced Practice Role of CRNAs in Ethical Issues

Although every nurse (as well as every healthcare professional) has an obligation to be an active participant in the resolution of clinical ethical situations, CRNAs, by virtue of their advanced practice role, have additional responsibilities. Bosek and Carpenter[1] proposed that advanced practice nurses need to develop additional proficiency in:

- Fostering decision-making skills in patients and their significant others, as well as in other healthcare professionals.
- Inviting divergent opinions and interpersonal discussions.
- Resolving commonly occurring ethical issues in their area of clinical specialty.
- Engaging in prospective planning regarding recurrent ethical issues in their clinical specialty.

Ethical Decision Making

Ethical Decision-Making Models

An assortment of ethical decision-making resources is available to help CRNAs resolve clinical ethical problems. A variety of ethical decision-making models and approaches exist.[2-4] Each model proposes a unique emphasis for guiding decision making, such as rights[5]; however, the majority of ethical decision-making models agree that the decision maker should: (1) identify the ethical dilemma, (2) identify and consider the pros and cons associated with each available option, (3) implement the selected option, and (4) evaluate the outcome and decision-making process.[6] These 4 steps are similar to the nursing process with the exception of identifying a goal.

Ethical Principles

Beauchamp and Childress[7] advocate the use of 4 key principles to guide ethical decision making. These 4 principles can serve as the goals for ethical decision making and could be prioritized as follows: autonomy, non-maleficence, beneficence, and justice. In Western societies, autonomy (self-determination that is free from coercion) is often considered the most important goal to be honored during ethical decision making. Nonmaleficence can be accomplished by implementing a specific action or by not performing a harmful act. Although nonmaleficence, or to "do no harm," is a fundamental goal guiding a healthcare practitioner's actions, non-maleficence may not be the patient's primary goal. For example, a fashion model made the autonomous decision that she would risk potentially dying (typically perceived as the ultimate of harms) rather than undergo a disfiguring surgery for appendicitis, which she believed would limit her career options.

Beneficence builds on the concept of nonmaleficence. The principle of beneficence requires that a positive action be implemented that will benefit the patient or bring about good. Thus, a CRNA is promoting beneficence when an anesthetic with antiemetic effects is used during induction. Finally, justice is concerned with equity or fairness in the distribution of scarce resources.[7] Many justice questions are societal questions (such as "Is there a universal right to healthcare?"). Although social justice questions are extremely important and affect individual ethical decision making, healthcare professionals should resist the temptation to resolve these social questions at an individual patient's bedside. Social justice issues cannot be resolved in a case-by-case manner; rather, these questions require the CRNA, through individual as well as professional organizational and political involvement,

to engage in community dialogues that can result in societal consensus and subsequent policy formation.

Evaluating Decision Making
Evaluation is an ongoing process that begins as soon as an option has been selected. The selected option is first evaluated for its potential to promote the identified values and ethical principles and then again after the ethical situation has been resolved to validate that the anticipated goals were achieved. During the evaluation phase, CRNAs should resist the temptation to claim that "this action just felt right or things feel good now, so it must have been the right thing to do." Doing the ethically appropriate thing does not mean that one's emotions will also feel good or positive. Often, implementing the ethically right option is an emotionally trying event. In addition, various participants in the ethical situation may evaluate outcomes differently because of differences in goals, values, and ethical commitments. Thus, at the end of any ethical situation, the outcomes should be evaluated from the identified decision maker's perspective and could include the following questions: "Were the identified goals achieved?" "Were the values and ethical priorities of the decision maker supported?" "Were any new ethical issues or questions raised as a result of implementing the chosen option?"

Decision-Making Resources
A variety of other ethical decision-making resources exist to facilitate CRNAs' ethical decision making. Institutional resources include policies and procedures, mission statements, and identified ethics mechanisms (either an ethics committee or an ethics consultant). Professional resources can be found through professional association

503

codes and position statements. For example, CRNAs should know the American Nurses Association (ANA) Code of Ethics for Nurses with Interpretive Statements,[8] the AANA Code of Ethics for the Certified Registered Nurse Anesthetist,[9] and the ANA Position Statement: Nurses' Participation in Capital Punishment.[10] Finally, a wide variety of ethical information can be found in the published or Internet media (see Key References at the end of this chapter).

Casuistry

Nursing is a science and an applied art. Similarly, healthcare ethics is both theoretical and an applied science. The issue becomes how CRNAs can best apply theoretical ethics content to clinical practice problems. Rather than using a principled or moral rule approach to ethics, this chapter will follow a casuistry ethics perspective. Proponents of casuistry ethics suggest that ethical reflection cannot be purely theoretical; rather, ethical reflection must consider the person's story and the contextual environment in which the scenario occurred. "What differentiates the new casuistry from applied ethics, then, is not the mere recognition that principles must eventually be applied, but rather a particular account of logic and derivation of the principles that we deploy in moral discourse."[11(p542)]

Scenario 1

Do-not-resuscitate (DNR) orders are a custom that Western society has promoted. In 1990, the Patient Self-Determination Act[12] legislated the patient's right to refuse treatment as well as the right to make an advance directive, such as a living will or durable power of attorney for healthcare. Since the advent of cardiopulmonary resuscitation (CPR), many acute care and long-term healthcare agencies have developed the custom of initiating CPR for all patients experiencing a respiratory and/or cardiac arrest unless otherwise stipulated by a physician's DNR order. However, the custom of writing DNR orders and/or a patient's refusal of life-sustaining treatment can create an ethical situation for CRNAs, whose personal and professional customs may be different. For example:

Mr Smith became ill while on vacation in another state. After being ill for 5 days, the patient sought medical care. He was diagnosed with a necrotic bowel and scheduled for immediate surgery. When assessed by the CRNA, the patient stated, "I have a living will and a durable power of attorney for healthcare on file at my doctor's office back home. If I'm bad, you let me go." The CRNA's immediate thought was "Nobody dies in my operating room if I can help it!"

The major ethical conflict in this scenario is the patient's autonomous refusal of life-sustaining treatment vs the CRNA's commitment to nonmaleficence. Maintaining Mr Smith's autonomy while doing no harm would be key goals for the decision-making process.

Nonmaleficence

Nonmaleficence is the concern for doing no harm or evil and is considered to be a foundational principle guiding actions by healthcare professionals. In the Hippocratic Oath, physicians pledge, "I will apply dietetic measures for the benefit of the sick according to my ability and judgment; I will keep them from harm and injustice."[13] Harm is a broad term that includes not just physical or psychological injury, but also threats to the individual's life goals.

Actions that inflict harm always require moral justification. Surgery and anesthesia can cause actual and potential harm to the patient but are morally justified by the premise of bringing about good for the patient by correcting an injury or illness. In other words, the potential for good (or beneficence) is perceived to outweigh the actual or potential harms associated with surgery and anesthesia. This tension between doing good and preventing harm is a key to understanding the CRNA's immediate response to Mr Smith's request to "let me go."

The CRNA's role during surgery is to maintain the patient's physical condition. The possibility exists for a patient receiving anesthesia to experience a life-threatening event related to hypotension, hypoxia, or a cardiac arrhythmia.[14] Thus, during a surgical intervention, the CRNA may be unable to discriminate when a life-threatening event is precipitated by an anesthetic agent or is the result of the patient's underlying illness. Based on the principle of nonmaleficence, many CRNAs believe that all actions must be taken to correct any life-threatening event occurring in the operating room.

Autonomy

The principle of autonomy, or patient self-determination, is a basic social value. An autonomous action is an act of intention that is free from coercion by others.

> Patients have the moral and legal right to determine what will be done with their own person; to be given accurate, complete and understandable information in a manner that facilitates an informed judgment; to be assisted with weighing the benefits, burdens, and available options in their treatment, including the choice of no treatment; to accept, refuse, or terminate treatment without deceit, undue influence, duress, coercion, or penalty;

and to be given necessary support throughout the decision-making and treatment process[8] (Provision 1.4).

Patients may communicate their values and autonomous decisions about life-sustaining treatment through the creation of a written advance directive.

Advance Directives

During the last 4 decades, medical technology has undergone explosive growth, especially in regard to life-sustaining technology, such as CPR, ventilators, feeding tubes, and renal dialysis. Inherent in these technological advancements are new problems associated with the ethical principle of respecting patient autonomy related to quality of life as well as the right to life vs the right to die. Thus, people are being encouraged to complete an advance directive.

An advance directive allows the person to communicate values and beliefs about healthcare decisions and life-sustaining treatment in the event that the person becomes unable to participate in healthcare decisions. Thus, as long as the person has decision-making capacity and is able to make healthcare decisions, the advance directive remains a secondary resource. The CRNA should engage the patient in further conversation if a discrepancy is noted between the patient's current decision(s) and the previously completed advance directive and should assist the patient to revise the advance directive as necessary.

In the United States, advance directives are legislated at the state level, and thus, the possibility exists that a specific action (eg, stopping tube feedings) may be legally possible in one state, but not possible in another. Nevertheless, states typically honor advance directives from other states in a

505

spirit of reciprocity, and when this is not possible, actions should be taken to promote the patient's transfer back to his or her home state. CRNAs working with patients from multiple states and CRNAs who are travelers or relocate to a different state for employment should think prospectively how these variances might affect their practice. There are 2 types of written advance directives: living wills and durable power of attorney for healthcare (DPOA-HC).

Living Wills

A living will, also called a directive to physicians, was first published in 1974 by the Euthanasia Educational Council, which later became the Concern for Dying and the Society for the Right to Die. Although originally not designed as a legal document, living wills have gained legal standing in many US states. A living will is an instructional advance directive that typically directs the physician:

> If at any time I should have an incurable and irreversible injury, disease, or illness judged to be a terminal condition by my attending physician who has personally examined me, and has determined that my death is imminent except for death-delaying procedures, I direct that such procedures which would only prolong the dying process be withheld or withdrawn, and that I be permitted to die naturally with only the administration of medication, sustenance, or the performance of any medical procedure deemed necessary by my attending physician to provide me with comfort care.[15]

A living will is a useful document for guiding healthcare decisions regarding resuscitation and withdrawal of treatment for persons with terminal illnesses (such as cancer) who lack decision-making capacity and do not have a significant other to serve as a surrogate decision maker. However, the living will has several limitations. First, the living will contains many ambiguous words or phrases that can be difficult to interpret. For example, at what point would the person be perceived to be imminently dying—when the person has 6 months, 6 weeks, 6 days, or 6 hours left to live? Second, the living will does not assist decision making for persons without decision-making capacity who are not terminally ill or imminently dying, but rather are in a persistent vegetative state or lack decision-making capacity because of illness such as head trauma or Alzheimer disease. Third, the living will is not designed to facilitate decisions related to the initiation of healthcare interventions; it is designed to direct the removal of death-delaying procedures. Finally, the completion of a living will may cause misperceptions for the patient and the healthcare team. For example, patients may inaccurately believe that completing a living will means that they will not receive cardiopulmonary resuscitation in the event of an arrest. Similarly, healthcare professionals may inaccurately assume that, because a patient has a living will, the patient would never want aggressive treatment. Therefore, the presence of a living will or any advance directive should trigger a conversation between the patient and the CRNA about the patient's healthcare wishes and goals related to the current medical need (surgery, pain management, or respiratory distress).

Durable Power of Attorney for Healthcare

A durable power of attorney for healthcare (DPOA-HC) is a more powerful advance directive and addresses many of the limitations inherent in the living will. The first DPOA-

506

HC was adopted in California in 1984. The DPOA-HC allows the person not only to refuse death-delaying procedures, but also to identify a surrogate decision maker and to specify which values and beliefs should be used to guide future healthcare decisions. In contrast with the living will, the DPOA-HC is not limited to when a person is imminently dying of a terminal illness. Therefore, the DPOA-HC may be used to guide healthcare decisions for any person who lacks decision-making capacity regardless of the cause or prognosis.

Although the Federal Patient Self-Determination Act of 1990[12] stipulates that all patients have the right to complete an advance directive, advance-directive legislation remains at a state level and, thus, the exact wording and/or scope may vary from state to state. Therefore, the possibility exists that Mr Smith's living will and DPOA-HC may not be legally binding in the state in which he is currently hospitalized. It therefore may be in Mr Smith's best interest to complete (while he still has decision-making capacity) a new DPOA-HC form for the state in which he is hospitalized. While Mr Smith remains able to participate in healthcare decision making, all efforts should be made to promote his autonomy and informed decision making about his healthcare choices, including the CRNA learning more about the content of these forms to better understand Mr Smith's healthcare goals. Thus, while Mr Smith possesses decision-making capacity he, rather than his DPOA-HC and living will, should be considered the primary source for decision making.

Values Clarification Documents

Occasionally individuals are reluctant or unable to complete an advance directive because they are uncertain what to select and,

thus, they benefit from engaging in a process of values clarification. Values clarification tools have been developed to assist individuals to clarify healthcare values and goals, to promote communication between patients and their families and healthcare professionals; and to augment existing advance directives. The Five Wishes form[14] has gained wide support from healthcare, legal, religious, and community organizations. The Five Wishes prompts the individual to think holistically about his or her wishes (personal, emotional, and spiritual in addition to medical) and "lets your family and doctor know:

- Which person you want to make healthcare decisions for you when you can't make them
- The kind of medical treatment you want or don't want
- How comfortable you want to be
- How you want people to treat you
- What you wish your loved ones to know"

As a result of its popularity and community support, the Five Wishes is now legally recognized in 42 states as meeting advance directive status.

Do-Not-Resuscitate Orders

The do-not- resuscitate order (DNR) order has become well accepted and widely used in Western hospitals. A DNR order is a medical order made by a physician and recorded in the patient's medical record to withhold resuscitation in the case of cardiac or respiratory arrest. Cardiopulmonary resuscitation (CPR) after a cardiac and/or respiratory arrest has become commonly used since its introduction in 1960[17,18]; however, CPR has both positive and negative potentials. The potential good, the sustaining of life, is obvious, but the potential

507

harms include anoxic encephalopathy, permanent ventilator dependence, or severe functional disability.[19,20] This negative side to CPR has brought experts in medicine, bioethics, and medical law together. Special orders, no CPR, no code, or, most commonly, DNR, have been established to ensure that CPR is not performed inappropriately. Many experts contend that a DNR order is fully compatible with aggressive care and should not imply that other life-sustaining treatment be withheld or withdrawn[7,21]; however, the presence of a DNR order creates ethical quandaries for anesthesia providers.[22] A DNR order prohibits the initiation of CPR, and it can also prohibit the use of intubation, mechanical ventilators, vasoactive drugs, and defibrillation,[23] which are interventions anesthesia providers may need to implement to provide safe and effective anesthesia.

Perioperative Do-Not-Resuscitate Orders

Do-not-resuscitate orders are often written for patients near the end of life in the event that a spontaneous (what some may refer to as a natural) cessation of respirations and/or circulation occurs.[23] This definition is effective for most medical patients; however, potential ethical questions can arise for the CRNA when a patient with an established DNR order opts for a surgical intervention. When an anesthetized patient experiences a respiratory or circulatory arrest, the cause of the arrest may not be readily known. For example, is the arrest the natural end of a terminal condition? Or is the arrest a consequence (foreseeable or unforeseeable) of an anesthetic agent or other medication?

If the perioperative team's primary ethical commitment is to prevent harm to the patient, resuscitation may be perceived by some to be an ethically mandatory act; however, this assumption may clash with the patient's previous autonomous decision to forgo resuscitation.[24] Some institutions have attempted to deal with this ethical quandary by establishing unilateral policies requiring established DNR orders to be suspended and all patients to be resuscitated during surgery; however, these policies are not perceived to be sensitive to cultural norms or patient autonomy. In response to this criticism, the American Society of Anesthesiologists[24] supports clarifying the patient's goals and expectations associated with resuscitation and has proposed 3 alternatives: (1) full attempt at resuscitation, (2) limited attempt at resuscitation defined with regard to specific procedures, or (3) limited attempt at resuscitation defined with regard to the patient's goals and values. Waisel[25] suggests that: "It is helpful to define a goal-directed approach on three axes: the burden that the patient is willing to accept, the benefit that the patient wants, and the likelihood of success."[25(p1)] These discussions should also consider whether a DNR order should be instituted and, if so, what process should be followed, for example, after discharge from postanesthesia recovery or after being weaned from the ventilator.[23]

Options for Scenario 1

Before identifying options, the CRNA should clarify Mr Smith's comments and related values. Is Mr Smith refusing all medical intervention or selected therapies? What does Mr Smith mean by "If I'm bad let me go"? Does "bad" refer to dying, a specific quality of life level, or seriousness of the injury? Does Mr Smith understand the technology (intubation, ventilator support, intravenous therapy, and anesthetic agents) that will be required to successfully correct his necrotic bowel? In addition, the institution's DNR policy should be reviewed. After Mr Smith's values and beliefs are validated, several options exist for resolving this ethical situation. Choices include:

- A DNR order written for the entire perioperative period (which may result in the CRNA refusing to provide anesthesia).
- Surgery with full resuscitation and a postoperative DNR order.
- Surgery with a limited resuscitation and a postoperative DNR order.
- Contacting the patient's primary care provider for more information and assistance in determining short-term and long-term treatment goals.
- No surgery.

Scenario 2

Nurse anesthetists may also find themselves involved in ethical conflicts with other members of the healthcare team.

Late one evening, a 20-year-old woman fell while roller blading and fractured her ankle. The on-call surgeon has spent 6 hours trying to fix the fracture, putting screws in and taking them out numerous times. The operating room walls are "papered" with 14 radiographs, and it is now early in the morning. The surgeon has contaminated the surgical field several times. The patient has been transferred from a spinal anesthetic to general anesthesia. The CRNA is now concerned that the woman is at risk for serious complications, including the possibility of losing her foot, if this surgeon continues to operate.

The ethical problem in this scenario involves the CRNA's obligation to advocate for the patient. Initially, the obligation to act as a patient advocate seems obvious; however, this CRNA is experiencing an ethical dilemma due to conflict between personal and professional values. Specifically, the CRNA is torn between the professional

obligation to promote a "good" outcome for the patient and the desire to avoid any personal harm to the CRNA's working relationship with the surgeon and within the institution. In this scenario, the CRNA's primary decision-making goal should be to promote a beneficent outcome for the patient with a secondary goal of doing no harm (nonmaleficence) to the CRNA's job security and to the various healthcare professional relationships and reputations involved in this scenario.

Beneficence

The principle of beneficence requires first that harm be avoided (the principle of nonmaleficence) and second that a benefit or good be created. Thus, beneficence is action-oriented and requires positive steps. The CRNA in the scenario was correctly acting to avoid harm by following the standards of practice for anesthesia as demonstrated by converting the patient to general anesthesia. However, the second component of the principle of beneficence requires the CRNA to purposefully act to cause good to occur. Good for this patient includes regaining full range of motion of her ankle. Since the CRNA cannot perform the surgical intervention, the CRNA will need to identify other ways to promote good for this patient, such as advocacy.

Advocacy

Both the AANA Code of Ethics[9] and the ANA Code of Ethics for Nurses[8] stipulate that nurses must act to safeguard patients from the incompetent practice of any healthcare provider. One way that a CRNA can safeguard the patient is by fulfilling the role of advocate. In fact, the AANA Code of Ethics states that advocating for the welfare of patients is a responsibility CRNAs must uphold. To be an advocate means to "plead the cause of another; an intercessor; defender."[26(p22)] This definition presumes that the advocate holds the belief that patients have rights that must be supported and that the patient's rights do in fact come before other priorities and obligations.[27]

Therefore, to act as an advocate, the CRNA must first know the patient's goals or cause. The ability to know and/or validate the patient's goals or cause is complicated in this case by the fact that the patient is under general anesthesia and, thus, unable to participate in decisions about her surgical treatment. Therefore, the CRNA's knowledge of the patient's goals is limited to preoperative assessment data and assumptions that may be universalized to all surgical patients, such as "patients who consent to a surgical procedure want their physical problem corrected to the fullest extent possible." Based on this assumption, the CRNA would be ethically justified to act on the belief that this particular patient also has a commitment to regaining optimal function of her ankle.

Second, the CRNA must identify to whom the intercession must be directed. In this scenario, the CRNA needs to intercede by verbally promoting the patient's cause to the surgeon. When promoting the patient's cause, the CRNA may need to create a distance between the patient and the source of harm. For example in this scenario, the CRNA could suggest that the surgeon needs a break and/or needs to seek consultation or assistance from an orthopedic surgeon. However, creating a distance between the patient and the perceived source of harm can be difficult during the perioperative phase because creating distance may result in the need to suspend the surgical procedure, which can be of equal or greater

threat to the patient's safety and recovery.

When intercession is insufficient to ensure the patient's rights are protected, the CRNA advocate will need to assume the client advocate role. The client advocate role builds on the CRNA's legitimate role and positional power as a member of the healthcare team.[27] The client advocate role may require the CRNA to work through the institutional hierarchy to gain political support for the patient's rights, as well as to identify supplemental resources that can be accessed to promote the patient's rights and to facilitate a beneficent outcome. For example, the CRNA could notify the surgeon's supervisor or the chief of orthopedic surgery about the patient's current status and the perceived need for immediate assistance. The ability to successfully implement the client advocate role is contingent upon the CRNA's professional reputation and clinical skills and judgment. In other words, to successfully fulfill the client advocate role, the CRNA must be able to capitalize on an established clinical expertise and dedication to patient safety and rights. Thus, prerequisites to being an advocate are recognized clinical expertise and an existing dedication to patient rights and beneficent care.

Impaired Practitioners

Unfortunately, the need for advocacy often occurs because a healthcare professional is incompetent or impaired. Healthcare professionals can be impaired from chemicals (drugs and alcohol); professional burnout or environmental factors, such as fatigue from working extended hours or short staffing patterns; or knowledge deficits related to working outside of their specialty areas.[28]

In this scenario, the surgeon may be experiencing a variety of environmental impairments, such as fatigue from a protracted surgery that is extending into the night[29] and possibly limited knowledge and experience regarding ankle orthopedics. CRNAs have an ethical obligation to work within their agencies and professional organization to enact policies and procedures that proactively address the antecedents of environmental impairment, as well as the stresses that result in the abuse of chemicals or professional burnout. In addition, CRNAs should be cognizant of institutional and state licensure policies for reporting healthcare professionals with chemical impairments. Finally, in the event that a CRNA experiences a chemical impairment, support is available through the AANA's Peer Assistance Advisors.[30]

Value Conflicts

Each CRNA holds a variety of professional as well as personal values. Curtin[5] defined values as "those assertions or statements that individuals make, either through their behavior, words, or actions, that define what they think is important and for which they are willing to suffer and even die—or perhaps to continue living."[31(p8)] Personal values are developed throughout one's life and are shaped by parents, family members, friends, teachers and school groups, and community and religious groups, in addition to both good and bad personal experiences.[32]

Professional values build upon an individual's personal values. CRNAs develop their professional values throughout their professional career. However, it is unclear whether professional educational programs can create an ethical practitioner with strong professional values if the person has a limited and/or superficial personal value system.

The CRNA in this scenario seems to be experiencing a conflict between professional and personal values. The CRNA appears to value professional skills and a commitment to helping patients and to potentially value advocacy. However, a commitment to acting on these professional values is potentially or actually threatening other key values. This CRNA may be thinking, "If I act on my professional values, I may be threatening my reputation as a team player. This surgeon is a powerful person in this institution. I'm not certain that I'm willing to risk my job and, thus, my family's financial security over this incident."

Before deciding how to act, the CRNA needs to undergo a process of values clarification. The CRNA seems to have already freely chosen a variety of values from existing alternatives. However, merely *choosing a value* is insufficient; the CRNA must also willingly share the values with others and consistently use the values to guide actions. Ideally, values clarification occurs within a group prior to the need to act on the value, for example during a staff meeting or in-service. However, this CRNA does not have the luxury of trying out the professional values first in a safe, nonthreatening environment since the CRNA is being forced to simultaneously share and act on these professional values. Thus, the process of clarifying values may create risks in addition to promoting self-actualization.[32]

Options for Scenario 2

Before problem solving begins, the CRNA should first clarify the professional and personal values influencing the CRNA's perception of the situation and willingness to intervene. In addition, the CRNA needs to have clearly identified and prioritized the ethical issues involved in this situation. How the agency customarily deals with issues of professional disagreement should also be considered. Ideally, this time of clarification

511

and prioritizing should bring the CRNA to the realization that a professional nurse anesthetist's primary professional obligation is to protect the patient from harm and to promote good whenever possible. This obligation is supported by professional as well as personal values regarding the value of human life and promoting autonomy by maintaining function and independence.

Thus, the CRNA has several options available, including:

- Address concerns directly to the surgeon about the actual and potential outcomes or harms and ask the surgeon to request assistance or consultation.
- Ask the circulating nurse for assistance and/or ideas for dealing with the situation.
- Notify the surgeon that the CRNA is calling in the orthopedic surgeon for consultation or assistance.
- Contact the on-call orthopedic surgeon for consultation or assistance without first notifying the surgeon.
- Seek consultation from the medical director of anesthesia regarding how to proceed.
- Notify the medical director of anesthesia on call of the CRNA's need to be removed from this case.
- Say nothing and allow the surgery to continue.

Moral Courage

Although the last 2 options (be removed from the case or say nothing) may address the CRNA's need to protect his or her professional relationships with the surgeon, these actions do not address the CRNA's ethical responsibility to minimize harm and promote good for the patient. In situations like this, the CRNA may need moral courage. "Moral courage is the individual's capacity to overcome fear and stand up for

his or her core values"[33(p131)] and "the willingness to risk shame and social disapproval for doing one's duty. It requires making a stand, often alone and in isolation."[34(p129)] In this scenario, moral courage might require the CRNA to identify the primary ethical obligations that need to be honored, for example, the need to advocate for the patient. Next, the CRNA should realistically reconsider his or her fear and rephrase as needed. Is it realistic to think that a surgeon would initiate a complaint against a CRNA who was advocating for a consultation? A positive outlook may be beneficial, but the CRNA must be prepared by clearly documenting the his or her actions as well as the actions and responses by other members of the surgical team. Furthermore, the CRNA would want to communicate concerns as well as seek support from the CRNA's supervisor and/or other CRNAs. Consistently acting on moral commitments will promote the CRNA's sense of moral integrity and, over time, will develop into ethical fitness supporting the CRNA's courage to act in future conflicts.[33,34]

Scenario 3

One of the hardest ethical situations a CRNA may face is the situation in which the CRNA's professional standard of practice and the CRNA's professional and personal values are challenged by another professional.

A CRNA was moonlighting at a surgical center. This center did therapeutic abortions. The first day, she used propofol and alfentanil for anesthesia with haloperidol for postoperative nausea. The second day, the owner of the center, who also is a CRNA, directed that propofol could not be used because the drug is too expensive. In addition, the owner didn't want the CRNA to change the circuits on the anesthesia machine between patients because the circuits were too expensive. The CRNA felt that she was being asked to compromise care to these women because of the financial cost.

Conscientious Refusal

"Conscience...is not a special moral faculty or self-justifying moral authority. It is a form of self-reflection on and judgment about whether one's acts are obligatory or prohibited, right or wrong, good or bad. It is an internal sanction that comes into play through critical reflection... Some ethical standards are sufficiently fundamental and powerful that violating them would diminish integrity and result in guilt and shame."[35(p38)]

Conflicts of conscience occur when a person is directed (often by someone with authority and power) to act against the person's standard of conduct, thus threatening the person's sense of integrity and self-worth. In the preceding scenario, this CRNA is not experiencing any conflicts of conscience related to participating in abortions. Rather, the CRNA is experiencing a conflict of conscience when the owner directs that the CRNA's standard of care is not obligatory and in fact is creating a financial harm to the surgical center, which would ultimately affect patient care by escalating surgical costs. When a conflict of conscience occurs, the CRNA must determine how to respond. Ultimately, the CRNA will have to decide whether to ignore the conflict of conscience (or in other words learn to live with the dissonance) or to express opposition to the direction causing the conflict.

During a conflict of conscience, CRNAs must be able to clearly describe the basis for refusing to comply. First, the CRNA may realize "I can't do that, because I could not live with myself if I were to do it."[36] This type of refusal is referred to as conscientious re-

fusal because it illustrates an insult to the individual's personal conscience. However, before making such a claim, the CRNA must be knowledgeable of how the state where the CRNA is practicing defines conscientious objection. For example, the Illinois Right of Conscience Act[37] defines conscience as "a sincerely held set of moral convictions arising from a belief in and relation to God, or which, though not so derived, obtains from a place in the life of its possessor parallel to that filled by God among adherents to religious faiths." Therefore, if the CRNA was employed in Illinois, the CRNA could not claim to have a conscientious objection because the CRNA was not acting to avert personal harm to his or her personal moral or religious convictions.

Rather, the CRNA is expressing a beneficent refusal. When claiming a beneficent refusal, the CRNA is attempting to avoid harm to the patient. Thus, the CRNA's objection to the owner's direction is based on professional knowledge and commitment to promoting the patient's welfare. An act of beneficent refusal may receive legal support from employment laws protecting the employee's right to decline to carry out acts required by an employer if such acts are inconsistent with current policies and professional codes.[36]

It is imperative that the CRNA use language accurately and be able to verbalize specific rationale for objecting. For example, a CRNA expressing a conscientious objection to participating in the termination of pregnancy would explain, "I believe that a fetus is a living being and I am commanded by God not to kill. Therefore, my conscience will not allow me to participate." In contrast, the CRNA in the preceding case would be expressing an objection based on beneficence when stating, "I cannot comply with your directive to reuse the anesthesia

513

circuits because the circuits would be contaminated and subsequently patients will be put at risk."

Justice

The CRNA could respond to the owner's request by stating, "It would not be fair to not change the circuits between patients." A similar claim could be made related to not providing propofol. But what does the CRNA mean by "fair"? If the use of the word fair by the CRNA means "harmful," then this would be another example of objection based on beneficence. However, if fair refers to justice and how scarce resources (money, time, and supplies) are distributed, then the CRNA would be basing the response on the principle of distributive justice.

Distributive justice is concerned with how scarce resources are used and distributed. The decision of how scarce resources should be distributed can be answered in a variety of ways. First, one would need to decide if the scarce resources should be distributed to each person equally or based on the person's need, merit, potential for or actual contribution(s) to society, or finally, based on free market price.[7]

Second, the principle of justice requires that equals should be treated equally. Therefore, the CRNA would need to determine if every woman treated at the surgical center was in fact equal to every other patient in terms of the need to be protected from infection and/or nausea. Assuming that every woman undergoing an elective termination of pregnancy is generally in normal health, the CRNA would be justified in determining that each woman needs equal protection from nosocomial infections. In addition, the CRNA would be hard-pressed to explain how the first patient of the day differs from the second patient of

the day, thus deserving of a new circuit when the remaining patients do not.

Finally, comparing the owner's perceived need for financial gain to the patient's need to be protected from infection seems ludicrous at best. First, the owner and the patients are not equals and, thus, should not be compared. Second, the needs being compared are not equal. Based on the principles of nonmaleficence and altruism, the patient's right to be free of harm should take precedence over any need the owner may have.

Options for Scenario 3

In this scenario, the CRNA has several options. She may choose to:

- Follow the owner's direction.
- Follow normal protocol for changing circuits.
- Provide care in a manner that does not require circuits to be used.
- Refuse to provide general anesthesia care.
- Perform assessments only.
- Perform local anesthesia.
- Refuse to work at this surgical center.

Other Ethical Issues CRNAs Experience

Many other ethical issues have been identified in the anesthesia literature about which CRNAs should become knowledgeable. In particular, CRNAs are becoming more involved in clinical research investigations. When engaged in research activities, the CRNA's ethical commitment to promote nonmaleficence toward the study's subjects must be nonnegotiable. Although each research study will have obtained institutional review board approval prior to beginning, the CRNA must remain vigilant in recognizing the potential for conflicts of interest that may threaten the subjects' rights and safety at any point during the research project.

Frequently occurring ethical issues that CRNAs have or may encounter include:

- Animal research requiring anesthesia[38,39]
- Obtaining of informed consent when the patient is a minor, emancipated, or mentally incompetent[40,41]
- Parental informed consent issues involving religious preferences, conflicts of interest, or inability to obtain care in emergency situations[42]
- Refusal of blood products by Jehovah's Witness patients[43]
- Euthanasia and assisted suicide[44]
- Terminal sedation[45,46]
- Provision of lethal injections for capital punishment[47]
- Publishing of case reports without consent by participants[48,49]
- Obligation to provide care to patients during a pandemic, such as severe acute respiratory syndrome (SARS) or influenza[50,51]
- Participation in cesarean deliveries for nonmedical reasons[52,53]
- Triage during natural disasters[54]
- Disclosure of errors[55,56]
- Management of pediatric chronic pain[57]
- Organ donation after determination of brain death[58]
- Maternal-fetal interventions[59]

The CRNA may become knowledgeable about ethical issues by learning about the various ethical positions and nuances and professional codes and standards and by engaging in personal and professional values clarification regarding these frequently occurring ethical issues in the perioperative setting. CRNAs may want to organize professional continuing education programs, brown bag discussions, journal club readings, and/or in-services as forums to encourage lifelong learning in addition to professional dialogue and debate on these frequently occurring ethical topics.

Summary

Nurse anesthetists experience a variety of ethical situations in the perioperative setting. Although a variety of decision-making models and resources are available to assist the CRNA in resolving these ethical situations, CRNAs need to consider each ethical issue as a unique situation involving specific values, customs, policies, and nuances. Thus, there is no one right answer that CRNAs can memorize for resolving clinical ethical situations. Rather, CRNAs need to develop expertise in assessing and discussing values and beliefs, identifying options, and communicating the ethical justifications for each option.

References

1. Bosek MS, Savage TA. Teachable moments: integrating ethics into clinical education. *Dean's Notes.* 1997;18(5): 1-4.

2. Devettere RJ. *Practical Decision Making in Health Care Ethics: Cases and Concepts.* 3rd ed. Washington DC: Georgetown University Press; 2000:1-25.

3. Husted JH, Husted GL. *Ethical Decision Making in Nursing and Health Care: The Symphonological Approach.* 4th ed. New York, NY: Springer Publishing Company, Inc; 2007:77.

4. Jonsen AR, Siegler M, Winslade WJ. *Clinical Ethics: A Practical Approach to Ethical Decisions in Clinical Medicine.* 6th ed. New York, NY: McGraw-Hill Medical; 2006:1-11.

5. Curtin L. No rush to judgment. In: Curtin L, Flaherty MJ, eds. *Nursing Ethics: Theories and Pragmatics.* Bowie, MD: Robert J. Brady Co; 1982:57-63.

515

6. Bosek MS, Savage TA. Ethics. In: Ignatavicius DD, Workman ML, Mishler MA, eds. *Medical-Surgical Nursing Across the Health Care Continuum.* 3rd ed. Philadelphia, PA: WB Saunders Company; 1999:75-91.

7. Beauchamp TL, Childress JF. *Principles of Biomedical Ethics.* 6th ed. New York, NY: Oxford University Press; 2008:12-19, 99-287.

8. American Nurses Association. Code of Ethics for Nurses With Interpretive Statements. Washington, DC: American Nurses Association; 2001.

9. American Association of Nurse Anesthetists. AANA Code of Ethics for the Certified Registered Nurse Anesthetist. Park Ridge, IL: American Association of Nurse Anesthetists; 2005.

10. American Nurses Association. Position Statement on Nurses' Participation in Capital Punishment. Kansas City, MO: American Nurses Association; 1994.

11. Arras JD. Getting down to cases: the revival of casuistry in bioethics. In: Monagle JF, Thomasma DC, eds. *Health Care Ethics: Critical Issues for the 21st Century.* 2nd ed. Gaithersburg, MD: Aspen Publishers, Inc; 1998:541-553.

12. *Omnibus Reconciliation Act.* Title IV. Section 4206, Congressional Record. October 26, 1990.

13. Temkin O, Temkin CL, eds. *Ancient Medicine: Selected Papers of Ladwig Edelstein.* Baltimore, MD: Johns Hopkins Press; 1967:6.

14. Aging With Dignity. Five Wishes. http://www.agingwithdignity.org/fw200 7.html. Accessed April 22, 2010.

15. *Illinois Living Will Act.* 755ILCS 35/1, et seq, 1992.

16. Sommer B. Patient health and safety. In: Waugaman WR, Foster SD, Rigor BM, eds. *Principles and Practice of Nurse Anesthesia.* 3rd ed. Saddle River, NJ: Prentice Hall Health; 1998:81-92.

17. Alzaga-Fernandez AG, Varon J. Open-chest cardiopulmonary resuscitation: past, present and future. *Resuscitation.* 2005;64(2):149-156.

18. Kouwenhoven WB, Jude JR, Knickerbocker GG. Landmark article July 9, 1960: closed-chest cardiac massage. *JAMA.* 1984;251(23):3133-3136.

19. Plunkett J. Resuscitation injuries complicating the interpretation of pre-mortem trauma and natural disease in children. *J Forensic Sci.* 2006:51(1): 127-130.

20. Thömke F, Marx JJ, Sauer O, et al. Observations on comatose survivors of cardiopulmonary resuscitation with generalized myoclonus. *BMC Neurol* (electronic journal). 2005;5:14.

21. The Hastings Center. *Guidelines on the Termination of Life-Sustaining Treatment and the Care of the Dying.* Bloomington, IN: Indiana University Press; 1987:46-52.

22. American Association of Nurse Anesthetists. Considerations for development of an anesthesia departmental policy on do-not-resuscitate orders. *AANA J.* 1994;62(5):397.

23. McBrien ME, Heyburn G. "Do not attempt resuscitation" orders in the peri-operative period. *Anaesthesia,* 2006;61(7):625-627.

24. American Society of Anesthesiologists. Ethical Guidelines for the Anesthesia Care of Patients With Do-Not-Resuscitate Orders. http://www.asahq.org/publicationsAnd Services/standards/09.pdf. Accessed April 22, 2010.

516

25. Waisel DB. Perioperative DNR orders: new options, greater flexibility. *ASA Newsletter.* 1999;63(4). http://www.asaweb.org/Newsletters/1999/04_99/Perioperative_0499.html. Accessed March 14, 2011.

26. *Funk & Wagnalls New International Dictionary of the English Language.* Comprehensive ed. Chicago, IL: World Publishers, Inc. 1996:22.

27. Bandman EL, Bandman B. Nursing Ethics: *Through the Life Span.* 4th ed. Upper Saddle River, NJ: Prentice Hall; 2002:22.

28. Carpenter M. The impaired nurse. *Medsurg Nurs.* 1994;3(2):139-141.

29. American Association of Nurse Anesthetists. Advisory Opinion 5.1: Patient Safety: Fatigue, Stress and Work Schedule Effects. Park Ridge, IL: American Association of Nurse Anesthetists. 2005. http://www.aana.com/. Accessed March 14, 2011.

30. American Association of Nurse Anesthetists. Position Statement Number 1.7: Substance Misuse and Chemical Dependency. Park Ridge, IL: American Association of Nurse Anesthetists. 2007. http://www.aana.com. Accessed March 14, 2011.

31. Curtin L. What are human rights? In: Curtin L, Flaherty MJ, eds. *Nursing Ethics: Theories and Pragmatics.* Bowie, MD: Robert J. Brady Co; 1982:1-16.

32. Steele SM, Harmon VM. *Values Clarification in Nursing.* 2nd ed. Norwalk, CT: Appleton & Lange; 1983:1-37.

33. Lachman VD. Moral courage: a virtue in need of development? *Medsurg Nurs.* 2007;16(2):131-133.

34. Clancy TR. Courage and today's nurse leader. *Nurs Admin.* 2003;27(2):128-132.

35. Beauchamp TL, Childress JF. *Principles of Biomedical Ethics.* 5th ed. New York: Oxford University Press; 2001:38.

36. Brushwood DB. Conscientious objection and abortifacient drugs. *Clin Ther.* 1993;15(1):204-212.

37. *Illinois Right of Conscience Act.* 745ILCS 70/1, et seq, 1977.

38. Arras M, Rettich A, Seifert B, Käsermann HP, Rülicke T. Should laboratory mice be anaesthetized for tail biopsy? *Lab Anim.* 2007;41(1):30-45.

39. Francione GL. The use of nonhuman animals in biomedical research: necessity and justification. *J Law Med Ethics.* 2007;35(2):241-248.

40. American Association of Nurse Anesthetists. Informed Consent in Anesthesia. Park Ridge, IL: American Association of Nurse Anesthetists. 2010. http://www.aana.com. Accessed April 22, 2010.

41. Tait AR, Voepel-Lewis T, Malviya S. Do they understand? part II: assent of children participating in clinical anesthesia and surgery research. *Anesthesiology.* 2003;98(3):609-614.

42. Hoehner PJ. Ethical aspects of informed consent in obstetric anesthesia—new challenges and solutions. *J Clin Anesth.* 2003;15(8):587-600.

43. Trovarelli T, Valenti J. The pregnant Jehovah's Witness: how nurse executives can assist staff in providing culturally competent care. *JONAS Healthc Law Ethics Regul.* 2005;7(4):105-109.

44. Dieterle JM. Physician assisted suicide: a new look at the arguments. *Bioethics.* 2007;21(3):127-139.

45. Boyle J. Medical ethics and double effect: the case of terminal sedation. *Theor Med Bioeth.* 2004;25(1):51-60.

517

46. van Delden JJ. Terminal sedation: source of a restless ethical debate. *J Med Ethics.* 2007;33(4):187-188.

47. Gawande A. When law and ethics collide—why physicians participate in executions. *N Engl J Med.* 2006;354 (12):1221-1229.

48. Beven JC, Hardy JF. Permission to publish case reports/case series [editorial]. *Can J Anaesth.* 2004;51(9): 861-866.

49. Tierney E. Consent for publication of a case report. *Anaesthesia.* 2004;59(8): 822-823.

50. Berlinger N, Moses, J. The five people you meet in a pandemic—and what they need from you today. 2007. http://www.thehastingscenter.org/ uploadedFiles/Publications/Special _Reports/Pandemic-Backgrounder-The-Hastings-Center.pdf. Accessed April 30, 2010.

51. Bevan JC, Upshur RE. Anesthesia, ethics, and severe acute respiratory syndrome. *Can J Anaesth.* 2003;50(10): 977-982.

52. Camann W. It is the right of every anaesthetist to refuse to participate in a maternal-request caesarean section. *Int J Obstet Anesth.* 2006;15(1):35-37.

53. Gass CW. It is the right of every anaesthetist to refuse to participate in a maternal-request caesarean section. *Int J Obstet Anesth.* 2006;15(1):33-35.

54. Tännsjö T. Ethical aspects of triage in mass casualty. *Curr Opin Anaesthesiol.* 2007;20(2):143-146.

55. Liang BA. To tell the truth: potential liability for concealing physician impairment. *J Clin Anesth.* 2007;19(8): 638-641.

56. Winslade W, McKinney EB. To tell or not to tell: disclosing medical error. *J Law Med Ethics.* 2006;34(4):813-816.

57. McGrath PA, Ruskin D. Caring for children with chronic pain: ethical considerations [editorial]. *Paediatr Anaesth.* 2007;17(6):505-508.

58. McIlvaine WB. Ethics and transplantation. *Semin Anesth Perioperative Med Pain.* 2004;21(1):6-11.

59. Brown SD, Truog RD, Johnson JA, Ecker JL. Do differences in the American Academy of Pediatrics and the American College of Obstetricians and Gynecologists positions on the ethics of maternal-fetal interventions reflect subtly divergent professional sensitivities to pregnant women and fetuses? *Pediatrics.* 2006;117(4):1382-1387.

518

Key References

1. Berlinger N, Moses J. The five people you meet in a pandemic—and what they need from you today. Garrison, NY: The Hastings Center. www.the hastingscenter.org. Accessed April 22, 2010.

2. McGraw KS. Should do-not-resuscitate orders be suspended during surgical procedures? *AORN J.* 1998; 67(4):794-799.

3. Parens E. *Surgically Shaping Children: Technology, Ethics, and the Pursuit of Normality.* Baltimore, MD: John Hopkins University Press; 2006.

4. Post SG. *The Encyclopedia of Bioethics,* 3rd ed. New York, NY: MacMillan Reference Books; 2003.

5. President's Commission for the Study of Ethical Problems in Medicine and Biomedical and Behavioral Research. Deciding to Forgo Life-Sustaining Treatment Decisions. Washington, DC: President's Commission; 1983.

6. Walters L. *Bibliography of Bioethics.* Washington, DC: Georgetown University, 1975.

Study Questions

You are scheduled to provide anesthesia during an emergent abdominal vascular surgery that often requires a minimum of 4 units of packed red blood cells. The patient Is a 35-year-old mother of 3 children under the age of 12 and is a professed Jehovah's Witness. The patient stated that she does not want to receive a blood transfusion (donor or via cell saver) under any circumstances.

1. What questions would you need to ask the patient to verify her refusal of blood transfusions during surgery?

2. What questions would you ask or actions would you take to verify that her refusal of a blood transfusion was a deep fundamental value for this patient and not just an attempt to please the elders of the church?

3. What professional and personal values are influencing how you view this case?

4. What is your agency's policy about refusal of blood by persons with expressed religious convictions?

5. Should the fact that this woman is the sole support for 3 minor children influence how you view this case?

6. What is your state's legal position about refusal of blood by persons with expressed religious convictions?

7. If the CRNA's goal is to do no harm, should the CRNA be concerned about potential spiritual harm as well as potential physical harm associated with administering blood products to a patient professing religious objections?

Index

A

AANA Ad Hoc Peer Assistance Advisory Committee, 473, 511

AANA Association Management Services, 52, 56-57
  Housing services, 57
  Insurance services, 56-57
  Publishing services, 56

AANA Foundation, 49-50, 52

AANA Insurance Services, 56-57

AANA Journal, 56

AANA Publishing, Inc, 56

AANA Wellness Program, 56, 473-474, 475

AANA. See American Association of Nurse Anesthetists.

ABNS. See American Board of Nursing Specialties under Credentialing and certification.

Accountability, 156-157

Accountable care organizations, 453

Act, definition, 370

Addiction, 472, 486-489
  Advocacy for impaired practitioners, 510-511
  Reentry into practice, 488-489
  Treatment and recovery, 488-489

Administrative management, 427-450
  Clinical sites, education, 448
  Code of conduct, 447
  Collaboration, 431
    Corporate culture, 432
    Hospital administrative structure, 431-435
  Community responsibilities, 448-449
  Conflict, 434-435
  Decision making, 430-431
  Financial management, 450-470
  Knowledge development, 432-433
  Managing professionals, 433
  Materials management, 438-439
    Case needs, 438

Surgeon preference, 438
    Mentoring, 444
    Operations management, 430-432
    Quality improvement, 439-441, 445-448
    Talent development and management, 444-445

Advanced practice, 97-101, 106, 107, 109, 110, 111, 114-115, 454

Advisory opinions, definition, 163

Advocacy, 18-19, 28, 34, 303-333, 509-511

Agency for Healthcare Research and Quality, 279-280, 281-282, 291

AHRQ. See Agency for Healthcare Research and Quality.

Algorithms, definition, 163

Amendment, definition, 370

American Association of Nurse Anesthetists, 41-52
  Advisory Opinion 5.1 on sleep deprivation and fatigue, 483
  Advocacy, professional, 28, 303-333
  Annual meetings, 59
  and Antitrust, 326-327
  Assemblies, 58-59
  Board of directors, 57
  Committees, 57-58
    Continuing education, 140, 144
  and Council on Surgical and Perioperative Safety, 282
  Councils, 52, 54-55, 122, 123
  and Education funding, 327-329
  Evidence-based practice, 155
  Federal political director program, 338
  Foundation. See AANA Foundation.
  and Healthcare policy, 335-372
  Healthcare reform, 253-254
  International Federation of Nurse Anesthetists, 65-67
  Membership, 44-46
    Benefits, 47-49
    Categories, 45, 46
    Services, 60
  Mission, values, philosophy, and objectives, 44, 45

521

523

528

531